Cardiology Research and Clinical Developments Series

HANDBOOK OF CARDIOVASCULAR RESEARCH

CARDIOLOGY RESEARCH AND CLINICAL DEVELOPMENTS SERIES

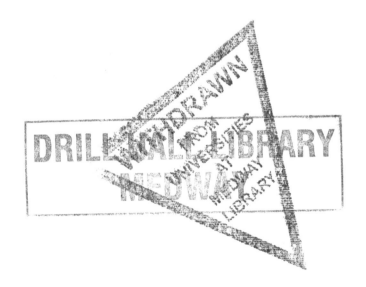

Cardiology Research and Clinical Developments Series

HANDBOOK OF CARDIOVASCULAR RESEARCH

JORGEN BRATAAS
AND
VIGGO NANSTVEIT
EDITORS

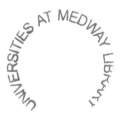

Nova Biomedical Books
New York

Library of Congress Cataloging-in-Publication Data

Handbook of cardiovascular research / editors, Jorgen Brataas and Viggo Nanstveit.
    p. ; cm.
 Includes bibliographical references and index.
 ISBN 978-1-60741-792-7 (hardcover)
 1. Heart--Pathophysiology. I. Brataas, Jorgen. II. Nanstveit, Viggo.
 [DNLM: 1. Cardiovascular Diseases. WG 120 H2359 2009]
 RC682.9.H36 2009
 616.1--dc22

               2009021233

Published by Nova Science Publishers, Inc. ✝ *New York*

Contents

Preface

Cardiovascular disease refers to the class of diseases that involve the heart of blood vessel. Most countries face high and increasing rates of cardiovascular disease. Each year, heart disease kills more Americans than cancer. It is the number one cause of death and disability in the U.S. and most European countries. The causes, prevention and/or treatment of all forms of cardiovascular disease are active fields of biomedical research. This book presents current research from around the world in this field.

Chapter I - Neurotensin is a tridecapeptide originally extracted from bovine hypothalamus by Carraway and Leeman (1973), and later found in a variety of peripheral tissues with the highest levels determined in the jejuno-ileal portion of the gastrointestinal tract. Neurotensin possess a broad spectrum of physiological activity, and could act as a neurotransmitter and neuromodulator in the central nervous system and as a local hormone in gastrointestinal tract. Importantly, there is increasing evidence to suggest that neurotensin plays a pivotal role in regulation of the cardiovascular system. Indeed, neurotensin-containing neural fibers are found in close contact with atrial and ventricular cardiomyocytes, sinoatrial and atrioventricular nodal cells, neurons of intracardiac ganglia, as well as coronary vessels in humans and various animal species. The density of neurotensin-immunoreactive myocardial innervation is reduced in cardiac disease. Neurotensin produces a variety of cardiovascular actions including potent effects on blood pressure, heart rate, myocardial contractility, coronary vascular tone, venous smooth muscle tone as well as regional blood flow in the gastrointestinal tract, skin and adipose tissue. Neurotensin also modifies the electrophysiological properties of the heart and exerts a protective effect in vagally-induced cardiac arrhythmias. Moreover, neurotensin could trigger cardiovascular reflexes by stimulating primary visceral afferents synaptically connected with preganglionic sympathetic neurons in the spinal cord. Neurotensin-induced cardiovascular effects are strongly influenced by species-dependent differences, and rapidly subjected to tachyphylaxis. Structural determinants of biological activity of neurotensin reside primarily in the C-terminal portion of its molecule. Indeed, C-terminal neurotensin hexapeptide fragment, neurotensin (8-13), is shown to be equipotent to intact neurotensin in eliciting cardiovascular effects, as well as in binding to the purified neurotensin receptor. In contrast, short N-terminal neurotensin fragments, neurotensin (1-6), (1-8) and (1-10), do not possess cardiovascular activity, and exhibit very low affinity for the neurotensin receptor.

Neurotensin-induced cardiovascular responses are mediated via direct activation of neurotensin receptors, as well as through stimulation of release of various endogenous biologically active substances such as histamine, serotonin, catecholamines and prostaglandins. To date, three subtypes of neurotensin receptors (NTS_1, NTS_2 and NTS_3) have been identified and found to be expressed in the brain and various peripheral tissues including the myocardium. NTS_1, a G-protein-coupled receptor with seven putative transmembrane domains, represents a high-affinity ($K_d \sim$ 0.1-0.3 nM) neurotensin binding site coupled to phospholipase C-inositoltrisphosphate transduction pathway. The NTS_1 receptor seems to play a pivotal role in the mechanism of neurotensin-induced cardiovascular responses, whereas a putative significance of NTS_2 and NTS_3 receptor subtypes remains to be determined.

Chapter II - Cardiovascular disease affects over 200 million people worldwide and accounts for nearly 30% of global mortality. Approximately 80% of these cardiovascular deaths occur in low and middle-income countries. By the year 2020, ischemic heart disease mortality in developing countries is predicted to increase by 120% for women and 137% for men [1]. In the United States alone, cardiovascular disease (CVD) affects over 37 million American women, representing over one third of the American female population, with coronary heart disease (CHD) affecting 5.9 million women. By age 55, the prevalence of cardiovascular disease in women exceeds that in men. Cardiovascular disease accounts for 1 in 2.5 female deaths compared to 1 in 30 deaths attributable to breast cancer. Despite the high prevalence and mortality rate of cardiovascular disease, only 13% of women consider it to be their greatest health risk [2]. While a recent survey of 1008 women found that the level of awareness regarding CVD mortality in women has nearly doubled since 1997, still only 55% of women recognize CVD as the leading cause of mortality in women. In addition, the survey found that the level of awareness in minorities continues to significantly lag behind the white population with only 38% of blacks and 34% of Hispanics recognizing the magnitude of the problem [3]. Although the past two to three decades has seen a decline in the overall mortality rate from CHD in men, the mortality rates for women have remained stable. The overall incidence of CHD in women has actually increased, as evidenced by a 47% increase in hospital discharges related to CHD [2, 4]. A prospective registry study of men and women who presented with an acute myocardial infarction found that women were at increased risk for 28-day case fatality (18.5% vs. 8.3%), 6-month mortality (28.5% vs. 10.8%) and readmission rates (23.3% vs. 12.2%) after a first myocardial infarction compared with men, independent of co-morbidities, coronary risk factors and the use of thrombolytics [5]. Not only did women in this study have a higher mortality from their first MI compared to men, it was also found that the median time between symptom onset and initial presentation to the hospital was on average one hour longer in women compared to men. Furthermore, the delay between the emergency room and admission to the coronary care unit was also on average over two hours longer in women than in men. The results from this registry were recently mirrored in the Euro Heart Survey of Stable Angina. This prospective observational trial found that women who presented with a new diagnosis of stable angina were less often referred for noninvasive or invasive studies and were less likely to undergo revascularization or given optimal secondary prevention medication even in the presence of confirmed obstructive coronary artery disease compared to men [6]. These studies highlight the discrepancies in the recognition and appropriate treatment of CHD in women as compared to men and underscore the importance of appropriately identifying women who are at risk for CHD. The aim of this report is to review the primary and secondary prevention measures that are unique to women and to examine the sensitivity and specificity of the current diagnostic modalities in detecting CHD in women.

Chapter III - Nowadays, there is no doubt that exposure to passive smoking, whatever it may be approached to be studied – and there are a lot of study approaches: clinical, biological, metabolic, epidemiologic, statistic and so on, that recognize different pathogenetic mechanisms of damage- leads to only one final result that is a reversibly functional harm of the heart and blood vessels following acute exposure, and pathologic alterations that become, in the long run, irreversible lesions of the above target organs after chronic exposure. Therefore, the American Heart Association has included passive smoking among the major risk factors for heart disease in both adults and children. However, our findings are able to demonstrate that cardiovascular damage from passive smoking could be considered more than a major risk factor for cardiovascular events, but particularly an etiologic factor of cardiovascular pathology.

The harm of the heart and blood vessels from passive smoking is the result of either an isolated action or combined action of some toxics contaminant indoor air by tobacco –and there are over 4,000 chemicals identified in cigarette smoking-. The majority of these have carcinogenic and/or negative cardiovascular effects in humans and animals. To what it concerns cardiovascular system, they may be classified into three groups: nicotine and its metabolites, carbon monoxide, and thiocyanates.

The degree of cardiovascular damage caused by passive smoking exposure depends by three factors- type of smoking, environment, and study subject - as well as by numerous variables which may be related to them. Exponential number of possibly numerous variables related to smoking, environment, and individuals permits to build a mathematical equation that quantify the level of damage as well as its exact reproducibility, as observed for a subject in one of our studies.

Either there is a functional damage particularly due to acute exposure or a pathologic damage which characterizes chronic exposure, the result of exposure to passive smoking varies widely in healthy individuals and in those individuals suffering from heart disease, especially ischemic heart disease.

The response to the harm can be of clinical type – signs of cardiac and/or blood vessel ischemic pathology which may be accompanied by arrhythmias and heart failure-, metabolic type – signs of altered oxygen transport and pro-thrombotic changes in coagulation-fibrinolysis cascade- and sympathetic type with changes in heart rate and blood pressure. Moreover, some special categories like women are influenced by their endocrine constellation. There is a different response in premenopausal women exposed to passive smoking who have an atherogenic response and in women after menopause who have an atherosclerotic response similar to that observed in men.

Genetic factors have also been demonstrate to influence cardiovascular response due to passive smoking with an increasing rate primarily for what involves the oxidative stress.

From these data, there is no doubt that passive smoking exposure demonstrates to be characterized by a major incidence of possible cardiovascular events acting, in this case, as a risk factor. However, exposure may be considered an etiologic factor of cardiovascular alterations since it leads, in the long run, to a damage of the heart and blood vessels also when intercurrent cardiovascular events can be lacking .

Chapter IV - The non-protein amino acid homocysteine (Hcy), a metabolite of the essential amino acid methionine, is implicated in the pathology of human cardiovascular and neurodegenerative diseases. In addition to its elimination by the remethylation and transsulfuration pathways, Hcy is also metabolized to the thioester Hcy-thiolactone in an error-editing reaction in protein biosynthesis when Hcy is mistakenly selected in place of methionine by methionyl-tRNA synthetase. In humans, the accumulation of Hcy-thiolactone can be detrimental because of its intrinsic ability to modify proteins by forming N-Hcy-protein adducts, in which a carboxyl group of Hcy is N-linked to ε-amino group of a protein lysine residue. N-linked Hcy occurs in each protein examined and constitutes a significant pool of Hcy in human blood. N-Hcy proteins are recognized as neo-self antigens and induce an auto-immune response. As a result, IgG and IgM anti-N-Hcy-protein auto-antibodies, are produced in humans. Serum levels of anti-N-Hcy-protein IgG auto-antibodies are positively correlated with plasma total Hcy, but not with plasma cysteine or methionine levels, which is consistent with the etiology of these auto-antibodies. In a group of male patients with stroke, the levels of anti-N-Hcy-protein IgG auto-antibodies and total Hcy are significantly higher than in a group of healthy subjects. In a group of male patients with angiographically documented coronary artery disease, seropositivity for anti-N-Hcy-protein IgG auto-antibodies occurs 5-times more frequently than in controls and is an independent predictor of coronary artery disease. These findings show that an auto-immune response against N-Hcy-proteins is a general feature of atherosclerosis and provide support for a hypothesis that N-Hcy-protein is a neo-self antigen, which contributes to immune activation, an important modulator of atherogenesis. Plasma Hcy lowering by folic acid administration leads to significant decreases in anti-N-Hcy-protein IgG auto-antibody levels in control subjects, but not in coronary artery disease patients. The results of these Hcy-lowering treatments suggest that, while primary Hcy-lowering intervention is beneficial, secondary Hcy-lowering intervention in coronary artery disease patients may be ineffective in reducing the advanced damage caused by Hcy, and may explain at least in part the failure of vitamin therapy to lower cardiovascular events in recent Hcy-lowering trials. Chronic activation of immune responses towards N-Hcy-protein associated with hyperhomocysteinemia over many years would lead to vascular disease.

Chapter V - Over the last decades, the survival of patients with systemic lupus erythematosus (SLE) has improved dramatically. Having improved treatment for active lupus disease, the challenge is now to understand and prevent the long-term complications of the disease, which may be due to the disease itself or the therapies used. To date, long-term complications of SLE are now considered to be important, including cardiovascular disease, osteoporosis and infections.

Cardiovascular disease in patients with SLE, including coronary artery disease, ischemic cerebrovascular disease, and peripheral vascular disease, is the result of premature atherosclerosis. Besides the traditional risk factors (like hypertension, hypercholesterolaemia and smoking), renal insufficiency, raised homocysteine levels, and the presence of anti-phospholipid, antibodies have been recognized as additional risk factors for cardiovascular disease in SLE. Recent studies have demonstrated that the nitric oxide pathway and its endogenous inhibitor asymmetric dimethylarginine may also be involved in the pathogenesis of cardiovascular organ damage in SLE. The metabolic syndrome and insulin resistance in SLE patients are current topics of research in this field.

Several studies have demonstrated a high prevalence of low bone mineral density in patients with SLE, especially in females. In the last few years, more attention is paid to osteoporotic fractures, one of the items of the organ damage index for SLE, and likely the most preventable form of musculoskeletal organ damage in SLE patients. Recent studies have demonstrated an increased frequency of symptomatic vertebral and nonvertebral fractures in patients with SLE. Moreover, a high prevalence of mostly asymptomatic vertebral fractures in patients with SLE was detected. These vertebral fractures were associated with previous use of intravenous methylprednisolone. The importance of identifying vertebral fractures in SLE patients is illustrated by the observed association between prevalent vertebral fractures and reduced quality of life as well as an increased risk of future vertebral and nonvertebral fractures in the general population.

Infection imposes a serious burden on patients with SLE. In case series, infectious complications were found in 25% to 45% of SLE patients, and infection as primary cause of death has been demonstrated in up to 50% of SLE patients. Defects of immune defence and treatment with corticosteroids and other immunosuppressive agents are supposed to play a role in the pathogenesis of infections in SLE. Recently, research has focused on the role of the lectin pathway of complement activation in the occurrence of infections in SLE.

In this review the results of recent studies on cardiovascular disease, osteoporosis and infectious complications in SLE will be discussed.

Chapter VI - Studies on the risk of coronary heart disease in persons exposed to environmental tobacco smoke have been conducted since mid eighties of the last century. Their results were published in numerous articles, including seven meta-analyses. The majority of them show that the risk of coronary artery disease is increased in passive smokers by about 20-30% in comparison with non-smoking controls. The effect is more significant that one might expect comparing the amounts of toxic substances aspirated by passive versus active smokers. This may result from increased levels of atherogenous substances in plasma, e.g. homocysteine and asymmetric dimethylarginine (an endogenous inhibitor of nitric oxide synthase) and from the weakened body self-defense due to decreased non-enzymatic antioxidants levels.

The purpose of the present study was the evaluation of the effects of passive smoking on the concentration of substances involved in pathogenesis of cardiovascular diseases, namely homocysteine, cysteine, asymmetric dimethylarginine, symmetric dimethylarginine and non-enzymatic antioxidants (α-tocopherol, γ-tocopherol, retinol).

Seventy-two men (mean age 39.3±2.7) years, were selected to the study. Non-smokers group included persons with plasma cotinine level not exceeding 10 ng/ml (31 men). Passive smokers group consisted of men with plasma cotinine level between 10 and 30 ng/ml (41 men). Plasma biochemical parameters were assessed with use of high performance liquid chromatotography. Plasma total homocysteine in passive smokers was statistically signifficantly higher than in non-smokers (10.17 versus 8.57 μmol/L). There was a significant positive correlation between plasma total homocysteine level and cotinine levels in passive smokers as well in the entire population. (r = 0.331; P = 0.034 and r = 0.332; P = 0.008, respectively). Plasma α-tocopherol levels in passive smokers were signifficantly lower than in non-smokers (12.31 versus 14.12 μg/ml). Both in passive smokers as well in the entire study population a significant negative correlation between cotinine and α-tocopherol levels in plasma was found (-0.378; P = 0.036 and –0.220; P = 0.046, respectively). The changes in concentration of the remaining biochemical parameters were insignificant and did not correlate with plasma cotinine level. The obtained results indicate that chronic exposure to environmental tobacco smoke may result in elevated total plasma homocysteine level and may affect the body anti-oxidative barrier by lowering plasma α-tocopherol level.

Chapter VII - The evidence obtained during more than last 10 years suggests that melatonin exerts some effects on the cardiovascular system. It is especially important in the case of elderly people, because of the increased incidence of both, acute and chronic heart diseases. In the course of aging concentrations of some of the hormones decrease, e.g., melatonin, dehydroepiandrosterone, eostrogensoestrogen, etc. It has been shown that melatonin concentration in serum and the level of its main metabolite 6-sulphatoxymelatonin in urine are lower in older people compared to younger population. The melatoninergic receptors demonstrated in vascular system are functionally associated with either vasoconstrictory,vasoconstrictory or vasodilatory effects of this pineal indoleamine. In the 90ties of the last century melatonin was established as a potent antioxidant. In the pathogenesis of some age-related diseases the generation of free radicals play an important role. Melatonin contributes to the general cardioprotection in rat models of oxidative stress induced by myocardial ischemia-reperfusion or adriamycin-induced cardiotoxicity. It has been shown that patients with coronary heart disease have a low melatonin production rate, especially those with the higher risk of cardiac infarction and/or of the sudden death. The suprachiasmatic nucleus and, possibly, the melatoninergic system may modulate cardiovascular rhythmicity. It has been shown, that melatonin may influence other age-related problems including hypercholesterolemia and hypertension. People with high levels of LDL-cholesterol and also those with hypertension have lower levels of melatonin compared to the population without lipid disturbance and with the normal blood pressure. It has been shown that melatonin suppresses the formation of cholesterol, reduces LDL oxidation and accumulation in the vascular system. The administration of melatonin decreases blood pressure to the normal levels.

It has been observed, that melatonin replacement therapy may decrease the incidence of sudden cardiac deaths, especially in elderly patients with deficiency of its endogenous level. This review summarises up-to-date knowledge about correlation between the cardiovascular system and melatonin.

Chapter VIII - The serotonin transporter (SERT) on the surface membrane of platelets is a primary and saturable mechanism for serotonin uptake from plasma. After the uptake of 5-hydroxytryptamine (5HT) by SERT, 5HT is stored in dense granules that are released following stimulation of platelet and other intravascular events. 5HT is a monoamine neurotransmitter that also functions as a vasoconstrictor during blood vessel injury and as a mitogen during early embryogenesis. Alterations in 5HT levels in the nervous system or blood plasma are associated with a number of neuropsychiatric disorders and cardiovascular disease.

The 5HT uptake capacity of platelets depends on the number of SERT molecules on the plasma membrane, which exhibits a biphasic relationship to plasma 5HT concentration. Specifically, the density of SERT molecules on the platelet surface is down-regulated when plasma 5HT is elevated, *in vitro* or *in vivo,* to a level that was observed during hypertension. Thus, high 5HT at high levels appears to limit its own uptake into platelets by down-regulating SERT, and results in a "platelet to plasma shift" in 5HT distribution.

In exploring the factors involved in the intracellular movement of SERT, the authors focused on the associations between platelet SERT, Rab4, and vimentin. Mechanistically, our studies investigate the link between elevated plasma 5HT and the intracellular tethering of SERT by Rab4, and the 5HT-mediated phosphorylation of vimentin that arrests SERT recycling on a paralyzed vimentin network. These novel findings support the hypothesis that high plasma 5HT leads to abnormalities in the platelet trafficking of SERT, which reduces the density of SERT molecules on the plasma membrane to deplete 5HT content.

Overall, the authors provide the first detailed information on the 5HT-mediated biochemical pathways that regulate the number of functional SERT molecules on the platelet surface. The importance of understanding the structure, function, and regulation of SERT is underscored by the observations that plasma 5HT may be elevated in the plasma, either locally or globally, during atherosclerosis, hypertension, stroke, and other cardiovascular diseases.

Chapter IX - *Context* Patients are frequently transferred during their care for acute myocardial infarction. The clinical risks and benefits associated with inter-hospital transfer have not been fully evaluated.

Objective: To compare and contrast the analytic methods used to handle transferred patients in previous acute myocardial infarction research.

Design: Systematic review of acute myocardial infarction literature over the past 10 years.

Main Outcomes: Benefits and risks of various methods used for handling transferred patients in acute myocardial infarction research

Results: Seven major methods for dealing with inter-hospital transfer emerged: 1) Count each hospitalization as a separate event. 2) Delete transferred patients from analysis. 3) Link the data from different hospitals and produce a record of the "episode" of acute myocardial infarction. 4) Analyze data on transferred patients the same as on non-transferred patients. 5) Transfer patients are the specific population of interest. 6) Diagnosis, treatment, outcomes are attributed to the index hospital. 7) Control for transfer in logistic regression modeling. Several studies included a combination of these methods.

Conclussion: Inter-hospital transfer in the care of acute MI is common and increasing. From a clinical standpoint, determining the patient most likely to benefit from inter-hospital transfer will help guide clinicians faced with this difficult decision. From a health services standpoint it is essential to understand the implications of using a particular method for handling transfer patients, the impact on data collection, the data lost, the appropriate analyses, and the generalizability of findings.

Chapter X - Cardiac transplantation of stem cells (SCs) has been shown to improve regional perfusion and systolic function of the failing heart after myocardial infarction (MI). However, once delivered to the heart, unlabeled cells cannot be visualized or tracked *in vivo*.

While iron oxide-labeled SCs can be detected by magnetic resonance imaging (MRI), this method is insensitive to a small number of cells, is hindered by the label dilution due to cell division and migration, and cannot distinguish live from dead cells.

The reporter gene approach is a promising method to track SC fate non-invasively.

Because the reporter probe is expressed only in living cells and is passed to daughter cells upon cell division without dilution, the sensitivity for *in vivo* detection is enhanced. Using a reporter system, multimodality (bioluminescence, fluorescence, and positron emission tomography (PET)) imaging permits longitudinal monitoring of the cell survival, homing, and proliferation, if the reporter gene is stably expressed.

The authors have adapted and validated the reporter gene method for *in vivo* monitoring of cardiac SC therapy in a large animal model of MI that would facilitate translational research.

Domestic pigs underwent a closed-chest, reperfused acute myocardial infarction (AMI), which mimics most human AMI, followed by percutaneous intramyocardial injections of autologous mesenchymal stem cell (MSC) transfected stably with a trifusion reporter gene containing the renilla luciferase (RL)-red fluoroscent protein (RFP)-herpes simplex truncated thymidine kinase (tTK, PET-reporter) (LV-RL-RFP-tTK).

The osteogenic, chondrogenic and adipogenic differentiation of the MSCs was not altered by transfection. Both cell viability and proliferation assays showed no significant difference between the nontransfected MSCs and LV-RL-RFP-tTK-MSCs. Serial PET imaging demonstrated focal [18F]-FHBG tracer uptake of the injured anterior myocardial wall accompanied by a pattern of intense tracer foci at the local injections of the LV-RL-RFP-tTK-MSCs when injected in 2 sites at 8 h post delivery. Ten days after LV-RL-RFP-tTK-MSC implantation, fluorescence confocal microscopy of the myocardium showed the presence of RFP+ cells in the area surrounding the intramyocardial injections. Analysis of luciferase enzyme activities revealed decreased level of expression of the RL gene in the myocardial injection sites, but increasing number of surviving cells in the remote organs at 8 days post-delivery. Fluorescence confocal microscopy confirmed the presence of RFP+ cells in a mediastinal lymph node, thereby validating the migration of the LV-RL-RFP-tTK-MSCs.

Chapter XI - While the full extent of the role that growth hormone (GH) and its effector Insulin-like growth factor 1 (IGF-1) play in the development and maintenance of cardiovascular morphology and function is debated, several conditions associated with altered GH activity have characteristic cardiovascular impairments.[1-3] The effects of GH therapy on cardiac function have been studied in the pediatric population, primarily in the setting of GH deficiency. For individuals whose circulating levels of GH are low, GH replacement therapy appears to improve cardiovascular health. GH therapy has also been shown to improve lean body mass and decrease percent body fat, which may further improve overall cardiovascular health. However, GH excess may lead to cardiac hypertrophy, as seen in acromegaly. GH therapy may also lead to reduced insulin sensitivity, a pre-diabetic state, in some individuals, particularly women with Turner syndrome. Thus, the systemic effects of GH therapy, specifically its effect on the cardiovascular system, vary by underlying condition.

Chapter XII - The neurohypophysial hormone oxytocin (OT) was the first peptide hormone to be chemically synthesized in biologically active form [1]. OT is synthesized primarily in magnocellular neurons in the paraventricular and supraoptic nuclei of the hypothalamus. It is also produced in peripheral tissues [2], including the heart [3]. In addition to OT effects on reproductive functions and induction of maternal behavior, it is involved in endocrine and neuroendocrine regulation of the heart, vasculature, and kidneys [4-6]. It has been reported that OT acts via neuroendocrine-endocrine-paracrine pathways to regulate blood volume via its natriuretic properties and to modulate blood pressure by stimulating the release of atrial natriuretic peptide (ANP) [4, 6]. In addition, it was demonstrated that in isolated, perfused hearts, an OT antagonist (OTA) blocks basal ANP release [4]. ANP induces vasorelaxation of coronary arteries, inhibition of L-type Ca^{2+} channels in the myocardium, and suppression of the renin-angiotensin system [7]. These effects are recognized as being protective to the cardiovascular system and are also induced by estrogen [8]. Empirical studies suggest that OT may affect or regulate the function of the heart through several different mechanisms.

Chapter XIII - Cardiomyopathies represent an heterogeneous group of inherited diseases, characterized by different signs and symptoms, natural history, and clinical outcome. The genetic knowledge regarding this class of diseases is rapidly growing in the last two decades. The genetics of cardiomyopathies has born in 1989 with a single gene theory (identification of beta myosin mutations in hypertrophic cardiomyopathy: one gene=one disese), but the complexity and wide heterogeneity of the disease has moved toward a different direction (sarcomeric genes in hypertrophic cardiomyopathy: many genes=one diseases; beta myosin as disease causing for hypertrophic, dilated, restrictive and noncompaction cardiomyopathy: one gene=many diseases or genocopies). Elucidation of the molecular basis of cardiomyopathies has led to a categorization of the phenotypes according to their genetic etiology. The American Hearth Association and the European Society of Cardiology have recently proposed a different scheme of classification based on a distinction between primary (genetic, mixed, non genetic types) and secondary cardiomyopathies, or between the familial and non familial types, respectively. The possibility of a different approach of intervention (i.e. enzyme replacement therapy in metabolic cardiomyopathies) underlies the need to make an early and precise etiologic diagnosis.

Family history, physical examination, electrocardiogram and non-invasive imaging techniques are the essential methods for a "first step" toward an etiologic diagnosis, followed by biochemical and, eventually, genetic investigations which can help the final discriminations between similar pathologic conditions (phenocopies).

Chapter XIV - Tako-tsubo cardiomyopathy (TC) is a recently described acute cardiac syndrome that mimics acute myocardial infarction and is characterized by ischemic chest symptoms, an elevated ST segment on electrocardiogram, increase levels of cardiac disease markers and transient left apical and middle ventricular walls disfunction (apical "ballooning"). In contrast to the acute coronary arterial syndromes (ACS), patients with TC have no angiographically detectable or nonobstructive coronary arterial disease [1].

This syndrome can be triggered by profound psychological stress and is also known as "stress cardiomyopathy" or "broken-heart syndrome" [2].

Chapter XV - Chest pain is one of the most frightening symptoms a person can have. It is sometimes difficult even for a doctor or other medical professional to tell what is causing chest pain and whether it is life-threatening.

Chest pain can be defined as discomfort or pain that you feel anywhere along the front of your body between your neck and upper abdomen.

Chapter XVI - Chronic heart failure(CHF) has emerged as a major worldwide epidemic. Recently, a fundamental shift in the underlying etiology of CHF is becoming evident, in which the most common cause is no longer hypertension or valvular disease, but rather long-term survival after acute myocardial infarction (AMI) [1,2].

The costs of this syndrome, both in economic and personal terms, are considerable [3]. American Heart Association statistics indicate that CHF affects 4.7 million patients in the United States and is responsible for approximately one million hospitalizations and 300,000 deaths annually.

The total annual costs associated with this disorder have been estimated to exceed $22 billion. The societal impact of CHF is also remarkable. Patients with CHF often suffer a greatly compromised quality of life. About 30% of diagnosed individuals (i.e.,1.5 million in U.S.) experience difficulty breathing with little or no physical exertion, and are very restricted in their daily functions. This forced sedentary lifestyle inevitably leads to further physical and mental distress.

The CHF problem is growing worse. While CHF already represents one of our greatest health care problems, it is expected to become even more severe in the future. By 2010, the number of patients suffering from HF will have grown to nearly 7 million, a more than 40% increase.

Coronary artery disease (CAD) is the cause of CHF in the majority of patients, and CHF is the only mode of CAD presentation associated with increasing incidence and mortality.

However, it is evident, running through the different therapeutical strategies of CHF, that the appropriate treatment of patients with ischemic heart failure is still unknown [4,5].

After myocardial infarction, injured cardiomyocytes are replaced by fibrotic tissue promoting the development of heart failure. Cell transplantation has emerged as a potential therapy and stem cells may be an important and powerful cellular source.

Chapter XVII - Among the more that a hundred known types of pain in the chest, angina ranks at the top of the list for seriousness as well as for reckless diagnosis -- too frequently diagnosed when absent and too dangerously when overlooked.. Failure to recognize it in an emergency facility leading to risky discharge becomes a source for both litigation and patient injury; faulty targeting the diagnosis for one of the many other sources becomes both expensive and provocative of unnecessary anxiety. The diagnosis is certain to be overlooked if all the sources fail to be considered.

Such oversight has been responsible for most of the treatment failures that have been encountered in my consultation practice. Identification of the specific cause for pain or distress in the chest in clinical practice is ordinarily more difficult than specific treatment. Proper recognition becomes the first step in clinical management; more than 100 different disorders have been identified to produce pain or discomfort in the chest.

Pain considered to arise within the chest may actually originate in the wall of the chest as well as in its viscera. It can also arise from disorders from within the head, neck, or abdomen. Diagnosis may ordinarily be fairly simply established when the significant details from the clinical history taking, from physical examination, and from laboratory investigation are adequately evaluated. Special investigations, ordinarily available in university and diagnostic centers, sometimes become essential; although details of the more readily available diagnostic facilities become more important safeguards for correct diagnosis than are the reports from referral centers.

Detailed analysis of the pain itself provides the essential guide through the perplexing labyrinth of a lot of possible causes. Unfortunately the patient readily abandons his essential leadership role through that labyrinth when forced into a rigid inquiry prematurely. With skill and experience, however, the patient can be enticed to go all the way through that labyrinth when the physician and patient work adequately together. Both must appreciate the diagnostic significance of the entire trip. The patient can ordinarily take the physician almost directly to the correct diagnosis. Even when the patient is personally mistaken at the outset, often fearfully mistaken, about the real significance of the symptoms, the diagnostic target cam still be struck by combined physician-and-patient skill.

Chapter XVII - Smoking cessation reduces both the mortality and re-infarction rate amongst smokers who have experienced a myocardial infarction (MI). Smoking cessation programs have tended to be conducted with post-operative or seriously ill patients. In this study, the authors examined the efficacy of a relapse prevention program for hospital cardiovascular patients who did not require operative procedures or extensive hospitalization. A pre-post, two groups, control trial involving 208 patients (103 in the intervention group) recruited from three coronary care units in large metropolitan hospitals was used to assess the effect of the intervention. Smoking status of self-reported quitters were verified using CO concentrations in expired air. Complete follow-up was obtained from 129 (62.0%) of initial participants. At three months after discharge, the self-report quite rate in the intervention group was 19.4%, significantly higher than in the control group (7.6%) (p = 0.046). This difference persisted at nine months after discharge, when the self reported quit rate was 27.3% in the intervention group and 12.9% in the control group (p = 0.043). A behavior-based smoking cessation program was effective for less serious cardiovascular patients and the effect persisted for nine months after discharge.

Chapter XIX - Apoptosis is implicated in wide variety of physiological and pathological processes, and the role of apoptosis in cardiovascular diseases is also becoming more evident. In this paper, the authors review the current literature on the known caspases and their role in the heart. The importance of the categories of initiator and effector caspases are well recognized in the heart and role of the inflammatory caspases is emerging. Furthermore, the authors present specific studies that are being done in our laboratory as well as others in elucidating the mechanism of inhibiting apoptosis in cardiac myocytes. The inhibition of apoptosis as a potential therapeutic tool is emerging for various forms of cardiovascular disease, and the inhibition of caspases is an important target for anti-apoptotic therapy in the heart.

Chapter XX - Oxidative stress seems to play a key-role in the pathogenesis of atherosclerosis. Agents that prevent LDL from oxidation have been shown to reduce initiation of atherosclerosis. Among these, the antioxidant micronutrients, including the carotenoids and vitamins C and E, have gained wide interest because of the potential for prevention of atherosclerotic vascular disease in humans. Lipid-soluble antioxidants present in LDL, including α-tocopherol (vitamin E), and water-soluble antioxidants present in the extracellular fluid, including ascorbic acid (vitamin C), inhibit LDL oxidation through an

LDL-specific antioxidant action. Moreover antioxidants present in the cells of the vascular wall decrease cellular production and release of reactive oxygen species (ROS), inhibit endothelial activation (expression of adhesion molecules and monocyte chemoattractants), and improve the biologic activity of endothelium-derived nitric oxide (EDNO) through a cell- or tissue-specific antioxidant action. [1] In the last decade many trials with antioxidants have been planned in patients with cardiovascular disease but the results are equivocal. The reason for the disappointing findings is unclear but one possible explanation is the lack of identification criteria of patients who are potentially candidates for antioxidant treatment. Several studies have been done in patients at risk of cardiovascular disease indicating that enhanced oxidative stress is associated with the presence of the classical risk factors for atherosclerosis, like diabetes, hypercholesterolemia, hypertension, smoking and obesity.

In this chapter the data so far reported will be analyzed to see if there is a clear support the hypothesis that patients at risk of cardiovascular may be candidates for antioxidant treatment.

Chapter XXI - During exercise cardiovascular apparatus operates some adjustments which aim at meeting the metabolic needs of exercising muscle. Both mechanical (skeletal-muscle and respiratory pumps) and nervous (centrally and peripherally originating) mechanisms contribute to regulate blood pressure and flow to the metabolic demand.

Concerning the nervous component of this regulation, there are several inputs of both central/cortical and peripheral/intravascular origin that converge to the brain-stem neurons controlling cardiovascular activity and regulate the hemodynamic responses to exercise on the basis of the motor strategy. Furthermore, evidences support the concept that also nervous signals of extravascular origin, i.e. arising from muscle mechano- and/or metabo- receptors, activate the same control areas on the basis of the muscle mechanical and metabolic involvement.

This review focuses on inputs arising from exercising muscles which modulate cardiovascular system in order to connect blood pressure and flow with the actual muscle mechanical status (muscle length and strain, and tissue deformation due to muscle movements) and metabolic condition (concentration of catabolites in the extra-cellular compartment produced by muscle activity).

It was reported that the stimulation of type I afferent nervous fibers from muscle receptors increases blood pressure through a mechanism of peripheral origin. Among sub-groups of type I afferents, indirect findings suggest that type Ib from Golgi tendon organs may contribute to the muscle-induced cardiovascular reflex. On the contrary, it appears that group Ia from muscle spindle primary ending and group II afferents are not involved in this reflex. Opposite, it seems ascertained that type III and IV afferent nervous fibers can be activated by exercise-induced mechanical and chemical changes in the extracellular environment into they are scattered. It is believed that type III afferents act mainly as "mechanoreceptors", as they respond to muscle stretch and compression occurring during muscle contraction, while type IV fibres act as "metaboreceptors", since they are stimulated by end-products of muscle metabolism. The activity of both type III and IV afferents can reflexely increase heart rate and systemic vascular resistance which, in turn, lead blood pressure to raise. Moreover, there are several growing evidences that also myocardial contractility, stroke volume and cardiac pre-load can be modulated by the activity of these reflexes of muscular origin.

These findings suggest that signals arising from exercising muscle act to regulate cardiovascular adjustments during exercise so that blood flow can be set to meet the muscle metabolic request.

In: Handbook of Cardiovascular Research
Editors: Jorgen Brataas and Viggo Nanstveit

ISBN 978-1-60741-792-7
© 2009 Nova Science Publishers, Inc.

Chapter I

Neurotensin: Physiological Properties and Role in Cardiovascular Regulation

Oleg Osadchii[1,2], Angela Woodiwiss[2] and Gavin Norton[2]
1. Normal Physiology Department, Kuban Medical Academy, Krasnodar, Russia
2. Cardiovascular Pathophysiology and Genomics Research Unit,
School of Physiology, University of the Witwatersrand, Medical School,
Parktown, Johannesburg, South Africa

Abstract

Neurotensin is a tridecapeptide originally extracted from bovine hypothalamus by Carraway and Leeman (1973), and later found in a variety of peripheral tissues with the highest levels determined in the jejuno-ileal portion of the gastrointestinal tract. Neurotensin possess a broad spectrum of physiological activity, and could act as a neurotransmitter and neuromodulator in the central nervous system and as a local hormone in gastrointestinal tract. Importantly, there is increasing evidence to suggest that neurotensin plays a pivotal role in regulation of the cardiovascular system. Indeed, neurotensin-containing neural fibers are found in close contact with atrial and ventricular cardiomyocytes, sinoatrial and atrioventricular nodal cells, neurons of intracardiac ganglia, as well as coronary vessels in humans and various animal species. The density of neurotensin-immunoreactive myocardial innervation is reduced in cardiac disease. Neurotensin produces a variety of cardiovascular actions including potent effects on blood pressure, heart rate, myocardial contractility, coronary vascular tone, venous smooth muscle tone as well as regional blood flow in the gastrointestinal tract, skin and adipose tissue. Neurotensin also modifies the electrophysiological properties of the heart and exerts a protective effect in vagally-induced cardiac arrhythmias. Moreover, neurotensin could trigger cardiovascular reflexes by stimulating primary visceral afferents synaptically connected with preganglionic sympathetic neurons in the spinal cord. Neurotensin-induced cardiovascular effects are strongly influenced by species-dependent differences, and rapidly subjected to tachyphylaxis. Structural determinants of biological activity of neurotensin reside primarily in the C-terminal portion of its molecule. Indeed, C-terminal neurotensin hexapeptide fragment, neurotensin (8-13), is shown to be equipotent to intact neurotensin in eliciting cardiovascular effects, as well as in binding to the purified neurotensin receptor. In contrast, short N-terminal neurotensin fragments, neurotensin (1-6), (1-8) and (1-10), do not possess cardiovascular activity, and exhibit very low affinity for the neurotensin receptor. Neurotensin-induced cardiovascular responses are mediated via direct activation of neurotensin receptors, as well as through stimulation of release of various endogenous biologically active substances such as histamine, serotonin, catecholamines and prostaglandins. To date, three subtypes of neurotensin receptors (NTS_1, NTS_2 and NTS_3) have been identified and found to be expressed in the brain and various peripheral tissues including the myocardium. NTS_1, a G-protein-coupled receptor with seven putative transmembrane domains, represents a high-affinity ($K_d \sim 0.1$-0.3 nM) neurotensin binding site coupled to phospholipase C-inositoltrisphosphate transduction pathway. The NTS_1 receptor seems to play a pivotal role in the mechanism of neurotensin-induced cardiovascular responses, whereas a putative significance of NTS_2 and NTS_3 receptor subtypes remains to be determined.

Introduction

Neurotensin (NT), a tridecapeptide with a broad spectrum of physiological activity, was originally extracted from the bovine hypothalamus [24] and later found in the bovine [108] and human [73] small intestine. Since the discovery of NT in 1973, rapid progress has been achieved in understanding various aspects related to NT function in the central nervous system and peripheral organs, as well as exploring the nature of the mechanisms involved in the physiological effects of NT in health and disease. The main focus of research in this area over the last 30 years has been on the mechanisms of central NT effects such as antinociception, hypothermia and various behavioural actions [45, 185, 233], as well as elucidating the role of NT in hormonal regulation of the digestive system [53] and proliferation of normal and cancerous cells [231]. The potential therapeutic relevance of these findings for the diagnosis and treatment of schizophrenia, cancer and obesity as well as for pain suppression has been recently reviewed [111, 233]. However, there has been much less attention given to the experimental findings demonstrating potent and diverse effects of NT on the cardiovascular system. In the present chapter we review the current knowledge related to the role of NT in various aspects of cardiovascular regulation, with a particular focus on the mechanisms mediating NT effects upon myocardial and vascular tissue. For systematic purposes, a detailed overview of NT effects upon the cardiovascular system will be preceded by a brief summary of the data related to the structural properties as well as the pharmacokinetics and metabolism of the NT molecule. We will also briefly discuss the results of some studies designed to evaluate concentrations of endogenous NT in blood plasma and its distribution profile in peripheral tissues and organs.

**Scheme 1. NT structure in humans and various animal species
(adapted from [207] with modifications)**

	1	2	3	4	5	6	7	8	9	10	11	12	13
Human, dog, rat, pig, bovine	pGlu –	Leu –	Tyr –	Glu –	Asn –	Lys –	Pro –	Arg –	Arg –	Pro –	Tyr –	Ile –	Leu
Guinea-pig	----	----	----	----	----	----	Ser	----	----	----	----	----	---
Possum	----	----	His	Val	----	----	Ala	----	----	----	----	----	---
Chicken	----	----	His	Val	----	----	Ala	----	----	----	----	----	---
Alligator, python	----	----	His	Val	----	----	Ala	----	----	----	----	----	---
Frog	----	Ala	His	Ile	Ser	----	Ala	----	----	----	----	----	---
Toad	----	Ala	Ile	Val	Ser	----	Ala	----	----	----	----	----	---

The interrupted lines indicate the presence of the same amino acid residue in NT structure. The underlined amino acid sequence represents a C-terminal portion of NT molecule responsible for NT receptor activation.

Neurotensin: Processing from a Precursor Molecule

NT is synthesized as a part of prohormone which also contains neuromedin N, a NT-like hexapeptide [235]. The NT/neuromedin N precursor is found in both the brain and various peripheral tissues including myocardium [34, 110] as well as in the human circulation [51], but the highest concentrations are measured in the jejuno-ileum part of the gastrointestinal tract [34, 110]. The NT/neuromedin N precursor is a polypeptide of 170 amino acids, with a structure that is 76% homologous in bovine, dogs and rats [107, 110, 207]. NT and neuromedin N are contained as adjacent sequences within the C-terminal of the precursor, and liberated in a 1:1 molar ratio following precursor processing by proprotein convertases [110]. The presence of the NT/neuromedin N precursor in various tissues accounts for a rapid (over seconds) and significant (by 25-200-fold) elevation of immunoreactive NT levels following the action of endogenous peptidases. In particular, large amounts of biologically active NT-related peptides are generated following the exposure of rat and chicken gastric tissue to aqueous acid, an effect accounted for by the proteolytic activity of pepsin-related enzymes (pepsin, cathepsin and renin) [29]. The presence of large (16-70 kDa) molecular weight protein substrates which can liberate immunoreactive NT upon pepsin treatment has also been shown to occur in a variety of feline tissues [32], as well as blood plasma of several mammalian species [31, 140, 220].

A biologically active NT derived from the precursor molecule is a 13 amino acid neuropeptide with a C-terminal portion that contains structural determinants primarily responsible for NT receptor activation (Scheme 1). The amino acid sequence of NT is similar in most mammalian species (Scheme 1). In the guinea-pig, however, Pro^7 is substituted for Ser in the NT molecule. In birds, reptiles and amphibian species the structure of NT is different from mammals due to the substitution of three-to-five amino acid residues in the N-terminal part of the NT molecule (Scheme 1). However, the amino acid sequence of the C-terminal portion of the NT molecule responsible for the physiological activity of this neuropeptide is highly conserved across species.

Pharmacokinetics and Metabolism

Exogenous NT is rapidly cleared from circulation upon intravenous administration as evidenced by significant peripheral arteriovenous extraction. The metabolic clearance rate and half-life time of NT determined in normal human subjects and two animal species are shown in table 1. Importantly, the C-terminal fragments of NT are metabolized significantly faster than the N-terminal fragments [5, 91, 121, 163, 218, 220].

The half-life of NT, as determined after incubating fresh human blood plasma with NT, is 226 min, which is significantly longer than the half-life found upon systemic infusions of intact NT in vivo (~1.4 min) [122]. Likewise, no N-terminal NT fragments are detected following a short-term (1-10 min) incubation of synthetic NT with rat blood [5]. These findings suggest that NT catabolism in vivo is mainly provided by tissue enzymes rather than peptidases present in blood plasma. In conscious sheep, the kidney, brain and gut are the major organs involved in the catabolism of intravenously injected synthetic NT [218].

Table 1. Parameters of NT pharmacokinetics

Species	Antibodies used	Clearance, ml/кg/min	Half-life, min	References
Human	N-terminal directed antisera	16±1	3.8±0.2	[19]
	C-terminal directed antisera	88±25	< 0.5	[219]
	N-terminal directed antisera	9.9±0.8	13.9±1.5	
	C-terminal directed antisera	36 (21-54)	1.7 (0.7-2.8)	[91]
	N-terminal directed antisera	11 (6.7-21.7)	8.3 (4.7-13.8)	
	C-terminal directed antisera	ND	1.4	[121]
	N-terminal directed antisera	ND	6.0	
Sheep	C-terminal directed antisera	25.8±3.2	2.1±0.3	[218]
	N-terminal directed antisera	12.8±1.4	6.3±0.5	
Rat	C-terminal directed antisera	ND*	0.55	[5, 220]
	N-terminal directed antisera	26.0±4.0	5.0	

ND, not determined. *No significant increase in C-terminal NT immunoreactivity in blood plasma was detected following intravenous infusion of intact NT.

Table 2. Plasma NT concentrations in humans and various animal species

Species	NT concentration, pM/l	References
Human		
healthy adults	14-65	[17-19, 26, 31, 33, 55, 74, 91, 97, 105, 121, 125, 130, 131, 163, 204, 217, 219]
healthy children of 1-14 years old	24	[16]
infants	29-48	[125]
pregnant women	29	[130]
Dog	2-40	[6, 26, 132, 139, 199]
Cat	25-30	[31, 61, 62]
Rabbit	37	[26]
Rat	20-48	[25, 26, 31, 200, 220, 230]
Bovine	15-25	[25, 26]
Frog *Xenopus laevis* *Rana catesbeiana* *Rana pipiens*	0.05-1.6 0.5 0.03-0.53	[28]

In humans, the liver and kidney are the two visceral organs primarily involved in NT catabolism [91, 219]. The NT molecule is catabolised by angiotensin-converting enzyme, neutral endopeptidase 24.11 (enkephalinase), endopeptidase 24.15 and endopeptidase 24.16 which cleave Arg^8-Arg^9, Pro^{10}-Tyr^{11} and Tyr^{11}-Ile^{12} bonds [13, 41, 110, 135, 136, 222]. The cleavage products detected following degradation of the intact NT are represented by free tyrosine, C-terminal dipeptide Ile^{12}-Leu^{13} as well as NT fragments such as NT_{1-7}, NT_{1-8}, NT_{1-10}, NT_{1-11} and NT_{11-13}. The overall rate of degradation of intact NT in a culture of human endothelial cells is 80 nM per 1 mg of protein per hour [144].

Blood Plasma Concentrations

Picomolar concentrations of endogenous NT are present in blood plasma (table 2) as well as cerebrospinal fluid [79, 216, 243] and human milk [50]. In rats, about 85% of the total plasma NT-like immunoreactivity is represented by N-terminal NT fragments such as NT_{1-8} (73%) and NT_{1-11} (11%), whereas only 15% is represented by intact NT [220]. In human blood plasma, the concentrations of N-terminal NT fragments are about 5-fold higher as compared to intact NT [163, 219].

No age- or gender-related differences have been found in fasting plasma NT levels in adult humans [163]. However, NT concentrations are reported to be higher in newborns as compared to adults, and full-termed infants have higher plasma NT levels as compared to preterm infants at birth [125].

NT concentrations in blood plasma are increased upon food intake. In humans, food intake elicits a biphasic elevation of NT concentrations which peaks at 20-30 and 90 min after the ingestion of a large meal, and enhanced blood plasma NT concentrations are maintained at least over 3 hours after ingestion [17, 55, 131, 204, 217]. Interestingly, the elevation of plasma NT concentration following food intake is faster and achieves a higher peak value in patients subjected to total or partial gastrectomy, an effect related to accelerated gastroduodenal passage of chyme [208]. Food intake-induced elevations of the total NT-like immunoreactivity in blood plasma is largely attributed to a significant (up to 10-fold) increase in concentrations of the stable N-terminal NT fragments such as NT_{1-8} and NT_{1-11} [74].

The increase in NT concentrations in blood plasma upon food intake is due to nutrient-induced stimulation of NT secretion by mucosal endocrine-like N-cells localised within the epithelial layer of small intestine [81, 167, 227]. Indeed, elevated NT concentrations in portal blood are found following perfusion of the isolated small intestine with solutions containing sodium oleate, bile acids or peptones in dogs [60], rats [49, 230] and cats [34]. A similar effect is observed following intraduodenal infusion of oleic acid in humans [105]. The most potent stimulant of NT secretion is fat, with a less significant effect produced by glucose [18, 49, 130]. NT secretion, however, is not affected by the intake of amino acids, coffee and alcohol [131]. During fasting, plasma NT levels are decreased below threshold of chromatographic detection.

Apart from a local stimulatory action of nutrients, NT secretion by N-cells is stimulated by some gastrointestinal hormones released into the portal circulation following food intake. In the isolated, vascularly perfused rat small intestine, a potent stimulation of NT secretion is induced by bombesin, calcitonin gene-related peptide, gastrin-releasing peptide, substance P and leu-enkephalin [48, 86, 200], whereas somatostatin exerts an inhibitory effect [54]. There is some evidence to suggest that the secretory activity of N-cells is stimulated by vagal nerve fibers. In particular, both basal and meal-stimulated NT concentrations in human blood plasma are reduced following the infusion of atropine, a muscarinic cholinergic receptor blocker, to healthy volunteers [55]. Consistently, NT secretion by rat N-cells is significantly increased by cholinergic agonists [86].

Increased basal plasma NT levels have been described in various types of pathology such as Parkinson's disease [214], diabetes mellitus [130], dumping syndrome in gasterectomized patients [18], and menopausal hot flashes in women [113]. Furthermore, plasma NT concentrations are markedly increased in patients with NT-secreting neuroendocrine tumors (neurotensinomas) localised in the liver, pancreas, stomach or prostate [33, 97]. Alternatively, an elevation of endogenous NT concentrations in blood plasma could result from a reduced degradation by renal and liver peptidases. In particular, elevated concentrations of NT are found in the systemic circulation in patients with liver cirrhosis [91] and chronic renal failure [219]. In rats subjected to bilateral nephrectomy, basal plasma NT concentrations have been reported to be 3-fold higher as compared to unoperated control rats, an effect associated with significantly reduced metabolic clearance rate of NT [220]. The clinical significance of these findings remains to be determined.

Tissue and Organ Distribution Profile

In rats, only about 10% of the total amount of NT-immunoreactive material is present in the brain, whereas 90% is distributed throughout a variety of peripheral tissues, with the highest amount (85%) found in the intestine [25]. In the brain, the highest concentrations of NT are found in the hypothalamus (60 pM/g) and pituitary gland (29 pM/g), and the lowest in the cerebellum (0.8 pM/g) [25].

In the rat gastrointestinal tract, the highest (50 pM/g) NT concentrations are found in the jejunum and ileum, whereas much lower (1-8 pM/g) concentrations are detected in the esophagus, stomach, duodenum and large intestine [25]. NT-immunoreactive cells (N-cells) have been found in the ileal mucosa of 13 animal species [81], being more abundant in non-mammalian vertebrates as compared to mammals [179]. In rats, the density of N-cells is about 150 cells per mm^2 of mucosal surface in terminal ileum [179]. These cells have triangular or slightly elongated shape, are located in the epithelium of the villi and crypts, and their apical pole reaches the gut lumen and constitutes part of the brush border ("open type" cells). NT is stored in round electron-dense secretory granules with an average diameter of about 260-290 nM, which are located in the basal portion of the N-cells [167, 179, 227].

In peripheral structures of the autonomic nervous system, NT is mainly localised in presynaptic terminals of preganglionic sympathetic nerves originating in the thoracic spinal cord [126, 182]. In cats, NT-containing sympathetic preganglionic neurons are mostly present in segments T4-T7 [115, 116]. The axons of these neurons project to the stellate ganglion, L7 ganglion of sympathetic chain, and coeliac ganglion [23, 126, 128, 129]. In the stellate ganglion, NT-containing nerve terminals are widespread and closely associated both with cardiac and non-cardiac sympathetic postganglionic neurons [23]. In guinea-pigs, a considerable number of NT-immunoreactive neural fibers are found in para- and prevertebral sympathetic ganglia [182]. NT-like immunoreactivity, however, is not found in perikarya of the principal ganglionic cells. In preganglionic sympathetic fibers, NT is subjected to anterograde axonal transport as evidenced by accumulation of NT-like immunoreactivity proximal to the ligation [126-128] as well as depletion of NT-like immunoreactivity following chronic decentralization of sympathetic ganglia [35].

With respect to endocrine glands, the highest NT levels are found in the adrenal glands where it is stored in the chromaffin granules present in a subpopulation of norepinephrine-containing cells [43, 65, 168, 187, 201, 229]. In cats, about 60-70% of norepinephrine-containing cells exhibit positive NT-like immunoreactivity. The highest adrenal NT concentrations were found in cat (64 pM/g), as compared to lower levels noted in bovine (6 pM/g), rat, guinea-pig and rabbit (1.3-2.1 pM/g) adrenal tissue [65]. In humans, the NT concentration in adrenal tissue is ~0.7 pM/g [201]. Importantly, NT could act as a neurotransmitter/neuromodulator regulating secretory function of chromaffin cells. Indeed, NT-immunoreactive fibers innervate norepinephrine-containing adrenal chromaffin cells in the cat [165], hamster [164] and frog [221]. Moreover, a stimulatory effect of NT on the release of catecholamines has been shown to occur in cultured bovine adrenal chromaffin cells [20].

High (50 Hz) frequency stimulation of the splanchnic nerve in cats induces a 3.6-fold increase of NT concentration in blood plasma collected from the adrenal vein, an effect antagonized by hexamethonium [62, 201]. Likewise, NT release from adrenal medulla has been demonstrated in stress models designed to stimulate the sympathoadrenal axis such as shock induced by splanchnic artery occlusion [62] and hemorrhagic hypovolemia [61]. In isolated, retrogradely perfused cat adrenal glands, NT secretion is stimulated by acetylcholine, nicotine or high potassium concentrations [43]. Both in vivo and vitro studies have shown that NT release from adrenal tissue occurs concurrently with catecholamines, enkephalins, neuropeptide Y and somatostatin [43, 61, 62, 201]. Taken together, these findings suggest that NT could act as an adrenal hormone involved in physiological responses to stress stimuli.

Cardiovascular Innervation

The presence of NT-immunoreactive neural fibers in the cardiovascular system of a variety of mammalian and non-mammalian species has been demonstrated in many studies (table 3).

Following the quantitative assessment of the total content of NT-like immunoreactive material in the heart of various species, the highest myocardial NT concentrations are found in the guinea-pig (3.1 pM/g) and hen (3.0 pM/g), followed by rat (2.2 pM/g), cat (1.0 pM/g), dog (0.8 pM/g) and human (0.8 pM/g) [201]. With regards to comparison of NT content in myocardium versus non-cardiac tissues, NT concentrations in rat atria and ventricles are found to be 1.8 and 2.3 pM/g, respectively, which is comparable to NT levels in rat liver, lung and oesophagus, but higher than NT concentrations in renal, duodenal and splenic tissue [67].

NT-Immunoreactive Cardiac Innervation

Using immunohistochemistry and radioimmunoassay, NT-containing fibers were found in close contact with atrial and ventricular cardiomyocytes as well as neurons of intracardiac ganglia localised in the vicinity of the sinoatrial node [59, 180, 181, 183, 184]. The NT-immunoreactive synaptic inputs to myocardial ganglionic cell bodies presumably mediate excitatory effects as evidenced by an increase in activity of right atrial neurons in the dog heart in situ following a local intra-arterial NT infusion [4]. In the rat [36], guinea-pig [181, 183] and rabbit [150] myocardium, NT levels are higher in the atria as compared to the ventricles, and higher NT concentrations are found in right atrium and ventricle as compared to the left side of the heart [149, 150]. A dense network of NT-containing fibers is found in the sinoatrial and atrioventricular node [181, 183, 184, 240] as well as in the bundle of His, where the density of NT-immunoreactive innervation is about 10-fold higher as compared to right atrial tissue [63]. In experiments conducted by our own group, NT was noted to be present at picomolar concentrations in both the rat ventricular myocardium and in samples obtained from the coronary effluent collected from isolated, perfused heart preparations from the rat [157]. These findings suggest that NT is stored in and could be released from neural terminals localised in rat myocardial tissue.

The origin of NT-immunoreactive cardiac innervation remains uncertain. The somata of NT-containing neurons whose axons project to cardiac structures seem to have extracardiac localization as no NT-like immunoreactivity is found in perikarya of intrinsic cardiac neurons [59, 78, 181].

Table 3. Distribution profile of NT-immunoreactive nerve fibers in myocardial tissue as determined by immunohistochemistry and radioimmunoassay

Species	Localization of NT-like immunoreactivity	References
Human	Cardiac ventricles, aorta, pulmonary vein and coronary vessels. No NT-immunoreactive fibers are found in atrial tissue and pulmonary artery.	[150, 180, 184]
Monkey	Sinoatrial node, intracardiac ganglia and coronary vessels. Coronary arteries are more densely innervated than veins.	[240]
Dog	Sinoatrial node, atrioventricular node, and coronary vasculature. In less amounts, NT-immunoreactive nerve fibers are found in close contact with atrial and ventricular cardiomyocytes, as well as in intracardiac ganglia.	[59, 240, 241]
Rabbit	Atrial tissue, aorta, pulmonary artery and vein. Lower NT levels are found in ventricular tissue.	[150]
Cat	Sinoatrial node, intracardiac ganglia and coronary vessels. Coronary arteries are more densely innervated than veins.	[240]
Rat	The highest NT levels are found in pulmonary vein, followed by right atrium and ventricle. In lower amounts, NT is present in aorta, left cardiac chambers and pulmonary artery.	[36, 149, 150, 241]
Guinea-pig	Sinoatrial node, atrioventricular node, the bundle of His, adventitia of the ascending aorta, aortic arch and pulmonary trunk. In coronary vasculature, arterial side is more densely innervated than veins. NT-containing nerve fibers are also found in intracardiac ganglia.	[63, 180, 181, 183, 240, 241]
Chicken	NT level in heart homogenates is found to be 3.0 ± 0.7 pM/g. NT-immunoreactive fibers are found to supply ascending aorta, coronary arteries and intracardiac ganglia.	[184, 201]
Quail	Small coronary arteries as well as atrial and ventricular cardiomyocytes.	[184]
Frog	NT level in heart homogenates is found to be 1.4 ± 0.1 pM/g. NT-immunoreactive fibers are associated with aortic trunk, coronary vasculature, atrial and ventricular cardiomyocytes.	[28, 67, 184]
Lizard	Adventitia of ascending aorta and coronary vessels, paravascular plexus, atrial and ventricular cardiomyocytes.	[184]
Australian lungfish, *Neoceratodus forsteri*	Sinus venosus, atrial myocytes, atrial ganglion cells.	[90]
Teleost bony fish, *Cottus scorpius*	Ventricular cardiomyocytes.	[184]

In the rat myocardium, NT-immunoreactive innervation is not affected by pretreatment with capsaicin, a neurotoxin targeting primary afferent sensory fibers, or 6-hydroxydopamine, an agent that destroys postganglionic sympathetic fibers [67]. Therefore, it is possible that NT is predominantly contained in cardiac preganglionic parasympathetic fibers [67]. However, to our knowledge, no studies assessing the effect of colchicine treatment and antibodies against choline acetyltransferase have been done to ascertain whether NT-immunoreactive fibers are related to cardiac parasympathetic innervation. Furthermore, there is no evidence to demonstrate the presence of NT-immunoreactivity in perikarya of cardiac preganglionic neurons in the dorsal motor nucleus of the vagus nerve [88]. Thus, the origin of a putative parasympathetic NT-immunoreactive innervation of the heart is uncertain.

NT-like immunoreactivity has not been found either in sympathetic or parasympathetic ganglionic cell bodies [126, 182, 184]. However, Weihe et al. have hypothesized that a fraction of ganglionic cells could contain a NT precursor polypeptide, a molecule which does not react with NT-specific antisera [241]. The NT-precursor may be delivered to presynaptic terminals of cardiac nerves by axonal transport and subjected there to enzymatic cleavage to produce the biologically active NT [241]. In support of this argument, high concentrations of NT precursor are found in cat myocardial tissue [34]. Nevertheless, further studies are required to assess this hypothesis.

NT-immunoreactive innervation is altered in cardiac disease. In rat model of monocrotaline-induced cardiac hypertrophy, endogenous NT levels are significantly decreased in all cardiac chambers, especially on the right side, and both cardiac and circulating NT concentrations are reduced with the transition from cardiac hypertrophy to heart failure [36].

NT-Immunoreactive Vascular Innervation

Numerous evenly distributed NT-containing fibers are detected in peri- and paravascular plexuses innervating coronary vessels [59, 181, 183, 240]. These fibers are found in all segments of coronary vasculature, but the coronary arteries are more densely innervated than the veins. Furthermore, NT-immunoreactive innervation of coronary vessels is more abundant in atria as compared to ventricles [184]. Numerous NT-containing neural fibers are also found in the adventitia of the ascending aorta, aortic arch, and pulmonary vein, whereas only scarce NT-immunoreactive innervation is detected in superior and inferior vena cava [149, 150, 181, 184].

NT-immunoreactive innervation has been found in large parietal and splachnic vessels in the guinea-pig and dog [184], with the density of innervation generally being higher in arteries as compared to veins. In large arteries, NT-containing neural fibers are mainly found at the adventitia-media border. NT-immunoreactive innervation is particularly pronounced in cortical arteries of the kidney, renal and intrapancreatic arteries, as well as in the arteries of the skin. However, very few NT-immunoreactive fibers are found in cerebral vessels [184]. Amongst venous vessels, only the portal vein exhibits relatively dense innervation by NT-immunoreactive fibers [184].

Vascular Effects of NT

Blood Pressure

The modulation of vascular smooth muscle tone is one of the typical physiological effects produced by NT, and this action was reported in the first publication describing the extraction procedure and biological activity of this neuropeptide [24]. Indeed, the name "NT" was originally derived from the potent vascular effects produced by this regulatory peptide extracted from the neural tissue. However, NT effect on systemic blood pressure is largely species-specific. In the rat [39, 44, 58, 138, 177, 190], dog [15, 52, 202] and rabbit [99], intravenous infusion of NT at nanomolar concentrations produces marked hypotensive effect lasting at least 40-60 min. The NT-induced hypotensive effect is rapidly subjected to tachyphylaxis thus enabling only one effective NT concentration to be tested in each animal. On the other hand, NT produces dose-dependent pressor effects in guinea-pigs [100, 143, 196, 197] and sheep [190]. In anesthetized rats [71, 101, 146, 148, 177, 191] and guinea-pigs [100, 143, 190], NT also elicits biphasic and triphasic variations (e.g. initial decrease followed by a transient increase and a further long-lasting decrease) of blood pressure. In humans, at physiological concentrations representing postprandial plasma NT levels, NT has no effect on blood pressure [18, 121, 124, 205, 219, 234], but produces a moderate pressor response following administration at a pharmacological ($\sim 10^{-5}$ M) dose [156].

Rat strain-related differences in NT effects upon blood pressure are noted in conscious animals. In particular, intravenous infusion of NT induces a marked fall in blood pressure in Sprague-Dawley rats [226] while producing pressor responses in Long Evans rats [10]. In anesthetized rats, the pattern of NT-induced changes in blood pressure could be influenced by the type of anesthetic employed. For instance, NT induces a uniform, prolonged hypotensive effect in urethane-anesthetized rats, whereas it elicits a biphasic response in rats anesthetized with sodium thiobutabarbitone, a decrease in blood pressure being preceded by a marked but transient pressor effect [39].

Hypotensive effects of NT in rats are abolished by H_1-histamine receptor antagonists or agents depleting histamine stores in mast cells such as compound 48/80 [39, 71, 146, 177, 190], as well as by SR 48692, a NT receptor antagonist [71, 212]. Consistently, NT exerts a direct, NT receptor-mediated stimulatory action on histamine release from isolated rat mast cells [14, 27, 30, 114, 118, 206, 215], an effect which will be discussed in more detail below. However, stimulation of endogenous histamine release seems to be only one of as a number of mechanisms mediating NT-induced vasodepressor responses. Indeed, NT-induced hypotension could be accounted for, at least in part, by an inhibitory NT effect on norepinephrine release from rat perivascular nerve fibers [232]. Furthermore, hypotensive effects of NT in anesthetized rats are strongly attenuated following acute bilateral nephrectomy as well as captopril or saralasin pretreatment [101, 190] indicating that NT could decrease the activity of renin-angiotensin system.

In anesthetized guinea-pigs, pressor effects of NT are completely abolished by ganglion blocking agents, reserpine or a mixture of α- and β-adrenoreceptor antagonists, thus indicating the involvement of a catecholamine-dependent mechanism [100]. Likewise, the hypertensive phase of a biphasic depressor-pressor NT effect is significantly reduced by adrenalectomy or α-adrenoreceptor antagonist administration in anesthetized ganglion-blocked rats [191]. There is some evidence to suggest that NT-induced sympathetic activation represents an indirect effect mediated by stimulation of substance P and/or calcitonin gene-related peptide release from capsaicin-sensitive sensory neurons coupled to spinal preganglionic sympathetic neurons [9, 10]. Indeed, sympathetically-mediated pressor effects produced by intravenous NT administration in anesthetized guinea-pigs [9, 197] and conscious, unrestrained Long Evans rats [10] are abolished by chronic pretreatment with capsaicin, a neurotoxin that depletes substance P and calcitonin gene-related peptide stores in primary sensory neurons. Consistently, NT has been shown to promote stimulus-induced release of substance P from the myenteric plexus of the guinea-pig small intestine [92]. Importantly, NT-induced pressor responses in guinea-pigs are inhibited by SR 48692, a NT receptor antagonist [143], suggesting that the functional NT receptor is located on capsaicin-sensitive sensory neurons involved in NT-induced sympathetic activation. The functional significance of these effects for reflex regulation of cardiovascular system will be discussed below.

It can be hypothesized that the potent stimulatory effects of NT upon release of various vasoactive endogenous neuromodulators could mask its own direct effect on vascular smooth muscle tone. However, NT has no effects on isolated rat [44] and rabbit [198] aortic strips, as well as the rabbit pulmonary artery [145] in in vitro studies. Likewise, only weak endothelium-dependent relaxation of the dog isolated carotid artery was elicited by NT at concentrations about two orders of magnitude higher than those of tachykinins, reference vasoactive peptides [46]. Furthermore, NT-induced vasodepressor responses in anesthetized rats were not affected by prior administration of L-NAME, an inhibitor of nitric oxide synthase [71]. Taken together, these findings suggest that a direct effect of NT on vascular smooth muscle tone does not significantly contribute to changes in blood pressure evoked by systemic NT administration.

Coronary Vascular Tone

NT induces coronary vasoconstriction in rats [171, 172, 176, 192], but evokes a dilation of coronary arteries in guinea-pigs [8] and dogs [15, 52]. On the other hand, NT has no effect on coronary vascular tone in the isolated, perfused rabbit heart [171]. In isolated, electrically-driven guinea-pig heart preparation, NT-induced coronary vasodilator effects were shown to be larger at high basal coronary perfusion pressures [8, 52]. The vasodilator effects were abolished by atropine but markedly potentiated by neostigmine, a cholinesterase inhibitor, indicating that NT actions on coronary arteries are mediated via stimulation of presynaptic acetylcholine release [8].

In the dog, NT has no effect on coronary blood flow upon systemic administration [6], but produces coronary vasodilation upon intracoronary injection, an effect significantly potentiated by captopril, an inhibitor of angiotensin-converting enzyme [15]. NT-induced coronary vasodilatation in anesthetized open-chest dogs is abolished by indomethacin thus suggesting that this effect is mediated by prostanoid products produced by cyclooxygenase [52]. Moreover, NT-induced effects on coronary vascular tone is abolished following gradual reduction of coronary perfusion pressure, an effect presumably related to preactivation of the prostaglandin system in the ischemic myocardium [52].

NT-induced coronary vasoconstriction in isolated, perfused rat heart preparation is abolished by the NT receptor antagonists, [D-Trp^{11}]-NT and [Tyr(Me)^{11}]-NT, but not by antagonists of angiotensin II, serotonin, H_1-histamine and α-adrenergic receptors, suggesting a direct, NT receptor-mediated effect on coronary vascular tone [176]. Interestingly, this effect is potentiated in hearts pretreated with compound 48/80 or dexamethasone [192] indicating that NT receptor-mediated coronary vasoconctrictor responses could be partially antagonized by concomitant NT-induced stimulation of histamine release from cardiac mast cells.

The hypotensive and coronary vasoconstrictor effects of NT in rats are markedly enhanced following 24-72 hours fasting [172], an effect related to reduction of plasma NT concentrations which presumably contributes to up-regulation of NT receptors in the cardiovascular system.

Gastrointestinal Blood Flow

NT reduces gastric mucosal blood flow in human subjects [56]. On the other hand, NT induces a significant dose-dependent increase in intestinal blood flow in rats [148], cats [77] and dogs [6, 112, 202], an effect related to reduced intestinal vascular resistance. In the dog, NT-induced increases in regional intestinal blood flow are observed in the muscular layer of the duodenum, jejunum, ileum and colon while mucosal blood flow is unchanged [6]. The intestinal vasodilation following systemic NT administration is induced at concentrations below those eliciting hypotension, suggesting that locally released NT could potentially act as a mediator of postprandial intestinal hyperemia. This function, however, seems not to be preserved in ischemic intestinal tissue. Indeed, NT aggravates the intestinal microcirculatory disturbances produced by local ischemia-reperfusion in rats [87].

NT increases pancreatic blood flow in the dog [112]. Consistently, NT-immunoreactive neural fibers are found in close contact with intrapancreatic vasculature in the dog [184].

Cerebral Blood Flow

NT, at pharmacological concentrations ($\sim 10^{-5}$ M), produces a significant contractile effect on isolated human cerebral arteries [242]. In this regard, the efficacy of NT is higher as compared to some reference vasoconstrictor agents such as norepinephrine, serotonin, arginine vasopressin and angiotensin II. On the other hand, perivascular infusion of NT over a wide range of concentrations has no effect on the smooth muscle tone of feline cerebral arteries in situ [238]. Likewise, intravenous NT infusion does not affect regional cerebral blood flow in anesthetized dogs [6].

Regional Blood Flow in other Areas

NT infusion produces cutaneous vasodilation in anesthetized rats [24], an effect mediated via stimulation of histamine release from skin mast cells [42]. NT also moderately increases perfusion medium flow in an intact, in situ perfused rat adrenal gland [89], but has no effect on regional blood flow in adrenal glands and kidney following intravenous administration in anesthetized dogs [6]. On the other hand, NT induces a delayed vasoconstriction in denervated subcutaneous adipose tissue in dogs [202, 203] and abdominal adipose tissue in humans [124], suggesting a physiological role of NT in the regulation of postprandial uptake of nutrients by adipose tissue.

NT induces a vasoconstrictor effect in the isolated, perfused rat hindquarter, an action antagonized by methysergide, a serotonin receptor blocker [102]. Consistently, NT elicits a prolonged vasoconstrictor effect in renal, superior mesenteric and hindquarter vascular beds upon systemic administration to conscious rats [10]. NT-induced vasoconstrictor responses are significantly reduced by α-adrenoreceptor blocker indicating an interacton between NT and the sympathetic nervous system.

Venous Smooth Muscle Tone

NT induces dose-dependent increases in basal tension, spontaneous contraction rate and peak phasic contraction of the longitudinal strips of the isolated rat portal vein [80, 188, 238]. In this regard, NT is more potent than substance P, bradykinin and norepinephrine, but less potent than angiotensin II [80]. NT-induced venoconstrictor effects are markedly inhibited by indomethacin, suggesting an involvement of prostaglandin-dependent mechanisms [188]. Consistently, NT induces prostacyclin release from endothelial cells of the human umbilical vein, as well as elevation of circulating 6-keto-prostaglandin $F_{1\alpha}$ levels in anesthetized rats [212]. Both NT-induced venoconstrictor responses [188, 189] and an increase in plasma levels of prostaglandin $F_{1\alpha}$ [212] are abolished by the selective NT receptor antagonists, [D-Trp^{11}]-NT, [Tyr(Me)^{11}]-NT and SR 48692. NT, however, has no detectable effect on the smooth muscle tone of the guinea-pig portal vein [238].

Cardiac Effects

Basal Heart Rate

NT induces a significant tachycardia in rats [10, 169, 190, 225], guinea-pigs [7, 100, 143, 169, 196, 197], cats [12, 152] and sheep [190]. In healthy human volunteers, NT has no effect on basal heart rate upon intravenous infusion at physiological (picomolar) concentrations [19, 121, 124, 205, 219], but produces a tachycardia following bolus injection at a pharmacological ($\sim$10^{-5} M) dose in patients with cardiac disease [156]. NT does not modify the rate of spontaneous contraction in isolated rabbit heart preparations [169, 202]. Furthermore, no consistent evidence is available to show reproducible chronotropic responses to NT in dogs. Indeed, although NT has no effect on basal heart rate upon systemic administration [202], it produces a modest bradycardia after intracoronary injection [15, 52] or marginal heart rate acceleration following injection into the intact sinus node artery in anesthetized, open chest dogs [186].

Interestingly, NT has been shown to modify basal heart rate in some non-mammalian animal species. In particular, an increase in heart rate follows systemic NT administration in the estuarine crocodile [98]. On the other hand, NT produces an atropine-dependent bradycardia in free-swimming, unanesthetized Australian lungfish [90]. NT has no effect upon basal heart rate in anesthetized hens [47].

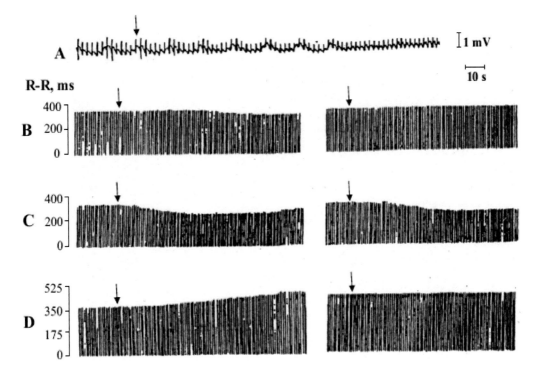

Figure 1. Modifications of the cardiac electrogram (panel A) and changes of the cardiac cycle length (R-R interval of the cardiac electrogram, ms) (panels B-D) following systemic administration of neurotensin and epinephrine in anesthetized cats. Neurotensin (4.0×10^{-8} M) and epinephrine (0.5×10^{-8} M) were administered as intravenous bolus injections. Arrows in all fragments indicate the moment of injection. Panel B: positive chronotropic response to neurotensin (left fragment) is subjected to rapid tachyphylaxis as evidenced by the lack of shortening of the cardiac cycle following the second neurotensin injection (right fragment). Panel C: positive chronotropic responses following the first (left fragment) and second (right fragment) epinephrine administration are very similar indicating the lack of tachyphylaxis. Panel D: neurotensin-induced effect is blunted (right fragment) after prior intravenous administration of propranolol (1.0 mg/kg), a β-adrenoreceptor blocker (left fragment). Note a reduction in the voltage of R waves on cardiac electrogram trace following neurotensin injection (panel A), and lengthening of the cardiac cycle following propranolol administration (panel D, left fragment). The time interval between two consequent injections of neurotensin (panel B) or epinephrine (panel C), as well as administrations of propranolol and neurotensin (panel D) was 15 min. A comparison of the mean values of variables characterising the dynamics of neurotensin- and epinephrine-induced chronotropic responses is given in table 4.

In guinea-pigs, heart rate acceleration induced by systemic NT administration in vivo [100] as well as in isolated, spontaneously beating heart [7] is not abolished by ganglion blocking agents or antagonists of β-adrenoreceptors, H_2-histamine and 5-HT receptors, thus indicating a direct effect of NT on the sinoatrial node. The magnitude of NT-induced positive chronotropic responses tends to be larger in heart preparations with lower basal rates of contraction [7]. On the other hand, NT-induced tachycardia in rats [10, 191], cats [152] (figure 1) and sheep [190] is abolished by β-adrenoreceptor blockers, reserpine pretreatment or adrenalectomy thus indicating that chronotropic responses to NT are mediated by the release of adrenal catecholamines. Indeed, plasma epinephrine levels are increased by ~4-fold following systemic NT administration in anesthetized rats, an effect suppressed by adrenalectomy [147].

Catecholamine-dependent tachycardia induced by NT in cats could be mediated by facilitation of sympathetic ganglionic transmission [11, 12, 23]. Indeed, NT is released by tonic firing of preganglionic sympathetic axons projecting to the stellate ganglion [128, 129]. Furthermore, a profound heart rate acceleration can be induced by close intra-arterial injection of NT into the decentralized stellate ganglion in anesthetized spinal cats [12]. NT-induced tachycardia is abolished by propranolol, a β-adrenoreceptor antagonist, as well as by section of the inferior cardiac nerve thus indicating that the NT effect is related to excitation of sympathetic postganglionic neurons [12].

Chronotropic responses elicited by equimolar concentrations of NT and epinephrine upon systemic administration in anesthetized cats are of a similar magnitude (table 4). However, both latency and duration of NT-induced chronotropic responses are longer as compared to epinephrine-induced effects (table 4). Moreover, in contrast to epinephrine-induced cardioaccelearation, the chronotropic responses to NT rapidly undergo tachyphylaxis (figure 1) lasting at least for two hours after systemic NT administration.

Table 4. Parameters of the positive chronotropic responses induced by NT and epinephrine in anesthetized cats

Agent used	Basal cardiac cycle length, ms	Peak shortening of the cardiac cycle, ms	Latency of chronotropic response, s	Time to peak of chronotropic response, s	Duration of chronotropic response, s
Neurotensin (n=7)	372.5±10.6	315.0±9.8*	25.4±5.1**	11.9±1.5	193.6±23.1**
Epinephrine (n=8)	368.8±18.1	293.8±13.5*	7.8±2.2	9.5±2.2	98.9±12.6

Both agents were infused intravenously at equimolar concentrations (~10^{-8} M) in anesthetized cats maintained on artificial lung ventilation. Cardiac cycle length (R-R interval of the cardiac electrogram) was recorded on a beat-to-beat basis. *$P<0.01$ vs. baseline cardiac cycle length; **$P<0.01$ vs. the same value after epinephrine infusion.

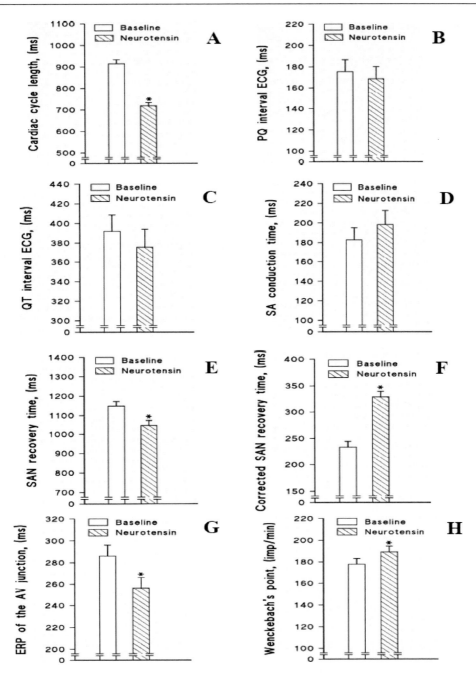

Figure 2. Effects of neurotensin on electrophysiological properties of the human myocardium. Electrophysiological parameters of the cardiac conduction system were determined in patients with cardiac disease (n=40) by programmed transesophageal atrial pacing. In recumbent patients, a bipolar electrode probe introduced intranasally into the esophagus towards the level of the left atrium was used to stimulate the myocardium with a series of rectangular pulses (10 ms, 12.8±2.3 mA). Neurotensin (~10^{-5} M) was administered as an intravenous bolus injection. ECG, electrocardiogram; SA, sinoatrial; SAN, sinoatrial node; ERP, effective refractory period; AV, atrioventricular. The corrected SAN time (panel F) was determined by subtracting the cardiac cycle length from the corresponding value of the SAN recovery time. *P<0.05 as compared to baseline value.

Cardiac Electrophysiology

In patients with cardiac disease, NT administered intravenously at a pharmacological concentration ($\sim 10^{-5}$ M) produces a variety of effects on electrophysiological properties of the cardiac conduction system [156]. In particular, NT reduces cardiac cycle (R-R interval ECG) duration, shortens the effective refractory period of the atrioventricular junction, as well as increases the value of Wenckebach's point following rapid atrial pacing (figure 2). Taken together, these findings indicate that NT exerts a positive chronotropic response associated with increases in myocardial excitability and atrioventricular conduction in the human heart, which is similar to the cardiac effects induced by sympathetic stimulation. Sinus node recovery time was slightly reduced upon NT administration, an effect largely attributed to a marked NT-induced shortening of the cardiac cycle. Indeed, an evaluation of the corrected sinus node recovery time (pre-automatic pause) revealed that a restoration of sinus node automaticity upon cessation of the rapid atrial pacing was significantly slowed following NT administration (figure 2, panel F). Further clinical studies are needed to examine whether a sustained elevation of endogenous plasma NT levels (e.g. in patients with NT-secreting neuroendocrine tumors) could potentially contribute to sinus node dysfunction.

Autonomic Regulation of the Heart

NT-induced stimulation of sinoatrial node automaticity contributes to reduction of the magnitude of cardioinhibitory responses induced by concomitant activation of parasympathetic nervous system. In anesthetized cats, NT reduces the magnitude of the lengthening of the cardiac cycle evoked by vagal stimulation [151-153, 155] and abolishes vagally-induced cardiac arrhythmias such as second degree atrioventricular block and isorhythmic atrioventricular dissociation [154] (figure 3). A relatively long latency of NT-induced antiarrhythmic effects (second degree atrioventricular block: 40.7 ± 4.6 s; atrioventricular dissociation: 58.7 ± 10.3 s) indirectly suggests that NT action is mediated via stimulation of the release of some endogenous substance with a cardiostimulatory profile of action. Interestingly, the modulatory influence of NT upon vagal chronotropic and arrhythmogenic effects is abolished both by [D-Trp^{11}]-NT, a competitive NT receptor antagonist, and by propranolol, a β-adrenoreceptor blocker. Thus, NT-induced reduction of the vagal cardioinhibitory effects in cats seems to be largely related to the cardiostimulatory action of endogenous catecholamines presumably released by NT upon systemic administration.

NT effects upon autonomic regulation of the heart are species-specific. Indeed, in contrast to potent modulation of parasympathetically-mediated cardiac responses in cats, NT has no effect on the negative chronotropic responses elicited by vagal stimulation in the dog [106]. Furthermore, NT does not modify the magnitude of maximal heart rate deceleration induced by parasympathetic activation following the Valsalva maneuver in human subjects [156].

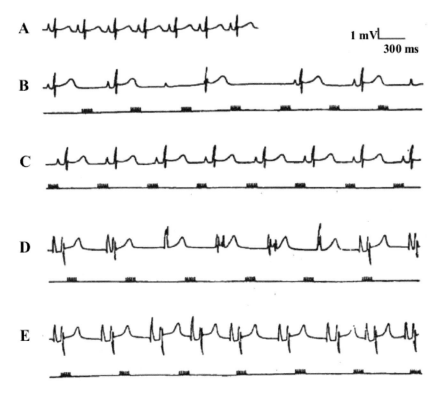

1 mV
300 ms

Figure 3. The impact of neurotensin on vagally-induced cardiac arrhythmias in anesthetized cats. Cardiac electrogram was recorded at baseline (panel A) and following stimulation of the right vagus nerve with bursts of six pulses (40 Hz, 2 ms, 2.5-4.0 V) (panels B-E) in anesthetized cats (n=14). Vagally-induced second degree atrioventricular (AV) block (panel B) and isorhythmic AV dissociation (panel D) were abolished following intravenous bolus neurotensin administration (4.0 x 10^{-8} M) (panels C and E, respectively).

Myocardial Contractility

NT at nanomolar concentrations increases contractility of isolated rat and guinea-pig atria [9, 143, 169, 173, 225]. On the basis of a comparison of pEC_{50} values, NT has been shown to be 20-30-fold more potent than epinephrine at eliciting atrial contractile responses, although inotropic efficacy of NT was lower than that of epinephrine. In rat atria, NT also potentiates norepinephrine-induced inotropic responses [225]. In isolated guinea-pig atria, positive inotropic and chronotropic effects of NT are preserved following blockade of β-adrenoreceptors, but significantly reduced by chronic pretreatment with capsaicin [9, 173] as well as after prior administration of SR 48692, a nonpeptide NT receptor antagonist [143]. Therefore, cardiostimulatory responses induced by NT in this experimental model are ascribed to NT receptor-mediated stimulation of substance P and/or calcitonin gene-related peptide release from cardiac capsaicin-sensitive afferent neurons [9]. Interestingly, contractile effects of NT in isolated guinea-pig atria are also reduced by prior somatostatin infusion [170], an effect presumably related to a reduced availability of the intracellular Ca^{2+} pool mobilized by NT to elicit the inotropic response.

NT exerts a potent contractile effect on the isolated rat ventricular myocardium (figure 4, panels A-B). On the basis of a comparison of pEC_{50} values, NT is ~four orders of magnitude more potent as an inotrope than norepinephrine, an endogenous sympathetic neurotransmitter (figure 5, lower panel). With regards to the efficacy of inotropic action, the maximal NT-induced contractile effects are equivalent in magnitude to those of norepinephrine in Sprague-Dawley (SD) rats, but lower than norepinephrine-induced responses in Wistar-Kyoto (WKY) rats (figure 5, upper panel). NT-induced inotropic responses in the rat left ventricle are largely attributed to the C-terminal portion of its molecule. Indeed, the effect of the C-terminal NT hexapeptide fragment, NT_{8-13}, on myocardial contraction is very similar to that of intact NT, whereas the N-terminal NT hexapeptide fragment, NT_{1-6}, has no effect on the isolated rat left ventricle [157].

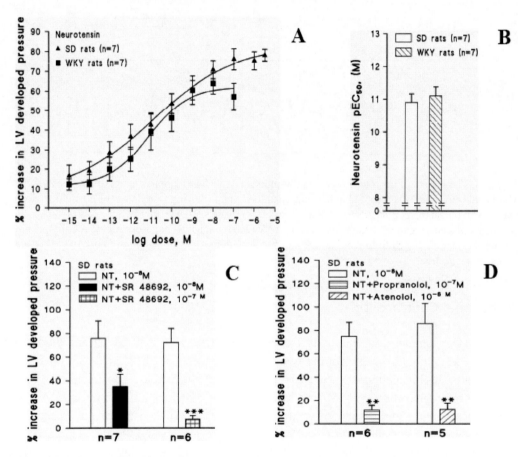

Figure 4. Neurotensin-induced positive inotropic responses in rat ventricular myocardium. % increase in left ventricular (LV) developed pressure was determined in isolated, perfused heart preparations of male Sprague-Dawley (SD) and Wistar-Kyoto (WKY) rats exposed to a wide range of neurotensin (NT) concentrations. Cumulative dose-response curves (panel A) and pEC_{50} values (panel B) are shown. Neurotensin (10^{-8} M)-induced inotropic responses were dose-dependently inhibited by SR 48692 (panel C), a specific neurotensin receptor antagonist, as well as by β-adrenoreceptor blockers (panel D), propranolol and atenolol. SR 48692 and β-adrenoreceptor blockers were infused for 10 min prior to NT administration. *P<0.05, **P<0.01, ***P<0.001 vs. basal value.

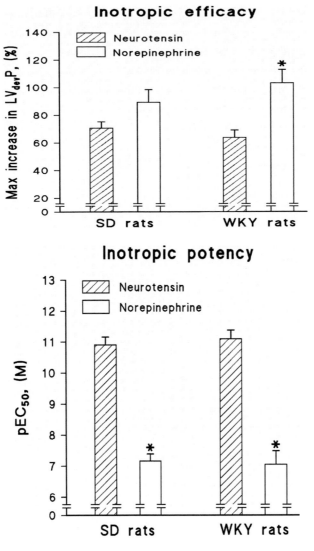

Figure 5. A comparison of neurotensin and norepinephrine inotropic efficacy (upper panel) and potency (lower panel) in the rat ventricular myocardium. The maximal (Max) increase in left ventricular developed pressure ($LV_{dev}P$) was elicited by neurotensin and norepinephrine at concentrations of 10^{-8} M and 10^{-5} M, respectively. Sample size: Sprague-Dawley (SD) rats: neurotensin (n=7), norepinephrine (n=8); Wistar-Kyoto (WKY) rats: neurotensin (n=7), norepinephrine (n=9). * $P<0.05$ vs. neurotensin value.

NT-induced contractile effects on the rat left ventricle are dose-dependently inhibited by SR 48692, a specific NT receptor antagonist (figure 4, panel C). Interestingly, NT-induced contractile effects are also abolished by β-adrenoreceptor blockers (figure 4, panel D), but are unaffected by antagonists of serotonin, histamine or angiotensin II receptors [157]. These findings suggest a pivotal role of sympathetic activation in NT-induced positive inotropic responses. Indeed, a significant elevation of norepinephrine concentrations in the coronary effluent is observed when isolated, perfused rat heart preparations are exposed to NT (figure 6, panel A). The magnitude of NT-induced stimulatory effect upon myocardial norepinephrine release is higher in SD as compared to WKY rats (figure 6, panel A).

Importantly, a strong positive correlation is noted between NT-induced stimulation of myocardial norepinephrine release and contractile responses to this neuropeptide (figure 6, panel B). Furthermore, like NT-induced ventricular contractile responses (figure 4, panel C), NT effects upon myocardial norepinephrine release are inhibited by SR 48692, a specific NT receptor antagonist (figure 6, panel A). Taken together, these findings indicate that NT-induced contractile responses in isolated rat ventricular tissue are largely mediated via presynaptic stimulation of norepinephrine release from myocardial adrenergic terminals. A complete abolishment of NT-induced inotropic responses by β-adrenoreceptor blockers (figure 4, panel D) suggests that NT produces no direct contractile effect on the rat ventricular myocardium.

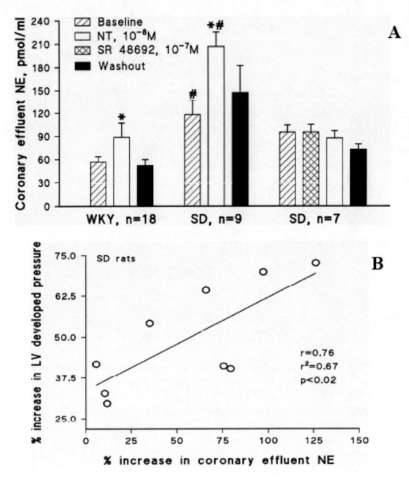

Figure 6. Stimulatory effects of neurotensin (NT) on myocardial norepinephrine (NE) release in Wistar-Kyoto (WKY) and Sprague-Dawley (SD) rats. Norepinephrine concentrations were determined by high-performance liquid chromatography in samples of coronary effluent collected from the isolated, perfused heart preparations. Neurotensin (10^{-8} M) effects on myocardial norepinephrine release were determined at baseline and after prior 10 min infusion of SR 48692, a specific neurotensin receptor antagonist (panel A). A positive correlation was found between neurotensin (10^{-8} M)-induced stimulation of myocardial norepinephrine release and neurotensin-induced left ventricular (LV) contractile responses (panel B). Panel A: *$P<0.05$ vs. basal value; #$P<0.05$ vs. corresponding value in WKY rats.

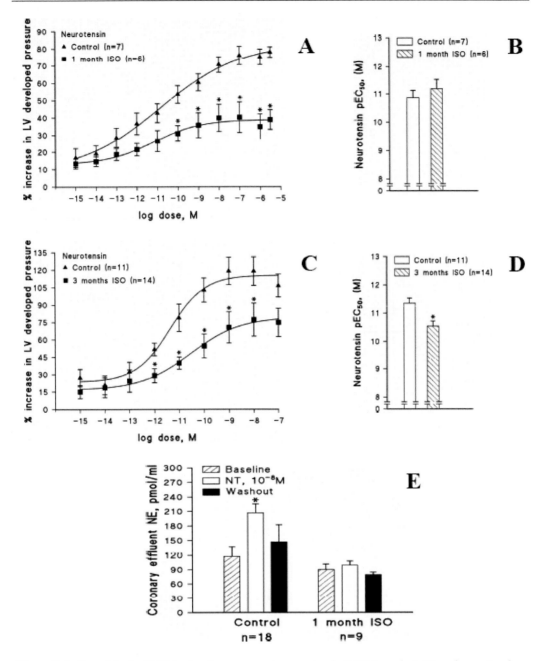

Figure 7. Left ventricular (LV) inotropic responses to neurotensin (NT) (panels A-D) and neurotensin-induced stimulation of myocardial norepinephrine (NE) release (panel E) in control and isoproterenol (ISO)-treated Sprague-Dawley rats. Isoproterenol, a β-adrenoreceptor agonist, was administered daily intraperitoneally at a dose of 0.05 mg/kg over 1 month (panels A-B) or 3 months (panels C-D) to male Sprague-Dawley rats. Control rats were injected with a similar (~0.2 ml) volume of saline vehicle. Isolated, perfused heart preparations were used to assess contractile responses to neurotensin. Cumulative dose-response curves (panels A, C) and pEC_{50} values (panels B, D) are shown. Neurotensin (10^{-8} M)-induced stimulation of myocardial norepinephrine release (panel E) was assessed by high-performance liquid chromatography measurements of norepinephrine concentrations in samples of coronary effluent. Panels A, C and D: *$P<0.05$ vs. corresponding value in control rats; panel E: *$P<0.05$ vs. baseline value.

NT effects on the ventricular myocardium are modified in cardiac disease [158, 159]. In particular, positive inotropic responses to NT are reduced over wide range of concentrations following sustained sympathetic activation produced by chronic administration of isoproterenol, a β-adrenoreceptor agonist, to rats (figure 7, panels A and C). Furthermore, the inotropic potency of NT as assessed by pEC_{50} values is decreased in rats with a cardiomyopathy induced by chronic (3 months) isoproterenol administration (figure 7, panel D). A downregulation of NT-induced contractile responses following chronic β-adrenoreceptor activation is attributed to a blunted stimulatory effect of NT upon myocardial norepinephrine release in isoproterenol-treated rats (figure 7, panel E).

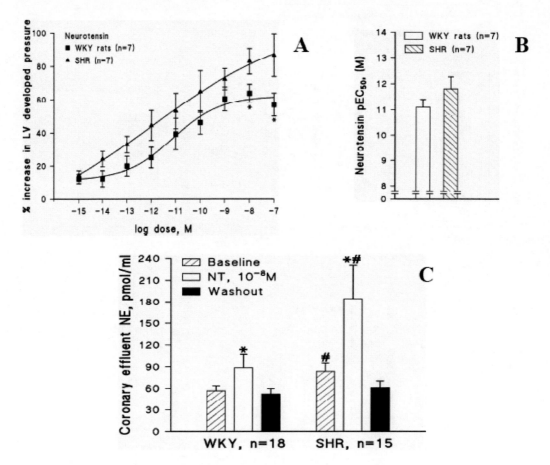

Figure 8. Left ventricular (LV) inotropic responses to neurotensin (NT) (panels A-B) and neurotensin-induced stimulation of myocardial norepinephrine (NE) release (panel C) in Wistar-Kyoto (WKY) and spontaneously hypertensive rats (SHR). Isolated, perfused heart preparations of young (6-8 months age) WKY rats and SHR were used to assess contractile responses to neurotensin. Cumulative dose-response curves (panel A) and pEC_{50} values (panel B) are shown. Neurotensin (10^{-8} M)-induced stimulation of myocardial norepinephrine release (panel C) was assessed by high-performance liquid chromatography measurements of norepinephrine concentrations in samples of coronary effluent. Panel A: *P<0.05 vs. corresponding value in SHR rats. Panel C: *P<0.05 vs. baseline value; # P<0.05 vs. corresponding value in WKY rats.

A different pattern of changes in myocardial contractile responses to NT is noted in compensated pressure-overload cardiac hypertrophy [158]. Specifically, the maximal ventricular inotropic responses to NT are increased in young spontaneously hypertensive rats as compared to normotensive control Wistar-Kyoto rats (figure 8, panel A). This change is associated with significant enhancement of NT-induced stimulation of the myocardial norepinephrine release (figure 8, panel C). The putative significance of these changes for the progression of the cardiac disease remains to be determined.

As with many other physiological effects of NT, its action on myocardial contractility is species-specific. In particular, in contrast to rat and guinea-pig, NT has no contractile effects on the dog [6, 52, 187], rabbit [169] and frog [225] atrial and ventricular myocardium.

Cardiovascular Reflexes

NT-immunoreactive fibers are involved in sensory innervation of the cardiovascular system. In particular, NT-immunoreactive nerve endings are found in the wall of guinea-pig carotid sinus where they are mostly distributed in adventitia and tunica media [68, 117]. These neural terminals have sensory origin as they degenerate after transection of the carotid sinus nerve. Moreover, retrograde tracing has revealed the presence of NT-like immunoreactivity in primary afferent neurons of the petrosal ganglion which projects to the carotid sinus [117]. In the rat brain stem, NT-containing cells are found in dorsomedial region of the nucleus of the tractus solitarius, which receives numerous synaptic inputs from afferent fibers of aortic nerves [88, 95]. Furthermore, NT-containing neural fibers are found in close contact with cardiac vagal preganglionic neurons in the lateral portion of the dorsal vagal nucleus at the level of the obex [88]. In rats, intracerebroventricular administration of NT elicits significant pressor [226] or depressor [190] responses presumably mediated via activation of specific NT binding sites found both in the nucleus of the tractus solitarius and dorsal vagal nucleus [104].

Collectively, these findings suggest an important role played by NT in cardiovascular reflexes originating in reponse to stimulation of arterial baroreceptors.

There is evidence to suggest that NT is also involved in cardiovascular reflexes originating in reponse to stimulation of primary afferents localised in some visceral organs. In particular, topical application of NT at picomolar concentrations on the epicardial surface of the left ventricle [194] or to serousal surface of abdominal organs (ileum, stomach or right hepatic lobe) [195] induces transient dose-dependent increases in blood pressure and heart rate in anesthetized guinea-pigs. These hemodynamic responses are significantly attenuated by ganglion blockers or α-adrenoreceptor antagonists thus indicating that these NT-induced effects are mediated via an increased sympathetic outflow. Furthermore, both NT-induced pressor effects and tachycardia are markedly suppressed by chronic pretreatment of guinea-pigs with capsaicin, suggesting an excitatory effect of NT upon sensory, substance P and calcitonin gene-related peptide-containing neurons [194, 195]. Importantly, NT-induced cardiovascular responses are also prevented by prior topical application of lidocaine, a local anesthetic, to the surface of the left ventricle or abdominal organs. Taken together, these findings suggest that NT could trigger cardiovascular reflexes by stimulating visceral capsaicin-sensitive primary afferents which activate preganglionic sympathetic neurons at the spinal cord via a substance P and/or a calcitonin gene-related peptide-dependent mechanism. Once activated, these neurons transmit impulses to para- and prevertebral ganglionic cells innervating the heart and vessels which ultimately results in a pressor effect and a tachycardia.

The afferent limb of these reflexes is provided by sympathetic rather than parasympathetic fibers as NT-induced cardiovascular responses are preserved after acute bilateral cervical vagotomy [194-196]. Importantly, cardiovascular responses following NT-induced activation of visceral afferents are accompanied by transient twitch-like contractions of the guinea-pig abdominal wall, an effect inhibited by pancuronium and morphine but potentiated by naloxone [196, 197]. Furthermore, both hemodynamic and abdominal motor responses elicited by NT are abolished by acute spinalization. Thus, NT-induced pressor effects and tachycardia could represent a cardiovascular component of the complex spinal nociceptive reflex originating in response to distension of hollow visceral organs, transient episodes of intestinal ischemia, or any other visceral nociceptive stimulus [196, 197].

Structural Determinants of Cardiovascular Activity of NT

The cardiovascular effects of NT are not modified by removal of the N-terminal sequence $pGlu^1-Leu^2-Tyr^3-Glu^4-Asn^5-Lys^6-Pro^7$ thus indicating that the major determinants of biological activity of this neuropeptide reside primarily in the C-terminal portion of its molecule. Indeed, the C-terminal NT hexapeptide, NT_{8-13}, has been shown to be equivalent to intact NT in eliciting vasodepressor responses [44], coronary vasoconstrictor effects [176], contractile effects on the isolated portal vein [189], as well as positive inotropic responses in the isolated atrial [173] and ventricular [157] myocardium. A shorter C-terminal NT fragment, NT_{9-13}, has only about 2% of intact NT potency but it still able to elicit the same maximum response at high concentrations, whereas the NT_{10-13} tetrapeptide is completely inactive. Therefore, the C-terminal sequence $Arg^9-Pro^{10}-Tyr^{11}-Ile^{12}-Leu^{13}-OH$ seems to be the minimum structure required for displaying cardiovascular activity of NT [173, 174, 176, 189].

These findings are consistent with NT structure-activity relationships determined in receptor binding studies. In particular, the C-terminal NT pentapeptide, NT_{9-13}, is the shortest C-terminal fragment exhibiting properties of a full agonist in binding with neuronal and extraneuronal NT receptors, whereby it possesses about 3% of the potency of intact NT [1, 69, 109, 133]. The addition of Arg^8 to this sequence yields a hexapeptide fragment, NT_{8-13}, which is as potent as intact NT in binding to NT receptors expressed in various cell lines [1, 37, 109, 211], or purified from newborn human [247] and mouse [133] brain tissue. On the other hand, the N-terminal NT fragments, NT_{1-6}, NT_{1-8} and NT_{1-10}, do not possess cardiovascular activity [157, 173, 174, 176, 189] and exhibit a very low affinity ($IC_{50} > 10$ μM) for the NT receptor in binding studies [247].

Of the C-terminal portion of NT molecule, amino acids Ile^{12} and Leu^{13} contribute mainly to the affinity of NT for its receptor, whereas the chemical groups responsible for NT receptor activation reside in the sequence Arg^9-Pro^{10}-Tyr^{11} [174]. Indeed, NT fragments missing Ile^{12} and Leu^{13} (NT_{1-12} and NT_{1-11}), although being less potent than intact NT, are able to elicit the same maximal contractile responses in isolated guinea-pig atria [173]. On the other hand, substitutions in positions 9, 10 and 11 yield NT analogues exhibiting a very low potency in eliciting cardiovascular effects [173, 174, 176, 189]. Amongst C-terminal amino acids, Tyr^{11} is particularly important for NT receptor activation [173, 176]. Indeed, NT analogues where Tyr^{11} is replaced with D-Tyr, D-Phe, Phe, Ala or Leu are three-four orders of magnitude less potent than the intact NT in eliciting positive inotropic responses in isolated guinea-pig atria [173, 174], coronary vasoconstrictor effect in isolated, perfused rat hearts [176] and contractile effects in the isolated rat portal vein [189]. Likewise, in contrast to intact NT, a NT analogue in which Tyr^{11} is replaced with D-Trp ([D-Trp^{11}]-NT), has no contractile effect on isolated rat ventricular myocardium [157], as well as basal heart rate and vagally-induced cardioinhibitory effects in anesthetized cats [151-155]. Consistently, [Phe^{11}]-NT and [D-Tyr^{11}]-NT analogues are several orders of magnitude less potent than intact NT in binding to NT receptors expressed in human umbilical vein endothelial cells [211]. These findings raise the possibility that the presence in position 11 of an aromatic residue with the L-configuration is important for NT binding with its receptor. Indeed, replacing Tyr^{11} with Trp, an aromatic residue with a longer side chain, yields a NT analogue, [Trp^{11}]-NT, which is equivalent to intact NT in eliciting cardiovascular responses in rats [176, 189].

Interestingly, NT analogues in which Tyr^{11} is substituted for $Tyr(Me)^{11}$ or D-Trp^{11} exhibit properties of competitive NT receptor antagonists at concentrations below 10^{-6} M while behaving like weak agonists at higher concentrations [176, 189]. NT receptor antagonist effects produced by these compounds have been shown in a number of studies (table 5). Importantly, [D-Trp^{11}]-NT and $Tyr(Me)^{11}$-NT antagonize coronary vasoconstrictor responses induced by native NT in isolated perfused rat hearts [175, 176] as well as its contractile effects on isolated rat portal vein [189], but has no effect on NT-induced positive inotropic responses in isolated guinea-pig atria [175]. Taken together, these findings raise the possibility that receptors underlying the influence of NT on the vascular smooth muscle tone are pharmacologically distinct from those mediating myocardial effects of NT, at least in rats.

Mechanisms of NT-Induced Cardiovascular Effects

NT Receptors

NT Receptor Subtypes and Specific Antagonists
To date, three subtypes of NT receptors (NTS_1, NTS_2 and NTS_3) have been identified [235]. All three NT receptor subtypes recognize the same C-terminal NT sequence, Arg^9-Pro^{10}-Tyr^{11}-Ile^{12}-Leu^{13}-OH. NTS_1 and NTS_2 are G-protein-coupled receptors with seven putative transmembrane domains, whereas the NTS_3 receptor is an intracellular NT binding site structurally identical to gp95/sortilin, a protein of ~95 kDa with a single transmembrane domain [166].

Table 5. Inhibition of NT-induced cardiovascular effects by selective NT receptor antagonists

Species	Preparation used/In vivo experiment	NT effect	NT receptor antagonist used	NT receptor antagonist dose	Reference
Rat	Isolated portal vein	Venoconstrictor effect	[D-Trp[11]]-NT	$4\text{-}11 \times 10^{-7}$ M	[188]
			[Tyr(Me)[11]]-NT	$10^{-7}\text{-}10^{-6}$ M	[189]
	Isolated, perfused heart	Coronary vasoconstrictor effect	[D-Trp[11]]-NT	$10^{-7}\text{-}10^{-6}$ M	[175]
			[Tyr(Me)[11]]-NT	$10^{-7}\text{-}10^{-6}$ M	[176]
		Positive ventricular inotropic responses	SR 48692	$10^{-8}\text{-}10^{-7}$ M	[157-159]
	In vivo experiment	Hypotensive effect	SR 48692	0.1-10 mg/kg orally, 1 hour before NT	[71, 212]
			SR 142948A	0.01-1.0 mg/kg orally, 1 hour before NT	[213]
		Increase in cutaneous vascular permeability	SR 48692	5.0 pM, intradermally	[138, 213]
			SR 142948A	0.01-1.0 nM, intradermally	[213]
Guinea-pig	Isolated atria	Positive chronotropic and inotropic effects	SR 48692	$IC_{50} \sim 10^{-9}$ M	[143]
	In vivo experiment	Pressor effect	SR 48692	6-400 µg/kg, i.v.	[143]
Cat	In vivo experiment	Tachycardia	[D-Trp[11]]-NT	4.0×10^{-8} M, i.v.	[152]
		Reduction of vagally-induced bradycardia	[D-Trp[11]]-NT	4.0×10^{-8} M, i.v.	[151, 153, 155]
		Protective effect in vagally-induced cardiac arrhythmias	D-Trp[11]]-NT	4.0×10^{-8} M, i.v.	[154]
Human	Endothelial cells of umbilical vein	Stimulation of phosphoinositide turnover, elevation of intracellular Ca^{2+} level, and stimulation of prostacyclin release	SR 48692	$IC_{50} \sim 41\text{-}86$ nM	[211-213]
			SR 142948A	$IC_{50} \sim 17\text{-}24$ nM	

To study putative physiological roles of NT receptors, two selective nonpeptide NT receptor antagonists, SR 48692 and SR 142948A, have been synthesized by Sanofi Research [70, 72]. Both compounds at nanomolar concentrations competetively inhibit ^{125}I-labeled NT binding to NT receptors of neural and extraneural localization as well as NT-induced changes in intracellular levels of the second messengers [70, 72, 94, 160, 211, 213]. While SR 48692 has a higher affinity for NTS_1 as compared to NTS_2 receptor subtypes, SR 142948A equally recognizes both NT receptor subtypes and therefore exhibits a wider spectrum of pharmacological activity than SR 48692 [72]. Furthermore, in receptor binding studies SR 142948A exhibits about a 60-fold higher affinity for the human NTS_1 receptor as compared to SR 48692 [213]. Importantly, in contrast to [D-Trp^{11}]-NT and Tyr(Me)^{11}-NT, NT analogues possessing properties of NT receptor antagonists, SR 48692 and SR 142948A do not exhibit an intrinsic activity even at concentrations about 100-fold higher than those required for 50% inhibition of NT receptor binding [71, 72, 143, 213].

Although expression of NTS_3 receptor mRNA has been found in mouse [85], rat [123] and human [166] myocardial tissue, the intracellular localization of this NT receptor subtype limits the chances of it being involved in NT-induced cardiac effects. Hence the functional significance of the other two NT receptor subtypes, NTS_1 and NTS_2, only will be discussed.

NTS₁ Receptor

The NTS_1 receptor, purified from human [247] and mouse [133] brain, is a polypeptide with an apparent molecular weight of 100 kDa that reperesents a high-affinity (K_d~0.1-0.3 nM) NT binding site coupled to phospholipase C via pertussis toxin-insensitive G-proteins [2, 22]. The NTS_1 receptor which was cloned for the first time by Tanaka et al. (1990) from the rat brain, has a structure that consists of 424 amino acids. A polypeptide chain of the human NTS_1 receptor cloned from the colonic adenocarcinoma cell line HT 29 includes 418 amino acids and exhibits a high degree of structural identity (84%) with the rat NTS_1 receptor [236]. NTS_1 receptor subtype mRNA expression has been found in rat myocardial tissue [228] as well as human umbilical vein and aortic endothelial cells [211]. Furthermore, a specific binding of ^{125}I-labeled NT has been demonstrated in human umbilical vein (K_d ~ 0.23 nM, B_{max} ~ 5500 sites/cell) and aortic endothelial cell monolayers (K_d ~ 0.6 nM, B_{max} ~ 32000 sites/cell) [211, 213].

Activation of the NTS_1 receptor expressed in various cells exerts a strong stimulatory influence on phosphatidylinositol turnover as evidenced by a transient elevation of intracellular inositol phosphate levels with a subsequent stimulation of Ca^{2+} release from intracellular stores (table 6). With regards to the cardiovascular system, there is a strong positive correlation between the dissociation constant of NT in binding experiments and EC_{50} values for stimulation of $^{45}Ca^{2+}$ efflux in human endothelial cells [211]. Furthermore, NT-induced Ca^{2+} mobilization in human umbilical vein endothelial cells is abolished by SR 48692 and SR 142948A, selective NT receptor antagonists [213], suggesting a specific NT receptor-mediated effect.

Activation of the NTS_1 receptor expressed in mouse neuroblastoma N1E115 cells produces a transient increase in intracellular cGMP levels [1, 3, 64, 160]. However, no changes in intracellular cGMP levels were noted following activation of NTS_1 receptors expressed in fibroblasts [37], colonic adenocarcinoma HT29 cells [2, 160] and Chinese hamster ovary cells [160] thus indicating that this NT receptor subtype is functionally coupled to guanylate cyclase only in neural tissue. Likewise, no consistent evidence is available to show the impact of NTS_1 receptor activation on adenylate cyclase activity. Indeed, an increase [160, 244], a decrease [1] as well as no change [2, 37, 66, 239] in intracellular cAMP levels has been found following NTS_1 receptor activation in different studies. Collectively, these findings suggest that NTS_1 receptor-mediated stimulation of phosphatidylinositol turnover rather than a change in intracellular levels of cyclic nucleotides is involved in the cardiovascular effects of NT.

NT effects on blood pressure, heart rate, myocardial contractility and phosphoinositide turnover in endothelial cells, are dose-dependently inhibited by SR 48692 (table 5), a NT receptor antagonist exhibiting a significantly higher affinity for the NTS_1 ($IC_{50} \sim 5.6$ nM) as compared to the NTS_2 ($IC_{50} \sim 300$ nM) receptor subtype [70]. These findings suggest that NT-induced cardiovascular responses are primarily mediated via an activation of the NTS_1 receptor subtype. This notion is also supported by results of studies designed to compare the relative potency of different NT receptor antagonists in abolishing NT-induced cardiovascular responses [213]. In particular, a higher affinity of SR 142948A as compared to SR 48692 for the NTS_1 receptor accounts for a significantly higher potency of SR 142948A in antagonizing NT effects on blood pressure and cutaneous vascular permeability in anesthetized rats, as well as Ca^{2+} levels and prostacyclin release from isolated human umbilical vein endothelial cells [213].

Table 6. Stimulation of phosphoinositide hydrolysis and intracellular Ca^{2+} mobilization following activation of NTS_1 receptor subtype

Species	Cell/tissue expressing NT receptor	NT dose	Reference
Human	Colonic adenocarcinoma HT29 cells	EC_{50} 3.5±0.5 nM	[2, 22, 160]
	Pancreatic cancer cells	10^{-12}-10^{-9} M	[93, 94]
	Umbilical vein and aorthic endothelial cells	3-100 nM	[211, 212]
Mouse	Neuroblastoma N1E115 cells	EC_{50} 0.46-0.9 nM	[3, 64, 96, 160, 223]
Rat	Brain slices	EC_{50} 224±18 nM	[66]
	Brain cortex neurons	10^{-6}-10^{-9} M	[210]
	Serosal mast cells	10^{-7} M	[14]
	Fibroblasts	EC_{50} 4.84 nM	[37]
	Pheochromacetoma cells	10^{-7} M	[83]
	CHO cells	EC_{50} 3.0 nM	[82, 84, 160, 239]

NTS$_2$ Receptor

The NTS$_2$ receptor subtype represents a low-affinity (K$_d$~3-5 nM) NT binding site sensitive to levocabastine, a histamine H$_1$ receptor antagonist, which competitively inhibit NT binding to NTS$_2$ [235]. A polypeptide chain of the brain NTS$_2$ receptor comprises 417 (mouse), 416 (rat) or 410 (human) amino acids (~46 kDa) and shows a high degree of structural homology to NTS$_1$ [40, 134, 237]. Expression studies has revealed the presence of low levels of NTS$_2$ receptor mRNA in rat [40] and human [237], but not in mice [134] myocardial tissue. Interestingly, expression of the NTS$_2$ receptor subtype in neonatal rat cardiomyocytes is enhanced upon long-term exposure to leukaemia inhibitory factor, a cytokine which belongs to the interleukin-6 family and which is involved in cardiac remodeling and the development of heart failure [57]. However, the functional significance of the myocardial NTS$_2$ receptor remains uncertain. Indeed, although NT specifically binds to recombinant human [237] and mouse [21] NTS$_2$ receptors expressed in CHO or HEK 293 cell lines, it does not elicit a physiological response as assessed by measurements of intracellular levels of second messengers. Furthermore, only small elevations of intracellular Ca^{2+} levels are elicited by very high (1 μM) NT concentrations upon activation of the rat NTS$_2$ receptor expressed in CHO cells [245]. In contrast, nonpeptide NTS$_1$ receptor antagonists, SR 48692 and SR 142948A, behave as potent agonists of the NTS$_2$ receptor, stimulating polyphosphoinositide hydrolysis and increasing intracellular Ca^{2+} levels [237, 245]. Surprisingly, these effects are fully antagonized by NT suggesting that some yet unidentified endogenous compound rather than NT could act as a natural agonist for the NTS$_2$ receptor [237, 245]. In the light of these findings, it is very unlikely that the NTS$_2$ receptor subtype is involved in NT-induced cardiovascular responses.

Stimulation of Endogenous Neurotransmitter/Neuromodulator Release

Histamine

NT could act as a modulator producing a potent stimulatory effect on the release of a variety of endogenous biologically active substances (table 7). Only those modulatory effects of NT that could contribute to the cardiovascular activity of this neuropeptide will be briefly discussed.

A number of cardiovascular effects produced by NT are mediated via stimulation of histamine release from mast cells. In particular, the histamine-releasing effect of NT accounts for vasodepressor responses, peripheral vasodilatation, increased capillary permeability and plasma extravasation following intravenous NT infusion in anesthetized rats [24, 27, 38, 42, 71, 77, 148, 137].

The stimulatory effect of NT on histamine release has been demonstrated using different experimental models. In anesthetized rats, intravenous NT infusion induces a transient, dose-dependent increase in plasma histamine levels which is abolished by pretreatment with compound 48/80, a mast cell degranulating agent [27, 147]. Furthermore, NT-induced stimulation of histamine release has been shown in the isolated, perfused rat heart [192, 193], hindquarter [102, 103], skin slices [42] as well as isolated mast cells [14, 27, 30, 114, 118, 206, 215]. On a molar basis, NT is 5-6 times as active as compound 48/80 in increasing histamine concentrations in coronary effluent collected from the isolated, spontaneously beating rat heart [192].

Table 7. Stimulatory effects of NT upon release of various endogenous biologically active substances from peripheral tissues

Endogenous substance released by NT	Species	Preparation used	NT dose	References
Histamine	Rat	Isolated, perfused heart	EC_{50} 0.34 nM	[192, 193]
		Isolated, perfused hindquarter	10^{-8}-10^{-6} g/ml	[103]
		Isolated, perfused skin slices	10^{-13}-10^{-6} M	[42]
		Blood samples collected from carotid artery	1 nM, i.v.	[27, 137, 147]
		Peritoneal mast cells	10^{-9}-10^{-5} M	[14, 27, 30, 118, 137, 206]
		Pleural mast cells	EC_{50} 3 x 10^{-8} M	[14, 114, 137]
	Human	Jejunal mast cells	10^{-9}-10^{-6} M	[215]
Norepinephrine	Rat	Perfused mesenteric arteries	10^{-6}-10^{-7} M	[232]
		Isolated, perfused heart	10^{-8} M	[157-159]
		Pheochromacetoma cells	EC_{50} 59 μM	[162]
Epinephrine	Rat	Samples of blood plasma	10^{-9} M, i.v.	[147]
Serotonin	Rat	Isolated, perfused hindquarter	5-15 x 10^{-7} /ml	[102]
		Peritoneal mast cells	3 μM	[30]
Acetylcholine	Guinea-pig	Myenteric plexus-longitudinal muscle strips of small intestine	3 pM-3 nM	[178, 246]
			10^{-10}-10^{-7} M	[141]
Prostaglandins	Rat	Samples of blood plasma	2-3 nM/kg, i.v.	[212]
	Human	Umbilical vein endothelial cells	EC50 14+1 nM	[212]
Substance P	Guinea-pig	Inferior mesenteric ganglion	5.0 x 10-6 M	[224]
		Myenteric plexus-longitudinal muscle strips of small intestine	60 nM	[92]
□-aminobutyric acid	Guinea-pig	Strips of ileum	10-10-10-7 M	[141]
Somatostatin	Rat	Samples of portal venous blood	3 □g/100 g BW, i.v.	[209]
			0.24-0.72 pM/kg/hr , i.v.	[76]
			7.2 nM/kg/hr, i.v.	[75]

NT-induced stimulation of histamine release is independent of heart rate and coronary perfusion pressure, but is suppressed in Ca^{2+}-free perfusion media [193]. There is some evidence to suggest that endogenous NT is involved in stress-induced stimulation of histamine release from cardiac mast cells [161]. Indeed, cardiac mast cell degranulation induced by acute immobilization stress in rats is completely abolished by pretreatment with SR 48692, a NT receptor antagonist [161].

In isolated serosal rat mast cells, the maximal amount of histamine released by NT constitutes about 20% of the total histamine content [114, 206]. However, mast cell degranulating capacity of NT is significantly reduced in Ca^{2+}- or glucose-free perfusion media [27, 30]. There is a strong evidence to suggest that the stimulatory effect of NT upon histamine release is mediated via activation of a mast cell NT receptor. Indeed, NT-induced elevation of plasma histamine levels [137], stimulation of histamine release from isolated rat mast cells [137, 206], as well as increases in cutaneous vascular permeability [137, 213] are blocked by the selective NT receptor antagonists, SR 48692, SR 142948A and [D-Trp^{11}]-NT. Consistently, a specific and reversible ^{125}I-NT binding (K_d=154 nM) has been found in rat mast cells [119]. These findings are supported by results of structure-activity studies demonstrating that the histamine releasing effect of NT requires a preserved integrity of the C-terminal portion of the NT molecule [103, 206]. Indeed, a replacement of Arg^8, Arg^9 or Tyr^{11} with various amino acids yields NT analogues exhibiting a very low potency at eliciting histamine release in the isolated, perfused rat hindquarter [103]. On the other hand, in rat mast cell binding studies, substitutions of N-terminal amino acids with their D-isomers has no significant impact on NT binding, whereas modifications performed within the C-terminal portion of NT, residues Pro^{10} through Leu^{13}, considerably reduces NT binding capacity [120].

C-terminal NT hexa- and pentapeptide fragments, NT_{8-13} and NT_{9-13}, are found to possess about 70% of the relative affinity for mast cell NT receptors as compared to intact NT [120].

Mast cell NT receptors are coupled with phospholipase C via pertussis toxin-sensitive G-proteins [14]. In isolated rat serosal mast cells, NT-induced stimulation of histamine release is accompanied by a rapid and transient increase in intracellular free Ca^{2+} and inositol trisphosphate levels [14]. These effects were suppressed by pretreatment with U-73122, an inhibitor of phospholipase C, as well as by pertussis toxin.

Serotonin

Serotonin is a mast cell mediator released in parallel fashion with histamine upon NT exposure. In isolated peritoneal rat mast cells, NT induces a prompt (within seconds) and dose-dependent concomitant liberation of histamine and serotonin, with both secretory effects being Ca^{2+}- and energy-dependent [30]. In isolated, perfused rat hindquarters, NT-induced stimulation of serotonin release is associated with a marked increase in vascular resistance [102]. Both serotonin releasing effect of NT and NT-induced vasoconstriction are inhibited by compound 48/80.

Catecholamines

NT induces a transient increase in plasma epinephrine concentrations following intravenous administration in anesthetized rats, an effect attenuated by adrenalectomy [147]. However, NT does not affect plasma norepinephrine concentrations. On the other hand, NT exerts a potent stimulatory effect on myocardial norepinephrine release in isolated, perfused rat heart preparations (figure 6, panel A) [157-159].

Prostaglandins

NT induces a dose-dependent prostacyclin release from human umbilical vein endothelial cells, an effect associated with a transient elevation of intracellular Ca^{2+} levels [212]. Furthermore, intravenous infusion of NT ~doubles circulating levels of 6-keto-prostaglandin $F_{1\alpha}$ in anesthetized rats, an effect accompanied by a significant fall in blood pressure [212]. All of these effects are abolished by nanomolar concentrations of SR 48692 and SR 142948A, nonpeptide NT receptor antagonists, suggesting a direct, high-affinity NT receptor-mediated stimulatory effect upon release of endogenous prostaglandins [212, 213]. A prostaglandin-dependent mechanism is also involved in NT-induced contractile effects on the isolated rat portal vein [188] as well as the NT-induced vasodilatory effects on the coronary vasculature in anesthetized dogs [52].

References

[1] Amar, S; Mazella, J; Checler, F; Kitabgi, P; Vincent, JP. (1985). Regulation of cyclic GMP levels by neurotensin in neuroblastoma clone N1E115. *Biochem. Biophys. Res. Commun., V.129,* 117-125.

[2] Amar, S; Kitabgi, P; Vincent, JP. (1986). Activation of phosphatidylinositol turnover by neurotensin receptors in the human colonic adenocarcinoma cell line HT29. *FEBS Lett., V.201,* 31-36.

[3] Amar, S; Kitabgi, P; Vincent, JP. (1987). Stimulation of inositol phosphate production by neurotensin in neuroblastoma N1E-115 cells: implication of GTP-binding proteins and relationship with the cyclic GMP response. *J. Neurochem., V.49,* 999-1006.

[4] Armour, JA (1996). Comparative effects of endothelin and neurotensin on intrinsic cardiac neurons in situ. *Peptides, V.17,* 1047-1052.

[5] Aronin, N; Carraway, RE; Ferris, CF; Hammer, RA; Leeman, SE. (1982). The stability and metabolism of intravenously administered neurotensin in the rat. *Peptides, V.3,* 637-642.

[6] Baca, I; Mittmann, U; Feurle, GE; Haas, M; Muller, Th. (1981). Effect of neurotensin on regional intestinal blood flow in the dog. *Res. Exp. Med. (Berl), V.179,* 53-58.

[7] Bachelard, H; St-Pierre, S; Rioux, F. (1985). The chronotropic action of neurotensin in the guinea-pig isolated heart. *Peptides, V.6,* 841-845.

[8] Bachelard, H; St-Pierre, S; Rioux, F. (1986). The coronary vasodilator effect of neurotensin in the guinea-pig isolated heart. *Peptides, V.7,* 431-435.

[9] Bachelard, H; St-Pierre, S; Rioux F. (1987). Participation of capsaicin-sensitive neurons in the cardiovascular effects of neurotensin in guinea-pigs. *Peptides, V.8,* 1079-1087.

[10] Bachelard, H; Gardiner, SM; Kemp, PA; Bennett, T. (1992). Mechanisms contributing to the regional haemodynamic effects of neurotensin in conscious, unrestrained *Long Evans* rats. *Br. J. Pharmacol., V.105,* 191-201.

[11] Bachoo, M; Ciriello, J; Polosa, C. (1987). Effect of preganglionic stimulation on neuropeptide-like immunoreactivity in the stellate ganglion of the cat. *Brain Res., V.400,* 377-382.

[12] Bachoo, M; Polosa, C. (1988). Cardioacceleration produced by close intra-arterial injection of neurotensin into the stellate ganglion of the cat. *Can. J. Physiol. Pharmacol., V.66,* 408-412.

[13] Barelli, H; Fox-Threlkeld JET; Dive, V; Daniel, EE; Vincent, JP; Checler, F. (1994). Role of endopeptidase 3.4.24.16 in the catabolism of neurotensin, in vivo, in the vascularly perfused dog ileum. *Br. J. Pharmacol., V.112,* 127-132.

[14] Barrocas, AM; Cochrane, DE; Carraway, RE; Feldberg, RS. (1999). Neurotensin stimulation of mast cell secretion is receptor-mediated, pertussis-toxin sensitive and requires activation of phospholipase C. *Immunopharmacol., V.41,* 131-137.

[15] Bauer, B; Neubauer, S; Spindler, M; Durr, R; Becker, HH; Ertl, G.(1995). Interference of angiotensin-converting enzyme inhibition with vasoactive peptides in the coronary circulation of dogs. *J. Cardiovasc. Pharmacol., V.25,* 756-762.

[16] Besterman, HS; Bloom, SR; Sarson, DL; Blackburn, AM; Johnston, DI; Patel, HR; Stewart, JS; Modigliani, R; Guerin, S; Mallinson, CN. (1978). Gut-hormone profile in coeliac disease. *Lancet, V.1,* 785-788.

[17] Blackburn, AM; Bloom, SR. (1979). A radioimmunoassay for neurotensin in human plasma. *J. Endocrinol., V.83,* 175-181.

[18] Blackburn, AM; Christofides, ND; Ghatei, MA; Sarson, DL; Ebeid, FH; Ralphs DN; Bloom, SR. (1980). Elevation of plasma neurotensin in the dumping syndrome. *Clin. Sci., V.59,* 237-243.

[19] Blackburn, AM; Fletcher, DR; Adrian, TE; Bloom, SR. (1980). Neurotensin infusion in man: pharmacokinetics and effect on gastrointestinal and pituitary hormones. *J. Clin. Endocrinol. Metab., V.51,* 1257-1261.

[20] Bommer, M; Herz, A. (1989). Neurotensin affects metabolism of opioid peptides, catecholamines and inositol phospholipids in bovine chromaffin cells. *Life Sci., V.44,* 327-335.

[21] Botto, JM; Chabry, J; Sarret, P; Vincent, JP; Mazella J. (1998). Stable expression of the mouse levocabastine-sensitive neurotensin receptor in HEK 293 cell line: binding properties, photoaffinity labeling, and internalization mechanism. *Biochem. Biophys. Res. Commun., V.243,* 585-590.

[22] Bozou, JC; Rochet, N; Magnaldo, I; Vincent, JP. (1989). Neurotensin stimulates inositol trisphosphate-mediated calcium mobilization but not protein kinase C activation in HT29 cells. *Biochem. J., V.264,* 871-878.

[23] Carbo, R; Zetina, ME; Corkidi, G; Morales, MA. (1997). Topographic relationship of neurotensin-containing axon terminals with cardiac and non-cardiac principal ganglion cells in the stellate ganglia of the cat. *Synapse, V.25,* 277-284.

[24] Carraway, R; Leeman, SE. (1973). The isolation of a new hypotensive peptide, neurotensin, from bovine hypothalami. *J. Biol. Chem., V.248,* 6854-6861.

[25] Carraway, R; Leeman, SE. (1976). Characterization of radioimmunoassayable neurotensin in the rat. *J. Biol. Chem., V.251,* 7045-7052.

[26] Carraway, R; Hammer, RA; Leeman, SE. (1980). Neurotensin in plasma: immunochemical and chromatographic character of acid/acetone-soluble material. *Endocrinology, V.107,* 400-406.

[27] Carraway, R; Cochrane, DE; Lansman, JB; Leeman, SE; Paterson, BM; Welch, H.J. (1982). Neurotensin stimulates exocytotic histamine secretion from rat mast cells and elevates plasma histamine levels. *J. Physiol., V.323,* 403-414.

[28] Carraway, R; Ruane, SE; Feurle, GE; Taylor, S. (1982). Amphibian neurotensin is not xenopsin: dual presence of neurotensin-like and xenopsin-like peptides in various amphibian. *Endocrinology, V.110,* 1094-1101.

[29] Carraway, RE. (1984). Rapid proteolytic generation of neurotensin-related peptides and biologic activity during extraction of rat and chicken gastric tissues. *J. Biol. Chem., V.259,* 10328-10334.

[30] Carraway, RE; Cochrane, DE; Granier, C; Kitabgi, P; Leeman, S; Singer, EA. (1984). Parallel secretion of endogenous 5-hydroxytryptamine and histamine from mast cells stimulated by vasoactive peptides and compound 48/80. *Br. J. Pharmacol., V.81,* 227-229.

[31] Carraway, RE; Mitra, SP; Ferris, CF. (1986). Pepsin treatment of mammalian plasma generates immunoreactive and biologically active neurotensin-related peptides in micromolar concentrations. *Endocrinology, V.119,* 1519-1526.

[32] Carraway, RE; Mitra SP. (1987).Precursor forms of neurotensin in cat: processing with pepsin yields NT-(3-13) and NT-(4-13). *Regul. Peptides, V.18,* 139-154.

[33] Carraway, RE; Mitra, SP; Feurle, GE; Hacki, W.H. (1988). Presence of neurotensin and neuromedin N within a common precursor from a human pancreatic neuroendocrine tumor. *J. Clin Endocrinol. Metab., V.66,* 1323-1328.

[34] Carraway, RE; Mitra, SP; Spaulding, G. (1992). Posttranslational processing of the neurotensin/neuromedin N precursor. *Ann. N.Y. Acad. Sci., V.668,* 1-16.

[35] Caverson, MM; Bachoo, M; Ciriello, J; Polosa, C. (1989). Effect of preganglionic stimulation or chronic decentralization on neurotensin-like immunoreactivity in sympathetic ganglia of the cat. *Brain Res., V.482,* 365-370.

[36] Ceconi, C; Condorelli, E; Quinzanini, M; Rodella, A; Ferrari, R; Harris P. (1989). Noradrenaline, atrial natriuretic peptide, bombesin and neurotensin in myocardium and blood of rats in congestive cardiac failure. *Cardiovasc. Res., V.23,* 674-682.

[37] Chabry, J; Labbe-Jullie, C; Gully, D; Patrick, K; Vincent, JP; Mazella, J. (1994). Stable expression of the cloned rat brain neurotensin receptor into fibroblasts: binding properties, photoaffinity labeling, transduction mechanisms, and internalization. *J. Neurochem., V.63,* 19-27.

[38] Chahl, L.A. (1979). The effect of putative peptide neurotransmitters on cutaneous vascular permeability in the rat. *Naunyn-Schmiedeberg's Arch. Pharmacol., V.309,* 159-163.

[39] Chahl, LA; Walker, SB. (1981). Responses of the rat cardiovascular system to substance P, neurotensin and bombesin. *Life Sci., V.29,* 2009-2015.

[40] Chalon, P; Vita, N; Kaghad, M; Guillemot, M; Bonnin, J; Delpech, B; Le Fur, G; Ferrara, P; Caput, D. (1996). Molecular cloning of a levocabastine-sensitive neurotensin binding site. *FEBS Lett., V.386,* 91-94.

[41] Checler, F; Kostolansca, B; Fox, J. (1988). In vivo inactivation of neurotensin in dog ileum: major involvement of endopeptidase 24.11. *J. Pharmacol. Exp. Ther.,* *V.244,* 1040-1044.

[42] Cochrane, DE; Emigh, C; Levine, G; Carraway, RE; Leeman, SE. (1982). Neurotensin alters cutaneous vascular permeability and stimulates histamine release from isolated skin. *Ann. N.Y. Acad. Sci., V.400,* 396-397.

[43] Corder, R; Mason, DF; Perrett, D; Lowry, PJ; Clement-Jones, V; Linton EA; Besser GM; Rees, LH. (1982). Simultaneous release of neurotensin, somatostatin, enkephalins and catecholamines from perfused cat adrenal glands. *Neuropeptides, V.3,* 9-17.

[44] Di Paola, ED; Richelson E. (1990). Cardiovascular effects of neurotensin and some analogues on rats. *Eur. J. Pharmacol., V.175,* 279-283.

[45] Dobner, PR; Deutch, AY; Fadel, J. (2003). Neurotensin: dual roles in psychostimulant and antipsychotic drug responses. *Life Sci., V.73,* 801-811.

[46] D'Orleans-Juste, P; Dion, S; Mizrahi, J; Regoli, D. (1985). Effects of peptides and non-peptides on isolated arterial smooth muscles: role of endothelium. *Eur. J. Pharmacol., V.114,* 9-21.

[47] Duke, GE; Carraway, RE; Raven, JA. (1993). Cardiovascular effects of neurotensin in anesthetized white leghorn hens. *Poult. Sci., V.72,* 1606-1610.

[48] Dumoulin, V; Dakka, T; Plaisancie, P; Chayvialle, JA; Cuber, JC. (1995). Regulation of glucagons-like peptide-1-(7-36) amide, peptide YY, and neurotensin secretion by neurotransmitters and gut hormones in the isolated vascularly perfused rat ileum. *Endocrinology, V.136,* 5182-5188.

[49] Dumoulin, V; Moro, F; Barcelo, A; Dakka, T; Cuber, JC. (1998). Peptide YY, glucagon-like peptide-1, and neurotensin responses to luminal factors in the isolated vascularly perfused rat ileum. *Endocrinology, V.139,* 3780-3786.

[50] Ekman, R; Ivarsson, S; Jansson, L. (1985). Bombesin, neurotensin and pro-gamma-melanotropin immunoreactants in human milk. *Regul. Peptides, V.10,* 99-105.

[51] Ernst, A; Hellmich, S; Bergmann, A. (2006). Proneurotensin 1-117, a stable neurotensin precursor fragment identified in human circulation. *Peptides, V.27,* 1787-1793.

[52] Ertl, G; Bauer, B; Becker H. (1993). Effects of neurotensin and neuropeptide Y on coronary circulation and myocardial function in dogs. *Am. J. Physiol., V.264,* H1062-H1068.

[53] Evers, BM. (2002). Endocrine gene neurotensin: molecular mechanisms and a model of intestinal differentiation. *World J. Surg., V.26,* 799-805.

[54] Ferris, CF; Parker, MC; Armstrong, MJ; Leeman, SE. (1985). Inhibition of neurotensin release by a cyclic hexapeptide analog of somatostatin. *Peptides, V.6,* 945-948.

[55] Fletcher, DR; Shulkes, A; Bladin, PH; Booth, D; Hardy, KJ. (1983). Cholinergic inhibition of meal stimulated plasma neurotensin-like immunoreactivity in man. *Life Sci., V.33,* 863-869.

[56] Fletcher, DR; Shulkes, A; Hardy, KJ. (1985). The effect of neurotensin and secretin on gastric acid secretion and mucosal blood flow in man. *Regul. Peptides, V.11,* 217-226.

[57] Florholmen, G; Andersson, KB; Yndestad, A; Austbo, B; Henriksen, UL; Christensen G. (2004). Leukaemia inhibitory factor alters expression of genes involved in rat cardiomyocyte energy metabolism. *Acta Physiol. Scand., V.180,* 133-142.

[58] Folkers, K; Chang, D; Humphries, J; Carraway, R; Leeman, SE; Bowers CY. (1976). Synthesis and activities of neurotensin, and its acid and amide analogs: possible natural occurrence of [Gln^4]-neurotensin. *Proc. Natl. Acad. Sci. USA, V.73,* 3833-3837.

[59] Forssmann, WG; Reinecke, M; Weihe, E. (1982). Cardiac innervation. In: Bloom SR, Polak JM, Lindenlaub E. *Systemic role of regulatory peptides.* Symposia Medica Hoechst 18. 329-349.

[60] Fujimura, M; Khalil, T; Sakamoto, T; Greeley, GH; Salter, MG; Townsend, CM; Thompson, JC. (1989). Release of neurotensin by selective perfusion of the jejunum with oleic acid in dogs. *Gastroenterology, V.96,* 1502-1505.

[61] Gaumann, DM; Yaksh, TL. (1988). Effects of hemorrhage and opiate antagonists on adrenal release of neuropeptides in cats. *Peptides, V.9,* 393-405.

[62] Gaumann, DM; Yaksh, TL; Tyce, GM; Stoddard, SL. (1989). Adrenal vein catecholamines and neuropeptides during splanchnic nerve stimulation in cats. *Peptides, V.10,* 587-592.

[63] Gerstheimer, FP; Simon, T; Kolb, J; Hopker, W; Metz, J. (1988). Computer-assisted morphometric study of the innervation of the guinea-pig heart. *Histochemistry, V.88,* 545-551.

[64] Gilbert, JA; McCormick, DJ; Pfenning, A; Kanba, KS; Enloe, LJ; Moore, A; Richelson, E. (1989). Neurotensin (8-13): comparison of novel analogs for stimulation of cyclic GMP formation in neuroblastoma clone N1E-115 and receptor binding to human brain and intact N1E-115 cells. *Biochem. Pharmacol., V.38,* 3377-3382.

[65] Goedert, M; Reynolds, GP; Emson PC. (1983). Neurotensin in the adrenal medulla. *Neurosci. Lett., V.35,* 155-160.

[66] Goedert, M; Pinnock, RD; Downes, CP; Mantyh, PW; Emson, PC. (1984). Neurotensin stimulates inositol phospholipid hydrolysis in rat brain slices. *Brain Res., V.323,* 193-197.

[67] Goedert, M; Sturmey, N; Williams, BJ; Emson, PC. (1984). The comparative distribution of xenopsin- and neurotensin-like immunoreactivity in *Xenopus laevis* and rat tissues. *Brain Res., V.308,* 273-280.

[68] Gorgas, K; Reinecke, M; Weihe, E; Forssman, WG. (1983). Neurotensin and substance P immunoreactive nerve endings in the guinea-pig carotid sinus and their ultrastructural counterparts. *Anat. Embryol., V.167,* 347-354.

[69] Granier, C; Van Rietschoten, J; Kitabgi, P; Poustis, C; Freychet, P. (1982). Synthesis and characterization of neurotensin analogues for structure/activity relationship studies. Acetyl-neurotensin-(8-13) is the shortest analogue with full binding and pharmacological Activities. *Eur. J. Biochem., V.124,* 117-125.

[70] Gully, D; Canton, M; Boigegrain, R; Jeanjean, F; Molimard, JC; Poncelet, M; Gueudet, C; Heaulme, M; Leyris, R; Brouard, A; Pelaprat, D; Labbe-Jullie, C; Mazella, J; Soubrie, P; Maffrand, JP; Rostene, W; Kitabgi, P; Le Fur, G. (1993). Biochemical and pharmacological profile of a potent and selective nonpeptide antagonist of the neurotensin receptor. *Proc. Natl. Acad. Sci. USA, V.90,* 65-69.

[71] Gully, D; Lespy, L; Canton, M; Rostene, W; Kitabgi, P; Le Fur, G; Maffrand JP. (1996). Effect of the neurotensin receptor antagonist SR 48692 on rat blood pressure modulation by neurotensin. *Life Sci., V.58,* 665-674.

[72] Gully, D; Labeeuw, B; Boigegrain, R., Oury-Donat, F; Bachy, A; Poncelet, M; Steinberg, R; Suaud-Chagny, MF; Santucci, V; Vita, N; Pecceu, F; Labbe-Jullie, C; Kitabgi, P; Soubrie, P; Le Fur, G; Maffrand, JP. (1997). Biochemical and pharmacological activities of SR 142948A, a new potent neurotensin receptor antagonist. *J. Pharmacol. Exp. Ther., V.280,* 802-812.

[73] Hammer, RA; Leeman, SE; Carraway, R; Williams, RH. (1980). Isolation of human intestinal neurotensin. *J. Biol. Chem., V.255,* 2476-2480.

[74] Hammer, RA; Carraway, RE; Leeman, SE. (1982). Elevation of plasma neurotensin-like immunoreactivity after a meal. *J. Clin. Invest., V.70,* 74-81.

[75] Hammer, RA; Fernandez, C; Ertan, A; Arimura, A. (1991). Anesthetic dependence of the inhibitory effect of neurotensin on pentagastrin-stimulated acid secretion in rats. A possible role for somatostatin. *Life Sci., V.48,* 333-339.

[76] Hammer, RA; Ochoa, A; Fernandez, C; Ertan, A; Arimura, A. (1992). Somatostatin as a mediator of the effect of neurotensin on pentagastrin-stimulated acid secretion in rats. *Peptides, V.13,* 1175-1179.

[77] Harper, SL; Barrowman, JA; Kvietys, PR; Granger, DN. (1984). Effect of neurotensin on intestinal capillary permeability and blood flow. *Am. J. Physiol., V.247,* G161-G166.

[78] Hassall, CJS; Burnstock, G. (1986). Intrinsic neurons and associated cells of the guinea-pig heart in culture. *Brain Res., V.364,* 102-113.

[79] Hedner, J; Hedner, T; Lundell, KH; Bissette, G; O'Connor, L; Nemeroff, CB. (1989). Cerebrospinal fluid concentrations of neurotensin and corticotrophin-releasing factor in pediatric patients. *Biol. Neonate, V.55,* 260-267.

[80] Helle, KB; Serck-Hanssen, G; Jorgensen, G; Knudsen, R. (1980). Neurotensin-induced contractions in venous smooth muscle. *J. Auton. Nerv. Syst., V.2,* 143-155.

[81] Helmstaedter, V; Taugner, C; Feurle, GE; Forssman, WG. (1977). Localization of neurotensin-immunoreactive cells in the small intestine of man and various mammals. *Histochemistry, V.53,* 35-41.

[82] Hermans, E; Maloteaux, JM; Octave, JN. (1992). Phospholipase C activation by neurotensin and neuromedin N in Chinese hamster ovary cells expressing the rat neurotensin receptor. *Mol. Brain Res., V.15,* 332-338.

[83] Hermans, E; Gailly, P; Octave, JN; Maloteaux, JM. (1994). Rapid desensitization of agonist-induced calcium mobilization in transfected PC12 cells expressing the rat neurotensin receptor. *Biochem. Biophys. Res. Commun., V.198,* 400-407.

[84] Hermans, E; Gailly, P; Gillis, JM; Octave, JN; Maloteaux, JM. (1995). Lack of rapid desensitization of calcium responses in transfected CHO cells expressing the rat neurotensin receptor despite agonist-induced internalization. *J. Neurochem., V.64,* 2518-2525.

[85] Hermey, G; Riedel, B; Hampe, W; Schaller, HC; Hermans-Borgmeyer, I. (1999). Identification and characterization of SorCS, a third member of a novel receptor family. *Biochem. Biophys. Res. Commun., V.266,* 347-351.

[86] Herrmann, C; Cuber, JC; Abello, J; Dakka, T; Bernard, C; Chayvialle, JA. (1991). Release of ileal neurotensin in the rat by neurotransmitters and neuropeptides. *Regul. Peptides, V.32,* 181-192.

[87] Heuser, M; Gralla, O; Pfaar, O; Nustede, R; Grone, HJ; Post, S. (2000). Differential effects of neurotensin and cholecystokinin on intestinal microcirculation after ischemia-reperfusion. *Langenbeck's Arch. Surg., V.385,* 357-362.

[88] Higgins, GA; Hoffman, GE; Wray, S; Schwaber, JS. (1984). Distribution of neurotensin-immunoreactivity within baroreceptive portions of the nucleus of the tractus solitarius and the dorsal vagal nucleus of the rat. *J. Comp. Neurol., V.226,* 155-164.

[89] Hinson, JP; Cameron, LA; Purbrick, A; Kapas, S. (1994). The role of neuropeptides in the regulation of adrenal vascular tone: effects of vasoactive intestinal polypeptide, substance P, neuropeptide Y, neurotensin, met-enkephalin and leu-enkephalin on perfusion medium flow rate in the intact perfused rat adrenal. *Regul. Peptides, V.51,* 55-61.

[90] Holmgren, S; Fritsche, R; Karila, P; Gibbins, I; Axelsson, M; Franklin, C; Grigg, G; Nilsson, S. (1994). Neuropeptides in the Australian lungfish *Neoceratodus forsteri*: effects in vivo and presence in autonomic nerves. *Am. J. Physiol., V.266,* R1568-R1577.

[91] Holst Pedersen, J; Andersen, HO; Olsen, PS; Henriksen, JH. (1989). Pharmacokinetics and metabolism of neurotensin in man. *J. Clin. Endocrinol. Metab., V.68,* 294-300.

[92] Holzer, P. (1984). Characterization of the stimulus-induced release of immunoreactive substance P from the myenteric plexus of the guinea-pig small intestine. *Brain. Res., V.297,* 127-136.

[93] Ishizuka, J; Townsend, CM; Thompson, JC. (1993). Neurotensin regulates growth of human pancreatic cancer. *Ann. Surg., V.217,* 439-446.

[94] Iwase, K; Evers, M; Hellmich, M; Kim, HJ; Higashide, S; Gully, D; Thompson, JC; Townsend, CM. (1997). Inhibition of neurotensin-induced pancreatic carcinoma growth by a nonpeptide neurotensin receptor antagonist, SR 48692. *Cancer, V.79,* 787-793.

[95] Jennes, L; Stumpf, WE; Kalivas, PW. (1982). Neurotensin: topographical distribution in rat brain by immunohistochemistry. *J. Comp. Neurol., V.210,* 211-224.

[96] Kanba, KS; Richelson, E. (1987). Comparison of the stimulation of inositol phospholipid hydrolysis and of cyclic GMP formation by neurotensin, some of its analogs, and neuromedin N in neuroblastoma clone N1E-115. *Biochem. Pharmacol., V.36,* 869-874.

[97] Kapuscinski, M; Shulkes, A; Read, D; Hardy, KJ. (1990). Expression of neurotensin in endocrine tumors. *J. Clin. Endocrinol. Metab., V.70,* 100-106.

[98] Karila, P; Axelsson, M; Franklin, CE; Fritsche, R; Gibbins, IL; Nilsson, S; Holmgren S. (1995). Neuropeptide immunoreactivity and co-existence in cardiovascular nerves and autonomic ganglia of the estuarine crocodile, *Crocodylus porosus*, and cardiovascular effects of neuropeptides. *Regul. Peptides, V.58,* 25-39.

[99] Kataoka, K; Taniguchi, A; Shimizu, H; Soda, K; Okuno, S; Yajima, H; Kitagawa. K. (1978). Biological activity of neurotensin and its C-terminal partial sequences. *Brain Res. Bull., V.3,* 555-557.

[100]Kerouac, R; Rioux, F; St-Pierre, S. (1981). Mechanism of neurotensin-induced pressor effect and tachycardia in guinea-pigs. *Life Sci., V.28*, 2477-2487.

[101]Kerouac, R; St-Pierre, S; Manning, M; Rioux, F. (1983). Partial blockade of neurotensin-induced hypotension in rats by nephrectomy, captopril and saralasin. Possible mechanisms. *Neuropeptides, V.3*, 295-307.

[102]Kerouac, R; St-Pierre, S; Rioux, F. (1984). Participation of mast cell 5-hydroxytryptamine in the vasoconstrictor effect of neurotensin in the rat perfused hindquarter. *Life Sci., V.34*, 947-959.

[103]Kerouac, R; St-Pierre, S; Rioux, F. (1984). Histamine release by neurotensin in the rat hindquarter: structure-activity studies. *Peptides, V.5*, 695-699.

[104]Kessler, JP; Beaudet, A. (1989). Association of neurotensin binding sites with sensory and visceromotor components of the vagus nerve. *J. Neurosci., V.9*, 466-472.

[105]Kihl, B; Rokaeus, A; Rosell, S; Olbe, L. (1981). Fat inhibition of gastric acid secretion in man and plasma concentrations of neurotensin-like immunoreactivity. *Scand. J. Gastroenterol., V.16*, 513-526.

[106]Kilborn, MJ; Potter, EK; McCloskey, DI. (1986). Effects of periods of conditioning stimulation and of neuropeptides on vagal action at the heart. *J. Auton. Nerv. Syst., V.17*, 131-142.

[107]Kislauskis, E; Bullock, B; McNeil, S; Dobner, PR. (1988). The rat gene encoding neurotensin and neuromedin N. *J. Biol. Chem., V.263*, 4963-4968.

[108]Kitabgi, P; Carraway, R; Leeman, SE. (1976). Isolation of a tridecapeptide from bovine intestinal tissue and its partial characterization as neurotensin. *J. Biol. Chem., V.251*, 7053-7058.

[109]Kitabgi, P; Poustis, C; Granier, C; Van Rietschoten, J; Rivier, J; Morgat, JL; Freychet, P. (1980). Neurotensin binding to extraneural and neural receptors: comparison with biological activity and structure-activity relationships. *Mol. Pharmacol., V.18*, 11-19.

[110]Kitabgi, P; De Nadai, F; Rovere, C; Bidard, JN. (1992). Biosynthesis, maturation, release and degradation of neurotensin and neuromedin N. *Ann. N.Y. Acad. Sci., V.668*, 30-42.

[111]Kitabgi, P. (2002). Targeting neurotensin receptors with agonists and antagonists for therapeutic purposes. *Curr. Opin. Drug Discov. Devel., V.5*, 764-776.

[112]Konturek, SJ; Jaworek, J; Cieszkowski, M; Pawlik, W; Kania, J; Bloom, SR. (1983).Comparison of effects of neurotensin and fat on pancreatic stimulation in dogs. *Am. J. Physiol., V.244*, G590-G598.

[113]Kronenberg, F; Carraway, RE. (1985). Changes in neurotensin-like immunoreactivity during menopausal hot flashes. *J. Clin. Endocrinol. Metab., V.60*, 1081-1086.

[114]Kruger, PG; Aas, P; Onarheim, J; Helle, KB. (1982). Neurotensin-induced release of histamine from rat mast cells in vitro. *Acta Physiol. Scand., V.114*, 467-469.

[115]Krukoff, TL; Ciriello, J; Calaresu, FR. (1985). Segmental distribution of peptide-like immunoreactivity in cell bodies of the thoracolumbar sympathetic nuclei of the cat. *J. Comp. Neurol., V.240*, 90-102.

[116]Krukoff, TL. (1987). Coexistence of neuropeptides in sympathetic preganglionic neurons of the cat. *Peptides, V.8*, 109-112.

[117]Kummer, W; Reinecke, M; Heym, C. (1991). Neurotensin-like immunoreactivity in presumptive baroreceptor neurons innervating the guinea-pig carotid sinus. *J. Auton. Nerv. Syst., V.35,* 107-116.

[118]Kurose, M; Saeki, K. (1981). Histamine release induced by neurotensin from rat peritoneal mast cells. *Eur. J. Pharmacol., V.76,* 129-136.

[119]Lazarus, LH; Perrin, MH; Brown, MR. (1977). Mast cell binding of neurotensin. I. Iodination of neurotensin and characterization of the interaction of neurotensin with mast cell receptor sites. *J. Biol. Chem., V.252,* 7174-7179.

[120]Lazarus, LH; Perrin, MH; Brown, MR; Rivier, JE. (1977). Mast cell binding of neurotensin. II. Molecular conformation of neurotensin involved in the stereospecific binding to mast cell receptor sites. *J. Biol. Chem., V.252,* 7180-7183.

[121]Lee, YC; Allen, JM; Uttenthal, LO; Walker, MC; Shemilt, J; Gill, SS; Bloom, SR. (1984). The metabolism of intravenously infused neurotensin in man and its chromatographic characterization in human plasma. *J. Clin. Endocrinol. Metab., V.45,* 45-50.

[122]Lee, YC; Uttenthal, LO; Smith, HA; Bloom, SR. (1986). In vitro degradation of neurotensin in human plasma. *Peptides, V.7,* 383-387.

[123]Lin, B; Pilch, PF; Kandror, KV. (1997). Sortilin is a major protein component of Glut4-containing vesicles. *J. Biol. Chem., V.272,* 25145-24147.

[124]Linde, B; Rosell, S; Rokaeus, A. (1982). Intravenous administration of (Gln^4)-neurotensin induces vasoconstriction in human adipose tissue. *Ann. N.Y. Acad. Sci., V.400,* 392-393.

[125]Lucas, A; Aynsley-Green, A; Blackburn, AM; Adrian, TE; Bloom, SR. (1981). Plasma neurotensin in term and preterm neonates. *Acta Paediatr. Scand., V.70,* 201-206.

[126]Lundberg, JM; Rokaeus, A; Hokfelt, T; Rosell, S; Brown, M; Goldstein, M. (1982). Neurotensin-like immunoreactivity in the preganglionic sympathetic nerves and in the adrenal medulla of the cat. *Acta Physiol. Scand., V.114,* 153-155.

[127]Maher, E; Bachoo, M; Cernacek, P; Polosa, C. (1991). Dynamics of neurotensin stores in the stellate ganglion of the cat. *Brain Res., V.562,* 258-264.

[128]Maher, E; Bachoo, B; Polosa, C. (1994). Role of neuron soma firing in the restoration of neurotensin store in sympathetic preganglionic neuron terminals after stimulus-evoked depletion. *Brain Res., V.640,* 126-130.

[129]Maher, E; Bachoo, B; Polosa, C. (1994). In vitro and in vivo evidence of neurotensin release from preganglionic axon terminals in the stellate ganglion of the cat. *Brain Res., V.640,* 131-135.

[130]Martinez, M; Hernanz, A; Grande, C; Pallardo, LF. (1993). Plasma molecular forms of gastrin, neurotensin and somatostatin in pregnancy and gestational diabetes after an oral glucose load or a mixed meal. *Regul. Peptides, V.47,* 73-80.

[131]Mashford, ML; Nilsson, G; Rokaeus, A; Rosell, S. (1978). The effect of food ingestion on circulating neurotensin-like immunoreactivity in the human. *Acta Physiol. Scand., V.104,* 244-246.

[132]Mashford, ML; Nilsson, G; Rokaeus, A; Rosell, S. (1978). Release of neurotensin-like immunoreactivity from the gut in anaesthetized dogs. *Acta Physiol. Scand., V.104,* 375-376.

[133] Mazella, J; Chabry, J; Zsurger, N; Vincent, JP. (1989). Purification of the neurotensin receptor from mouse brain by affinity chromatography. *J. Biol. Chem., V.264*, 5559-5563.

[134] Mazella, J; Botto, JM; Guillemare, E; Coppola, T; Sarret, P; Vincent, JP. (1996). Structure, functional expression, and cerebral localization of the levocabastine-sensitive neurotensin/neuromedin N receptor from mouse brain. *J. Neurosci., V.16*, 5613-5620.

[135] McDermott, JR; Virmani, MA; Turner, JD; Kidd, AM. (1986). Peptidases involved in the catabolism of neurotensin: inhibitor studies using superfused rat hypothalamic slices. *Peptides, V.7*, 225-230.

[136] Mentlein, R; Dahms, P. (1994). Endopeptidases 24.16 and 24.15 are responsible for the degradation of somatostatin, neurotensin and other neuropeptides by cultivated rat cortical astrocytes. *J. Neurochem., V.62*, 27-36.

[137] Miller, LA; Cochrane, DE; Carraway, RE; Feldberg, RS. (1995). Blockade of mast cell histamine secretion in response to neurotensin by SR 48692, a nonpeptide antagonist of the neurotensin brain receptor. *Br. J. Pharmacol., V.114*, 1466-1470.

[138] Miller, VM; Hoffman, AM; South, FE. (1981). Cardiovascular responses to neurotensin in the Genus marmota. *Fed. Proc., V.40*, 581.

[139] Mogard, M; Bottcher, W; Kauffman, GL; Washington, J; Walsh, JH. (1986). Neurotensin-like immunoreactivity released into the portal vein by duodenal acidification in the dog. *Scand. J. Gastroenterol., V.21*, 97-103.

[140] Mogard, MH; Kobayashi, R; Lee, TD; Chen, CF; Hagiwara, M; Leung, F; Reeve, JR; Shively, JE; Walsh, JH. (1987). Neurotensin-like immunoreactivity generated by pepsin from human plasma and gastric tissue. *Regul. Peptides, V.18*, 221-232.

[141] Nakamoto, M; Tanaka, C; Taniyama, K. (1987). Release of γ-aminobutiric acid and acetylcholine by neurotensin in guinea-pig ileum. *Br. J. Pharmacol., V.90*, 545-551.

[142] Nicholls, DP; Riley, M; Elborn, JS; Stanford, CF; Shaw, C; McKillop, JM; Buchanan, KD. (1992). Regulatory peptides in the plasma of patients with chronic cardiac failure at rest and during exercise. *Eur. Heart J., V.13*, 1399-1404.

[143] Nisato, D; Guiraudou, P; Barthelemy, G; Gully, D; Le Fur, G. (1994). SR 48692, a non- peptide neurotensin receptor antagonist, blocks the cardiovascular effects elicited by neurotensin in guinea-pigs. *Life Sci., V.54*, 95-100.

[144] Norman, MU; Reeve, SB; Dive, V; Smith, AI; Lew, RA. (2003). Endopeptidases 3.4.24.15 and 24.16 in endothelial cells: potential role in vasoactive peptide metabolism. *Am. J. Physiol., V.284*, H1978-H1984.

[145] Obara, H; Kusunoki, M; Mori, K; Mikawa, K; Iwai, S. (1989). The effects of various peptides on the isolated pulmonary artery. *Peptides, V.10*, 241-243.

[146] Oishi, M; Inagaki, C; Fujiwara, M; Takaori, S; Yajima, H; Akazawa ,Y. (1981). Possible mechanisms of the triphasic effects of neurotensin on the rat blood pressure. *Jap. J. Pharmacol., V.31*, 1043-1049.

[147] Oishi, M; Ishiko, J; Inagaki, C; Takaori, S. (1983). Release of histamine and adrenaline in vivo following intravenous administration of neurotensin. *Life Sci., V.32*, 2231-2239.

[148] Onarheim, J; Helle, KB; Jorgensen, G. (1982). Neurotensin-induced increase in intestinal blood flow in the anesthetized rat. *Acta Physiol. Scand., V.114*, 505-511.

[149] Onuoha, GN; Alpar, EK; Chukwulobelu, R; Nicholls, DP. (1999). Distributions of VIP, substance P, neurokinin A and neurotensin in rat heart: an immunocytochemical study. *Neuropeptides, V.33,* 19-25.

[150] Onuoha, GN; Nicholls, DP; Alpar, EK; Ritchie, A; Shaw, C; Buchanan, K. (1999). Regulatory peptides in the heart and major vessels of man and mammals. *Neuropeptides, V.33,* 165-172.

[151] Osadchii, OE; Pokrovskii, VM; Kurzanov, AN. (1993). Modulatory action of neurotensin on the parasympathetic regulation of cardiac rhythm. *Bull. Exp. Biol. Med., V.115,* 453-455.

[152] Osadchii, OE; Pokrovskii, VM; Kompaniets, OG; Kurzanov, AN. (1996). A comparative evaluation of the cardiotropic effects of neurotensin and adrenaline in cats. *Fiziol. Zh. Im. I M Sechenova, V.82,* 104-110.

[153] Osadchii, OE; Pokrovskii, VM; Kompaniets, OG; Kurzanov, AN. (1997). The effect of neurotensin and adrenaline on sinus arrhythmia induced by vagus nerve stimulation. *Bull. Exp. Biol. Med., V.123,* 494-497.

[154] Osadchii, OE; Pokrovskii, VM; Kompaniets, OG; Kurzanov, AN. (1997). Protective effect of neurotensin in vagal arrhythmias. *Bull. Exp. Biol. Med., V.124,* 495-497.

[155] Osadchii, OE; Pokrovskii, VM. (1999). The dynamics of the chronotropic effect evoked by a single vagal stimulus in cats under the action of met-enkephalin and neurotensin. *Ross. Fiziol Zh Im I M Sechenova, V.85,* 547-53.

[156] Osadchii, OE; Kanorskii, SG; Pokrovskii, VM; Kurzanov, AN; Skibitskii, VV. (2001). The effect of regulatory peptides upon electrophysiological properties of the human heart. *Human Physiol., V.27,* 105-110.

[157] Osadchii, O; Norton, G; Deftereos, D; Badenhorst, D; Woodiwiss, A. (2005). Impact and mechanisms of action of neurotensin on cardiac contractility in the rat left ventricle. *Eur. J. Pharmacol., V.520,* 108-117.

[158] Osadchii, O; Norton, G; Deftereos, D; Badenhorst, D; Woodiwiss, A. (2006). Neurotensin-induced myocardial noradrenergic effects in spontaneously hypertensive rats. *J. Cardiovasc. Pharmacol., V.47,* 221-227.

[159] Osadchii, O; Norton, G; Deftereos, D; Muller, D; Woodiwiss, A. (2006). Impact of chronic β-adrenoceptor activation on neurotensin-induced myocardial effects in rats. *Eur. J. Pharmacol.,V.553,* 246-253.

[160] Ouru-Donat, F; Thurneyssen, O; Gonalons, N; Forgez, P; Gully, D; Le Fur, G; Soubrie P. (1995). Characterization of the effect of SR 48692 on inositol monophosphate, cyclic GMP and cyclic AMP responses linked to neurotensin receptor activation in neuronal and non-neuronal cells. *Br. J. Pharmacol., V.116,* 1899-1905.

[161] Pang, X; Alexacos, N; Letourneau, R; Seretakis, D; Gao, W; Boucher, W; Cochrane, DE; Theoharides, TC. (1998). A neurotensin receptor antagonist inhibits acute immobilization stress-induced cardiac mast cell degranulation, a corticotrophin-releasing hormone-dependent process. *J. Pharmacol. Exp. Ther., V.287,* 307-314.

[162] Park, TJ; Kim, KT. (2003). Activation of B2 bradykinin receptors by neurotensin. *Cell. Signal., V.15,* 519-527.

[163] Pedersen, JH; Fahrenkrug, J. (1986). Neurotensin-like immunoreactivities in human plasma: feeding responses and metabolism. *Peptides, V.7,* 15-20.

[164] Pelto-Huikko, M; Salminen, T; Partanen, M; Toivanen, M; Hervonen, A. (1985). Immunohistochemical localization of neurotensin in hamster adrenal medulla. *Anat. Rec., V.211,* 458-464.

[165] Pelto-Huikko, M; Salminen, T; Hervonen, A. (1987). Localization of enkephalin- and neurotensin-like immunoreactivities in cat adrenal medulla. *Histochemistry, V.88,* 31-36.

[166] Petersen, CM; Nielsen, MS; Nykjar, A; Jacobsen, L; Tommerup, N; Rasmussen, HH; Roigaard, H; Gliemann, J; Madsen, P; Moestrup, SK. (1997). Molecular identification of a novel candidate sorting receptor purified from human brain by receptor-associated protein affinity chromatography. *J. Biol. Chem., V.272,* 3599-3605.

[167] Polak, JM; Sullivan, SN; Bloom, SR; Buchan, AM; Facer, P; Brown, MR; Pearse, AG. (1977). Specific localization of neurotensin to the N cell in human intestine by radioimmunoassay and immunocytochemistry. *Nature, V.270,* 183-184.

[168] Polak JM; Bloom, SR. (1982). The central and peripheral distribution of neurotensin. *Ann. N.Y. Acad. Sci., V.400,* 75-93.

[169] Quirion, R; Rioux, F; Regoli, D. (1978). Chronotropic and inotropic effects of neurotensin on spontaneously beating auricles. *Can. J. Physiol. Pharmacol., V.56,* 671-673.

[170] Quirion, R; Regoli, D; Rioux, F; St-Pierre, S. (1979). An analysis of the negative inotropic action of somatostatin. *Br. J. Pharmacol., V.66,* 251-257.

[171] Quirion, R; Rioux, F; Regoli, D; St-Pierre, S. (1979). Neurotensin-induced vessels constriction in perfused rat hearts. *Eur. J. Pharmacol., V.55,* 221-223.

[172] Quirion, R; Rioux, F; St-Pierre, S; Regoli, D. (1979). Increased sensitivity to neurotensin in fasted rats. *Life Sci., V.25,* 1969-1973.

[173] Quirion, R; Regoli, D; Rioux, F; St-Pierre, S. (1980). The stimulatory effects of neurotensin and related peptides in rat stomach strips and guinea-pig atria. *Br. J. Pharmacol., V.68,* 83-91.

[174] Quirion, R; Regoli, D; Rioux, F; St-Pierre, S. (1980). Structure-activity studies with neurotensin: analysis of positions 9, 10 and 11. *Br. J. Pharmacol., V.69,* 689-692.

[175] Quirion, R; Rioux, F; Regoli, D; St-Pierre, S. (1980). Selective blockade of neurotensin-induced coronary vessel constriction in perfused rat hearts by a neurotensin analogue. *Eur. J. Pharmacol., V.61,* 309-312.

[176] Quirion, R; Rioux, F; Regoli, D; St-Pierre, S. (1980). Pharmacological studies of neurotensin, several fragments and analogues in the isolated perfused rat heart. *Eur. J. Pharmacol., V.66,* 257-266.

[177] Quirion, R; Rioux, F; Regoli, D; St-Pierre, S. (1980). Compound 48/80 inhibits neurotensin-induced hypotension in rats. *Life Sci., V.27,* 1889-1895.

[178] Rakovska, AD. (1993). Functional and neurochemical evidence that neurotensin-induced release of acetylcholine from Auerbach's plexus of guinea-pig ileum is presynaptically controlled via alpha 2-adrenoceptors. *Neurochem. Res., V.18,* 737-741.

[179] Reinecke, M; Almasan, K; Carraway, R; Helmstaedter, V; Forssmann, WG. (1980). Distribution patterns of neurotensin-like immunoreactive cells in the gastrointestinal tract of higher vertebrates. *Cell Tissue Res., V.205,* 383-395.

[180]Reinecke, M; Weihe, E; Carraway, RE; Forssmann, WG. (1981). Localization of neurotensin-immunorectivity in the heart by immunohistochemistry and radioimmunoassay. *Acta Anat., V.III,* 123-124.

[181]Reinecke, M; Weihe, E; Carraway, RE; Leeman, SE; Forssmann, WG. (1982). Localization of neurotensin immunoreactive nerve fibers in the guinea pig heart: evidence derived by immunohistochemistry, radioimmunoassay and chromatography. *Neuroscience, V.7,* 1785-1795.

[182]Reinecke, M; Forssmann, WG; Thiekotter, G; Triepel, J. (1983). Localization of neurotensin-immunoreactivity in the spinal cord and peripheral nervous system of the guinea-pig. *Neurosci. Lett., V.37,* 37-42.

[183]Reinecke, M; Forssmann, WG. (1984). Regulatory peptides of autonomic nerves in the guinea-pig heart. *Clin. Exp. Hypertens. A., V.6,* 1867-1871.

[184]Reinecke, M. (1985). Neurotensin. Immunohistochemical localization in central and peripheral nervous system and in endocrine cells and its functional role as neurotransmitter and endocrine hormone. *Progr. Histochem. Cytochem., V.16,* 1-173.

[185]Richelson, E; Boules, M; Fredrickson, P. (2003). Neurotensin agonists: possible drugs for treatment of psychostimulant abuse. *Life Sci., V.73,* 679-690.

[186]Rigel, DF. (1988). Effects of neuropeptides on heart rate in dogs: comparison of VIP, PHI, NPY, CGRP, and NT. *Am. J. Physiol., V.255,* H311-H317.

[187]Rigel, DF; Grupp, IL; Balasubramaniam, A; Grupp, G. (1989). Contractile effects of cardiac neuropeptides in isolated canine atrial and ventricular muscles. *Am. J. Physiol., V.257,* H1082-H1087.

[188]Rioux, F; Quirion, R; Leblanc, MA; Regoli, D; St-Pierre, S. (1980). Possible interactions between neurotensin and prostaglandins in the isolated rat portal vein. *Life Sci., V.27,* 259-267.

[189]Rioux, F; Quirion, R; Regoli, D; Leblanc, MA; St-Pierre, S. (1980). Pharmacological characterization of neurotensin receptors in the rat isolated portal vein using analogues and fragments of neurotensin. *Eur. J. Pharmacol., V.66,* 273-279.

[190]Rioux, F; Kerouac, R; Quirion, R; St-Pierre, S. (1982). Mechanisms of the cardiovascular effects of neurotensin. *Ann. N.Y. Acad. Sci., V.400,* 56-74.

[191]Rioux, F; Kerouac, R; St-Pierre, S. (1982). Analysis of the biphasic depressor-pressor effect and tachycardia caused by neurotensin in ganglion-blocked rats. *Neuropeptides, V.3,* 113-127.

[192]Rioux, F; Kerouac, R; St-Pierre, S. (1984). Neurotensin stimulates histamine release from the isolated, spontaneously beating heart of rats. *Life Sci., V.35,* 423-431.

[193]Rioux, F; Kerouac, R; St-Pierre, S. (1985). Characterization of the histamine-releasing effect of neurotensin in the rat heart. *Peptides, V.6,* 121-125.

[194]Rioux, F; Bachelard, H; Barabe, J; St-Pierre, S. (1986). The cardiovascular response to epicardial application of neurotensin in guinea-pigs. *Peptides, V.7,* 1087-1094.

[195]Rioux, F; Lemieux, M; Kerouac, R; Bernoussi, A; Roy, G. (1989). Local application of neurotensin to abdominal organs triggers cardiovascular reflexes in guinea-pigs: possible mechanisms. *Peptides, V.10,* 647-655.

[196]Rioux, F; Lemieux, M. (1992). Hemodynamic and abdominal motor reflexes elicited by neurotensin in anaesthetized guinea-pigs. *Br. J. Pharmacol., V.106,* 187-195.

[197]Rioux, F;.Pare, D. (1983). Cardiovascular and abdominal motor responses evoked by intravenous neurotensin in guinea-pigs. *Peptides, V.14,* 227-234.

[198]Rokaeus, A; Burcher, E; Chang, D; Folkers, K; Rosell, S. (1977). Actions of neurotensin and (Gln^4)-neurotensin on isolated tissues. *Acta Pharmacol. Toxicol., V.41,* 141-147.

[199]Rokaeus, A. (1981). Studies on neurotensin as a hormone. *Acta Physiol. Scand., V.501, Suppl.,* 1-62.

[200]Rokaeus, A; Yanaihara, N; McDonald, TJ. (1982). Increased concentration of neurotensin-like immunoreactivity in rat plasma after administration bombesin and bombesin-related peptides. *Acta Physiol. Scand., V.114,* 605-610.

[201]Rokaeus, A; Fried, G; Lundberg, JM. (1984). Occurrence, storage and release of neurotensin-like immunoreactivity from the adrenal gland. *Acta Physiol. Scand., V.120,* 373-380.

[202]Rosell, S; Burcher, E; Chang, D; Folkers, K. (1976). Cardiovascular and metabolic actions of neurotensin and (Gln^4)-neurotensin. *Acta Physiol. Scand., V.98,* 484-491.

[203]Rosell, S; Rokaeus, A; Chang, D; Folkers, K. (1978). Indirect vascular actions of (Gln^4)- neurotensin in canine adipose tissue. *Acta Physiol. Scand., V.102,* 143-147.

[204]Rosell, S; Rokaeus, A. (1979). The effect of ingestion of amino acids, glucose and fat on circulating neurotensin-like immunoreactivity in man. *Acta Physiol. Scand., V.107,* 263-267.

[205]Rosell, S; Thor, K; Rokaeus, A; Nyquist, O; Lewenhaupt, A; Kager, L; Folkers, K. (1980). Plasma concentration of neurotensin-like immunoreactivity and lower esophageal sphincter pressure in man following infusion of (Gln^4)-neurotensin. *Acta Physiol. Scand.,* V.109, 369-375.

[206]Rossie, SS; Miller, RJ. (1982). Regulation of mast cell histamine release by neurotensin. *Life Sci., V.31,* 509-516.

[207]Rostene, WH; Alexander, MJ. (1997). Neurotensin and neuroendocrine regulation. *Front. Neuroendocrinol., V.18,* 115-173.

[208]Sagor, GR; Ghatei, MA; McGregor, GP; Mitchenere, P; Kirk, RM; Bloom, SR. (1981). The influence of an intact pylorus on postprandial enteroglucagon and neurotensin release after upper gastric surgery. *Br. J. Surg., V.68,* 190-193.

[209]Saito, H; Saito, S. (1980). Effects of substance P and neurotensin on somatostatin levels in rat portal plasma. *Endocrinology, V.107,* 1600-1605.

[210]Sato, M; Shiosaka, S; Tohyama, M. (1991). Neurotensin and neuromedin N elevate the cytosolic calcium concentration via transiently appearing neurotensin binding sites in cultured rat cortex cells. *Devel. Brain Res., V.58,* 97-103.

[211]Schaeffer, P; Laplace, MC; Savi, P; Pflieger, AM; Gully, D; Herbert, JM. (1995). Human umbilical vein endothelial cells express high affinity neurotensin receptors coupled to intracellular calcium release. *J. Biol. Chem., V.270,* 3409-3413.

[212]Schaeffer, P; Laplace, MC; Prabonnaud, V; Bernat, A; Gully, D; Lespy, L; Herbert, J M. (1997). Neurotensin induces the release of prostacyclin from human umbilical vein endothelial cells in vitro and increases plasma prostacyclin levels in the rat. *Eur. J. Pharmacol., V.323,* 215-221.

[213] Schaeffer, P; Laplace, M; Bernat, A; Prabonnaud, V; Gully, D; Lespy, L; Herbert, JM. (1998). SR 142948A is a potent antagonist of the cardiovascular effects of neurotensin. *J. Cardiovasc. Pharmacol., V.31,* 545-550.

[214] Schimpff, RM; Avard, C; Fenelon, G; Lhiaubet, AM; Tenneze, L; Vidailhet, M; Rostene, W. (2001). Increased plasma neurotensin concentrations in patients with Parkinson's disease. *J. Neurol. Neurosurg. Psych., V. 70,* 784-786.

[215] Selbekk, BH; Flaten, O; Hanssen, LE. (1980). The in vitro effect of neurotensin on human jejunal mast cells. *Scand. J. Gastroenterol., V.15,* 457-460.

[216] Sharma, RP; Janicak, PG; Bissette, G; Nemeroff, CB. (1997). Cerebrospinal fluid concentrations and antipsychotic treatment in schizophrenia and schizoaffective disorder. *Am. J. Psych., V.154,* 1019-1021.

[217] Shulkes, A; Chick, P; Wong, H; Walsh, JH. (1982). A radioimmunoassay for neurotensin in human plasma. *Clin. Chim. Acta., V.125,* 49-58.

[218] Shulkes, A; Fletcher, DR; Hardy, KJ. (1983). Organ and plasma metabolism of neurotensin in sheep. *Am. J. Physiol., V.245,* E457-62.

[219] Shulkes, A; Bijaphala, S; Dawborn, JK; Fletcher, DR; Hardy KJ. (1984). Metabolism of neurotensin and pancreatic polypeptide in man: role of the kidney and plasma factors. *J. Clin. Endocrinol.Metab., V.58,* 873-879.

[220] Shulkes, A; Englin, I; Read, D; Hardy, KJ. (1987). Neurotensin metabolism in the rat: contribution of the kidney. *Peptides, V.8,* 961-965.

[221] Sicard, F; Vaudry, H; Braun, B; Chartrel, N; Leprince, J; Conlon, JM; Delarue, C. (2000). Immunohistochemical localization, biochemical characterization, and biological activity of neurotensin in the frog adrenal gland. *Endocrinology, V.141,* 2450-2457.

[222] Skidgel, RA; Engelbrecht, S; Johnson, AR; Erdos, EG. (1984). Hydrolysis of substance P and neurotensin by converting enzyme and neutral endopeptidase. *Peptides, V.5,* 769-776.

[223] Snider, RM; Forray, C; Pfenning, M; Richelson, E. (1986). Neurotensin stimulates inositol phospholipid metabolism and calcium mobilization in murine neuroblastoma clone N1E-115. *J. Neurochem., V.47,* 1214-1218.

[224] Stapelfeldt, WH; Szurszewski, JH. (1989). Neurotensin facilitates release of substance P in the guinea-pig inferior mesenteric ganglion. *J. Physiol., V.411,* 325-345.

[225] Stene-Larsen, G; Helle, KB. (1979). Inotropic and chronotropic effects of neurotensin in the rat atrium and of physalaemin in the auricles of *R.esculenta. Comp. Biochem. Physiol., V.64,* 279-283.

[226] Sumners, C; Phillips, MI; Richards, EM. (1982). Central pressor action of neurotensin in conscious rats. *Hypertension, V.4,* 888-893.

[227] Sundler, F; Alumets, J; Hakanson, R; Carraway, R; Leeman, SE. (1977). Ultrastructure of the gut neurotensin cell. *Histochemistry, V.53,* 25-34.

[228] Tanaka, K; Masu, M; Nakanishi, S. (1990). Structure and functional expression of the cloned rat neurotensin receptor. *Neuron, V.4,* 847-854.

[229] Terenghi, G; Polak, JM; Varndell, IM; Lee, YC; Wharton, J; Bloom, SR. (1983). Neurotensin-like immunoreactivity in a subpopulation of noradrenaline-containing cells of the cat adrenal gland. *Endocrinology, V.112,* 226-233.

[230] Theodorsson-Norheim, E; Al-Saffar, A; Saria, A; Rosell, S. (1985). The effect of nephrectomy and ureter ligation on plasma neurotensin-like immunoreactivity levels in the conscious rat. *Acta Physiol. Scand., V.123,* 269-272.

[231] Thomas, RP; Hellmich, MR; Townsend, CM; Evers, BM. (2003). Role of gastrointestinal hormones in the proliferation of normal and neoplastic tissues. *Endocr. Rev., V.24,* 571-599.

[232] Tsuda, K; Masuyma, Y. (1993). Effects of neurotensin on norepinephrine release in blood vessels of spontaneously hypertensive rats. *Am. J. Hypertens., V.6,* 473-479.

[233] Tyler-McMahon, BM; Boules, M; Richelson, E. (2000). Neurotensin: peptide for the next millennium. *Regul. Peptides, V.93,* 125-136.

[234] Unwin, RJ; Calam, J; Peart, WS; Hanson, C; Lee, YC; Bloom, SR. (1987). Renal function during bovine neurotensin infusion in man. *Regul. Peptides, V.18,* 29-35.

[235] Vincent, JP; Mazella, J; Kitabgi, P. (1999). Neurotensin and neurotensin receptors. *Trends Pharmacol. Sci., V.20,* 302-309.

[236] Vita, N; Laurent, P; Lefort, S; Chalon, P; Dumont, X; Kaghad, M; Gully, D; Le Fur, G; Ferrara, P; Caput, D. (1993). Cloning and expression of a complementary DNA encoding a high affinity human neurotensin receptor. *FEBS Lett., V.317,* 139-142.

[237] Vita, N; Oury-Donat, F; Chalon, P; Guillemot, M; Kaghad, M; Bachy, A; Thurneyssen, O; Garcia, S; Poinot-Chazel, C; Casellas, P; Keane, P; Le Fur, G; Maffrand, JP; Soubrie, P; Caput, D; Ferrara, P. (1998). Neurotensin is an antagonist of the human neurotensin NT_2 receptor expressed in Chinese hamster ovary cells. *Eur. J. Pharmacol., V.360,* 265-272.

[238] Wagner, F; Wahl, M. (1986). Effects of neurotensin in feline pial arteries, guinea-pig ileum and portal vein of rat and guinea-pig. *Arch. Int. Pharmacodyn. Ther., V.282,* 240-251.

[239] Watson, MA; Yamada, M; Yamada, M; Cusack, B; Veverka, K; Bolden-Watson, C; Richelson, E. (1992). The rat neurotensin receptor expressed in Chinese hamster ovary cells mediates the release of inositol phosphates. *J. Neurochem., V.59,* 1967-1970.

[240] Weihe, E; Reinecke, M. (1981). Peptidergic innervation of the mammalian sinus nodes: vasoactive intestinal polypeptide, neurotensin, substance P. *Neurosci. Lett., V.26,* 283-288.

[241] Weihe, E; Reinecke, M; Forssmann, WG. (1984). Distribution of vasoactive intestinal polypeptide-like immunoreactivity in the mammalian heart. Interrelation with neurotensin- and substance P-like immunoreactive nerves. *Cell Tissue Res., V.236,* 527-540.

[242] White, RP; Robertson, JT. (1987). Pharmacodynamic evaluation of human cerebral arteries in the genesis of vasospasm. *Neurosurgery, V.21,* 523-531.

[243] Widerlov, E; Lindstrom, LH; Besev, G; Manberg, PJ; Nemeroff, CB; Breese, GR; Kizer, JS; Prange, AJ. (1982). Subnormal cerebrospinal fluid levels of neurotensin in a subgroup of schizophrenic patients: normalization after neuroleptic treatment. *Am. J. Psych., V.139,* 1122-1126.

[244] Yamada, M; Yamada, M; Watson, MA; Richelson, ER. (1993). Neurotensin stimulates cyclic AMP formation in CHO-rNTR-10 cells expressing the cloned rat neurotensin receptor. *Eur. J. Pharmacol., V.244,* 99-101.

[245] Yamada, M; Yamada, M; Lombet, A; Forgez, P; Rostene, W. (1998). Distinct functional characteristics of levocabastine sensitive rat neurotensin NT_2 receptor expressed in Chinese hamster ovary cells. *Life Sci., V.62,* PL 375-380.

[246] Yau, WM; Verdun, PR; Youther, ML. (1983). Neurotensin: a modulator of enteric cholinergic neurons in the guinea-pig small intestine. *Eur. J. Pharmacol., V.95,* 253-258.

[247] Zsurger, N; Mazella, J; Vincent, JP. (1994). Solubilization and purification of a high affinity neurotensin receptor from newborn human brain. *Brain Res., V.639,* 245-252.

In: Handbook of Cardiovascular Research
Editors: Jorgen Brataas and Viggo Nanstveit

ISBN 978-1-60741-792-7
© 2009 Nova Science Publishers, Inc.

Chapter II

Frontiers in Women's Cardiovascular Health Prevention: What Have We Learned So Far?*

Rebecca M. Scandrett and Sandip K. Mukherjee
Yale School of Medicine, CT USA

Introduction

Cardiovascular disease affects over 200 million people worldwide and accounts for nearly 30% of global mortality. Approximately 80% of these cardiovascular deaths occur in low and middle-income countries. By the year 2020, ischemic heart disease mortality in developing countries is predicted to increase by 120% for women and 137% for men [1]. In the United States alone, cardiovascular disease (CVD) affects over 37 million American women, representing over one third of the American female population, with coronary heart disease (CHD) affecting 5.9 million women. By age 55, the prevalence of cardiovascular disease in women exceeds that in men. Cardiovascular disease accounts for 1 in 2.5 female deaths compared to 1 in 30 deaths attributable to breast cancer. Despite the high prevalence and mortality rate of cardiovascular disease, only 13% of women consider it to be their greatest health risk [2]. While a recent survey of 1008 women found that the level of awareness regarding CVD mortality in women has nearly doubled since 1997, still only 55% of women recognize CVD as the leading cause of mortality in women. In addition, the survey found that the level of awareness in minorities continues to significantly lag behind the white population with only 38% of blacks and 34% of Hispanics recognizing the magnitude of the problem [3]. Although the past two to three decades has seen a decline in the overall

---

* A version of this chapter was also published in *Exercise and Women's Health: New Research*, edited by Laura T. Allerton and Gloria P. Rutherfode published by Nova Science Publishers, Inc. It was submitted for appropriate modifications in an effort to encourage wider dissemination of research.

mortality rate from CHD in men, the mortality rates for women have remained stable. The overall incidence of CHD in women has actually increased, as evidenced by a 47% increase in hospital discharges related to CHD [2, 4]. A prospective registry study of men and women who presented with an acute myocardial infarction found that women were at increased risk for 28-day case fatality (18.5% vs. 8.3%), 6-month mortality (28.5% vs. 10.8%) and readmission rates (23.3% vs. 12.2%) after a first myocardial infarction compared with men, independent of co-morbidities, coronary risk factors and the use of thrombolytics [5]. Not only did women in this study have a higher mortality from their first MI compared to men, it was also found that the median time between symptom onset and initial presentation to the hospital was on average one hour longer in women compared to men. Furthermore, the delay between the emergency room and admission to the coronary care unit was also on average over two hours longer in women than in men. The results from this registry were recently mirrored in the Euro Heart Survey of Stable Angina. This prospective observational trial found that women who presented with a new diagnosis of stable angina were less often referred for noninvasive or invasive studies and were less likely to undergo revascularization or given optimal secondary prevention medication even in the presence of confirmed obstructive coronary artery disease compared to men [6]. These studies highlight the discrepancies in the recognition and appropriate treatment of CHD in women as compared to men and underscore the importance of appropriately identifying women who are at risk for CHD. The aim of this report is to review the primary and secondary prevention measures that are unique to women and to examine the sensitivity and specificity of the current diagnostic modalities in detecting CHD in women.

Hormone Replacement Therapy

Chapter 1 - Proposed Mechanism for Estrogen's Cardiovascular Protection

The role of estrogen replacement therapy (ERT) and combined estrogen/progestin hormone replacement therapy (HRT) in the primary and secondary prevention of CHD has been an issue of debate for the past several decades. Given that estrogen is believed to be a cardioprotective agent, it is no surprise that the rates of coronary heart disease in postmenopausal women are two to three times greater than in premenopausal women of the same age [2] (2). In the basic science arena researchers have demonstrated that estrogen has systemic effects as well as direct effects on the vasculature. These systemic effects of estrogen include alteration in lipoprotein profiles, changes in the coagulation, fibrinolytic and antioxidant systems, as well as production of other vasoactive substances [7]. Activation of estrogen receptors located in hepatic tissue results in alteration of expression of apoprotein genes which in turn results in a decrease in total cholesterol and low-density lipoprotein (LDL) cholesterol, an increase in high density lipoprotein (HDL) cholesterol and triglyceride levels, and a decrease in serum Lp(a) lipoprotein. These effects of estrogen on lipid concentrations have been demonstrated in several large-scale clinical trials. In the Postmenopausal Estrogen/Progesterone Interventions (PEPI) trial [8, 9] orally administered estrogen was shown to decrease LDL by about 15%, increase HDL level by about 15% and increase triglyceride level by about 20-25% in postmenopausal women. In addition to its effects on lipids, estrogen has been shown to regulate the hepatic expression of fibrinogen and the anticoagulant proteins antithrombin III and protein S, and to have direct effects on vascular cells and tissues [7]. Estrogen has both rapid effects on the vasculature, resulting in vasodilatation and increase in nitric oxide production, as well as long term effects mediated through its receptors, α and β, resulting in alterations in gene expressions that decrease atherosclerosis, decrease vascular injury, decrease smooth muscle cell growth and increase endothelial cell growth. In addition to the above beneficial effects in preventing atherosclerosis, estrogen has also been shown to have a proinflammatory effect as reflected in the increase in C-reactive protein (CRP) levels that is observed in subjects treated with HRT [10, 11]. Based on these effects of estrogen on the vasculature, coagulation milieu, and cholesterol profile, it is not surprising that the initial observational studies found a protective effect of ERT/HRT in postmenopausal women.

Chapter 2 – Data from Randomized Control Trials: Why Placebo Matters

The role for ERT and HRT was initially supported by numerous observational epidemiological studies. A meta-analysis of these initial studies published from 1970 through the 1990s showed a significant reduction (35-40%) in risk of CHD in women taking HRT[12]. Based on these observational data, the use of HRT/ERT in the primary and secondary prevention of CHD in women was the standard of care until 1998 when results from large, randomized control trials contradicted the findings from observational studies. The largest of the secondary prevention trials was the Heart and Estrogen/Progestin Replacement Study (HERS) [13]. This study evaluated the hypothesis that treatment with HRT (conjugated equine estrogen [CEE] and medroxyprogesterone [MPA]) would reduce future CHD events in postmenopausal women with documented CHD. In contrast to findings from observational studies, the authors found that after a mean follow-up of 4.1 years, there was no difference in recurrent CHD events between the treatment group and the control group (relative hazard (RH) 0.99, 95% CI 0.80 to 1.22). The post-hoc time trend analysis showed a 52% increase in CHD events during the first year of HRT use compared to placebo (95% CI 1.01-2.29) and a trend towards a decrease in CHD events in years 3 and 4 (RH 0.87, 95% CI 0.55-1.37; RH 0.67, 95% CI 0.43 – 1.04, respectively) [13] (13). In order to explore whether the beneficial effects of HRT would be recognized with longer follow-up, the participants in HERS who continued the assigned study drug after completion of the initial trial (93% agreed to continue to be followed) were followed for another 2.7 years. After a total of 6.8 years of follow-up there was still no significant difference in recurrent CHD events between the HRT group and the placebo group [14].

Chapter 3 - Does the Type of HRT or the Method of Delivery Matter in Secondary Prevention? No

Once HERS and HERS II proved that combined estrogen plus progestin did not successfully reduce recurrent CHD events, it was hypothesized that perhaps progestin attenuated the beneficial effects of estrogen and that estrogen alone would prove to be beneficial. In a test of this hypothesis, a study of 1,017 postmenopausal women aged 50-69 years who had survived their first myocardial infarction were randomized to receive either estradiol valerate (E2) or placebo and then followed for two years. The frequency of reinfarction or cardiac death did not differ between the two groups after 24 months of follow-up [15]. Similarly, in a study of transdermal estrogen delivery in 255 postmenopausal women with known CHD, there was no difference in recurrent CHD between the treatment arms and there was a non-significant trend towards increased CHD events in the HRT groups compared to placebo in the first two years of treatment [16].

Chapter 4 - Is There a Role of HRT in the Primary Prevention of CHD?

A potential explanation for the lack of benefit of ERT/HRT in the secondary prevention trials was the delay in pharmacotherapy. It has been postulated that estrogen is only effective at preventing the development of atherosclerosis in healthy women. Once atherosclerosis is established, estrogen is ineffective at preventing its progression. This hypothesis, however, did not hold true when tested in a large randomized control clinical trial. The Women's Health Initiative [17, 18] evaluated the role of HRT (CEE plus MPA) and ERT (CEE) on the primary prevention of CHD. Over 16,000 generally healthy postmenopausal women ranging in age from 50 to 79 years old were randomly assigned to HRT or placebo and were followed for a mean of 5.2 years. The authors actually found a trend towards an increase in CHD events with an adjusted hazard ratio for CHD in the HRT group 1.24 (95% CI 1.00-1.54), with the greatest amount of risk occurring in the first year after randomization with a hazard ratio of 1.81 (95% CI 1.09-3.01). A subgroup analysis of women stratified according to years since menopause, however, revealed a non-significant trend towards a reduction in CHD in women with less than 10 years since menopause (HR 0.89, 95% CI 0.5-1.7). Over 10,000 women with a hysterectomy were randomized into the estrogen-alone trial and were followed for an average of 6.8 years [19]. As with the HRT trial, there was no significant difference between the ERT group and the placebo group in CHD event rate (HR 0.91, 95% CI 0.75 – 1.12).

Chapter 5 - Why Did ERT/HRT Fail? Unanswered Questions and Future Trials

Regardless of the type of estrogen used, the method of hormone delivery or the combination of hormone replacement with estrogen and progestin, no significant benefit in CHD prevention was found in the aforementioned randomized trials. Many theories have been set forth to explain the significant discrepancy between observational and placebo controlled trials. One possible explanation is that the women in the observational trials who took HRT /ERT were a healthier cohort than those women who did not take HRT/ERT (selection bias). Another theory is that women in the observational studies on HRT/ERT were followed more closely than women not on HRT/ERT (prevention bias) [8] The pro-inflammatory effect of HRT as reflected in the increase in C-reactive protein seen in women taking HRT [10] has been proffered as an explanation for the early increased risk of CHD events that was observed in both the HERS trial and in the Women's Health Initiative.

Table 1. Hormone Replacement Therapy and Cardiovascular Outcomes

Study	Published	# Subjects	Endpoint	Follow-Up Time	Intervention	Results
Observational Studies						
Nurse's Health Study	*NEJM.* 1996; 335: 453-61	59,337 postmenopausal women free of CVD at study entry	CVD = nonfatal MI, fatal coronary disease, CABG/PTCA, fatal or nonfatal CVA	16 years	Estrogen Estrogen + Progestin	RR 0.60 (0.43-0.83) RR 0.39 (0.19-0.78)
	Ann Int Med. 2001; 135: 1-8.	2,489 postmenopausal women with previous MI or documented CAD	Non-fatal MI or coronary death	20 years	Estrogen alone OR estrogen + progestin	RR 0.65 (0.45-0.95)
Effect on Cholesterol and Inflammatory Markers						
PEPI	*JAMA;* 1995; 273: 199-208	875 healthy postmenopausal women	HDL-c SBP Insulin Fibrinogen	3 years	1) placebo 2) CEE 3) CEE + MPA cyclic 4) CEE + consecutive MPA 5) CEE + MP	CEE alone: Inc. HDL 5.6 mg/dL (5.4-6.7), dec. LDL 14.5 mg/dL (12.1-16.8) MPA regimens: Inc. HDL 1.2-1.6 mg/dL, Dec. LDL 16.5-17.7 mg/dL CEE + MP: Inc HDL 4.1 mg/dL, Dec LDL 14.8 mg/dL (12-17) No effect on insulin, sbp or fibrinogen
	Circ. 1999; 100: 717-722	365 healthy postmenopausal women	CRP E-selectin	3 years	As above	All active treatment groups: CRP inc. 85% E-selectin decreased by 18%
Women's Health Study	*Circ.* 1999; 100: 713-716	493 healthy women	CRP		Any HRT regimen	CRP 2x higher among women on HRT compared to no HRT (0.27 vs. 0.14 mg/dL, p = 0.001)

Table 1. (Continued)

Study	Published	# Subjects	Endpoint	Follow-Up Time	Intervention	Results
Primary Prevention Randomized Control Clinical Trials						
EPAT	*Ann Int Med.* 2001; 135: 939-953	222 healthy women	Carotid intima-media thickness	2 years	17β-E_2 or placebo	Less progression in E_2 group c/t placebo (-0.0017 vs. 0.0036 mm/yr) Avg. rates of progression did not differ in patient who also took lipid lowering meds
WHI	*NEJM.* 2003; 349: 523-534	16,608 healthy postmenopausal women	1) CHD = nonfatal MI and CHD death 2) Invasive breast ca	5.2 years (stopped early 2° risks exceeding benefits)	CEE + MPA vs. placebo	CHD: RR 1.24 (1.00-1.54) 1st year CHD: RR 1.81 (1.09-3.01) Menopause < 10 yrs CHD: RR 0.89 (0.5-1.7)
	JAMA. 2004; 291: 1701-1712	10,739 women with hysterectomy	CHD = nonfatal MI or CHD death	6.8 yrs	CEE vs. placebo	CHD: 0.91 (0.75-1.12) 1st year CHD: 1.16
Secondary Prevention Randomized Clinical Control trials						
HERS	*JAMA.* 1998; 280: 605-613	2,763 postmenopausal women with intact uterus and history of CAD	1° endpoint: nonfatal MI or CHD death 2° endpoint: revascularization, UA, cholesterol, CVA/TIA, PAD, all cause mortality	4.1 years	CEE + MPA or placebo	No difference in 1° or 2° endpoints 1° endpoint: RR 0.99 (0.80-1.22) 1st yr RR: 1.52 (1.01-2.29) Year 3 RR: 0.87 (0.55-1.37) Year 4 RR: 0.67 (0.43-1.04)
HERS–II	*JAMA.* 2002; 288: 49-57.	2,321 of original HERS participants	1° endpoint: nonfatal MI or CHD death	6.8 years	CEE + MPA or placebo (open label)	RR 1.00 (0.77-1.29)
PHASE	*BJOG.* 2002; 109: 1056-1062.	255 postmenopausal women with angiographically proven CAD	CHD death, nonfatal MI, hospitalization for UA	30.8 months	Transdermal 17β E_2 or 17β E_2 + norethisterone or placebo	HRT/ERT vs. placebo RR 1.29 (0.84-1.95)

Table 1. (Continued)

Study	Published	# Subjects	Endpoint	Follow-Up Time	Intervention	Results
ESPRIT	*Lancet.* 2003; 360: 2001-2008	1,017 women who survived first MI	Reinfarction of cardiac death and all-cause mortality	2 years	Oral estradiol vs. placebo	Reinfarction/CHD death RR 0.99 (0.7-1.41) All cause mortality RR 0.79 (0.5-1.27)
ERA	*NEJM.* 2000; 343:522-529	309 women with angiographically confirmed CAD	Mean minimal coronary artery diameter	3.2 ± 0.6 years	CEE or CEE + MPA or Placebo	No difference between treatment groups
WELL-HART	*NEJM.* 2003; 349: 535-545.	226 postmenopausal women with at least 1 coronary lesion	% coronary stenosis (QCA)	3.3 years	Usual care or 17β E_2 or 17β E_2 + MPA (all groups LDL < 130 mg/dL)	No difference in change in % stenosis between groups

Finally, in the randomized trials, the average time between menopause and enrollment in the studies ranged from 16 years to over 20 years. The initiation of hormone or estrogen therapy at this late stage may not truly represent a physiologic replacement and may contribute to lack of benefit in both primary and secondary prevention of CHD. The delay in HRT/ERT may have allowed subclinical atherosclerosis to develop and may have reduced the cardiovascular benefits of estrogen. The trend toward a reduction in CHD events in the subgroup analysis in the Women's Health Initiative of women who began HRT/ERT within 10 years of menopause [17] as well as a series of experiments in primates which showed a benefit of ERT on atherogenesis progression only when started immediately post oophorectomy [20] lends support to this theory. These observations have kept the door open for a possible role of HRT in primary prevention in women at the inception of menopause and is the basis for the ongoing Kronos Early Estrogen Prevention Study (KEEPS) [21]. For now, however, there is no clear role of HRT or ERT for either primary or secondary prevention of CHD in postmenopausal women. A summary of the aforementioned trials can be found in Table 1.

Obesity

Over the last 20 years obesity has become a pandemic, affecting over half of women in the United States -- an increase of over 30% in the past three decades [22]. Furthermore the rate of obesity is increasing more rapidly in women than men. In addition to being linked to several CHD risk factors (namely hypertension, diabetes, dyslipidemia, hyperinsulinemia, and increased levels of procoagulant and proinflammatory markers), obesity has also been shown to be an independent risk factor for CHD in women. In the Nurses Health Study,

115,818 women aged 30 to 55 years who were free of CHD at study entry were followed for 14 years. The investigators found not only a significant increase in the relative risk for CHD events in the group with the highest body mass index (BMI), but also an increase risk in CHD with modest increases in BMI (multivariate RR for BMI 23-24.9: 1.46, BMI 25-28.9: 2.06, BMI >29: 3.56) [23]. In addition, the authors found that women who gained more than 5 kg compared to their weight at age 18 years were at increased risk for CHD events (gain 5-7.9 kg multivariate RR: 1.25, gain 8-10.9 kg multivariate RR: 1.65, gain 11-19 kg multivariate RR: 1.92, gain >20 kg multivariate RR: 2.65). A recent re-analysis of 20-year follow-up data from the Nurses Health Study reinforces the above findings, showing that both obesity and inactivity are strong independent predictors of CHD events in women [24].

The question of how adipose distribution affects CHD risk has also been raised. It has been shown that abdominal adiposity is independently linked to significant metabolic abnormalities (insulin resistance, elevated triglycerides, hypertension, glucose intolerance and diabetes) and is an independent risk factor for CHD in men and possibly in women. Using a subset of women from the Nurses Health Study, Rexrode et al examined the impact of abdominal adiposity (as measured by waist hip ratio [WHR] and waist circumference) on the incidence of CHD over 8 years of follow-up. When controlled for BMI, WHR and waist circumference were independent predictors of CHD events. In women with a WHR of 0.88 or higher, the RR was 3.25 compared with women with a WHR < 0.72. Similarly, a waist circumference of > 96.5 cm had a RR of 3.06 when compared to women with a waist circumference of < 71.1 cm. This increase in risk remained significant even when adjustment for biological mediators was performed and when results were stratified by BMI (RR for BMI < 25 and WHR > 0.88: 3.54), suggesting that abdominal adiposity is a strong independent predictor of CHD in women regardless of BMI [25].

Abdominal adiposity is 1 of 5 clinical criteria for metabolic syndrome. It has been suggested that the effect of obesity on CHD risk in women observed in the Nurses Health Study was actually a surrogate for the increased risk associated with the metabolic syndrome. In order to address this theory, Kip et al evaluated the prevalence of CHD and subsequent development of CHD events over 3.5 years in a group of 780 women with suspected myocardial ischemia enrolled in the Women's Ischemia Syndrome Evaluation (WISE) study [26]. Women were classified by their BMI and as being either dysmetabolic or metabolically normal. Although the authors found a strong correlation between the metabolic syndrome and obesity, only the metabolic syndrome was associated with significant underlying CAD, death or major adverse cardiovascular events (HR 2.01 death, HR 1.88 MACE). In fact, normal weight women (BMI < 25) who were dysmetabolic had the highest rate of MACE (25% 3 year event rate) and death (13.4% 3 year event rate). These findings suggest that screening women for metabolic syndrome, even women with normal BMI (< 25), may prove a useful intervention in the primary prevention of CHD events. This study, however, did not assess whether measurements of abdominal adiposity were independent predictors of MACE when metabolic status was also accounted for. See Table 2 for ideal weight and body measurement goals.

Diet and Lifestyle

The ideal diet for primary and secondary prevention of CHD in women has been an issue of much debate over the past several decades. The recommendation of the traditional high carbohydrate, low fat diet espoused for the prevention of CHD is now being questioned. It has now been shown that this diet reduces levels of HDL and increases triglyceride levels, both of which independently increase the risk of CHD in women. In addition, the growth in popularity of high fat diets, such as the South Beach Diet and the Atkins diet, has made the question of diet in the prevention of CHD an even more pressing issue for physicians.

Table 2. Weight and Body Measurement Goals

Weight and Body Measurement Goals

1. BMI < 23

2. WHR < 0.72 (waist measured at the level of the umbilicus, hips measured at the largest circumference)

3. Waist circumference < 71.1 cm (measured at the level of the umbilicus)

Using the Nurse's Health Study database Hu et al examined the role of dietary intake of specific types of fat on risk of CHD. While a higher total fat intake was associated with an increased risk of CHD over 14 years of follow-up, this association almost disappeared when one accounted for confounders such as smoking, alcohol use, vigorous exercise and vitamin E supplementation (relative risk 1.02 for an increase of 5% in energy obtained from total fat as compared with the equivalent energy obtained from carbohydrates). However, a comparison of the different types of fat as percentage of total energy intake revealed that replacing 5% of energy from saturated fat with energy from unsaturated fats was associated with a 42% lower risk of CHD events. This reduction in CHD events was larger than the one observed when carbohydrates replaced saturated fat or trans unsaturated fat in the diet [27]. Further exploring the role of carbohydrates on CHD risk, Liu et al examined the role of glycemic load on CHD risk in women enrolled in the Nurse's Health Study. After accounting for possible confounding clinical and dietary factors, they found that women who had diets with the highest glycemic load had a relative risk for CHD events of 1.98 compared to the women with the lowest glycemic load. The adverse effect of a high glycemic load was observed in women of all body weights; however, the effect was most evident in women with average or above average BMIs [28]. As fruits and vegetables represent examples of foods high in fiber and a low glycemic index, it would follow from these observations that women with diets high in fruits and vegetables would have a lower risk of CHD. Data from the Nurse's Health Study and the Health Professionals' Follow-Up support this observation. Compared to women who ate fewer than three servings of fruit and vegetables a day, women who consumed more than eight servings a day had a 20% lower risk of CHD events over 14 years of follow-up. The lowest risk of CHD events were observed in women who consumed green leafy vegetables, cruciferous vegetables and vitamin C-rich fruits and vegetables [29]. However, the authors estimated that in order for one woman to avoid a coronary heart disease event, 1,443 people would have to increase their consumption of fruits and vegetables by one serving a day for 12 years. To further evaluate the role of fiber in the prevention of CHD in women, Wolk et al looked at 68,782 women aged 37 to 64 years who were free of CHD, diabetes and hyperlipidemia at study entry over 10 years. After accounting for possible confounders, they found that women with the highest intake of total fiber had a nonsignificant trend towards lower CHD events (RR 0.77, 95% CI 0.57-1.04, p = 0.07). However, when the sources of fiber were evaluated independently (cereal, fruit, vegetable), women with the highest intake of cereal fiber had a 34% reduction in CHD events over 10 years (RR 0.66, 95% CI 0.49-0.88, p < .001). The relationship with cereal fiber was strongest in women who were nonsmokers, BMI < 25, and those in the lowest tertile of saturated and trans unsaturated fat. Interestingly, consumption of vegetable and fruit fiber was not significantly associated with risk of CHD. The beneficial effect of fiber on CHD risk may be explained in part by its role in reducing total and LDL cholesterol via increased bile acid excretion and decreased hepatic synthesis of cholesterol. Fiber may also play a role in delaying absorption of macronutrients, which would lead to decreased insulin sensitivity and lower triglyceride levels [30].

While these studies suggest a role of individual foods and nutrients in the reduction of CHD in women, they do not address how overall eating patterns affect the incidence of CHD. In an effort to answer this question Fung et al evaluated the diet patterns of women in the Nurse's Health Study. Comparing a prudent diet (characterized by high intakes of fruits, vegetables, legumes, fish, poultry and whole grains) to a Western diet (characterized by higher intakes of red and processed meats, sweets and desserts, French fries and refined grains) they found that women in the highest quintile of the prudent diet had a relative risk of 0.76 for CHD events over 10 years compared to those in the lowest quintile. In contrast, those in the highest quintile of the Western diet had a relative risk of 1.46 compared to those in the lowest quintile [31]. This study supports the role of a diet high in polyunsaturated fat, high in fiber, and low in foods with a high glycemic index in the primary prevention of CHD in women.

Although the recently published Women's Health Initiative Dietary Modification Trial which compared a diet low in fat and high in fruit, vegetable and fiber intake to a standard diet on CVD risk in healthy postmenopausal women did not support these observational findings [32], the secondary prevention Lyon Diet Heart Study did find a similar decrease in subsequent cardiac events and mortality in men and women who followed a Mediterranean diet with a high amount of α linolenic acid compared to the standard recommended low fat post-MI diet following a first myocardial infarction (RR 0.28, p = 0.0001) [33]. The suboptimal reduction in fat intake in the study group (only a 8% reduction in total fat intake) in the Women's Health Initiative rendered the study with inadequate power to detect a true difference in CVD outcomes between the groups (power estimation of about 40%). Therefore the conclusions from this study regarding the utility of a low fat diet in the primary prevention of CVD must be viewed with caution. Based on the observational data and the date from the Lyon Diet Heart Study, it appears that a Mediterranean type diet that is high in fiber, low in foods with a high glycemic index, low in trans-fatty acids and saturated fats and high in polyunsaturated fat would be beneficial in the primary and secondary prevention of CHD events in women of all weights.

Exercise – How Much and How Often?

The role of exercise and the type of exercise (walking versus vigorous exercise) in the prevention of CHD in women is somewhat controversial. Although there have not been randomized control trials, data from the Nurse's Health Study and the Women's Health Initiative Observational study have shed some light on this topic. Manson et al evaluated the role of walking versus vigorous exercise in the primary prevention of CHD in women over 8 years of follow-up. When adjusting for potential clinical confounders, the authors found a strong positive relationship between increased physical activity and reduced risk of the CHD events. There were significant 34% reduction in CHD events in women who exercised for more than 10.5 MET-hours per week (equivalent of $\geq$ 3 hours per week of brisk walking or 1.5 hours per week of vigorous exercise). This decrease in risk was found regardless of BMI, smoking status and family history of premature coronary artery disease. A similar reduction in risk was observed in women who only participated in walking (no vigorous activity) with a relative risk of 0.70 in women with a walking score of 3.9 to 9.9 MET-hours per week (equivalent to 1 to 2.9 hours of walking per week at a brisk pace) and a relative risk of 0.60 in women who walked for more than 5 hours per week. Walking pace, in addition to total time walking, also emerged as an independent predictor of CHD events. The magnitude of risk reduction was similar with brisk walking and with vigorous exercise if the total energy expenditures were roughly equivalent [34]. Similar reductions were seen in CHD risk when diabetic women from the Nurse's Health Study were evaluated separately (50% reduction in CHD events in the women who exercise > 7 MET-hours per week compared to < 1 MET-hour per week) [35]. Investigators from the Women's Health Initiative also addressed the role of the walking and vigorous exercise in the prevention of CHD in a more ethnically diverse population of postmenopausal women. Paralleling the results from the Nurse's Health Study, a risk reduction of about 30% was seen in the women with the highest energy expenditure, regardless if the activity was walking or vigorous exercise. In addition, the authors found that longer duration of sitting was associated with a substantially increased risk of cardiovascular events (RR 1.68 for women who sit for 16 hours a day compared to women who sit for less than 4 hours a day). These changes in cardiovascular risk were seen in all women, regardless of race, BMI or age [36]. From these observational studies, it is reasonable to recommend moderate intensity exercise (walking briskly 3 hours per week or vigorous exercise for 1.5 hours per week) to women of all races, body weights and age, in an effort to reduce the risk of CHD. The use of a pedometer to measure the number of steps walked may be a useful objective barometer of exercise and may help facilitate the development of an exercise goals for women.

What Does It All Mean?

When evaluating lifestyle as a whole, Stampfer et al found that women who adhered to a "low risk" lifestyle (defined as not currently smoking, BMI less than 25, consuming at least a half an alcoholic beverage a day, engaging in moderate to vigorous physical activity for at least 30 minutes a day, and being in the highest 40 percent of the cohort in consumption of cereal fiber, marine n-3 fatty acids, folate, ratio of polyunsaturated to saturated fats, lack of consumption of trans fat and low glycemic load) had a significantly reduced risk of CHD events compared to those who did not adhere to such a lifestyle (RR 0.17). This model suggested that 82% of the CHD events in this large cohort of women could have been prevented if all women had followed a low risk lifestyle [37]. See Table 3 for a summary of recommended diet and lifestyle modifications.

Table 3. Diet and Exercise Recommendations

Diet and Exercise Recommendations
1. Diet with a low glycemic load (glycemic load = glycemic index%/100 gm of carbohydrate)
2. Diet low in saturated ($\leq$ 11% of total energy intake)
3. Diet low in trans-unsaturated fats ($\leq$ 2% of total energy intake)
4. Diet high in polyunsaturated fats ($\geq$ 6% of total energy intake)
5. >8 servings of fruits and vegetables a day
6. >5 servings of fish per week
7. Diet high in cereal fiber (> 4 g/day)
8. Brisk walking 3 hr/wk OR vigorous exercise 1.5 hr/wk (at least 30 min of moderate exercise per day, 5 days a week)

Dietary and Vitamin Supplements

Is There a Role for Anti-Oxidant Vitamin Supplements in the Primary or Secondary Prevention of CHD in Women?

As with the debate over hormone replacement therapy in the primary and secondary prevention of CHD in women, the role of antioxidant vitamins has been investigated over the past two decades. The initial data from a large, prospective cohort study suggested a modest benefit of Vitamin E in the reduction of primary cardiovascular events in women. Like estrogen, Vitamin E had a plausible biological basis in which it was postulated it could prevent atherosclerosis. This theory was based on the hypothesis that oxidative modification of low-density lipoprotein initiates atherosclerosis and the idea that anti-oxidant vitamins, such as Vitamin E, could inhibit this lipid peroxidation thereby preventing the development or progression of atherosclerosis and CHD [38]. Observational data from the Nurses Health Study and Iowa Women's Study initially supported this hypothesis [39, 40]. However, the positive benefit of vitamin E supplements noted in observational studies has not been supported by subsequent randomized placebo-controlled clinical trials. Although the Cambridge Heart Antioxidant Study (CHAOS) [41] suggested a beneficial effect on the secondary prevention of CHD, subsequent trials of Vitamin E or combinations of antioxidant vitamins (vitamin E and C) in the secondary prevention of CHD have not shown a similar benefit. The GISSI-Prevenzione trial [42], the Heart Protection Study (HPS) [43] and the WAVE trial [44] found no benefit in the secondary prevention of CHD events or in the angiographic progression of coronary atherosclerosis. In secondary analysis of the GISSI-Prevenzione trial, the authors did find a significant 20% reduction in all cardiovascular deaths

(RR 0.80, 95% CI 0.65-0.99) and a 35% reduction in sudden cardiac deaths (RR 0.65, 95% CI 0.48-0.89). The ability to apply these results to a female population, however, is limited because of the low proportion of women (15% in CHAOS, 19% in GISSI, 25% in HPS) in the majority of these trials.

Similarly, the data for the role of vitamin E supplements in the primary prevention of CHD in women has also not been born out in randomized placebo-controlled studies. The HOPE and HOPE-TOO trials evaluated the role of 400 IU of Vitamin E from natural sources in the prevention of myocardial infarction (MI), stroke and death from cardiovascular causes over 4.5 years and 7 years of follow-up, respectively, in 2,545 women and 6,996 men who were at high risk for cardiovascular disease. These studies found no benefit of Vitamin E on the reduction of cardiovascular events (RR 1.05, 95% CI 0.95-1.16, p = 0.33). In subgroup analysis there was no difference in primary outcome when evaluating only the female subjects [45, 46]. Likewise, the Primary Prevention Project, a randomized controlled study of 4,495 high risk patients (2583 women) comparing placebo to 300 mg of synthetic Vitamin E supplementation on the rate of cardiovascular death, non-fatal MI and nonfatal stroke over a mean of 3.6 years of follow-up also found no benefit to Vitamin E supplementation (RR 1.07, 95% CI 0.74 – 1.56). This study, however, did not include a subgroup analysis based on gender [47].

The Women's Health Study evaluated the role of high dose vitamin E (600 IU every other day) in the primary prevention of CVD and cancer in 39,876 low risk women over ten years of follow-up. The authors found a non-significant 7% reduction in major cardiovascular events (non-fatal MI, non-fatal stroke, cardiovascular death) at the end of the trial (RR 0.93, 95% CI 0.82-1.05, p = 0.26). Although vitamin E had no effect on total MI or stroke, they did find a significant 24% reduction in cardiovascular death in the vitamin E group (RR 0.76, 95% CI 0.59-0.98), which was largely attributable to fewer sudden deaths in the vitamin E group. They also found a significant reduction in major cardiovascular events in the subgroup of women aged 65 years or older (RR 0.74, 95% CI 0.59-0.93, p=0.009) [48], suggesting a possible role in the primary prevention of CHD events in this elderly subset of women.

While the data regarding the use of antioxidant vitamins, specifically vitamin E, in the primary and secondary prevention of CHD have been contradictory; the bulk of the data does not support the use of vitamin E in the prevention of CHD in women. Randomized controlled trials have failed to show a significant benefit of any single vitamin supplement or combination of supplements in either the primary or secondary prevention of CHD death or non-fatal MI. In fact, several meta-analyses of the role of antioxidant vitamins in the prevention of CHD have failed to show a consistent benefit of antioxidant vitamins [38, 49] and at this point in time they should not be recommended for the primary or secondary prevention of CHD in women.

Is There a Role for Folic Acid or Vitamin B6 in the Prevention of CHD in Women?

Plasma homocysteine has been shown to be a strong, independent predictor of cardiovascular disease in both men and women. From country to country, there is a variation in homocysteine levels and with increasing levels of homocysteine there is a greater risk of cardiovascular mortality. The correlation between homocysteine and CVD mortality (r = 0.71) suggests that homocysteine may play an important role in determining CVD mortality between different populations [50]. Several plausible mechanisms by which homocysteine could increase risk of CHD (direct toxicity to endothelial cells, increased coagulation, decreased endothelial reactivity, and stimulation of smooth muscle cell proliferation [51]) have been previously elucidated.

Folate and vitamin B6 are important cofactors in the metabolism of homocysteine and changing the intake of folic acid and vitamin B6 can modify homocysteine levels. Accordingly, studies have shown that low dietary intake of vitamin B6 is also associated with increased risk of cardiovascular disease. Based on these observations, some investigators have hypothesized that lowering levels of homocysteine via folate and vitamin B6 supplementation would translate into a reduction in cardiovascular events. Support for this hypothesis in women was initially offered from observations from the Nurse's Health Study [51]. The authors found that the multivariate relative risk of CHD in the highest quintile of folate consumption (≥545 μg folate) was 0.69 (95% CI 0.55-0.87). The authors reported an 11% relative risk reduction of CHD events for each 200 μg increase in folate intake. Similar to folate intake, there was a 33% multivariate relative risk reduction in the women with the highest intake of vitamin B6 (median intake 4.6 mg) (RR 0.67, 95% CI 0.53-0.85) and a relative risk of 0.83 for each 2 mg increase in vitamin B6 consumption (95% CI 0.74-0.94). Because of the high correlation between folate and vitamin B6 intake (Spearman r = 0.77), the ability to assess the independent effects of the individual vitamins was limited.

The concern that the observed relation of homocysteine and vitamin B6/folate to CHD risk may actually represent unrecognized confounders rather than a true causal relationship has led to the development of randomized clinical trials. Therefore, in order to better understand the role of folate and vitamin B6 in the secondary prevention of cardiovascular disease, the NORVIT investigators [52] randomized 3,749 patients (26% women) who had had an MI within the past 7 days, into four groups; folate (0.8 mg/day) plus vitamin B6 (40 mg/day), folate, vitamin B6, or placebo. These subjects were followed for an average of 3.5 years and were monitored for nonfatal and fatal MI and stroke. The investigators found that although the folate groups lowered plasma homocysteine levels by 28% (no significant change in homocysteine levels in the vitamin B6 group), there was no difference in the combined primary endpoint (folate RR 1.1, 95% CI 0.9-1.3, p = 0.3; vitamin B6 RR 1.1, 95% CI 1.0-1.3, p = 0.09). The authors found a trend towards increased risk in primary endpoint (MI and stroke) when folate and vitamin B6 were given in combination (RR 1.2, 95% CI 1.0-1.4, p = 0.03). The preliminary results from this study do not support a role for folate or vitamin B6 in the secondary prevention of CHD and suggest that these interventions may in fact be harmful. The role of these vitamins in the primary prevention of CHD, however, is still a question. Until a randomized, clinical trial addresses this issue, the routine use of these supplements in primary prevention of CHD in women is not recommended.

Is There a Role for Fish Oil (Omega-3 Fatty Acid) Supplementation in the Prevention of CHD in Women?

The observation that populations with a high intake of fish have a lower rate of cardiovascular disease initially led to the hypothesis that fish consumption may have a protective effect for atherosclerosis. Some of the proposed biological mechanisms that would explain this observation are: reducing susceptibility of the heart to ventricular arrhythmias, antithrombogenic properties of fish oil, lowering triglyceride levels, retardation of atherosclerotic plaque growth via reduced adhesion molecule expression, reducing platelet derived growth factor, acting as an anti-inflammatory mediator, and promoting nitric-oxide induced endothelial relaxation [53]. Several epidemiological prospective studies in men have lent support to this hypothesis. In the 30-year follow-up of the Chicago Western Electric Study, men who consumed 35 g or more of fish daily compared to those who ate none had a significant reduction in CHD death (RR 0.62) [53]. Similar risk reductions were also observed in women in the Nurse's Health Study cohort [54]. Using multivariate analysis the authors found that the risk of major CHD events in the women who consumed fish ≥5 times per week compared to the women who never ate fish was 0.69 (95% CI 0.52-0.93). They even found a 21% risk reduction in the women who only ate fish 1-3 times per month compared to those who ate fish < 1 time per month (RR 0.79, 95% CI 0.64-0.97). In addition, a similar reduction in CHD events was seen in the women who were in the highest quintile of omega-3 fatty acid supplement intake (0.24% of energy) compared to the lowest quintile (0.03% of energy), with a multivariate relative risk of 0.69 (95% CI 0.57-0.84). Although this epidemiologic data is compelling, to date there are no randomized controlled clinical trials to support the role of fish or fish oil in the primary prevention of CHD events in women. Currently the JELIS investigators [55] are following 10,796 postmenopausal women and 4,204 men who were free of CHD, in a trial of eicosapentaenoic acid (EPA), a component of fish oil, in addition to treatment with a statin in hyperlipidemic patients for 5 years. The primary end-points in this trial are major coronary events (sudden cardiac death, fatal and nonfatal MI, unstable angina, and coronary revascularization). The initial results of this trial, which were presented at the American Heart Association scientific session in 2005, revealed a 19% risk reduction in major cardiovascular events (RR 0.81, 95% CI 0.69-0.95) in the group treated with EPA plus statin therapy compared to statin therapy alone, and a 24% risk reduction in unstable angina (RR 0.76, 95% CI 0.62- 0.95).

In contrast to the dirth of data from randomized controlled trials on the role of fish oil in the primary prevention of CHD, there have been several observational trials as well as randomized controlled clinical trials showing a benefit of fish oil on the secondary prevention of CHD events. An observational trial of atherosclerosis progression in postmenopausal women revealed that the consumption of ≥ 2 servings of fish per week compared with < 2 servings per week was associated with significantly smaller increases in the percentage of stenosis (4.54 ± 1.37% versus – 0.06 ± 1.59%, p < 0.05) in diabetic women and fewer new stenoses (21% versus 34%, p = 0.02) [56]. Randomized clinical control trials have also supported the role of fish oil in the secondary prevention of CHD events. The first such trial, the DART trial [57], was published in 1989 and evaluated the role n-3 polyunsaturated fatty acids (PUFA) on the recurrence rate of CHD events over a 2 year period in men with a recent MI. This study found a 29% reduction in total mortality and in CHD deaths in the group who increased their dietary intake of n-3 PUFA to 0.5-1 g/day. The GISSI-Prevenzione trial [42], evaluated the role of n-3 PUFA and vitamin E in the secondary prevention of CHD events in 11,324 men and women (about 15% women). The authors found a 15% relative risk reduction in the rate of death, non-fatal MI and non-fatal stroke over 3.5 years of follow-up in the n-3 PUFA supplement group (RR 0.85, 95% CI 0.74-0.98). In secondary analysis the reduction in fatal events was almost entirely accounted for by a reduction in cardiovascular deaths (30% reduction in cardiovascular deaths, 95% CI 0.56-0.87). The low number of female subjects participating in these trials limits the applicability of the results to women.

Although the data is limited in women at this time, it is reasonable to recommend the use of n-3 omega fatty acids for the secondary prevention of CHD events in women who have recently had an MI. The recent results from the JELIS study also supports the recommendation of adding fish oil to the treatment of hyperlipidemics in the primary prevention of CHD events.

Aspirin Use in Women

The Debate over Aspirin in the Primary Prevention of CHD in Women

The role of aspirin in the secondary prevention of cardiovascular events is well established in both men and women. The role of aspirin in the primary prevention of cardiovascular disease in women, on the other hand, is not as clear. The Physician's Health Study, which was the first trial to uncover a significant 44% reduction in first myocardial infarction with aspirin use only included men in its subject population. Subsequent trials, however, have included women as well as men in their study population. The Hypertension Optimal Treatment Study (HOT) [58] evaluated the effect of blood pressure control and 75 mg of aspirin on the rate of major cardiovascular events (namely CV death, MI, stroke) in 9,907 men and 8,883 women over 3.8 years of follow-up. The authors found a significant 42% reduction in first MI in men (RR 0.58, 95% CI 0.41-0.81), which was similar to the results from the Physician's Health Study. However, there was only a non-significant 19% reduction in first MI in women (RR 0.81, 95% CI 0.49-1.31). In addition, there was a significant increase in non-fatal major bleeding in women randomized to aspirin therapy (2.7/1000 patient-years versus 1.3/1000 patient-years, p = 0.006). The Primary Prevention Project (47) evaluated the effect of 100 mg of aspirin on subsequent major cardiovascular events (cardiovascular death, non-fatal MI and non-fatal stroke) over 3.6 years of follow-up in 4,495 subjects (57% women) who had at least one cardiovascular risk factor. This study found a non-significant 29% reduction in combined endpoint (RR 0.71, 95% CI 0.48-1.04) and a significant reduction in cardiovascular death (RR 0.56, 95% CI 0.31-0.99). There was not a significant difference, however, in the rate of myocardial infarction (RR 0.69, 95% CI

0.38-1.23). The authors report that the direction and the size of the effects of aspirin on all of the predefined endpoints were similar in men and women when evaluated separately. This data, however, was not presented in the paper. The data from these two trials present a less than convincing argument for the use of aspirin in the primary prevention of MI in women.

The Women's Health Study [59] sought to finally answer this question. This study enrolled 39,876 women who were free of cardiovascular disease and had low risk cardiovascular profiles. The subjects were randomized to low dose aspirin (100 mg every other day) or to placebo and were followed for 10 years for a first cardiovascular event (non-fatal MI, non-fatal stroke or death from cardiovascular cause). The investigators found a non-significant 9% risk reduction in major cardiovascular events (RR 0.91, 95% CI 0.80-1.03), with no significant effect on fatal or non-fatal MI (RR 1.02, 95% CI 0.84-1.25). The authors did find, however, a significantly higher rate of bleeding complications in the aspirin group as compared to placebo (bleeding requiring transfusion RR 1.40, 95% CI 1.07-1.83, p 0.02). When evaluating the subgroup of women over the age of 65, however, they did find a significant reduction in major cardiovascular events (RR 0.74, 95% CI 0.59-0.92) and in MI (RR 0.66, 95% CI 0.44-0.97).

Based on these data there does not appear to a clear role for aspirin in the primary prevention of cardiovascular disease in women in the low-risk female population. There may be a benefit in the elderly female population. However, given the risk of bleeding complications, this needs to be further evaluated with a large-scale trial dedicated to answering this question.

Cholesterol and Inflammatory Biomarkers of CHD in Women

The Optimal Lipid Levels in Women for the Prevention of CHD

The role of LDL cholesterol in the development of atherosclerosis has been well established. However, the best lipid parameter for predicting CHD events in women continues to be an issue of some debate. In a nested case-control study from the Nurse's Health Study cohort [60], Shai et al preformed a multivariate assessment of the role of each lipid parameter in predicting future CHD events (non-fatal MI and fatal CHD) over 8 years of follow-up. In women without prior history of CHD, they found that an LDL cholesterol level of 132 mg/dL conferred a relative risk of future CHD events of 1.9 (95% CI 1.1-3.5) with 1 standard deviation (SD = 36 mg/dL) increase in LDL conferring a 40% increase in CHD risk (RR 1.4, 95% CI 1.1-1.7). LDL levels, however, did not completely predict CHD risk in women. In fact, one standard deviation (17 mg/dL) increase in HDL conferred a relative risk of CHD events of 0.5 (95% CI 0.4-0.7). Using the lipid index of total cholesterol/HDL-c provided an even better assessment of future CHD risk with one standard deviation corresponding to a relative risk of 1.8 (95% CI 1.5-2.1). When adding all of the lipid parameters to a step-wise model of CHD prediction (after accounting for age and smoking status), HDL-c was the primary contributor to the prediction model raising the ROC from 0.69 to 0.70, with LDL raising the ROC further to 0.72, suggesting that measurements of both LDL and HDL are essential in the prediction of CHD events. A similar contribution to the prediction model was seen when the ratio of total cholesterol/HDL was added (ROC increased to 0.72). This ratio reflects the proportion of atherogenic to antiatherogenic lipid fractions and appears to be a powerful tool for predicting CHD in postmenopausal women.

From this data it follows that lowering LDL cholesterol and raising HDL cholesterol should play a role in CHD prevention in women. Accordingly, the data from secondary prevention trials of statin therapy has shown reduced risks of CHD events in women placed on statin therapy. In subgroup analysis of the 4S trial [61], 827 postmenopausal women with known CHD and moderate hypercholesterolemia were randomized to either 20 mg of simvastatin or placebo and were followed over a mean of 5.4 years. They were monitored for all-cause mortality, CHD mortality, major coronary events (CHD death and non-fatal MI) and other acute atherosclerotic events. After 6 weeks of treatment the investigators found a mean 28% reduction in total cholesterol, 40% reduction in LDL cholesterol and 8% increase in HDL. They reported significant reductions in major coronary events (RR 0.66, 95% CI 0.48-0.91, $p = 0.12$), nonfatal MI (RR 0.64, 95% CI 0.47-0.98, $p = 0.011$), and revascularizations (RR 0.51, 95% CI 0.30-0.86, $p = 0.012$). These risk reductions were similar to those seen in the male population from the study. Because of the small number of events in women they did not find a significant decrease in overall or CHD mortality. A similar reduction in risk in CHD death and nonfatal MI was shown in the female subjects from the CARE trial [62]. This trial randomized 576 postmenopausal women (out of a total of 4,159 subjects) with a history of recent MI and an average cholesterol level (total cholesterol of < 240 mg/dL and LDL level between 115 to 174 mg/dL) to 40 mg of pravastatin or placebo. The subjects were followed for 5 years and were monitored for cardiac events. Similar to the 4S trial, the women treated with pravastatin had an average 20% reduction in total cholesterol level, a 28% reduction in LDL cholesterol and a 4% increase in HDL cholesterol levels. Women in the study experienced an overall risk reduction in combined coronary events of 46% (RR 0.54, 95% CI 0.48 – 0.78, $p = 0.001$) compared to a 20% reduction in events in men. In secondary analyses there were also significant reductions in nonfatal MI (RR 0.49, 95% CI 0.26 – 0.92, $p = 0.028$), and in revascularization rates (RR 0.47, 95% CI 0.30 – 0.74, $p = 0.001$) in the pravachol treatment group. The PROVE-IT –TIMI 22 trial [63], which included 22% women as subjects, has shown a significant reduction in recurrent CHD events in patients with a recent myocardial infarction who were treated with statins and achieved a mean LDL level of less than 70 mg/dL (2.7 vs. 4.0 events per 100 person years, $p = 0.008$). Based on observational and clinical trial data, the goal LDL in women with a history of CHD or diabetes should be ≤ 70 mg/dL.

Are There Other Markers of Inflammation That Are Predictive of CHD Events in Women?

In addition to LDL and HDL cholesterol, recent data has shown that various markers of inflammation are potent predictors of CHD events in women as well. Women in general have higher CRP levels compared to men [64] and black women have significantly higher CRP levels than white, Hispanic or Asian women [65]. These higher CRp levels may provide insight into the pathogenesis of angina in women with nonobstructive coronary disease and further aid in assessing CHD risk in women. Using the Nurse's Health Study cohort as a patient population, Ridker et al performed a nested-case control study to evaluate the role of inflammatory markers in the prediction of cardiovascular events (defined as death from CHD, nonfatal MI or stroke, or need for coronary revascularization) over 3 years of follow-up [66]. Four markers of inflammation (hs-CRP, serum amyloid A, IL-6, and sICAM-1) were univariate predictors of cardiovascular risk. Of these 4 markers, hs-CRP was the strongest predictor of future CHD events (RR 4.4, 95% CI 2.2-8.9 of highest [8.5 mg/L] to lowest [0. 6 mg/L] quartile) and the only independent predictor in multivariate analysis (RR associated with an increase of one quartile 1.5, 95% CI 1.1-2.1). In addition, they found that hs-CRP, IL-6, and amyloid A improved the prediction of cardiovascular events over the use of lipids alone. In fact when the authors performed a subgroup analysis of women with LDL < 130 mg/dL they found that the adjusted relative risk of cardiovascular events increased about 39% with each increase in quartile for hs-CRP (95% CI 13% to 89%, p= 0.03). In a subsequent analysis of the entire Nurse's Health Study cohort (27,939 women), Ridker et al compared the prognostic value of LDL cholesterol compared to CRP in the prediction of cardiovascular events over 8 years of follow-up [67]. Although CRP and LDL were both strong, independent predictors of cardiovascular events, the highest quintile of CRP (> 4.19 mg/L; RR 2.3, 95% CI 1.6-3.4) was a stronger predictor of events than the highest quintile of LDL (>153.9 mg/dL; RR 1.5, 95% CI 1.1-2.0). LDL and CRP, however, were not well correlated suggesting that each measurement identified different high-risk groups. Screening for both markers provided better information than either measurement alone. Additionally they reported that 77% of first cardiovascular events occurred in women with an LDL less than 160 mg/dL and 46% occurred in women with LDL less than 130 mg/dL. The addition of CRP measurements would have helped to identify at risk women that were missed by the standards set by the National Cholesterol Education Program. A prospective, randomized control study of the use of rosuvastatin in the primary prevention of cardiovascular disease in patients with low LDL cholesterol levels (<130 mg/dL) and elevated CRP levels ($\geq$ 2 mg/L) is currently underway in the JUPITER trial [68]. Results of this study should be known in the next several years and should help in setting guidelines for the optimal management of women with normal LDL cholesterol levels but elevated CRP levels.

Diagnosis and Prognosis

Exercise Treadmill Testing – The Basics

Women generally manifest CHD about 10 years later than men (2), present more commonly with atypical chest pain or dyspnea, and have a lower prevalence of luminal obstructive coronary disease by angiography. However, when women do present with obstructive coronary disease, they have higher morbidity and mortality rates compared to age-matched men. It is therefore imperative not only to find effective primary and secondary prevention measures in women, it is also important to appropriately identify and risk stratify women with CHD. Historically, the non-invasive diagnostic work-up in women has been underutilized secondary to a lack of physician confidence in the accuracy of the test results [69]. While exercise stress testing is the most commonly used non-invasive diagnostic modality for detecting coronary artery disease in men, many studies have demonstrated a low sensitivity and specificity of exercise treadmill testing in women. In a meta-analysis of 19 studies of exercise stress tests in 3,721 women, the mean sensitivity was 61%, mean specificity 70%, positive likelihood ratio (LR) 2.25 and negative LR 0.55. This is compared to a mean sensitivity of 68% and specificity of 77% in a meta-analysis of exercise testing in 24,074 men [70]. In fact, women are 5 to 20 times more likely to have a false positive exercise ECG compared to men.

Why Is Exercise Treadmill Testing Less Accurate in Women?

Several mechanisms for the reduced specificity of exercise ECG testing in women have been proposed. These mechanisms include a lower achieved workload, the digoxin-like effect of estrogen, an inappropriate catecholamine response to exercise in women, a higher incidence of mitral valve prolapse, and different chest wall anatomy [68]. In addition, it is important to note that the standards for abnormal exercise ECG test were developed in a male population. In order to better elucidate the role of estrogen and progesterone on the sensitivity and specificity of the exercise ECG to detect CAD in postmenopausal women, Bokhari et al retrospectively examined the ability of exercise ECG to detect CAD in 140 postmenopausal women who were either on ERT, HRT or no hormone therapy. Myocardial perfusion imaging (MPI) was the gold standard for comparison. When comparing women on ERT to HRT to no hormone therapy, they found that there was no significant difference in sensitivity (56% vs. 57% vs. 54%). However, there was a significant decrease in specificity in women on ERT alone compared to women on no hormone therapy or on combined estrogen/progestin therapy (46% vs. 78% vs. 80%, respectively) [71]. These finding support the observation that estrogen leads to an unacceptably high rate of false positives, which is counterbalanced by the addition of progesterone.

Does Perfusion Imaging Improve Diagnostic Accuracy in Women?

As a result of the high false positive rate in exercise ECG testing in women, various imaging modalities have been evaluated in the diagnosis and risk stratification of CHD in women. Myocardial perfusion imaging has been shown to have a significantly higher sensitivity and specificity for detecting CAD in men. However the small size of the left ventricle in women and breast artifact have led to some doubt regarding its utility in women. In an effort to evaluate the utility of MPI in the diagnosis of CAD in women, Taillefer et al compared the diagnostic accuracy of Tl-201 and Tc-99m sestamibi SPECT imaging in detecting CAD in 85 women with suspected CAD who were already scheduled for coronary angiography [72]. This study revealed that the overall sensitivity for detection of CAD (≥50% stenosis) was 75% for Tl-201 and 71.9% for Tc-99m sestamibi with a specificity of 61.9% vs. 85.7%, respectively (p = 0.07). For the detection of stenosis ≥70% the sensitivity was 84.3% vs. 80.4% and the specificities were 58.8% vs. 82.4%, for Tl-201 and Tc-99m respectively (p =0.01). The use of gated SPECT Tc-99m imaging resulted further improvement in the specificity of the test for detecting both ≥50% and ≥70% stenoses as compared to Tl-201 (70.6% vs. 94.1% p=0.002 and 67.2% vs. 92.2% p=0.004, respectively).

The addition of myocardial perfusion imaging to treadmill testing provides for a significant improvement in both the sensitivity and specificity in the detection of CAD in women regardless of the imaging agent used. However, for the greatest specificity Tc-99m gated SPECT imaging appears to be the ideal imaging agent.

How Does Stress Echocardiography Compare with ETT?

Exercise echocardiography has also been shown to be an accurate modality to non-invasively diagnose CAD in men. There have, however, been conflicting reports regarding its utility in women, with specificities ranging from 46% to 93% [73]. In order to determine whether there is a cost efficient role for exercise echocardiography in the detection of CAD in women (defined as ≥50% occlusion of a major epicardial artery), Marwick et al evaluated 161 women referred for exercise echocardiography and coronary angiography for an evaluation of cardiac symptoms. This study found that the sensitivity of exercise echocardiography for detecting CAD was 80%, the specificity was 81%, the positive predictive value was 71% and the negative predictive value was 87%. Compared to the exercise ECG, stress echocardiography had significantly higher specificity (80% vs. 56% p ≤ 0.0004), accuracy (81% vs. 64% p < 0.005), and positive predictive value (74% vs. 54%, p < 0.05) whereas the sensitivity (81% vs. 77%, p = 0.5) and the negative predictive value (86% vs. 78%, p = 0.19) were comparable (71). The authors concluded that exercise echocardiography was a cost efficient initial first test for the detection of coronary artery disease, especially in women with an intermediate pre-test probability of CAD.

Based on these studies it is clear that exercise ECG is a less than ideal test for detecting CAD in women, with a very high false positive rate which leads in turn to many unnecessary invasive coronary angiograms. The addition of Tc-99m sestamibi or echocardiography to exercise ECG provides for an effective and cost efficient way to diagnose women with suspected CAD without a high rate of false positives.

Is There a Role for Electron Beam Tomography in the Detection of CAD in Women?

Although myocardial perfusion imaging and stress echocardiography greatly increased the specificity of stress testing over exercise ECG, the sensitivity did not substantially improve. Electron beam tomography (EBT) has been offered as a possible non-invasive modality that would improve the sensitivity of detection of CAD in women. Budoff et al established the sensitivity, specificity and predictive value of EBT in 387 symptomatic women and 733 symptomatic men, using coronary angiography as the gold standard (significant CAD defined as a stenosis > 50%) [74]. Using a coronary calcium score cut-off of zero, the authors found that the sensitivity of EBT in detecting significant CAD in both men and women was 96%. The specificity, however, was significantly higher in women (57% vs. 41%, $p < 0.001$). By using a receiver operator curve (ROC) the authors found that using a calcium score cutoff of 34 yielded the optimal sensitivity (81%) and specificity (81%).

Although EBT using a calcium score cutoff of 34 does offer a modest advantage in sensitivity over myocardial perfusion imaging, the specificity is still less than that seen in Tc-99m gated SPECT imaging or stress echocardiography. A combination of EBT and stress imaging may offer the best combination of sensitivity and specificity for non-invasively detecting CAD in women. See table 4 for a summary of these non-invasive diagnostic modalities.

Table 4. Stress Testing and Cardiac Imaging in Women

Test	Sensitivity	Specificity
ETT	61%	70%
Tl-201 MPI	75%	61.9%
Tc-99m MPI	71.9%	85.7%
Gated-Tc-99m MPI	n/a	94.1%
Exercise echo	80%	81%
EBT (cutoff 34)	81%	81%

What Is the Prognostic Utility of Stress Testing in Women?

Both myocardial perfusion imaging as well as stress echocardiography have been evaluated for their roles in risk stratification of women with suspected CAD. Hachamovitch et al explored the gender related differences in the prognostic value of exercise dual isotope stress testing in identifying men and women at risk for cardiac death or nonfatal myocardial infarction [75]. The authors retrospectively studied 2,742 men and 1,394 women for a mean 20 ± 5 months for the above endpoints. The women included in this study were significantly older, had more atypical symptoms and had more cardiac risk factors compared to the men who more frequently had a history of prior myocardial infarction and more frequently presented without symptoms. The overall event rates were similar between the men and the women (3.5% vs. 3.2% $p = NS$). The authors found that the event rate in both men and women increased as a function of the perfusion scan abnormality. Women with a definitely abnormal scan, however, had a greater than twofold higher event rate compared to men with a similar scan result (13.9% vs. 6.6% $p = 0.001$). Accordingly, the perfusion scan result was better able to risk stratify women than men. The odds ratio for an event with an abnormal versus a normal scan in women was 22.8, as compared to the odds ratio of 4.4 for men ($p < 0.0001$). This effectiveness was independent of patient characteristics and ECG test results. The nuclear scan information added 17% and 37% additional prognostic information in men and women, respectively.

In order to address the question of whether pharmacologic perfusion imaging adds incremental prognostic value over clinical predictors, Berman et al retrospectively examined the rate of cardiac death over a follow-up of 27 ± 8.8 months in 2,656 women and 2,677 men who had undergone adenosine dual isotope MPI [76]. Cardiac death occurred in 4.4% of women and 6.1% of men over the follow-up time period. Similar to the results in exercise MPI, the annual rate of cardiac death rose as a function of worsening sum stress score. With a normal scan the annual mortality rate was 0.6% and 0.9% for men and women respectively, while a severely abnormal scan conferred an annual cardiac mortality rate of 5.5% in men and 7.0% in women ($p < 0.001$). As in exercise myocardial perfusion imaging, the scan data added incremental prognostic value to the clinical predictors of cardiac death.

Exercise and dobutamine stress echocardiography have also been proven beneficial in risk stratifying both men and women. In a study of 3,322 men and 2,476 women who were prospectively followed for 3.2 years, exercise induced wall motion abnormality on exercise echocardiogram was independently associated with increased risk of cardiac events (defined as nonfatal myocardial infarction and cardiac death) with a relative risk in women 1.49 (95% CI 1.14-1.94, p 0.003) and a relative risk in men 1.53 (95% CI 1.32-1.77, p = 0.0001) [77]. These results were confirmed in a long-term prospective study in 4,234 women and 6,898 men. In both exercising patients and patients who underwent dobutamine stress echocardiography, extent of ischemia was an independent predictor of time to cardiac death, with a relative risk of 1.45 (95% CI 1.20-1.74, $p < 0.0001$) in exercising patients and a relative risk of 1.27 per vascular territory in patients undergoing dobutamine stress (95% CI 1.07-1.52, p = 0.007).

Based on these studies both exercise and pharmacologic myocardial perfusion imaging and stress echocardiography are valuable tools in women for risk stratification. The choice of imaging modality will need to be based on each individual woman's risk factors and body habitus.

Conclusion

Cardiovascular disease in women is a health problem of epidemic proportions throughout the world. The battle to properly diagnose, treat and prevent CVD in women is just beginning. While the majority of the data we have to guide our diagnostic and treatment decisions are based on trials done primarily in men, there is an emerging database that specifically addresses these important issues in women. In fact, a recent series of articles published in the Journal of American College of Cardiology have focused on the gender differences in the presentation, diagnosis and pathophysiology of CHD [78, 79]. Based on the data available to date several primary and secondary prevention strategies should be implemented in women. Women should be counseled about the importance of diet and exercise in the prevention of CHD. They should be encouraged to maintain a BMI less than 23, a waist to hip ratio of less than 0.72 and a waist circumference of less than 71 cm. In order to achieve these beneficial physical dimensions, women should be encouraged to eat a diet high in cereal fiber, foods with a low glycemic index and high in polyunsaturated fat. The consumption of trans-fatty acids and saturated fats should be avoided. Women of all sizes should be encouraged to walk briskly 3 hours per week or exercise vigorously for 1.5 hours per week. LDL cholesterol and HDL cholesterol, in addition to the index of total cholesterol/HDL and CRP levels should be used to guide statin therapy to optimize primary and secondary risk reduction of CHD in women. Currently, there is no role for postmenopausal hormone replacement, antioxidant vitamins or folate/Vitamin B6 therapy in either the primary or secondary prevention of CHD in women. In addition, aspirin should not be recommended for the primary prevention in low risk women but can be supported in diabetics, high-risk patients or in elderly women. There appears to be a role for fish oil supplementation in both the primary and secondary prevention of CHD in women. As ongoing and future trials in women are completed, novel approaches tailored towards eradicating the epidemic of CHD in women appears likely.

References

[1]   A Race Against Time: The Challenge of Cardiovascular Disease in Developing Economies. Available at: http://www.earthinstitute.columbia.edu/news/2004/images/raceagainsttime_FINAL_410404.pdf. Accessed January 15, 2006.

[2]   *Heart Disease and Stroke Statistics – 2005 Update*. American Heart Association.

[3]   Mosca L, Mochari H, Christian A et al. National Study of Women's Awareness, Preventive Action, and Barriers to Cardiovascular Health. *Circulation*. 2006; 113: 525-534.

[4]   Rich-Edwards JW, Manson JE, Hennekens CH, and Buring JE. The Primary Prevention of Coronary Heart Disease in Women. *N. Eng. J. Med*. 1995; 332(26): 1758-1766.

[5]   Marrugat J, Sala J, Masia R et al. Mortality Differences Between Men and Women Following First Myocardial Infarction. *JAMA*. 1998;280(16):1405-9.

[6]   Daly C, Clemens F, Lopez-Sendon JL et al. Gender Differences in the Management and Clinical Outcome of Stable Angina. *Circulation*. 2006; 113: 490-498.

[7]   Mendelsohn ME and Karas RH. The Protective Effects of Estrogen on the Cardiovascular System. *N. Eng. J. Med*. 1999; 340 (23): 1801-11.

[8]   The Postmenopausal Estrogen/Progesterone Interventions (PEPI) Trial: the Writing Group for the PEPI trial. Effects of Estrogen or Estrogen/Progestin regimens on heart disease risk factors in postmenopausal women. *JAMA*. 1995; 273: 199-208.

[9]   Mosca L, Collin P, Herrington DM et al. Hormone Replacement Therapy and Cardiovascular Disease. A Statement for Healthcare Professionals From the American Heart Association. *Circulation*. 2001; 104: 499-503.

[10]   Cushman M, Legault C, Barrett-Connor E et al. Effect of Postmenopausal Hormones on Inflammation-Sensitive Proteins. The PEPI Study. *Circulation*. 1999; 100: 717-722.

[11]   Ridker PM, Hennekens CH, Rifai N, Buring JE, and Manson JE. Hormone Replacement Therapy and Increased Plasma Concentration of C-Reactive Protein. *Circulation*. 1999; 100: 713-716.

[12]   Low AK, Russell LD, Holman HE et al. Hormone Replacement Therapy and Coronary Heart Disease in Women: A review of the evidence. *Am. J. Med. Sci*. 2002; 324 (4): 180-4.

[13] Hulley S, Grady D, Bush T et al. Randomized Trial of Estrogen Plus Progestin for Secondary Prevention of Coronary Heart Disease in Postmenopausal Women. *JAMA*. 1998; 280: 605-613.

[14] Grady D, Herrington D, Bittner V et al for the HERS Research Group. Cardiovascular Disease Outcomes During 6.8 Years of Hormone Therapy. Heart and Estrogen/Progestin Replacement Study Follow-Up (HERS II). *JAMA*. 2002; 288(1): 49-57.

[15] The ESPRIT Team. Oestrogen therapy for prevention of reinfarction in postmenopausal women: a randomized placebo controlled trial. *Lancet.* 2002; 360: 2001-8.

[16] Clarke SC, Kelleher J, Lloyd-Jones H, Slack M, Schofield PM. A study of hormone replacement therapy in postmenopausal women with ischaemic heart disease: the Papworth HRT Atherosclerosis Study. *BJOG*. 2002; 109: 1056-62.

[17] Manson JE, Hsia J, Johnson KC et al for the Women's Health Initiative Investigators. Estrogen plus Progestin and the Risk of Coronary Heart Disease. *N. Eng. J. Med.* 2003; 349: 523-34.

[18] Writing Group for the Women's Health Initiative Investigators. Risks and Benefits of Estrogen Plus Progestin in Healthy Postmenopausal Women. *JAMA*. 2002; 288(3): 321-333.

[19] The Women's Health Initiative Steering Committee. Effects of Conjugated Equine Estrogen in Postmenopausal Women with Hysterectomy. *JAMA*. 2004; 291(14): 1701-1712.

[20] Miller VM, Clarkson TB, Harman M et al. Women, hormones, and clinical trials: a beginning, not an end. *J. Appl. Physiol.* 2005; 99: 381-383.

[21] Harman SM, Brinton A, Cedars M et al. KEEPS: The Kronos Early Estrogen Prevention Study. *Climacteric.* 2005; 8: 3-12.

[22] Pradhan AD, Skerrett PJ, and Manson JE. Obesity, diabetes, and coronary risk in women. *J. Cardiovasc. Risk.* 2002; 9: 323-330.

[23] Willett WC, Manson JE, Stampfer MJ et al. Weight, Weight Change, and Coronary Heart Disease in Women: Risk Within the 'Normal' Weight Range. *JAMA*. 1995; 273(6): 461-465.

[24] Li TY, Manson JE, Willett WC et al. Obesity as Compared with Physical Activity in Predicting Risk of Coronary Heart Disease in Women. *Circulation.* 2006; 113: 499-506.

[25] Rexrode KM, Carey VJ, Hennekens CH et al. Abdominal Adiposity and Coronary Heart Disease in Women. JAMA. 1998; 280: 1843-1848.

[26] Kip KE, Marroquin OC, Kelley DE et al. Clinical Importance of Obesity versus the Metabolic Syndrome in Cardiovascular Risk in Women. A report from the Women's Ischemia Syndrome Evaluation (WISE) Study. *Circulation.* 2004; 109:706-713.

[27] Hu FB, Stampfer MJ, Manson JE et al. Dietary Fat Intake and the Risk of Coronary Heart Disease in Women. *N. Eng. J. Med.* 1997; 337: 1491-1499.

[28] Liu S, Willett WC, Stampfer MJ et al. A prospective study of dietary glycemic load, carbohydrate intake and risk of coronary heart disease in US women. *Am. J. Clin. Nutr.* 2000; 71: 1455-1461.

[29] Joshipura KJ, Hu FB, Manson JE et al. The Effect of Fruit and Vegetable Intake on Risk for Coronary Heart Disease. *Ann. Intern. Med.* 2001; 134:1106-1114.

[30] Wolk A, Manson JE, Stampfer MJ et al. Long-term Intake of Dietary Fiber and Decreased Risk of Coronary Heart Disease Among Women. *JAMA.* 1999; 281(21): 1998-2004.

[31] Fung TT, Willett WC, Stampfer MJ, Manson JE, Hu FB. Dietary Patterns and the Risk of Coronary Heart Disease in Women. *Arch. Intern. Med.* 2001;161: 1857-1862.

[32] Howard BV, Van Horn L, Hsia J et al. Low-Fat Dietary Pattern and Risk of Cardiovascular Disease. The Women's Health Initiative Randomized Controlled Dietary Modification Trial. *JAMA.* 2006; 295: 655-666.

[33] De Lorgeril M, Salen P, Martin JL et al. Mediterranean Diet, Traditional Risk Factors, and the Rate of Cardiovascular Complications After Myocardial Infarction. *Circulation.* 1999; 99: 779-785.

[34] Manson JE, Hu FB, Rich-Edwards JW et al. A Prospective Study of Walking as Compared with Vigorous Exercise in the Prevention of Coronary Heart Disease in Women. *N. Eng. J. Med.* 1999; 341:650-658.

[35] Hu FB, Stampfer MJ, Solomon C et al. Physical Activity and Risk for Cardiovascular Events in Diabetic Women. *Ann. Intern. Med.* 2001; 134: 96-105.

[36] Manson JE, Greenland P, LaCroix AZ et al. Walking Compared with Vigorous Exercise for the Prevention of Cardiovascular Events in Women. *N. Eng. J. Med.* 2002; 347: 716-725.

[37] Stampfer MJ, Hu FB, Manson JE, Rimm EB, Willett WC. Primary Prevention of Coronary Heart Diase in Women through Diet and Lifestyle. *N. Eng. J. Med.* 2000; 343: 16-22.

[38] Morris CD, Carson S. Routine Vitamin Supplementation to Prevent Cardiovascular Disease: A Summary of the Evidence for the U.S. Preventive Services Task Force. *Ann. Intern. Med.* 2003; 139: 56-70.

[39] Stampfer MJ, Hennekens CH, Manson JE et al. Vitamin E Consumption and the Risk of Coronary Disease in Women. *N. Eng. J. Med.* 1993; 328: 1444-1449.

[40] Kushi LH, Folsom AR, Prineas RJ et al. Dietary Antioxidant Vitamins and Death from Coronary Heart Disease in Postmenopausal Women. *N. Eng. J. Med.* 1996; 334: 1156-1162.

[41] Stephens NG, Schofield PM, Cheeseman K, Mitchinson MJ, Brown, MJ. Randomised controlled trial of vitamin E in patients with coronary disease: Cambridge Heart Antioxidant Study (CHAOS). *Lancet.* 1996; 347: 781-786.

[42] GISSI-Prevenzione Investigators. Dietary supplementation with n-3 polyunsaturated fatty acids and vitamin E after myocardial infarction: results of the GISSI-Prevenzione trial. *Lancet.* 1999; 354: 447-455.

[43] Heart Protection Study Collaborative Group. MRC/BHF Heart Protection Study of antioxidant vitamin supplementation in 20,536 high-risk individuals: a randomized placebo-controlled trial. *Lancet.* 2002; 360: 23-33.

[44] Waters DD, Alderman EL, Hsia J et al. Effects of Hormone Replacement Therapy and Antioxidant Vitamin Supplements on Coronary Atherosclerosis in Postemenopausal Women. A randomized controlled trial. *JAMA.* 2002; 288: 2432-2440.

[45] The Heart Outcomes Prevention Evaluation Study Investigators. Vitamin E Supplementation and Cardiovascular Events in High Risk Patients. *N. Eng. J. Med.* 2000; 342:154-60.

[46] The HOPE and HOPE-TOO Trial Investigators. Effects of Long-term Vitamin E Supplementation on Cardiovascular Events and Cancer. JAMA. 2005; 293:1338-1347.

[47] Collaborative Group of the Primary Prevention Project. Low-dose aspirin and vitamin E in people at cardiovascular risk: a randomized trial in general practice. *Lancet.* 2001; 357:89-95.

[48] Lee IM, Cook NR, Gaziano JM et al. Vitamin E in the Primary Prevention of Cardiovascular Disease and Cancer. The Women's Health Study: A Randomized Controlled Trial. *JAMA.* 2005; 294: 56-65.

[49] Eidelman RS, Hollar D, Hebert PR, Lamas GA, Hennekens CH. Randomized Trials of Vitamin E in the Treatment and Prevention of Cardiovascular Disease. *Arch. Intern. Med.* 2004; 164: 1552-1556.

[50] Alfthan G, Aro A, Gey KF. Plasma homocysteine and cardiovascular disease mortality. Lancet. 1997; 349: 397.

[51] Rimm EB, Willett WC, Hu FB et al. Folate and Vitamin B6 from Diet and Supplements in Relation to Risk of Coronary Heart Disease Among Women. *JAMA.* 1998; 279: 359-364.

[52] NORVIT study group. Randomised trial of homocysteine-lowering with B vitamins for secondary prevention of cardiovascular disease after acute myocardial infarction. *The Norwegian Vitamin Study* (NORVIT). European Society of Cardiology Meeting. 2005.

[53] Kris-Etherton PM, Harris WS, Appel LJ. Fish Consumption, Fish Oil, Omega-3Fatty Acids and Cardiovascular Disease. *Circulation.* 2002; 106: 2747-2757.

[54] Hu FB, Bronner L, Willett WC et al. Fish and Omega-3 Fatty Acid Intake and Risk of Coronary Heart Disease in Women. *JAMA.* 2002; 287: 1815-1821.

[55] Yokoyama M, Origasa H. Effects of eicosapentaenoic acid on cardiovascular events in Japanese patients with hypercholesterolemia: rationale, design, and baseline characteristics of the Japan EPA Lipid Intervention Study (JELIS). *Am. Heart J.* 2003; 146: 613-620.

[56] Erkkila AT, Lichtenstein AH, Mozaffarian D, Herrington DM. Fish intake is associated with a reduced progression of coronary artery atherosclerosis in postmenopausal women with coronary artery disease. *Am. J. Clin. Nutr.* 2004; 80: 626-632.

[57] Schmidt EB, Arnesen H, Christensen JH et al. Marine n-3 polyunsaturated fatty acids and coronary heart disease. Part II: clinical trials and recommendations. *Thrombosis Research.* 2005; 115: 257-262.

[58] Kjeldsen SE, Kolloch RE, Leonetti G et al. Influence of gender and age on preventing cardiovascular disease by antihypertensive treatment and acetylsalicylic acid. The HOT study. *J. of Hypertension.* 2000; 18: 629-642.

[59] Ridker PM, Cook NR, Lee IM et al. A Randomized Trial of Low-Dose Aspirin in the Primary Prevention of Cardiovascular Disease in Women. *N. Eng. J. Med.* 2005; 352: 1293-1304.

[60] Shai I, Rimm EB, Hankinson SE et al. Multivariate Assessment of Lipid Parameters as Predictors of Coronary Heart Disease among Postmenopausal Women: Potential Implications for Clinical Guidelines. *Circulation.* 2004; 110: 2824-2830.

[61] Miettinen TA, Pyorala K, Olsson AG et al. Cholesterol Lowering Therapy in Women and Elderly Patients with Myocardial Infarction or Angina Pectoris. *Circulation.* 1997; 96: 4211-4218.

[62] Lewis SJ, Sacks FM, Mitchell JS et al. Effect of Pravastatin on Cardiovascular Evetns in Women After Myocardial Infarction: The Cholesterol and Recurrent Events (CARE) Trial. *J. Am. Coll. Cardiol.* 1998; 32: 140-146.

[63] Ridker PM, Cannon CP, Morrow D et al. C-Reactive Protein Levels and Outcomes after Statin Therapy. *N. Eng. J. Med.* 2005; 352: 20-28.

[64] Wong ND, Pio J, Valencia R, Thakal G. Distribution of C-reactive protein and its relation to risk factors and coronary heart diease risk estimation in the National Health and Nutrition Survey (NHANES) III. *Prev. Cardiol.* 2001; 4: 109-114.

[65] Albert MA, Glynn RJ, Buring J, Ridker PM. C-reactive protein levels among women of carious ethnic groups living in the United States (from the Women's Health Study). *Am. J. Cardiol.* 2004; 93: 1238-1242.

[66] Ridker PM, Hennekens CH, Buring JE, Rifal N. C-Reactive Protein and Other Markers of Inflammation in the Prediction of Cardiovascular Disease in Women. *N. Eng. J. Med.* 2000; 342:836-843.

[67] Ridker PM, Rifal N, Rose L, Buring JE, Cook NR. Comparison of C-Reactive Protein and Low-Density Lipoprotein Cholesterol Levels in the Prediction of First Cardiovascular Events. *N. Eng. J. Med.* 2002; 347:1557-1565.

[68] Ridker PM on behalf of the JUPITER study group. Rosuvastatin in the Primary Prevention of Cardiovascular Disease Among Patients with Low Levels of Low-Density Lipoprotein Cholesterol and Elevated High-Sensitivity C-Reactive Protein: Rationale and Design of the JUPITER trial. *Circulation.* 2003; 108: 2292-2297.

[69] Bigi R, Cortigiani L. Stress testing in women: sexual discrimination or equal opportunity? *European Heart Journal.* 2005; 26:423-425.

[70] Kwok Y, Kim C, Grady D, Segal M, Redberg R. Meta-Analysis of Exercise Testing to Detect Coronary Artery Disease in Women. *Am. J. Cardiol.* 1999;83: 660-666.

[71] Bokhari S, Bergmann SR. The Effect of Estrogen Compared to Estrogen Plus Progesterone on the Exercise Electrocardiogram. *J. Am. Coll. Cardiol.* 2002; 40: 1092-1096.

[72] Taillefer R, DePuey G, Udelson JE et al. Comparative Diagnostic Accuracy of Tl-201 and Tc-99m Sestamibi SPECT Imaging (perfusion and ECG-Gated SPECT) in Detecting Coronary Artery Disease in Women. *J. Am. Coll. Cardiol.* 1997; 29:69-77.

[73] Marwick TH, Anderson T, Williams MJ et al. Exercise Echocardiography Is an Accurate and Cost-Efficient Technique for the Detection of Coronary Artery Disease in Women. *J. Am. Coll. Cardiol.* 1995; 26: 335-341.

[74] Budoff MJ, Shokooh S, Shavelle RM, Kim T, French WJ. Electron beam tomography and angiography: sec differences. *Am. Heart J.* 2002; 143: 877-882.

[75] Hachamovitch R, Berman DS, Kiat H et al. Effective Risk Stratification Using Exercise Myocardial Perfusion SPECT in Women: Gender-Related Differences in Prognostic Nuclear Testing. *J. Am. Coll. Cardiol.* 1996; 28:34-44.

[76] Berman DS, Kang X, Hayes SW et al. Adenosine Myocardial Perfusion Single-Photon Emission Computed Tomography in Women Compared with Men. Impact of Diabetes Mellitus on Incremental Prognostic Value and Effect on Patient Management. *J. Am. Coll Cardiol.* 2003: 41: 1125-1133.

[77] Arruda-Olsen AM, Juracan EM, Mahoney DW et al. Prognostic Value of Exercise Echocardiography in 5,798 Patients: Is there a gender difference? *J. Am. Coll. Cardiol.* 2002; 39:625-631.

[78] Shaw LJ, Merz NB, Pepine CJ et al. Insights from the NHLBI-Sponsored Women's Ischemia Syndrome Evaluation (WISE) Study. Part I: Gender Differences in Traditional and Novel Risk Factors, Symptom Evaluation, and Gender-Optimized Diagnostic Strategies. *J. Am. Coll. Cardiol.* 2006; 47: 4S-20S.

[79] Merz NB, Shaw LJ, Reis SE et al. Insights from the NHLBI-Sponsored Women's Ischemia Syndrome Evaluation (WISE) Study. Part II: Gender Differences in Presentation, Diagnosis, and Outcome with regard to Gender-Based Pathophysiology of Atherosclerosis and Macrovascular and Microvascular Coronary Disease. *J. Am. Coll. Cardiol.* 2006; 47: 21S-29S.

In: Handbook of Cardiovascular Research
Editors: Jorgen Brataas and Viggo Nanstveit

ISBN 978-1-60741-792-7
© 2009 Nova Science Publishers, Inc.

Chapter III

Passive Smoking Exposure and Cardiovascular Health[*]

Aurelio Leone[†]

Cardio-thoracic Department University of Pisa, Italy
Former Director Department of Internal Medicine
City Hospital Massa and Carrara, Italy

Abstract

Nowadays, there is no doubt that exposure to passive smoking, whatever it may be approached to be studied – and there are a lot of study approaches: clinical, biological, metabolic, epidemiologic, statistic and so on, that recognize different pathogenetic mechanisms of damage- leads to only one final result that is a reversibly functional harm of the heart and blood vessels following acute exposure, and pathologic alterations that become, in the long run, irreversible lesions of the above target organs after chronic exposure. Therefore, the American Heart Association has included passive smoking among the major risk factors for heart disease in both adults and children. However, our findings are able to demonstrate that cardiovascular damage from passive smoking could be considered more than a major risk factor for cardiovascular events, but particularly an etiologic factor of cardiovascular pathology.

The harm of the heart and blood vessels from passive smoking is the result of either an isolated action or combined action of some toxics contaminant indoor air by tobacco – and there are over 4,000 chemicals identified in cigarette smoking-. The majority of these have carcinogenic and/or negative cardiovascular effects in humans and animals. To

---

[*] A version of this chapter was also published in *Passive Smoking and Health Research,* edited by Nivek A. Jeorgensen published by Nova Science Publishers, Inc. It was submitted for appropriate modifications in an effort to encourage wider dissemination of research.

[†] Address for mail: Dr. Aurelio Leone; Via Provinciale 27; 19030 Castelnuovo Magra (SP); Italy ; Phone: +390187676346 ; FAX: +390187676346; e-mail: reliol@libero.it.

what it concerns cardiovascular system, they may be classified into three groups: nicotine and its metabolites, carbon monoxide, and thiocyanates.

The degree of cardiovascular damage caused by passive smoking exposure depends by three factors- type of smoking, environment, and study subject - as well as by numerous variables which may be related to them. Exponential number of possibly numerous variables related to smoking, environment, and individuals permits to build a mathematical equation that quantify the level of damage as well as its exact reproducibility, as observed for a subject in one of our studies.

Either there is a functional damage particularly due to acute exposure or a pathologic damage which characterizes chronic exposure, the result of exposure to passive smoking varies widely in healthy individuals and in those individuals suffering from heart disease, especially ischemic heart disease.

The response to the harm can be of clinical type – signs of cardiac and/or blood vessel ischemic pathology which may be accompanied by arrhythmias and heart failure-, metabolic type – signs of altered oxygen transport and pro-thrombotic changes in coagulation-fibrinolysis cascade- and sympathetic type with changes in heart rate and blood pressure. Moreover, some special categories like women are influenced by their endocrine constellation. There is a different response in premenopausal women exposed to passive smoking who have an atherogenic response and in women after menopause who have an atherosclerotic response similar to that observed in men.

Genetic factors have also been demonstrate to influence cardiovascular response due to passive smoking with an increasing rate primarily for what involves the oxidative stress.

From these data, there is no doubt that passive smoking exposure demonstrates to be characterized by a major incidence of possible cardiovascular events acting, in this case, as a risk factor. However, exposure may be considered an etiologic factor of cardiovascular alterations since it leads, in the long run, to a damage of the heart and blood vessels also when intercurrent cardiovascular events can be lacking .

Keywords: Passive Smoking, Heart, Blood vessels, special population

Introduction

Nowadays, there is no doubt that exposure to passive smoking, whatever it may be the approach to be studied – and there are a lot of study approaches: clinical, biological, metabolic, epidemiologic, statistic, and other which recognize different pathogenetic mechanisms of damage – leads to only one result which is a reversibly functional harm of the heart and blood vessels following acute exposure, and pathologic alterations that become, in the long run, irreversible lesions of the above target organs after chronic exposure [1–7]. Therefore, the American Heart Association has included passive smoking among the major risk factors for heart disease in both adults and children [6].

No country is free from this problem, which plagues developing and developed countries alike, although with different results due to different lifestyles and diffusion of antismoking campaigns. Passive smoking influences negatively the health of both adults and children particularly following chronic exposure.

Chemically, environmental tobacco smoke is probably the main pollutant of indoor air acting in different places: workplaces, public buildings in some countries, business offices, and home. The chemical mixture of passive smoking consists of three main components: the constituents of that phase defined as sidestream smoke, that defined as mainstream smoke and, finally, that defined as vaporphase. Sidestream smoke contains greater concentration of many smoke constituents since it is unfiltered by the cigarette filter due to the fact that they do not pass into. Nicotine in the gaseous phase, and therefore easily spreading, and carbon monoxide are particularly present in sidestream phase. The mainstream smoke contains prevailingly nicotine in a particulate phase. Mainstream smoke is inhaled and exhaled particularly by the smokers making stronger the action of active smoking on themselves. Finally, vaporphase is constituted by those cigarette components in different mixture concentrations – nicotine, carbon monoxide, thiocyanates- that diffuse through cigarette paper into the environment [7].

Exposure to passive smoking is currently defined either as an exposure to sidestream smoke from burning cigarettes or as an exposure to mainstream smoke. Both sidestream smoke and mainstream smoke contain those toxic substances - in a large number – which lead to cardiovascular damage due to the fact that the pollutants stagnate in the environment even after the consumption of smoked cigarettes, and spread out surrounding environment by their gaseous phase . Usually, the particles of sidestream smoke are smaller than those of mainstream smoke so that they can be inhaled more deeply into the lungs [8]. From this way, harmful components of passive smoking reach blood flow and target organs.

The harm of the heart and blood vessels from passive smoking is the result of either an isolated action or combined action of particularly some active pollutants derived from burned tobacco. Burned tobacco contains over 4,000 chemicals [9]. The majority of these pollutants has carcinogenic and/or negative effects on the heart and blood vessels in humans and animals. Briefly, those pollutants which involve cardiovascular system can be classified into three groups as listed in Table 2.

Passive smoking damages cardiovascular system by biochemical pollutants which act as a major risk factor. However, in my opinion, passive smoking is particularly an etiologic factor of cardiovascular disease since cardiovascular patholgy is absolutely the final way of the exposure. The purpose of the article is to demonstrate this statement without any doubt as well as to describe the type of those alterations which, usually, affect cardiovascular system following exposure to passive smoke.

Table 1.Passive smoking pollutants and their phases

Phases	Pollutants	Damage
1. Sidestream Smoke	Gaseous nicotine Carbon monoxide	Smokers (increase active smoking damage), and people living with him.
2. Mainstream Smoke	Carbon monoxide Nicotine in particles	Environment and its residents
3. Vapor Phase	Carbon monoxide Nicotine (Gaseous and Particulate) Thiocyanates	Environment and its residents

Table 2. Potential chemical markers mainly derived from burned tobacco

1. Nicotine and its metabolites
2. Carbon monoxide
3. Thiocyanates

Table 3. Classification of risk factors derived from a statistical analysis

1. Risk factors strongly related to increased incidence of disease:	
a) their removal:	real decrease in incidence of the disease
b) unable to be removed:	no decrease in incidence of the disease (further study needing to change this pattern)
2. Risk factors probably related to increased incidence of disease:	
a) their removal:	possible decrease in incidence of the disease (further study needing to clarify this pattern)
b) unable to be removed:	no decrease in incidence of the disease (no further study)

What is a Risk Factor and what is an Etiologic Factor?

Two most important factors allow to interpret the probable incidence of occurence for every disease. They are known respectively as 1. Risk factor , that is today carefully considered to assess the incidence of a disease and then set up preventive measures, and 2. Etiologic factor which is the cause of a disease, the occurence of which is the result of its strength and potential charge.

The concept that some abnormal symptoms or diseases recognize a causal factor is as ancient as medical history [10]. In more modern terms, there are two major classes of etiologic factors: genetic and acquired factors. They relate strongly to the disease that are able to "cause". However, the occurence of specific abnormal symptoms derives from the power inherent these causal factors.

It is superfluous to underline that the level, power, and duration of the etiologic factors determine different patterns of illness severity.

On the contrary, the concept of risk factor completely differs from that of etiologic factor. A risk factor (Table 3) provides the global burden of disease by the analysis of a lot of events which involve socioeconomic states, geographic characteristics, lifestyle, age and gender of the studied piopulation. The examined data are deriving from epidemiologic studies, and there is no link cause-effect between a risk factor and occurence of disease that, on the contrary, has strongest links with own etiologic factor. Therefore, a risk factor relates with statistical methodologies, while an etiologic factor with biolgical and pathological patterns.

Analysis of risk factors for passive smoking has been able to establish that the risk of death from cardiovascular disease rise by up to 30 percent among those people who are chronically exposed to environmental tobacco smoke at home or work [11]. It is also estimated that about 35,000 non smokers die from cardiovascular events each year as a result of passive smoking [12].

Therefore, it is important to know how a risk factor acts on a particular disease in a large series of studies as well as in a largest number of subjects with different origin and lifestyle. It is necessary to assess the possibility of its removal for reducing the incidence- but not causing the diseappearance of a disease as well as intercurrent related events, making any effort to obtain that.

Therefore, exposure to passive smoking shoud be avoided if this factor is believed to be a risk factor, but absolutely forbidden if a leading role as a causal factor of cardiovascular damage can be demonstrated.

Coronary Heart Disease (CHD) and Passive Smoking: Epidemiologic Studies

The link between environmental tobacco smoke and CHD is difficult to interpret. Several reports have been published on the relationship that relates passive smoking to the appearance of major non-fatal or fatal cardiovascular events [12-31]. The majority of these studies concerns fatal coronary events in non-smoking women exposed at home to chronic smoke from their husbands' cigarettes as well as events in people at work. Statistical significance is differently analyzed in these studies which, however, lead to the conclusion of an important cardiovascular damage from environmental tobacco smoke, although showing various facets.

Three studies [13, 18, 20] demonstrated a strong relationship between passive smoking and CHD that was statistically significant at a P level less than 0.05, whereas others [32] at a P level less than 0.01, statistically different values but, in any case, all considered of relevant significance. The last study interested only women married to men who were smoking at least 20 cigarettes per day. Moreover, an excellent study performed on subjects undergone exposure to passive smoking reported a 71 percent increase in risk of CHD (P less than 0.05) among women exposed to environmental tobacco smoke.

Layard and LeVois [30, 34] conducted two studies that demonstrated no clear relationship between women exposed to passive smoking and CHD, whereas different conclusions reached Steenland et al. [21] using a statistically different method by the analysis of a different type of chronic exposure and study of subgroups. LeVois and Layard defined exposure that of a marriage to someone who was a past or current smoker, whereas Steenland et al. separeted out current smokers from past smokers.

Furthermore, there was a subgroup analysis including only those subjects who gave their responses on the smoking status of the spouse in agreement with self-report from that spouse. In this analysis, never-smoking males married to women who were smokers at the entry into the study had a relative risk of fatal CHD with a P less than 0.05, and never-smoking women married to smoker men showed the same statistically significant difference (P less than 0.05).

Also in the workplaces different observations were seen. Some reports [25] did not find relationship between exposure to passive smoking and CHD in workplaces, whereas others [19] found a demonstrable increase of CHD after exposure to passive smoking particularly in women who were not exposed at home. These reports, however, permit to underline that differences in indoor spaces, which may depend by their characteristics and types of exposure, may often lead to not unanimous observations. An accurate analysis of 12 epidemiological studies was conducted by Wells [4].He analysed heart disease mortality as an end-point for men and women separately since cardiovascular risk is different for the two sexes and, therefore, the effects of passive smoking could differ. The breakdown and reorganizing the above studies according to different statistical methods allowed to conclude that the risk of an increase in CHD was high when studied population underwent chronic exposure to passive smoking. Other studies which examined non fatal cardiovascular events [18, 22, 25–26, 28] could reach the conclusion that an elevation in risk for cardiovascular events was certainly demonstrable.

All these observations would seem to indicate that case-control and cross-sectional studies do not provide unanimous findings on the relationship between passive smoking and CHD. There are disagreements about the specific events that characterize home and workplace exposure. From the examined studies it seems that home exposure to environmental tobacco smoke is associated with an increased risk of CHD rather than workplace exposure. That could be probably due to the longer time that smoker individuals spend at home with much more exposure of home livings to smoke.

However, it is to be observed that the different case-control studies, cross-sectional studies, and meta-analysis studies conducted on the relationship between passive smoking and CHD are inconsistent with the fact that they measure obtained results with different statistical methods and different population lifestyle. In presence of a reproducible mathematical model the findings could reach different conclusions.

Finally, progression of coronary artery stenoses, acute myocardial infarction, angina, ventricular arrhythmias, and other malignant electrocardiographic changes [28, 34–35] (Table 4) are heart alterations that can follow passive smoking exposure.

In conclusion, the fact that the risk to increase CHD or cardiovascular intercurrent events has been documented by studies conducted in different countries with different socioeconomic characteristics and lifestyle – and therefore it does not relate itself to these factors – as well as the high magnitude of the degree of risk shown permits the statement that passive smoking causes heart disease [6].

**Table 4. Ischemic heart alterations due to passive smoking
as described from epidemiologic studies**

Myocardial Infarction
Angina
Ventricular Arrhythmias
Atrial fibrillation
Malignant Electrocardiographic Changes
Coronary Atherosclerosis

Impairment of pre-existing Heart Failure

Effects of Passive Smoking on the Arterial Wall

Cigarette smoking has been shown to be one of the major predictors of atherosclerotic plaque progression [36]. Such a progression has also been well documented after chronic exposure to environmental tobacco smoke.

In one of the largest study [37], carotid artery intimal-medial thickness (IMT) was followed over a three-year period in black and white men and women, aged from 45 to 65 years, enrolled for the Atherosclerosis Risk in Communities Study (ARIC) by using B-mode vascular ultrasonography to measure carotid wall thickness. Increase in artery wall thickness was deemed to be the result of atherosclerotic plaque progression. There were 10,914 enrolled participants, being 4,298 of these (39%) exposed to environmental tobacco smoke. Some had been past smokers, others had never smoked. Compared to non-smokers never exposed to passive smoking, cigarette smokers had about a 50 percent increase in IMT, while the same parameter increased only 20 per cent for those exposed to environmental tobacco smoke. There was a gradient in IMT from never smokers not exposed to passive smoking, never smokers exposed, past smokers and current smokers. Among non-smoking men exposed to environmental tobacco smoke, there was a significant IMT increase that was proportional to the hours per week of exposure. Some categories – diabetics and hypertensive subjects - were showing a greater impact from both active and passive smoke.

A critical question that arises from this study is whether IMT measurement by ultrasonography is a surrogate marker to establish the progression of atherosclerosis [38]. Whatever the limit in IMT measurements is, it is undeniable that methodologic procedures were applied to all studied subjects and, therefore, differences in IMT existed among subjects with different habits of exposure to different types of smoking.

Moreover, there are other studies [39–40] that correlate IMT measurement with the prevalence of atherosclerosis in other arteries. In over 1,000 men Salonen and Salonen observed that each millimeter increase in carotid artery IMT increased the risk of intercurrently acute coronary events 2.14-fold. Also Bots et al. reached similar results. Each 0.16 millimeter in IMT carotid increase caused a rose in risk of myocardial infarction of about 43 percent. Therefore, one can deduce that changes in IMT induced by environmental tobacco smoke exposure can be evidence of artery atherosclerosis progression, including atherosclerosis of coronary arteries.

Table 5. Main pathologic mechanisms due to passive smoking action that cause arterial wall damage

Endothelial dysfunction
Platelet activation and adhesiveness
Thrombi formation
Coagulation-fibrinolysis cascade
Atherogenic lipid components

Free radicals

The mechanism by which passive smoking induces arterial wall changes is not yet completely demonstrated, although a lot of studies [41–50] would seem to involve endothelium, platelets, coagulation-fibrinolysis cascade, and adrenergic stimulation. Not only studies on chronic exposure to passive smoking, but also experimental studies of healthy and diseased subjects undergone acute exposure help to clarify the mechanisms of arterial wall damage (Table 5).

Endothelium changes due to environmental tobacco smoke have to be briefly discussed.

During recent years, it has been well seen that vascular endothelium has a pivotal role in maintain vascular tone [51]. Findings lead to establish that endothelial dysfunction is an early marker of impending atherosclerosis. Papers [42, 47–50] indicate clearly that there is a strong relationship between environmental tobacco exposure and endothelial dysfunction with impaired endothelium-dependent vasodilation in healthy people. A normal response in endothelium-dependent vasodilation is a good marker of endothelium integrity that is related to release of endothelium-derived nitric oxide. This chemical plays an important role in maintaining endothelium homeostasis. Nitric oxide release is impaired by atherosclerotic progression, smoking and, probably, other major coronary risk factors [7, 52–53]. Endothelial dysfunction with impaired endothelium- dependent vasodilation due to passive smoking exposure of healthy volunteers was very recently found by Giannini et al. [54].

Also changes in platelet function and characteristics play a strong role in activating those complex mechanisms that are involved in arterial wall damage by passive smoking.

Passive smoking activates platelets, which increase the likelihhod of thrombi formation to which coagulation-fibrinolysis system changes actively contribute. The final step of this combined action is a progression of atherosclerosis [50, 55–57] with arterial lumen reduction for increase in size of the atherosclerotic plaque which is, also, a consequence, of the action of other factors particularly atherogenic lipids and some free radicals that passive smoking releases into the environment.

Detrimental effects of environmental tobacco smoke on arterial wall have been attributed to toxic chemicals in burned tobacco. Endothelial dysfunction may be a consequence of carbon monoxide in sidestream smoke, benzopyrene and gaseous nicotine [58]. Such chemicals, however, may act also directly on the structure of the arterial wall together with some coagulation factors. So doing, a strong interaction of different pathogenetic mechanisms activates and maintains arterial damage.

Previous findings would seem to suggest that smoke-related endothelial dysfunction is potentially reversible after withdrawal from active or passive smoking [59–60].These studies reinforce the importance to avoid passive smoking exposure in an attempt to reduce the burden of arterial wall damage, the progression of which leads to appearance of lesions at a different stage, fresh lesions superimposed to old alterations of the atherosclerotic plaque until the plaque undergoes rupture with possibly severe complications particularly of ischemic type for the heart and brain.

Clinical and Experimental Studies.
Types of Damage from Passive Smoking

A large series of clinical and experimental studies conducted in both humans and animals after exposure to environmental tobacco smoke permits to define the type of damage (Table 6) that may affect cardiovascular system.

Observations about passive smoking as a factor, which causes cardiovascular damage, have appeared in the last thirty years. Indoor atmosphere and confined spaces often are polluted by tobacco smoke which is inhaled involuntarily by both smokers and nonsmokers. The smokers increase, although slightly, the damage caused by their active smoking, whereas the nonsmokers are damaged heavily against their will.

Experimental and clinical studies conducted on humans and animals following acute or chronic exposure to environmental tobacco smoke allow to confirm the harmful effects on the heart and blood vessels.

Acute exposure to passive smoking (from 20 minutes to 8 hours) can result in a decrease in platelet sensitivity to prostacyclin, leading to increased occurence of thrombosis, a strong effect of carboxyhemoglobin on blood oxygen transport, which induce significant myocardial and endothelial damage [61].

Table 6. Effects of passive smoking exposure and type of cardiovascular damage

Acute exposure	
1. Impaired cardiac performance (transient)	-healthy subjects: functional damage (diminished exercise tolerance)
	-ischemic subjects:functional damage (diminished exercise tolerance, ventricular arrhythmias)
2. Endothelial dysfunction (transient)	-healthy subjects: functional damage (impaired endothelium-dependent vasodilation)
	-ischemic subjects: functional damage (impaired endothelium-dependent vasodilation) anatomical damage (impaired endothelium-independent vasodilation)
Chronic exposure	
1. Myocardial infarction:	clinical damage
	anatomical damage
2. Atherosclerosis progression:	anatomical damage
3. Heart failure progression:	clinical damage
4. Arrhythmias:	functional damage
	clinical damage
5. Hypertension:	clinical damage
	anatomical damage

Also cardiac performance with diminished exercise tolerance [1] during acute exposure to environmental tobacco smoke was impaired in both healthy individuals and individuals suffering from a pre-existing myocardial infarction, although with different responses. Healthy individuals showed prolonged time to recovery pre-exercise heart rate, whereas survivors of an acute myocardial infarction had prolonged time to recovery pre-exercise heart rate but also a significant reduction of peak exercise power and ventricular arrhythmias. Higher post-exercise concentration of plasma-carbon monoxide and markedly lower expired-carbon monoxide concentration characterized post-myocardial infarction patients . Then survivors of infarction, who, usually, have hemodynamic impairment [62], must absolutely avoid indoor spaces polluted by cigarette smoke.

Endothelium-dependent coronary artery dilation is impaired in passive smoker women [47]. That should prove that the well characterized endothelial dysfunction in active smokers may occur in passive smokers as well.

Another acute effect of passive smoking on heart function is mediated by a complex set of events due to carbon monoxide inhalation. Indoor polluted by carbon monoxide from passive smoking has a level of this gas usually ranging from 3 ppm (part per million air) to 25 ppm , and exposure to 10 ppm over 8 hours results in 1.4% of the blood hemoglobin occupied as carboxyhemoglobin [29]. Carbon monoxide diminishes the transport of blood oxygen , increases heart rate to maintain an adequate oxygen supply, can cause lifethreating arrhythmias, and worsens the degree of myocardial ischemia [34, 63]. Otsuka and coworkers [48] examined the acute effects of exposure to passive smoking on coronary circulation using coronary flow velocity reserve as a measure of endothelial function in the coronary circulation, studing 30 Japanese men. Coronary flow velocity reserve was significantly higher in nonsmokers at baseline than in active smokers. However, 30 minute passive smoke exposed men, caused coronary endothelal dysfunction. Endothelial dysfunction assessed by ultrasonography was described in other systemic arteries in different studies [42, 47, 49 – 50, 54].

Chronic exposure to environmental tobacco smoke include a large series of studies [64 – 76] that prove undoubtedly negative effects on cardiovascular system, particularly due to the levels of carboxyhemoglobin. The great majority of patients examined in these studies showed important impairment of those symptoms which characterized their disease, particularly chest pain from angina pectoris and pre-existing myocardial infarction. Such an impairment well correlated to carboxyhemoglobin levels as well as artery endothelial dysfunction that is recognized to initiate the development of an atherosclerotic plaque. A dose-response relationship was found to exist between the degree of passive smoking exposure and amount of endothelial dysfunction. HDL-cholesterol levels in children exposed to passive smoke from their parents were lower than those of children who did not undergo passive smoking exposure. Similar results were found in adults regularly exposed to environmental tobacco smoke in the workplaces [77].

Finally, passive smoking increases blood viscosity and hematocrit because of the relative hypoxia induced by chronic carbon monoxide exposure [78]. Also some factors of coagulation fibrinolysis cascade, particularly fibringen, increase their blood concentration [79–83] activating the via-thrombus formation.

Also other experimental studies conducted on animals exposed to environmental tobacco smoke showed an increased cardiovascular damage. Infarct size of rats undergone to a 35-minute occlusion of the left coronary artery increased in a dose-dependent manner after passive smoking exposure without threshold effect [84].

A lot of biochemical, metabolic, and structural alterations from passive smoking have been described [85–87], some of these well documented and some to be yet under control.

Prolonged exposure of animals to carbon monoxide has been shown to induce ultrastructural changes in myocardium with mitochondria damage, focal areas of myocardial necrosis at a different stage, interstitial fibrosis, perivascular infiltrates and punctate hemorrhage. Autophagocytosis and pigmented deposits were also described.

Experimental pathological alterations due to environmental tobacco smoke are summarized in Table 7. All these alterations impair heavily cellular function being, in the long run, the base to develop an irreversible damage.

Assessing the type of cardiovascular damage from passive smoking has been wrongly overlooked in many findings. On the contrary, we believe that its recording and understanding allow to deduce significant data on those pathologic mechanisms that cause cardiovascular damage.

Four types of cardiovascular damage are a consequence of acute or chronic exposure to passive smoking: a functional damage, that, usually, involves acute exposure; a clinical damage that is often observed following chronic exposure or acute exposure of subjects chronically exposed; an anatomical damage that is typical of the chronic exposure; and a different combination among the above damages.

Functional damage , usually following acute exposures, is transient and recognizes autonomic system involvement as a main pathogenetic factor [88–91]. Some parameters rather than others are interested negatively by functional damage: heart rate, systolic blood pressure, exercise tolerance, cardiac rhythm with possible development of ventricular arrhythmias. Also the increased levels of catecholamines share to maintain the damage. Functional damage is especially harmful for those subjects suffering from ischemic heart disease as well as for those who undergo chronic exposure, being autonomic system and catecholamines factors, in themselves, able to have spontaneously detrimental effects on heart and blood vessels.

Table 7. Pathologic and ultrastructural alterations of myocardium due to chronic passive smoking exposure – Experimental observations in animals

1. Changes in mitochondria function (respiratory change imbalance; cristae amputation)
2. Focal areas of myocardial cells necrosis at a different stage
3. Perivascular infiltrates (intramural myocardial vessels)
4. Punctate hemorrhage (into myocardial cells)
5. Interstitial fibrosis
6. Myocardial fiber swelling
7. Lysosomal autophagocytosis
8. Myocardial cardiomyopathy

Clinical damage affects particularly those individuals undergone chronic exposure. Symptoms of myocardial ischemia, particularly angina pectoris, myocardial infarction and arrhythmias, may be worsened by this type of damage. It is often associated with an anatomical damage that may act as an underlying disease. Also the association with a transiently functional damage, that may appear after acute environmental tobacco smoke exposure of subjects chronically exposed, worsens clinical damage of those individuals with symptoms related to coronary and cerebrovascular disease.

Finally, anatomical damage is the final and unavoidable result of chronic exposure to passive smoking. Its development is usually late but progressive untill to reach the characteristic of irreversibily.

Stable alterations that accompany anatomical damage involve more often coronary arteries, systemic arteries causing hypertension and cerebrovascular disease, and myocardium. In several cases alterations support the presence of clinical symptoms, the impairment of which, may be an useful, even if indirect, sign to follow-up further worsening and progression of anatomical damage.

Experimental studies previously examined in the present article would demonstrate undoubtedly that carbon monoxide plays a strong role in causing, maintaining, and worsening anatomical damage.

Carboxyhemoglobin concentration over 1.41% seems to be level that determines impairment of individual homeostasis as shown in figure 1.

Factor that supports anatomical damage is a progression of atherosclerotic alterations with, initially, endothelial dysfunction, an early key following acute environmental tobacco smoke exposure, platelet aggregation and fibrinogen changes. As one can see, there are all those factors that are involved in the pathogenesis of cardiovascular damage due to passive smoking, and anatomical damage is the final and heaviest result of their harmful action.

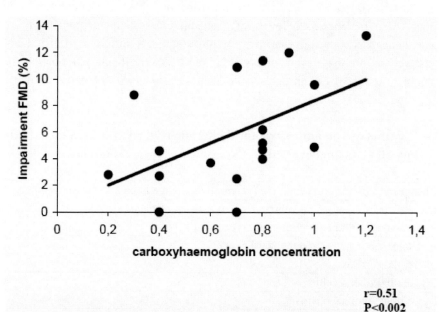

r=0.51
P<0.002

Figure 1.

One must assume that the development of an anatomical damage is a constant result of chronic passive smoking exposure, leading to consider environmental tobacco smoke more than a simple cardiovascular risk factor.

Biochemical Markers of Cardiovascular Damage from Passive Smoking

Adverse effects on the heart and blood vessels are mediated through the action of the many chemical components that are usually concentrated and condensed into burned tobacco mixture.

Cardiovascular effects of biochemical markers of tobacco smoke are difficult to distinguish if they are the result of active or passive smoke exposure, as being their action similar for the two types of exposure and consequently the concentration of toxic metabolites and duration of exposure, which are often unknown, determine the level of damage.

Three main smoking markers are usually used as an indicator of both active and environmental tobacco smoke exposure in different epidemiological surveys [92–93] because of their toxicity and laboratory assessment. They are blood carboxyhemoglobin, cotinine, a metabolite of nicotine, and thiocyanates. These markers are characterized by a different half-life that is about 5 hours for carboxyhemoglobin, 16 hours for cotinine, and 6.5 days for thiocyanates. The different chemicals' half-life permits to recognize smoke exposure of an individual although the economically high costs limit a large-scale use. Of these markers, therefore, the most specific cotinine is dosed even if it is of difficult assay.

Nicotine and Cotinine

Nicotine and cotinine are the most important markers in assessing smoking habit and exposure to environmental tobacco smoke.

Nicotine is metabolised to cotinine for its great majority in the liver. Both these compounds, which may be in different chemical phase in burned tobacco, can cause heart and blood vessel alterations that are followed by failure of vascular reconstrution particularly after chronic exposure. One can measure these markers in blood samples and urine (Table 8). Cotinine concentrations are found also in saliva where can also be measured, although with difficult techniques.

The concentrations of these chemicals in individuals are a consequence of both active smoking and air pollution. Biochemical concentrations of nicotine and cotinine as well as other toxic substances permit to identify those individuals who are exposed to tobacco smoke, but provide poor reflection of smoking habit and level of cardiovascular damage [94].

Table 8. Biochemical marker concentrations and methods
for assessing smoking exposure

Chemicals	Concentration	Usual Measuring
Nicotine	Blood, Liver, Urine	Serum, Urine
Cotinine	Blood, Liver, Urine, Saliva	Urine
Carbon Monoxide	Blood, Expired Air	Blood
Thiocyanates	Blood	Serum

Dosimetry of smoking constituents indicated that a low nicotine delivery, as it is a concentration of less than 0.6 mg per cigarette, usually induces an active smoker to draw larger puffs volumes (up to 55 ml / puff), or to inhale more deeply, or to puff more frequently [95]. On the contrary, nonsmokers exposed involuntarily to environmental tobacco smoke have their harm depending from blood concentrations reached by smoking indoor pollutants.

Cotinine, a major metabolite of nicotine, is used more widely than nicotine as a metabolic marker to dose since its concentration in the urines is a well defined parameter for measuring tobacco smoke exposure [96–99].

Different methods are used to quantify cotinine concentrations. Of wide use [100–103], gas chromatography and HPLC coupled or not with mass spectroscopy are preferred in a large majority of laboratories. However, these methods cannot be used in a large-scale because they need specialized laboratories and have high costs. Other methods [104–106], used not only for tobacco metabolite measures but also for detecting immunologic responses of several diseases in a single individual, - RIA, ELISA, and Fluorescence Polarisation Immunoassay – cannot be used on large – scale to measure cotinine concentrations because they also require specialized chemical structures.

Urinary cotinine concentrations are statistically higher (P less than 0.001) in children after their exposure to smoking as well as in pregnant women who were passively exposed to cigarette smoke [107–108]. Moreover, urinary levels of cotinine increased when exposure was increased.

Limit to evaluate cotinine concentrations is the difficulty – as it is a matter – to use a large-scale detection.

Carbon Monoxide

Carbon monoxide is a gas quickly absorbed into the blood and then reducing blood capacity to carry oxygen to the whole body. Inhalation of carbon monoxide has the same effects on active or passive smokers, depending its effects from the concentrations reached into the blood [2]. Carbon monoxide toxicity is due primarily to its strong bond with hemoglobin that produces carboxyhemoglobin. However, also the direct effects of carbon monoxide - as it is – on the heart and blood vessels must be well keept in mind because of their potential toxicity.

Since carbon monoxide is an extremely volatile gas, its potential toxicity is proportionally correlated with indoor cubic space, resulting, therefore, more harmful for individual in home and closed workplaces than that in open workplaces polluted by the gas.

The affinity of hemoglobin for carbon monoxide is about 240 times that of its affinity for oxygen, and carboxyhemoglobin levels into the blood are the close result of environmental tobacco smoke.

Biochemical monitoring of carbon monoxide inhalation from burned tobacco can be well measured by the dosage of carboxyhemoglobin.

Carboxyhemoglobin may be satisfactory measured in an arterial blood sample or, more easily, in a venous blood sample that must be collected in a closed container containing dry sodium heparine or disodium ethylene-diaminotetracetic acid (EDTA) as anticoagulant. Blood samples may be also stored for several days prior to analysis in a darkly cold container (4° C) and then measured by spectrophotometric methods [109–112]. So doing, a lot of samples may be simultaneously analysed with a sensible reduction of the costs.

Another approach to the determination of exposure to carbon monoxide is the analysis of the gas in expired air. This determination may be useful when individuals undergo acute exposure [1].

Increased coronary blood flow [113-115] is the response of the heart to mild carbon monoxide exposure, although, also in these circumstances, there is a well documented increase in carboxyhemoglobin concentration. Such a behaviour has been seen in both humans and, experimentally, dogs. However, animal long-term exposure induced pathological changes in the heart with an impairment of cardiovascular function [116].

In conclusion, carbon monoxide toxicity either following acute exposure or chronic exposure to environmental tobacco smoke is due particularly to tissue hypoxia that is a consequence of the much higher affinity for hemoglobin than that of oxygen. Cardiovascular damage involves with a major incidence coronary and carotid arteries reaching myocardial necrosis and brain ischemia in a few cases.However, transient evidence of cardiac toxicity does not result usually in long-term alterations, having been possible an heart transplantation from a victim of carbon monoxide poisoning [117].

Thiocyanates

Thiocyanates are a group of chemical compounds that have toxic action on several body organs [118–120]. They inhibit mitochondrial ferricytochrome oxidase and other enzyme systems and hence block electron transport resulting in reduced oxidative metabolism and oxygen utilization, decreased ATP production and lactic acidosis. The impairment of respiratory cellular chain induces tissue hypoxia or worsens a pre-existing hypoxia.

Burned tobacco commonly releases thiocyanates. People who smoke or undergo environmental tobacco smoke exposure may reach a mean level of thiocyanates into the blood of about 0.4 mcg/ ml. These levels increase two to two times and half the concentrations measured for non exposed individuals.

Thiocianates in serum have been monitored in the past to assess both smoke exposure and effectiveness of smoking cessation programs spread by some antismoking campaigns.

Actually, their measurements have been replaced by the dosage of nicotine and , usually, cotinine in the urines. Furthermore, there are some foods (milk, almonds, garlic, onion, leek, cabbage, and cauliflower) which determine a mild increase in serum concentration of thiocyanates and such a fact contributes to make difficult to distinguish what of the thiocyanate increased concentrations is due to smoke exposure or eaten foods.

Therefore, heavy limits reduce the measurements of these chemical compounds in the serum of individuals exposed to passive smoking.

In conclusion, biochemical markers of tobacco smoke could be most useful in assessing the level of environmental tobacco smoke exposure, but difficulties arise in carrying out their use on large- scale.

Several factors limit their epidemiological use: lower socio-economic levels of some classes of population who avoid a large-scale screening, highest costs of the screening, lifestyle and habit of nonsmoker individuals who, due to the fact that they are nonsmokers, overlook the potential harm that passive smoking may induce, limited number of specialized laboratories to dose biometabolites of tobacco smoke.

A large number of other chemical compounds derived from burned tobacco, which pollute the environment, have harmful effects for exposed humans. However, they are particularly carcinogens as well as damaging respiratory system or other body organs. Among these, one can find greater amount of ammonia, 2 naphtylamine, N-nitrosamine, and benzo-anthracene and benzo-pyrene in sidestream smoke.

Women, Children, and Passive Smoking

In our opinion, some important data should be well known to establish exactly the relationship between environmental tobacco smoke exposure and female gender. The analysis of heart and blood vessel damage provides observations arising from epidemiological studies of women exposed not only at home but also in workplaces. The risk for cardiovascular events in women differs from that in men, being in some age lower and in some heavier than that in men. Such a behaviour depends closely by the endocrine constellation of female gender.

Physiologically, sexual hormone constellation seems to protect pre-menopausal women from cardiovascular attacks, unless in a limited number of events [121–125]. Post-menopausal woman increases its cardiovascular risk, statistically, from two to three folds when compared with pre-menopausal state. However, opinions about that are not yet unanimous. A critical question, yet without a clear answer, is: why and how woman' endocrine constellation protects from the major coronary risk factors, smoking included, whereas smoking together with oral contraceptive use or ovarian disorders may lead to heavy cardiovascular damage, as it has been documented in our previous studies [123, 125]?.

Briefly [123, 125], one of the cases observed had exertional angina and silent myocardial ischemia assessed by Holter monitoring. This woman, 35 year-old, used oral contraceptives and was also an heavy active smoker. This patient was admitted to the Coronary Care Unit for unconsciousness due to ventricular fibrillation. After repeated direct-current cardioversion that restored sinus rhythm, acute myocardial infarction was seen at the electrocardiogram. The patient died four days later, and autopsy showed a massive transmural myocardial infarction and severe coronary narrowings.

Another smoker woman with ovarian disorders due to irregularity of estro-progesterone production developed myocardial infarction complicated by postinfarction aneurysm. She underwent successful cardiac surgery and then stopped smoking.

Estrogens usually protect woman against cardiovascular events.

In pre-menopausal women, the risk of cardiovascular events followed to oral contraceptive use is not due to atherogenesis progression but to an altered thrombogenesis caused by changes in serum lipoproteins, procoagulant substances, and platelet aggregation and adhesiveness [126].

Combined oral contraceptives can cause a state of increased coagulability that is most harmful in those women who smoke, since smoking also increases the risk of thrombogenesis. However, the most serious complications of smoking and oral contraceptive association are the thromboembolic and hemorrhagic phenomena particularly located in myocardium and coronary arteries, cerebrovascular arteries, pulmonary arteries with pulmonary embolism, and systemic veins.

The majority of reports on cardiovascular events due to smoking in women concerns active smokers. However, since the severity of damage is strickly related to the number of cigarettes smoked, and then to the blood levels reached by toxic biometabolites of smoking, there is to believe that we can transfer the results of active smoking to those of passive smoking comparing blood concentrations of toxic compounds.

However to confirm that, there are a lot of epidemiological studies on women who had been exposed to environmental tobacco smoke with development of cardiovascular damage depending from the type of exposure and premenopausal or postmenopausal status.

Data, which were statistically analyzed using effective methods, show an increased incidence of cardiovascular risk in nonsmoker women exposed to passive smoking, particularly at home but also in workplaces, with the appearance and/or impairment of symptoms related to ischemic pathology [16, 20–23, 25–26, 29-30]. Cardiac pathology consisting in an appearance or impairment of angina as well as electrocardiographic alterations with increased heart rate has been described more frequently. It is known that lowering heart rate is correlated with the reduction in cardiovascular mortality and in total mortality in the patients with pre-existing myocardial infarction and heart failure as well as with sudden death lower mortality as compared to higher heart rate [127–129].

The results of a previously longitudinal study [130] that involved white and black men and women aged from 18 years and 30 years without any history of cardiovascular disease allowed to conclude that those subjects who had increased heart rate impaired cardiovascular function and underwent intercurrently cardiovascular events with a major incidence as compared to those individuals without heart rate increase. Therefore, increased heart rate was considered an independent risk factor for cardiovascular disease, and, consequently, those factors like passive smoking exposure which may cause an increase of heart rate influence negatively the heart and blood vessels.

In nonsmoker women exposed to passive smoking where particularly heart rate increased, the epidemiological studies showed in a large majority symptoms statistically related to ischemic heart disease.

Such a fact would be a further indirect but significant confirmation that women exposed to passive smoking could have a progression in atherosclerotic lesions.

Since hormone constellation lowers in postmenopausal women, they have a response of atherogenic type - and, therefore, similar to that in men - to smoking exposure instead of thrombogenic type like that of premenopausal women. The difference in two types of response is of particular importance, being the atherogenic response to smoking due only to exposure of the woman, whereas thrombogenic response often needs woman exposure added to another factor like oral contraceptive use, that lead and increase cardiovascular risk. We must know this basic concept to well understand the reasons that cause cardiovascular damage in different age women.

Also blood pressure of nonsmoker women exposed to passive smoke show some suggestive changes. Both the systolic and diastolic blood pressures are higher when women live in a home polluted by environmental tobacco smoke [131]. Therefore exposure of nonsmoker women to environmental tobacco smoke cannot be regarded as a safe involuntary habit.

Also children exposure is useful to analyze, although the results may be susceptible of inaccuracies because they derive in a large majority from parental interviews , which may give information bias [132–133].

Children who are exposed to passive smoking, however, are suffering particularly from respiratory symptoms [134] more than cardiovascular symptoms. Among respiratory symptoms, asthma and respiratory infections [135] are prevailing in children of parents who smoke compared to those living with nonsmoking parents. Moreover, there is a significant relationship between the incidence of respiratory diseases and number of cigarettes smoked indoors.

Since environmental tobacco smoke exposure causes particularly those cardiovascular alterations which are related to a progression of the atherosclerosis, it is easy to understand the reasons of the lack of a clearly described impairment of heart and blood vessel function in children where atherosclerosis is, usually, yet far to develop due the fact of youngest age of this category of subjects. Moreover, doubts exist about published data that have been collected via parents' questionnaire, and have used merely general questions such as the presence or absence of smokers in the household, number of cigarettes smoked, mean duration of exposure, and characteristics of indoor spaces where children live. However, children exposed to tobacco smoke [133] have been distinguished, and may be distinguished, from non-exposed by the measurements of urinary cotinine concentrations. As we know, this procedure should be an effective method in limited numbers of subjects, since there are heavy difficulties, as mentioned above, to dose the biometabolite on large-scale. However, exposure of children to environmental tobacco smoke must be avoided due to the consistent increase in cardiovascular risk documented in adults.

How to Build a Mathematical Model

Building a mathematical model is the only way to characterize , quantify, and reproduce an experimental finding. Only the reproducibility of a study can confirm its validation as well as objectify obtained results.

Critical question that arises is: can we build a mathematical model to assess cardiovascular damage from passive smoke exposure as well as its reproducibility, and how?

Statistical and epidemiological studies analyze usually subjects who differ from themselves for a lot of habits, although the great number of individuals included into the study sample can lead to conclusions characterized –in case of similar responses – by statistical validation. However, there exists the probability that an incorrect analysis of statistical methods [136–138] can reach unreliable results. Another important aspect of statistical methods is to reach a clearly numerical presentation of the results as well as their correct interpretation. Incorrect interpretations of the results can lead to erroneous conclusions. Fortunately, the progresses in the study of statistical methodologies, reduce the errors of interpretation, although some limits are, nowadays, yet recognized particularly in collecting material which depends from interpretation, that could vary, of single researchers engaged in the same research. Moreover, statistical studies can provide effective data on the characteristics of a phenomenon even if they often fail to reproduce it exactly for the whole studied population. Recording too much information as a purpose of statistical studies on large-scale leads often to confusion in evaluating the results with care [139].

Reproducibility of almost similar results must be the objective of a finding to remove not unanimous opinions. Cardiovascular damage from environmental tobacco smoke exposure could be characterized by such an aspect. We reached [140] this result with an important finding, although limited to a single subject.

Briefly, in 1989 a 58-year-old man first presented with an anterior myocardial infarction at the Coronary Care Unit of the Hospital. Six months later, coronary angiography showed that the left anterior descending artery was totally occluded. Patient refused cardiac surgery for arterial revascularization. However, serial exercise testings performed according to the method of Fletcher and Schlant [141] did not show ischemic and/or arrhythmic alterations. Furthermore, the patient was asymptomatic when beta-blocker therapy (propranolol 120 mg/daily) was administered. Five years later, the patient gave his informed consent to undergo a study into the effects of passive smoking according to a modification of a method of Leone et al. [1].

He underwent 4 sessions of exercise stress testing on a bicycle ergometer, during which he was exposed alternatively to a smoke-free environment and an environment polluted with 30 to 35 parts per million air carbon monoxide concentration derived from burned tobacco. Plasma carboxyhemoglobin concentration measured before and after exercise was similar for the two pre-exposure and increased, but similar, during the two post-exposure to passive smoking. Electrocardiogram recordings during both sessions in the smoke-free environment showed a mild sinus tachycardia. During the two exercises in the polluted environment, similar and quantitatively same bigeminal ectopic beats occurred which necessitated the stopping of exercise. Therefore, this post-myocardial infarction patient showed exactly reproducible life-threatening ventricular arrhythmias when exercising in a same smoke-environmen polluted by carbon monoxide.

Therefore, the different opinions about the risk to the cardiovascular system following smoking exposure is the consequence of a wrong approach to the problem because of findings conducted without same experimental procedures.

Several variables may interfer with the experimental procedures. Some of these are related to passive smoking characteristics, some to the environment, and some to the exposed subjects. Table 9 shows some of those factors which contribute to make the variables difficult to standardize. Moreover, we can liste only some of these factors, but, obviously, there are a lot that may modify starting characteristics to assess cardiovascular damage from smoking.

Table 9. Variables to assess the damage from passive smoking

1. Passive smoking	
	Duration of exposure (acute, chronic)
	Chemicals concentration
	Type of inhalation
	Type of damage (functional, clinical, anatomical)
	Others
2. Indoor characteristics	
	Climate and Temperature
	Cubic metres
	Ventilation
	Workplace
	Home
	Others
3. Exposed subjects	
	Age
	Sex
	Socio-economic status
	Drug use
	Health status
	Risk factors associated
	Others

However, indicating the variables by the letters a, b, and c as well as n as being equal to the number of possible factors of each variable, we can build a mathematical equation that quantify exactly cardiovascular damage from passive smoking:

$$P = \frac{(na + nb + nc)^n}{n\,(abc)}$$

where P is the possibility of the mathematical combinations.

The large number of possible combinations may lead to different results in the findings.

However, when we standardize these variables, as shown in the case of our observation [140], cardiovascular damage may be exactly quantified as the result of the level of smoking exposure as well as indoor space and exposed population characteristics. Therefore, we can discuss about the degree of cardiovascular damage reached by an exposed subject, but we cannot deny the evidence that it occurs.

In exactly experimental procedures, cardiovascular damage due to environmental tobacco smoke is every time reproducible with the same characteristics. Therefore, building a mathematical model to assess those factors, which can act to reproduce the damage, has particular significance for understanding how to carry out effective preventive measures.

Conclusion

Passive smoking, as Glantz and Parmley stressed on their excellent publication on JAMA, causes heart disease [6]. Authors, also, underline the different ability of heart and blood vessels to adapt to changes due to smoking exposure . Active smokers – at least, we believe, before the appearance of an anatomical damage - adapt their cardiovascular system continuously to tobacco chemicals since they smoke daily. On the contrary, exposed to passive smoking do not have the benefit of cardiovascular adaptation, so that the effects of passive smoking on nonsmokers are much greater than on smokers. This difference, probably, is due to two reasons. Firstly, nonsmokers' heart and blood vessels have not attempted to adapt to the chemicals in secondhand smoke. Secondly, cardiovascular system is extremely sensitive to chemicals of secondhand smoke, and some toxics in environmental tobacco smoke have higher concentrations than those in smoke inhaled by smokers, although others have lower concentrations [142–143].

Using different statistical methodologies, several findings demonstrate undoubtedly the harmful effects of smoking exposure for cardiovascular system. As mentioned, particularly ischemic alterations due to endothelial dysfunction and atherosclerotic plaque progression result to be the target of the constituents of burned tobacco.Also an adrenergic stimulation [144] mediated by nicotine plays an important role in maintain cardiovascular damage. Different responses observed in clinical or experimental findings are the consequence of a different type of exposure whether for duration or chemicals concentration in the environment.

Some comments need the experimental findings conducted in animals, that show damages to cardiovascular system after exposure to tobacco smoke, to better clarify the harm of passive smoking. It is to believe that the results obtained, generally attributed to cigarette smoke without any detail about the type of smoking, are indeed related to passive smoking as being the consequence of animals exposure to an experimental indoor space polluted by cigarette smoking in almost all cases. To stick to the exact meaning of the word, these findings should be considered as conducted in passive smoke. They provide results of severe cardiovascular impairment without any doubt.

From the analysis of the provided data, there is evidence of the risk related to exposure to passive smoke. Different authors have estimated a number of deaths due to passive smoking ranging from 30,000 to 60,000 subjects [2, 4, 16, 145] annually in the United States.

In short, a worthwhile mention about recent observations that seem to link circulating endothelial progenitor cells and biochemical markers of cigarette smoking is to be pointed out, although conclusive results cannot be yet reached.

Circulating endothelial progenitor cells are a cell population [146–151] that have the capacity to circulate, proliferate, and differentiate into mature endothelial cells although they have not yet acquired characteristic mature endothelial markers or formed lumen. These precursor cells participate actively in postnatal neovascularization and reendothelialization.

Nicotine and the complex of its metabolites seem to influence both number and activity of circulating endothelial progenitor cells with augmentation and enhanced functional activity of them at relatively low concentrations, while citotoxicity was observed at higher metabolite concentrations [152]. Since nicotine is an active metabolite of the exposure to passive smoking, we can deduce that exposure to environmental tobacco smoke may interfer negatively with the activity of the circulating endothelial progenitor cells reducing the processes of cardiovascular revascularization. However, further studies need to confirm this hypothesis.

By the analysis of the several reports, passive smoking has to be considered an etiologic factor of cardiovascular disease since it leads, in the long run, to the evident development of cardiovascular pathology, although different levels of damage due to numerous factors may be observed. Moreover, passive smoking exposure is common and often unavoidable so that strong efforts need in an attempt to protect children, workers, and generally, all exposed individuals. The simplest way to reach an effective result is to prohibit indeed smoke in schools, workplaces, and public buildings [153–155] by environmental policy interventions that may have greater impact if they are carried out over multiple setting.

Finally, a newer and intriguing field of research concerns the relationship between passive smoking and genetics of the cardiovascular system [156]. Genetic variation in genes involved particularly in oxidative stress may determine a change of the homeostatic response in an environment polluted by cigarette smoking for increased oxidative burden. Many examples of gene-environment interactions exist and these may influence oxidative stress and subsequent cardiovascular disease. Clearly, large prospective findings are required to explore these in detail.

Appendix

Passive smoking, Involuntary smoking, Environmental tobacco smoke (ETS), and Secondhand smoke have the same meaning and may be used alternatively in a scientific article.

References

[1]   Leone A, Mori L, Bertanelli F, Fabiano P, Filippelli M. Indoor passive smoking: its effects on cardiac performance. *Int. J. Cardiol.* 1991; 8: 247 – 52.

[2]   Glantz SA, Parmley WW. Passive smoking and heart disease : epidemiology, physiology, and biochemistry. *Circulation* 1991; 83: 1 – 12.

[3]   Leone A. The heart: a target organ for cigarette smoking. *J. Smoking-Related Dis.* 1992; 3: 197 –201.

[4]   Wells AG. Passive smoking as a cause of heart disease. *J. Am. Coll. Cardiol.* 1994; 24: 546 – 54.

[5]   Leone A. Cigarette smoking and health of the heart. *J. Roy. Soc. Health* 1995; 115: 354 – 5.

[6]   Glantz SA, Parmley WW. Passive smoking and heart disease. *JAMA* 1995; 273: 1047 – 53.

[7]   Kritz H, Schmid P, Sinzinger H. Passive smoking and cardiovascular risk. *Arch. Intern. Med.* 1995;155: 1942 – 8.

[8]   US Department of Health and Human Services. The health consequences of involuntary smoking. A Report of the General Surgeons; Rockville, Md. *Office on Smoking and Health* DHHS Publication 1981; n° (CDC) 87-8398.

[9]   Byrd JC. Environmental tobacco smoke. *Medical and legal issues.* Medical Clinics of North America 1992; 76: 377 – 97.

[10] Majno G. *The Healing Hand.* Cambridge,MA, Harvard University Press, 1975: 43.

[11] He J, Vupputury S, Allen K, Prerost MR, Hughes J, Whelton PK. Passive smoking and the risk of coronary heart disease- A meta-analysis of epidemiologic studies . *N. Engl. J. Med.* 1999; 340 (12): 920.

[12] World Health Organization. The World Health Report 2002: *Reducing risks, promoting healthy life.* Geneva 2002: WHO.

[13] Doll R, Peto R. Mortality in relation to smoking: 20 years' observations on male British doctors. *Br. Med. J.* 1976; 25 (2): 1525 – 36.

[14] Sherman CB. Health effects of cigarette smoking. *Clin. Chest. Med.* 1991; 12 (4): 643 – 58.

[15] Giovino GA. Epidemiology of the tobacco use in the United States. *Oncogene* 2002; 21: 7326 – 39.

[16] Steenland K. Passive smoking and the risk of the heart disease. *JAMA* 1992; 267: 94 – 9.

[17] Lee PN, Chamberlain J, Alderson MR. Relationship of passive smoking to risk of lung cancer and other smoking-associated diseases. *Br. J. Cancer* 1986; 54: 97 – 105.

[18] Hole DJ, Gillis CR, Chopra C, Hawthorne WM. Passive smoking and cardiorespiratory health in a general population in the west of Scotland. *Br. Med. J.* 1989; 299: 423 – 7.

[19] Kawachi I, Colditz GA, Speizer FE, Manson JE, Stampfer MJ, Willet WC, et al. A prospective study of passive smoking and coronary heart disease. *Circulation* 1997; 95: 2374 – 9.

[20] Helsing K, Sandler D, Comstock G, Chee E. Heart disease mortality in nonsmokers living with smokers. *Am. J. Epidemiol.* 1988; 127: 915 – 22.

[21] Steenland K, Thun M, Lally C, Heath C Jr. Environmental tobacco smoke and coronary heart disease in the American Cancer Society CPS-II cohort. *Circulation* 1996; 94: 622 – 8.

[22] Sandler DP, Comstock JW, Helsing KJ, Shore DL. Death from all causes in non-smokers who lived with smokers. *Am. J. Public Health.* 1989; 79: 163 - 7.

[23] Svendsen KH, Kuller LH, Martin MJ, Ockene JK.Effects of passive smoking in the multiple risk factor intervention trials. *Am. J. Epidemiol.* 1987; 126: 783 – 95.

[24] Garland C, Barret-Connor E, Suarez L, Criqui MH, Wingard DL. Effects of passive smoking on ischemic heart disease mortality of nonsmokers. *Am. J. Epidemiol.* 1985; 121: 645 – 50.

[25] He Y, Li L, Wang Z, Zheng X, Jia G. Women's passive smoking and coronary heart disease. *Chin. J. Prev. Med.* 1989; 23: 19 – 22.

[26] Humble C, Croft J, Gerber A, Casper M, Hames CG, Tyroler HA. Passive smoking and 20-year cardiovascular disease mortality among nonsmoking wives, Evans County, Georgia. *Am. J. Public Health.* 1990; 80: 599 – 601.

[27] Muscat JE, Wynder EL. Exposure to environmental tobacco smoke and the risk of heart attack. *Int. J.Epidemiol.* 1995; 24: 715 – 9.

[28] La Vecchia C, D'Avanzo B, Franzosi MG, Tognoni G. Passive smoking and the risk of acute myocardial infarction. *Lancet* 1993; 341: 505 – 6.

[29] He Y, Lam TH, Li LS, Du RY, Jia GL, Huang JY, et al. Passive smoking at work as a risk factor for coronary heart disease in Chinese women who have never smoked. *Br. Med. J.* 1994; 308: 380 – 4.

[30] Layard MW. Ischemic heart disease and spousal smoking in the National Mortality Followback Survey. *Regular Toxicol. Pharmacol.* 1995; 21: 180 – 3.

[31] He Y, Lam TH, Li LS, Li LS, Du RY, Jia GL, et al. The number of stenotic coronary arteries and passive smoking exposure from husband in lifelong non-smoking women in Xi'an, China. *Atherosclerosis* 1996; 127 (2): 229 – 38.

[32] Hirayama T. Passive smoking (letter). *NZ. Med. J.* 1990; 103: 54.

[33] LeVois ME, Layard MW. Publication bias in the environmental tobacco smoke/coronary heart disease epidemiologic literature. *Regular Toxicol. Pharmacol.* 1995; 21: 184 – 91.

[34] Leone A. Cardiovascular damage from smoking: a fact or belief? *Int. J. Cardiol.* 1993; 38: 113 – 7.

[35] Leone A. Relationship between cigarette smoking and other coronary risk factors in atherosclerosis: risk of cardiovascular disease and preventive measures. *Curr. Pharm. Design.* 2003; 9 (29): 2417 – 23.

[36] Howard G, Burke GL, Szklo M, Tell GS, Eckfeldt J, Evans G, et al. Active and passive smoking are associated with increased carotid wall thickness. *Arch. Intern. Med.* 1994; 154: 1277 – 82.

[37] Howard G, Wagenknecht LE, Burke GL, Diez-Roux A, Evans GW, McGovern P, et al. Cigarette smoking and progression of atherosclerosis; The atherosclerosis risk in communities (ARIC) study. *JAMA* 1998; 279: 119 – 24.

[38] Werner RM, Pearson TA. What is so passive about passive smoking? Secondhand smoke as a cause of atherosclerotic disease. *JAMA* 1998; 279: 157 – 8.

[39] Salonen JT, Salonen R. Ultrasonography assessed carotid morphology and risk of coronary heart disease. *Arterioscler. Thromb. Vasc. Biol.* 1991; 11: 1245 – 9.

[40] Bots ML, Hoes AW, Koudstaal PJ, Hofman A, Grobbee DE. Common carotid intima-media thickness and risk of stroke and myocardial infarction: the Rotterdam Study . *Circulation* 1997; 96: 1432 – 7.

[41] Mikhailidis DP, Barradas MA, Nystrom ML, Jeremy JY. Cigarette smoking increases white blood cells aggregation in whole blood. *J. Roy. Soc. Med.* 1993; 86 (11): 680 – 1.

[42] Celermajer DS, Adams MR, Clarkson P, Robinson J, McRedie R, Donald A, et al. Passive smoking and impaired endothelium-dependent arterial dilatation in healthy young adults. *N. Engl. J. Med.* 1996; 334: 150 – 4.

[43] Stefanidis C, Vlachopoulos C, Tsiamis E. Unfavorable effects of passive smoking in aortic function in men. *Ann. Intern. Med.* 1998; 128: 426 – 34.

[44] Neufeld EJ, Mietus-Snyder M, Beiser AS, Baker AL, Newburger JW. Passive cigarette smoking and reduced HDL cholesterol levels in children with high risk lipid profiles. 1997; 96: 1403 – 7.

[45] Zhu BQ, Sun YP, Sievers RE, Isenberg WM, Glantz SA, Parmley WW. Passive smoking increases experimental atherosclerosis in cholesterol fed rabbits. *J. Am. Coll. Cardiol.* 1993; 21: 225 – 32.

[46] Penn A. Butadiene, a vaporphase component of environmental tobacco smoke, accelerates atherosclerotic plaque development. *Circulation* 1996; 93: 552P.

[47] Sumida H, Watanabe H, Kugiyama K, Ohgushi M, Matsumura T, Yasue H. Does passive smoking impair endothelium-dependent coronary artery dilation in women? *J. Am. Coll. Cardiol.* 1998; 31: 811 – 5.

[48] Otsuka R, Watanabe H, Hirata K, Tokai K, Muro T, Yoshiyama M, et al. Acute effects of passive smoking on the coronary circulation in healthy young adults. *JAMA* 2001; 286: 436 – 41.

[49] Celermajer DS, Sorensen KE, Gooch VM, Spiegelhalter DJ, Miller OL, Sullivan ID, et al. Non-invasive detection of endothelial dysfunction in children and adults at risk of atherosclerosis. *Lancet* 1992; 340: 1111 – 5.

[50] Davis J, Shelton L, Watanabe I, Arnold J. Passive smoking affects endothelium and platelets. *Arch. Intern. Med.* 1989; 149; 386 – 9.

[51] Deedwania PC. Endothelium: a new target for cardiovascular therapeutics. *J. Am. Coll. Cardiol.* 2000; 35: 67 – 70.

[52] Kugiyama K, Yasue H, Okomura K, Ogawa H, Fujimoto K, Nakao K, et al. Nitric oxide activity is deficient in spasm arteries of patients with coronary spastic angina. *Circulation* 1996; 94: 266 – 72.

[53] Penn A, Chen LC, Snyder CA. Inhalation of steady-state sidestream smoke from cigarettes promotes atherosclerotic plaque development. *Circulation* 1994; 90: 1363 – 7.

[54] Giannini D, Leone A, Di Bisceglie D, Nuti M, Strata G, Buttitta F, et al. The effects of acute passive smoke exposure on endothelium-dependent brachial artery dilatation in healthy individuals. *Angiology* 2005, (in press).

[55] Sinzinger H, Kefalides A. Passive smoking severely decreases platelet sensitivity to antiaggregatory prostglandins. *Lancet* 1982; 2: 392 – 3.

[56] Burghuber O, Punzengruber C, Sinzinger H, Haber P, Silberbauer K. Platelet sensitivity to prostacyclin in smokers and non-smokers. *Chest* 1986; 90: 34 – 8.

[57] Leone A. Biochemical markers of cardiovascular damage from tobacco smoke. *Curr. Pharm. Design.* 2005; 11: 2199 – 208.

[58] Taylor AE, Johnson DC, Kazemi H. Environmental tobacco smoke and cardiovascular disease: a position paper from the Council on Cardiopulmonary and Critical Care , American Heart Association. *Circulation* 1992; 86: 699 – 702.

[59] Celermajer DS, Sorensen KE, Georgakopoulos D. Cigarette smoking is associated with dose-related and potentially reversible impairment of endothelium-dependent dilation in healthy young adults. *Circulation* 1993; 88: 2149 – 55.

[60] Raitakari OT, Adams MR, McRedie RJ, Griffiths KA, Celermajer DS. Passive-smoke related arterial endothelial dysfunction is potentially reversible in healthy young adults. *Ann. Intern. Med.* 1999; 130: 578 – 81.

[61] Leone A, Giannini D, Bellotto C, Balbarini A. Passive smoking and coronary heart disease. *Current Vascular Pharmacology* 2004; 2: 175 – 82.

[62] Mori L, Bertanelli F, Fabiano P, Battaglia A, Leone A. Indoor passive smoking and cardiac performance: mechanisms able to cause heart failure. *J. Smoking-Related Dis.* 1993; 4 (3): 213 – 7.

[63] Leone A, Bertanelli F, Mori L, Fabiano P, Battaglia A. Features of ischaemic cardiac pathology resulting from cigarette smoking. *J. Smoking-Related Dis.* 1994; 5 (2): 109 – 14.

[64] Valkonen M, Kuusi T. Passive smoking induces atherogenic changes in low-density lipoprotein. *Circulation* 1998; 97: 2012 – 6.

[65] Strachan DP. Predictors of death from aortic aneurysm among middle-aged men: the Whitehall study. *Br. J. Surg.* 1991; 78: 401 – 4.

[66] Tribble DL, Giuliano LJ, Fortman SP. Reduced plasma ascorbic acid concentrations in nonsmokers regularly exposed to environmental tobacco smoke. *Am. J. Clin. Nutr.* 1993; 58: 886 – 90.

[67] Ayres SM, Mueller HS, Gregory JJ, Giannelli S Jr, Penny JL. Systemic and myocardial hemodynamic responses to relatively small concentrations of carboxyhemoglobin (COHB). *Arch. Environ. Health.* 1969; 18 (4): 699 – 709.

[68] Aronow WS, Rokaw SN. Carboxyhemoglobin caused by smoking nonnicotine cigarettes. Effects in angina pectoris. *Circulation* 1971; 44 (5): 782 – 8.

[69] Aronow WS, Harris CN, Isbell MW, Rokaw SN, Imparato B. Effect of freeway travel on angina pectoris. *Ann. Intern. Med.* 1972; 77 (5): 669 – 76.

[70] Anderson EW, Andelman RJ, Strauch JM, Fortuin NJ, Knelson JH. Effect of low-level carbon monoxide exposure on onset and duration of angina pectoris. A study in ten patients with ischemic heart disease. *Ann. Intern. Med.* 1973; 79 (1): 46 – 50.

[71] Aronow WS, Isbell MW. Carbon monoxide effect on exercise-induced angina pectoris. *Ann. Intern. Med.* 1973; 79 (3): 392 – 5.

[72] Aronow WS. Aggravation of angina pectoris by two percent carboxyhemoglobin. *Am. Heart. J.* 1981; 101 (2): 154 – 7.

[73] Sheps DS, Adams KF Jr, Bromberg PA, Goldstein GM, O'Neil JJ, Horstman D, et al. Lack of effect of low levels of carboxyhemoglobin on cardiovascular function in patients with ischemic heart disease. *Arch. Environ. Health* 1987; 42 (2): 108 – 16.

[74] Adams KF, Koch G, Chatterjee B, Goldstein GM, O'Neil JJ, Bromberg PA, et al. Acute elevation of blood carboxyhemoglobin to 6% impairs exercise performance and aggravates symptoms in patients with ischemic heart disease. *J. Am. Coll. Cardiol.* 1988; 12 (4): 900 – 9.

[75] Sheps DS, Herbst MC, Hinderliter AL, Adams KF, Ekelund LG, O'Neil JJ, et al. Production of arrhythmias by elevated carboxyhemoglobin in patients with coronary artery disease. *Ann. Intern. Med.* 1990; 113 (5): 343 – 51.

[76] Leone A, Bertanelli F, Mori L, Fabiano P, Bertoncini G. Ventricular arrhythmias by passive smoke in patients with pre-existing myocardial infarction. *J. Am. Coll. Cardiol.* 1992; 19; 256A.

[77] White JR, Criqui M, Kulk JA, Froeb HF, Sinsheimer PJ. Serum lipoproteins in non smokers chronically exposed to tobacco smoke in the workplace. 8th World Conference on Tobacco or Health, 1992.

[78] Benowitz NL. Nicotine and coronary heart disease. *Trends Cardiovasc. Med.* 1991; 1: 315 – 21.

[79] Miyaura S, Eguchi H, Johnston JM. Effect of a cigarette smoke extract on the metabolism of the proinflammatory autacoid, platelet-activating factor. *Circ. Res.* 1992; 70: 341 – 7.

[80] Imaizumi TA, Satoh K, Yoshida H, Kawamura Y, Hiramoto M, Takamatsu S. Effect of cigarette smoking on the levels of platelet-activating factor-like lipid(s) in plasma lipoproteins. *Atherosclerosis* 1991; 87: 47 – 55.

[81] Meade TW, Imeson J, Stirling Y. Effects of change in smoking and other characteristics on clotting factors and the risk of ischemic heart disease. *Lancet* 1987; 2: 986 – 8.

[82] Kannel WB, D'Agostino RB, Belanger AJ. Fibrinogen, cigarette smoking, and the risk of cardiovascular diseases: Insights from the Framingham Study: *Am. Heart J.* 1987; 113: 1006 – 10.

[83] Stone MC, Thorpe JM. Plasma-fibrinogen- a major coronary risk factor. *JR. Coll. Gen. Pract.* 1985; 35: 565 – 9.

[84] Zhu B-Q, Sun Y-P, Sievers RE, Glantz SA, Parmley WW, Wolfe CL. Exposure to environmental tobacco smoke increases myocardial infarct size in rats. *Circulation* 1994; 89: 1282 – 90.

[85] Kjeldsen K, Thomsen H, Astrup P. Effects of carbon monoxide on myocardium: ultrastructural changes in rabbits after moderate, chronic exposure. *Circ. Res.* 1974; 34: 339 – 48.

[86] Thomsen H, Kjeldsen K. Threshold limit for carbon monoxide-induced myocardial damage. *Arch. Environ. Health.* 1974; 29: 73 – 80.

[87] Lough J. Cardiomyopathy produced by cigarette smoke. *Arch. Pathol. Lab. Med.* 1978; 102: 377 – 80.

[88] Westfall T, Cipolloni P, Edmundowicz A. Influence of propranolol on hemodynamic changes and plasma catecholamine levels following cigarette smoking and nicotine. *Proc. Soc. Exp. Biol. Med.* 1966; 123: 174 – 9.

[89] White S, McRitchie R. Nasopharingeal reflexes: integrative analysis of evoked respiratory and cardiovascular effects. *Aust. J. Exp. Biol. Med. Sci.* 1973: 51: 17 – 31.

[90] McMurray RG, Hicks LL, Thompson DL. The effects of passive inhalation of cigarette smoke on exercise performance. *Eur. J. Appl. Physiol.* 1985; 54: 196 – 200.

[91] Leone A. Il fumo di sigaretta: un potente fattore di rischio cardiovascolare. *Il Cuore* 1991; 5: 573 – 80.

[92] Greenberg RA, Haley NJ, Ersel RA, Loda FA. Measuring the exposure of infants to tabacco smoke. *N. Engl. J. Med.* 1984; 310: 1075 – 8.

[93] Strachan DP, Jarvis MJ, Feyerabend C. Passive smoking, salivary cotinine concentrations and middle ear effusion in 7-year-old children. *Br. Med. J.* 1989; 289: 1549 – 52.

[94] Worrel PC, Edwards R, Powell JT. Smoking markers as a reflection of smoking habit. *J. Smoking-Related Dis.* 1995; 6: 89 – 97.

[95] Herning RI, Jones RT, Bacham J, Mines AH. Puff volumes increases when low-nicotine cigarettes are smoked. *Br. Med. J.* 1981; 283: 187 – 9.

[96] Apselhoff G, Ashton HM, Friedman H, Gerber N. The importance of measuring cotinine levels to identify smokers in clinical trials. *Clin. Pharmacol. Ther.* 1994; 56: 460 – 2.

[97] Benowitz NL. Cotinine as a biomarker of environmental tobacco smoke exposure. *Epidemiol. Rev.* 1996; 18: 188 – 204.

[98] Jarvis MJ, Tunstall-Pedoe H, Feyerabend C, Vesey C, SaloojeeY. Comparison of tests used to distinguish smokers from nonsmokers. *Am. J. Public. Health.* 1987; 77: 1435 – 8.

[99] Benowitz NL, Jacob P. Nicotine and cotinine elimination pharmacokinetics in smokers and non smokers. *Clin. Pharmacol. Ther.* 1993; 53: 316 – 23.

[100] Feyerabend C, Russel MAH. A rapid gas-liquid chromatographic method for the determination of cotinine and nicotine in biological fluids. *J. Pharm. Pharmacol.* 1999; 42: 450 – 2.

[101] Lequang Thuan NT, Migueres ML, Roche D, Roussel G, Mahuzier G, et al. Elimination of caffeine interference in HPLC determination of urinary nicotine and cotinine levels. *Clin. Chem.* 1989; 35: 1456 – 9.

[102] James H, Tibazi Y, Taylor R. Rapid method for the simultaneous measurement of nicotine and cotinine in urine and serum by gas-chromatography-mass spectrometry. *J. Chromatogr. B.* 1998; 708: 87 – 93.

[103] Tuomi T, Johnson T, Reijula K. Analysis of nicotine, 3-hydroxycotinine, cotonine, and caffeine in urine of passive smokers by HPLC-tandem mass spectrometry. *Chem.* 1999; 45: 2164 – 72.

[104] Langone JJ, Gjika HB, Van Vunakis H. Nicotine and its metabolites. Radioimmunoassay for nicotine and cotinine. *Biochemistry* 1973; 12: 5025 – 30.

[105] Langone JJ, Cook G, Bjercke R, Lifshitz MH. Monoclonal antibody ELISA for cotinine in saliva and urine on active and passive smokers. *J. Immunol. Methods.* 1988; 114: 74 – 8.

[106] Ekemin SA, Coxon RE, Colbert DL, Landon J, Smith DS. Urinary cotinine fluoroimmunoassay for smoking status screening adapted to an automated analyser. *Analyst* 1992; 117: 697 – 9.

[107] Roche D, Callais F, Reungoat P, Momas I. Adaptation on an enzyme immunoassay to assess urinary cotinine in nonsmokers exposed to tobacco smoke. *Clin. Chem.* 2001; 47: 950 – 2.

[108] Spierto FW, Hannon WH, Kendrick JS, Bernert JT, Pirkle J, Gargiullo P. Urinary cotinine levels in women enrolled in a smoking cessation study during and after pregnancy. *J. Smoking-Related Dis.* 1994; 5: 65 – 76.

[109] Drabkin DL, Austin JH. Spectrophotometric studies. II. Preparation from washed blood cells; nitric oxide hemoglobin and sulfhemoglobin. *J. Biol. Chem.* 1935; 112: 51 – 65.

[110] Malenfant AL, Gambino SR, Waraska AJ, Roe EL. Spectrophotometric determination of hemoglobin concentration and percent oxyhemoglobin and carboxyhemoglobin saturation. Clin. Chem. 1968; 14: 162 – 71.

[111] Small KA, Radford EP, Frazier JM, Rodkey FL, Collison HA. A rapid method for simultaneous measurement of carboxy and methemoglobin in blood. *J. Appl. Physiol.* 1971; 31: 154 – 60.

[112] Lily REC, Cole PV, Hawkins LH. Spectrophotometric measurements of carboxyhemoglobin. *Br. J. Ind. Med.* 1972; 29: 454 – 7.

[113] Permutt S, Fahri L. Tissue hypoxia and carbon monoxide. In: *Effects of chronic exposure to low levels of carbon monoxide on human health , behaviour, and performance.* National Academy of Sciences, National Academy of Engineering, Washington DC, 1969; 18 – 24.

[114] Adams JD, Erickson HH, Stone HL. Myocardial metabolism during exposure carbon monoxide in the conscious dog. *J. Appl. Physiol.* 1973; 34: 238 – 42.

[115] Horwath SM, Raven PB, Dahms TE, Gray DJ. Maximal aerobic capacity at different levels of carboxyhemoglobin. *J. Appl. Physiol.* 1975; 38: 300 – 3.

[116] Lewey FH, Drabkin DD. Experimental chronic carbon monoxide poisoning of dogs. *Am. J. Med. Sci.* 1944; 208: 502 – 11.

[117] Roberts JR, Bain M, Klachko MN, Seigel EG, Wason S. Successful heart transplantation from a victim of carbon monoxide poisoning. *An. Emerg. Med.* 1995; 26: 652 – 5.

[118] Apple FS. Serum thiocyanate concentrations in patients with normal or impaired renal function receiving nitroprusside. *Clin. Chem.* 1996; 42: 1878 – 9.

[119] De la Higuera AJ. Determination of serum thiocyanate in patients with thyroid disease using a modification of the Aldridge method. *J. Anal. Toxicol.* 1994; 18: 58 – 9.

[120] Olea F, Parras P. Determination of serum levels of dietary thiocyanate. *J. Anal. Toxicol.* 1992; 16: 258 – 60.

[121] Consensus: *Estrogen use and postmenopausal women.* National Institutes of Health Consensus Development Conference Summary 1979; 2: 8 (A consensus on the state of the heart as relates to risks and benefits).

[122] Mishell Dr Jr. Contraception. In: De Groot LJ et al., *Endocrinology*, Vol 3 ; Grune-Stratton, New York,1979 ; 1435 – 50.

[123] Leone A, Lopez M. Role du tabac et de la contraception orale dans l'infarctus du myocarde de la femme. Description d'un cas. *Pathologica* 1984 ; 76 : 493 – 8.

[124] Rosemberg L, Slone D, Shapiro S, Kaufman DW, Stolley PD, Miettinen OS. Non contraceptive estrogens and myocardial infarction in young women. *JAMA* 1980; 244: 339 – 42.

[125] Leone A, Lopez M. Oral contraception, ovarian disorders and tobacco in myocardial infarction of woman. *Pathologica* 1986; 78: 237 – 42.

[126] Foster DC. Low-dose monophasic and multiphasic oral contraceptives: a review of potency, efficacy, and side effects. *Semin. Reprod. Endocrinol.* 1989; 7: 205 – 212.

[127] Habib GB. Is heart rate a risk factor in the general population? *Dialogues in Cardiovascular Medicine* 2001; 6: 25 – 31.

[128] Purcel H. Is heart rate a prognostic factor for cardiovascular disease? *Dialogues in Cardiovascular Medicine* 2001; 6: 32 – 36.

[129] Castelli WP, Levy D, Wilson PWF, Kannel W. Sudden death: The view from Framingham. In: Kostis JB and Sanders M eds. *The prevention of sudden death.* E Wiley-Liss, New York 1990; 1 – 8.

[130] Zhang J, Kesteloot H. Anthropometric, lifestyle, and metabolic determinants of resting heart rate. A population study. *Eur. Heart J.* 1999; 20: 103 – 10.

[131] Matanoski G, Kanchanaraksa S, Lantry D, Chang Y. Characteristics of nonsmoking women in NHANES I and NHANES II. Epidemiologic follow-up study with exposure to spouses who smoke. *Am. J. Epidemiol.* 1995; 142: 149 – 57.

[132] Rubin DH, Damus C. The relationship between passive smoking and child health: methodologic criteria applied to prior studies. *Yale J. Biol. Med.* 1988; 61: 401 – 11.

[133] Bakoula CG, Kafritsa YJ, Kavadias GD, Lazopoulou DD, Theodoridou MC, et al. Objective passive-smoking indicators and respiratory morbidity in young children. *Lancet* 1995; 346: 280 – 1.

[134] Shima M, Adachi M. Effects of environmental tobacco smoke on serum levels of acute phase proteins in schoolchildren. *Preventive Medicine* 1996; 25: 617 – 24.

[135] Rossier ML, Fernandez Vega M, Villalba Caloca J, Letama C M, Flores Sanchez S. Frequency of acute respiratory infections in children of parents who smoke and children of nonsmoking parents. In *Tobacco and Health*, K Slama ed, Plenum Press, New York 1995; 537 – 9.

[136] Schor S, Karten I. Statistical evaluation of medical journal manuscripts. *JAMA* 1966; 195: 1123 – 8.

[137] Gore SM, Jones IG, Rytter EC. Misuse of statistical methods: critical assessement of articles in BMJ from January to March 1976. *Br. Med. J.* 1977; i: 85 – 7.

[138] White SJ. Statistical errors in papers in the British Journal of Psychiatry. *Br. J. Psychiatry.* 1979; 135: 336 – 42.

[139] Wright P, Haybittle J. Design of forms for clinical trials. *Br. Med. J.* 1979; ii: 650 – 1.

[140] Leone A. Passive smoking causes cardiac alterations in post-MI subjects. *Int. J. Smoking Cessation.* 1996; 3 (4): 42 – 3.

[141]Fletcher GF, Schlant RC. The exercise test. In : Schlant RC, Alexander WR eds., *Hurst's the heart*. 8th edn, New York 1994; 423 – 40.

[142]US Dept of Health and Human Services. The health consequences of involuntary smoking: *A Report of the Surgeon General*. Office on Smoking and Health, Centers for Disease Control, Public Health Service, 1986. Document DHHS (CDC); 87 – 8398.

[143]National Research Council Committee on Passive Smoking. *Environmental Tobacco Smoke: Measuring Exposures and Assessing Health Effects*. Washington D.C.: National Academic Press; 1986.

[144]Winniford MD, Wheelan KR, Kremers MS, Ugolini V, van den Berg Jr E, Niggemann EH, et al. Smoking-induced coronary vasoconstrition in patients with atherosclerotic coronary artery disease: evidence for adrenergically mediated alterations in coronary artery tone. *Circulation* 1986; 73: 662 – 7.

[145]Wells AJ. An estimate of adult mortality in the United States from passive smoking. *Environ. Int.* 1988; 14: 249 – 65.

[146]Asahara T, Murohara T, Sullivan A, Silver M, van der Zee R, Li T, et al. Isolation of putative endothelial progenitor cells for angiogenesis. *Science* 1997; 275: 964 – 7.

[147]Hill JM, Zalos G, Halcox JP, Schenke WH, Waclawiw MA, Quyyumi AA, et al. Circulating endothelial progenitor cells, vascular function, and cardiovascular risk. *N. Engl. J. Med.* 2003; 348: 593 – 600.

[148]Walter DH, Ritting K, Bahlmann FH, Kirchmair R, Silver M, Murayama T, et al. Statin therapy accelerates reendothelization: a novel effect involving mobilization and incorporation of bone-marrow derived endothelial progenitor cells. *Circulation* 2002; 105: 3017 – 24.

[149]Murohara T, Ikeda H, Duan J, Shintani S, Sasaki K, Eguchi H, et al. Transplanted cord blood-derived endothelial progenitor cells augment postnatal neovascularization. *J. Clin. Invest.* 2000; 105: 1527 – 36.

[150]Kocker AA, Schuster MD, Szabolcs MJ, Takuma S, Burkhoff D, Wang J, et al. Neovascularization of ischemic myocardium by human bone-marrow-derived angioblasts prevents cardiomyocyte apoptosis, reduces remodeling and improves cardiac function. *Nat. Med.* 2001; 7: 430 – 6.

[151]Grant MB, May WS, Caballero S, Brown GA, Guthrie SM, Mames RN, et al. Adult hematopoietic stem cells provide functional hemangioblast activity during retinal neovascularization. *Nat. Med.* 2002; 8: 607 – 12.

[152]Wang XX, Zhu JH, Chen JZ, Shang YP. Effects of nicotine on the number and activity of circulating endothelial progenitor cells. *J. Clin. Pharmacol.* 2004; 44: 881 – 9.

[153]Secondhand smoke: is it a hazard? *Consumer. Rep.* 1995; 60: 27 – 33.

[154]Woodruff T, Rosebrook B, Pierce J, Glantz S. Lower levels of cigarette consumption found in smoke-free workplaces in California. *Arch. Intern. Med.* 1993; 153: 1485 – 93.

[155]Siegel M. Involuntary smoking in the restaurant workplace: a review of employee exposure and health effects. *JAMA* 1993; 270: 490 – 3.

[156]Armani C, Landini L Jr, Leone A. Molecular and biochemical changes of the cardiovascular system due to smoking exposure. Curr Pharm Design 2009; 15: 1038 – 53.

In: Handbook of Cardiovascular Research
Editors: Jorgen Brataas and Viggo Nanstveit

Chapter IV

The Origin and Role of N-Homocysteinylated Proteins in Human Cardiovascular Disease[*]

Hieronim Jakubowski[†]

Department of Microbiology and Molecular Genetics, UMDNJ-New Jersey Medical
School, International Center for Public Health, Newark, NJ 07101, USA
Institute of Bioorganic Chemistry,
Polish Academy of Sciences, Poznań, Poland

Abstract

The non-protein amino acid homocysteine (Hcy), a metabolite of the essential amino acid methionine, is implicated in the pathology of human cardiovascular and neurodegenerative diseases. In addition to its elimination by the remethylation and transsulfuration pathways, Hcy is also metabolized to the thioester Hcy-thiolactone in an error-editing reaction in protein biosynthesis when Hcy is mistakenly selected in place of methionine by methionyl-tRNA synthetase. In humans, the accumulation of Hcy-thiolactone can be detrimental because of its intrinsic ability to modify proteins by forming *N*-Hcy-protein adducts, in which a carboxyl group of Hcy is *N*-linked to ε-amino group of a protein lysine residue. *N*-linked Hcy occurs in each protein examined and constitutes a significant pool of Hcy in human blood. *N*-Hcy proteins are recognized as neo-self antigens and induce an auto-immune response. As a result, IgG and IgM anti-*N*-Hcy-protein auto-antibodies, are produced in humans. Serum levels of anti-*N*-Hcy-protein IgG auto-antibodies are positively correlated with plasma total Hcy, but not with plasma cysteine or methionine levels, which is consistent with the etiology of these auto-

---

[*] A version of this chapter was also published in *Autoantibodies Research Progress*, edited by Quentin P. Dubois published by Nova Science Publishers, Inc. It was submitted for appropriate modifications in an effort to encourage wider dissemination of research.

[†] Corresponding author: Hieronim Jakubowski, Department of Microbiology and Molecular Genetics UMDNJ-New Jersey Medical School International Center for Public Health 225 Warren Street Newark, NJ 07101-1709, USA, Phone: 973-972-4483 Fax: 973-972-8981 E-mail:jakubows@umdnj.edu

antibodies. In a group of male patients with stroke, the levels of anti-*N*-Hcy-protein IgG auto-antibodies and total Hcy are significantly higher than in a group of healthy subjects. In a group of male patients with angiographically documented coronary artery disease, seropositivity for anti-*N*-Hcy-protein IgG auto-antibodies occurs 5-times more frequently than in controls and is an independent predictor of coronary artery disease. These findings show that an auto-immune response against *N*-Hcy-proteins is a general feature of atherosclerosis and provide support for a hypothesis that *N*-Hcy-protein is a neo-self antigen, which contributes to immune activation, an important modulator of atherogenesis. Plasma Hcy lowering by folic acid administration leads to significant decreases in anti-*N*-Hcy-protein IgG auto-antibody levels in control subjects, but not in coronary artery disease patients. The results of these Hcy-lowering treatments suggest that, while primary Hcy-lowering intervention is beneficial, secondary Hcy-lowering intervention in coronary artery disease patients may be ineffective in reducing the advanced damage caused by Hcy, and may explain at least in part the failure of vitamin therapy to lower cardiovascular events in recent Hcy-lowering trials. Chronic activation of immune responses towards *N*-Hcy-protein associated with hyperhomocysteinemia over many years would lead to vascular disease.

Keywords: autoantibodies; atherosclerosis; coronary artery disease; Hyperhomo-cysteinemia; homocysteine thiolactone hypothesis; protein N-homocysteinylation; stroke

Introduction

Cardiovascular disease is a major cause of morbidity and mortality in industrial nations.

Despite advances in our understanding of cardiovascular disease, traditional risk factors such as hyperlipidemia, hypertension, smoking, and diabetes do not accurately predict cardiovascular events and over half of all coronary events occur in persons without overt hyperlipidemia [1; 2; 3; 4]. Thus, a search continues for new markers and strategies to guide the development of novel antiatherosclerotic therapies beyond low-density lipoprotein (LDL) cholesterol reduction. Although atherosclerosis has been viewed as a lipid storage disease [5], the growing body of evidence suggests that inflammation participates in all stages of atherosclerosis from the initial lesion to the end-stage thrombotic complications [2; 6; 7; 8; 9; 10; 11]. The principal culprits responsible for the initiation of inflammation appear to be proteins modified by products of lipid peroxidation or by glucose, particularly oxidized or glycated LDL. Modified LDL induces both innate and adaptive immune responses, and autoantibodies against modified LDL are present in atherosclerotic plaques and in circulation [12; 13]. Among other inducers of inflammation is homocysteine (Hcy) [14], a non-traditional risk factor for vascular disease [15]. A mechanism by which Hcy induces an adaptive immune response is a topic of this chapter.

Severe hyperhomocysteinemia secondary to mutations in the *CBS*, *MTHFR*, or *MS* gene causes pathologies in multiple organs, including the cardiovascular system and the brain, and leads to premature death due to vascular complications [16; 17; 18]. McCully observed advanced arterial lesions in children with inborn errors in Hcy metabolism and proposed that Hcy causes vascular disease [19]. Although severe hyperhomocysteinemia is rare, mild hyperhomocysteinemia is quite prevalent in the general population and is associated with an increased risk of vascular [20] and neurological complications [21; 22], and predicts mortality in heart disease patients [23]. The strongest evidence that Hcy plays a causal role in atherothrombosis comes from the studies of severe genetic hyperhomocysteinemia in humans and the finding that Hcy-lowering by vitamin-B supplementation greatly improves vascular outcomes in CBS-deficient patients [16; 17; 18]. For example, untreated CBS-deficient patients suffer 1 vascular event per 25 patient-years [16] while vitamin-B-treated CBS-deficient patients suffer only 1 vasular event per 263 patient-years (relative risk 0.091, p<0.001) [18]. Hcy-lowering therapy started early in life also prevents brain disease from severe MTHFR deficiency [24]. Furthermore, studies of genetic and nutritional hyperhomocysteinemia in animal models also provide a strong support for a causative role of Hcy [14; 25; 26]. In humans, lowering plasma Hcy by vitamin-B supplementation improves cognitive function in the general population [27] and leads to a 21-24% reduction of vascular outcomes in high risk stroke patients [28; 29], but not in myocardial infarction (MI) patients [29; 30]. Hcy-lowering trials are currently ongoing, and the results of these trials are required before making recommendations on the use of vitamins for prevention of vascular disease [31].

Atherosclerosis, a disease of the vascular wall, is initiated by endothelial damage. Endothelial dysfunction, immune activation, and thrombosis, characteristic features of vascular disease [8], are all observed in hyperhomocysteinemia in humans [16] and experimental animals [26]. The degree of impairment in endothelial function during hyperhomocysteinemia is similar to that observed with hypercholesterolemia. Multiple mechanisms, such as protein homocysteinylation, unfolded protein response, decreased bioavailability of nitric oxide, oxidative stress, altered cellular methylation and epigenetic regulation, and the induction of innate and adaptive immune responses appear to contribute to Hcy pathobiology in cardiovascular disease [14; 25; 26; 32; 33; 34; 35; 36; 37]. The Hcy-thiolactone hypothesis [36] [37a, 37b] states that metabolic conversion of Hcy to Hcy-thiolactone, catalyzed by methionyl-tRNA synthetase (MetRS) (*Eq.* 1), followed by protein N-homocysteinylation by Hcy-thiolactone (*Eq.* 2), causes a variety of pathophysiological consequences including protein [38] and cell damage [39; 40; 41], enhanced thrombosis [42; 43], and induction of auto-immune responses [14; 35; 36]. In this chapter, I will discus the mechanism of formation of *N*-Hcy-proteins, new neo-self antigens derived from Hcy, summarize evidence for their presence in the human body, and describe their antigenic properties and emerging evidence for an important role of anti-*N*-Hcy-protein autoantibodies in vascular disease.

Overview of Homocysteine Metabolism

Homocysteine (Hcy) is a sulfur-containing amino acid that is found as an intermediary metabolite in all living organisms. In mammals Hcy is formed from dietary methionine (Met) as a result of cellular methylation reactions [16]. In this pathway, dietary Met is taken up by cells and then activated by ATP to yield S-adenosylmethionine (AdoMet), a universal methyl donor (Figure 1). As a result of the transfer of its methyl group to an acceptor, AdoMet is converted to S-adenosylhomocysteine (AdoHcy). The reversible enzymatic hydrolysis of AdoHcy is the only known source of Hcy in the human body. Levels of Hcy are regulated by remethylation to Met, catalyzed by the enzyme Met synthase (MS), and transsulfuration to cysteine, the first step of which is catalyzed by the enzyme cystathionine β-synthase (CBS). The remethylation requires vitamin B_{12} and 5,10-methyl-tetrahydrofolate (CH$_3$-THF), generated by 5,10-methylene-THF reductase (MTHFR). The transsulfuration requires vitamin B_6.

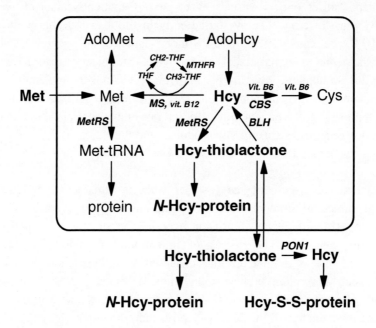

Figure 1. Neo-self antigen, protein N-linked Hcy (N-Hcy-protein), is a byproduct of Hcy metabolism in humans.

Table 1. Physical-chemical properties of L-Hcy-thiolactone and L-Hcy [46]

Property	L-Hcy-thiolactone	L-Hcy
Chemical character	Aminoacyl-thioester	Mercaptoamino acid
UV spectrum	Yes, λ_{max} = 240 nm, ε = 5,000 M^{-1} cm^{-1}	No significant absorption at λ >220nm
Stability at 37°C, $t_{0.5}$ phosphate-saline human serum	~30 h ~1 h	2 h 2 h
pK_a of amino group	6.67 [a]	9.04, 9.71 [b] 9.02, 9.69 (thiol group) [b]

Table 1. (Continued)

Property	L-Hcy-thiolactone	L-Hcy
Chemical reactivity	Acylates amino groups of protein lysine residues [c] Reacts with aldehydes to afford tetrahydrothiazines [a] Resistant to oxidation Base-hydrolyzed to Hcy	Condenses to Hcy-thiolactone Reacts with aldehydes to afford tetrahydrothiazines [a] Oxidized to disulfides Reacts with nitric oxide to afford S-nitroso-Hcy [d]

[a] Ref. [63], [b] Ref. [64], [c] Ref. [38; 50], [d] Ref. [65].

A fraction of Hcy is also metabolized by MetRS to a thioester, Hcy-thiolactone (Figure 1), in an error-editing reaction in protein biosynthesis when Hcy is mistakenly selected in place of Met [44; 45; 46; 47; 48]. The flow through the Hcy-thiolactone pathway is increased by a high-Met diet [49], inadequate supply of CH_3-THF [49; 50; 51], or impairment of re-methylation or trans-sulfuration reactions by genetic alterations of enzymes, such as CBS [49; 50; 52; 53], MS [52; 53], and MTHFR [49]. Because of its exceptionally low pK_a value (Table 1), Hcy-thiolactone is neutral at physiological pH and thus can diffuse out of the cell (Figure 1) and accumulate in the extracellular fluids [49; 50; 51; 54; 55]. Hcy-thiolactone is hydrolyzed to Hcy by intracellular [56] and extracellular Hcy-thiolactonases [57; 58; 59; 60], previously known as bleomycin hydrolase (BLH) and paraoxonase 1 (PON1), respectively. Because of the oxidative environment in the blood, extracellular Hcy forms disulfides, mostly with serum proteins [38; 57] such as albumin [34] and globulins [61], and only ~1% of plasma total Hcy exists in a free reduced form in humans [62]. Furthermore, as discussed in a greater detail in the following sections of this chapter, Hcy-thiolactone reacts spontaneously with proteins, forming N-Hcy-proteins (Figure 1), which are recognized as neo-self antigens by the immune system.

The Mechanism of Protein N-Homocysteinylation

Fundamental physical-chemical properties of Hcy (Table 1) underlie its ability to undergo metabolic conversion to Hcy-thiolactone. During protein biosynthesis Hcy is often mistakenly selected in place of Met by MetRS and metabolized to Hcy-thiolactone in an error-editing reaction according to Equation (1) [44; 55; 66].

$$\text{MetRS} + \text{Hcy} + \text{ATP} \overset{-PP_i}{\Longleftrightarrow} \text{MetRS} \bullet \text{Hcy} \sim \text{AMP} \overset{-AMP}{\Longrightarrow} \text{Hcy-thiolactone} + \text{MetRS} \quad (1)$$

It should be noted that the high energy of the anhydrate bond of ATP is conserved in the thioester bond of Hcy-thiolactone, which is responsible for the chemical reactivity of Hcy-thiolactone (Table 1). Thus, Hcy-thiolactone spontaneously modifies proteins by forming *N*-Hcy-protein adducts, in which Hcy is *N*-linked to the ε-amino group of protein lysine residues as shown in Equation (2) [38; 46; 50].

$$(2)$$

These two reactions, studied extensively *in vitro* in model systems and *ex vivo* in cultured cells [38; 46; 47; 48; 50], are relevant *in vivo*, as demonstrated in humans and mice [49; 53; 54; 61; 67]. Protein N-homocysteinylation is a novel example of protein modification reaction that expands the biological repertoire of known protein modifications by other metabolites, such as glucose, products of lipid peroxidation, or certain drugs, such as penicillin or aspirin [38]. These protein modification reactions have two common aspects: a) each involves protein lysine residues as sites of modifications, and b) are linked to human pathological conditions, including diabetes, vascular disease, Alzheimer's disease, or drug allergy or intolerance [38]. The primary focus of this chapter is on the mechanism of generation of protein N-linked Hcy epitopes in humans and their immunogenic properties.

The Molecular Mechanism of Hcy-Thiolactone Synthesis

In living organisms, the formation of Hcy-thiolactone is a consequence of error-editing reactions of aminoacyl-tRNA synthetases [44; 45; 47; 48; 68; 69; 70; 71]. Because of its similarity to protein amino acids Met, leucine, and isoleucine, the non-protein amino acid Hcy poses a selectivity problem in protein biosynthesis. Indeed, Hcy enters the first step of protein biosynthesis and forms Hcy-AMP with methionyl-, leucyl-, and isoleucyl-tRNA synthetases [72] [72a]. However, misactivated Hcy is not transferred to tRNA [65], and thus cannot enter the genetic code. Instead, Hcy-AMP is destroyed by editing activities of these aminoacyl-tRNA synthetases [44; 66], as shown in Equation (1). Hcy editing is universal, occurs in all organisms investigated, including bacteria [53; 72; 73; 74] [72a], yeast [52; 53; 75], plants [76], mice [36; 49], and humans [36; 49; 53; 54; 67], and prevents direct access of Hcy to the genetic code [44; 45; 46; 47; 48].

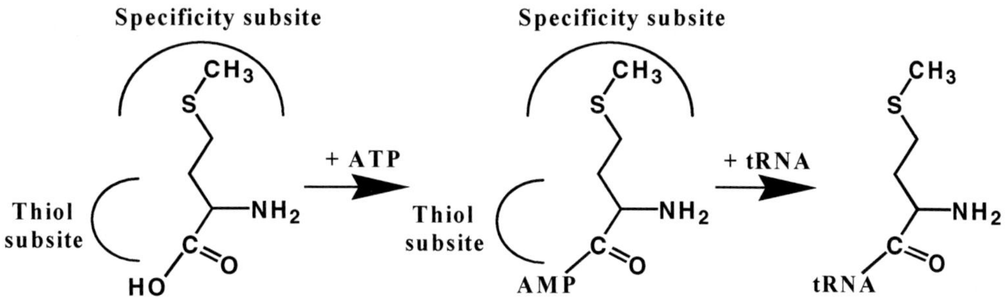

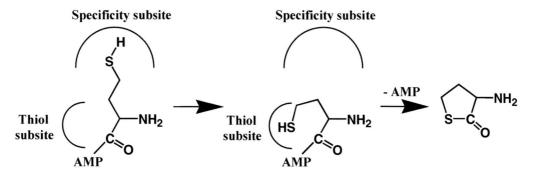

Figure 2. The aminoacylation of tRNA with Met catalyzed by MetRS.

Figure 3. The formation of Hcy-thiolactone during Hcy editing catalyzed by MetRS.

Although studied in several systems [77], molecular mechanism of Hcy editing is best understood for *E. coli* MetRS [78; 79; 80]. The Hcy editing reaction occurs in the synthetic/editing active site [78]], whose major function is to carry out the synthesis of Met-tRNA [80]. Whether an amino acid completes the synthetic or editing pathway is determined by the partitioning of its side chain between the specificity and thiol-binding sub-sites of the synthetic/editing active site [79]. A sub-site that binds carboxyl and α-amino groups of cognate or non-cognate substrates does not appear to contribute to specificity [78].

Methionine completes the synthetic pathway because its side chain is firmly bound by the hydrophobic and hydrogen bonding interactions with the specificity sub-site (Figure 2). Crystal structure of MetRS-Met complex [80] reveals that hydrophobic interactions involve side chains of Tyr15, Trp253, Pro257, and Tyr260; Trp305 closes the bottom of the hydrophobic pocket, but is not in the contact with the methyl group of the substrate methionine. The sulfur of the substrate methionine makes two hydrogen bonds: one with the hydroxyl of Tyr260 and the other with the backbone amide of Leu13.

The non-cognate substrate Hcy, missing the methyl group of methionine, cannot interact with the specificity sub-site as effectively as cognate methionine does. This allows the side chain of Hcy to move to the thiol-binding sub-site, which promotes the synthesis of the thioester bond during editing (Figure 3). Mutations of Tyr15 and Trp305 affect Hcy/Met discrimination by the enzyme [78]. Asp52, which forms a hydrogen bond with the α-amino group of the substrate methionine, deduced from the crystal structure of MetRS·Met complex [80], is involved in the catalysis of both synthetic and editing reactions, but does not contribute to substrate specificity of the enzyme. The substitution Asp52Ala inactivates the synthetic and editing functions of MetRS [65; 78; 79].

Futrhermore, the thiol-binding sub-site also supports the ability of MetRS to edit in trans, *i.e.*, to catalyze thioester bond formation between a thiol and the cognate methionine (Figure 4). With CoA-SH or cysteine as a thiol substrate, MetRS catalyzes the formation of Met-*S*-CoA thioesters [81] and Met-Cys di-peptides [79], respectively. The formation of Met-Cys di-peptide proceeds *via* a Met-*S*-Cys thioester intermediate, which spontaneously rearranges to the Met-Cys di-peptide. Remarkably, the formation of Met-Cys di-peptide as a result of editing in trans, is as fast as the formation of Hcy-thiolactone during Hcy editing.

Hcy-Thiolactone is Synthesized by Methionyl-tRNA Synthetase in Human Cells

As discussed above, the biosynthesis of Hcy-thiolactone *via* the Hcy editing pathway has been originally discovered in microorganisms, such as *Escherichia coli* [73] and the yeast *Saccharomyces cerevisiae* [52]. The first indication that Hcy-thiolactone is a significant component of Hcy metabolism in mammals, including humans, came with the discovery that Hcy-thiolactone is synthesized by cultured mammalian cells, such as human cervical carcinoma (HeLa), mouse adenocarcinoma (RAG), and Chinese hamster ovary (CHO) [55]. We also demonstrated that a temperature-sensitive MetRS mutant of CHO cells fails to synthesize Hcy-thiolactone at the non-permissive temperature, which indicates that MetRS is involved in Hcy-thiolactone formation in CHO cells [55].

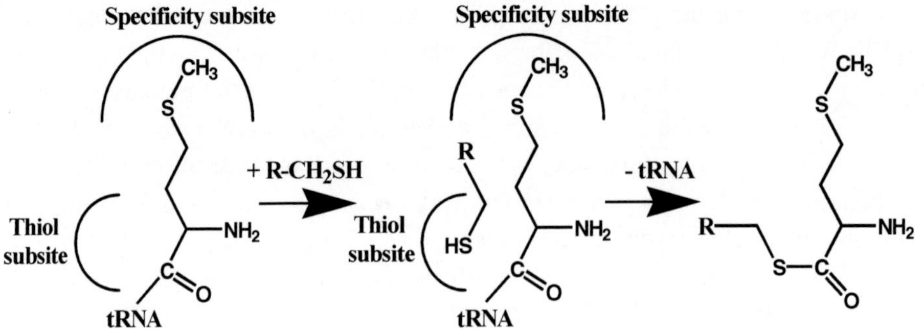

Figure 4. Editing in *trans*: The formation of methionyl thioesters catalyzed by MetRS.

Subsequent work has shown that human diploid fibroblasts in which Hcy metabolism has been deregulated by mutations in the *CBS* gene produced more Hcy-thiolactone than wild type fibroblasts [50]. Furthermore, supplementation of CBS-deficient and wild type human fibroblasts, and human breast cancer (HTB-132) cells with the anti-folate drug aminopterin, which prevents remethylation of Hcy to methionine by methionine synthase, greatly enhances Hcy-thiolactone synthesis. In general, human cancer cells produce more Hcy-thiolactone than normal cells [50; 55; 69].

Further experiments with cultured human umbilical vein vascular endothelial cells (HUVEC) suggest that Hcy-thiolactone synthesis is important in human vascular tissues [51].

These experiments have shown that in the presence of physiological concentrations of Hcy, methionine, and folic acid, HUVEC efficiently metabolize Hcy to Hcy-thiolactone. The extent of Hcy-thiolactone synthesis in human endothelial cells is directly proportional to Hcy, and inversely proportional to methionine, concentrations, consistent with the involvement of MetRS.

Although folates are utilized in Hcy metabolism and DNA synthesis, it appears that folic acid limitation predominantly impacts Hcy metabolism, but not DNA metabolism, in endothelial cells. For example, physiological levels of folic acid (26 nM) present in the M199 media used in our studies are insufficient for transmethylation of Hcy to methionine and, as a result, Hcy is mostly converted to Hcy-thiolactone, while very little methionine is synthesized in these cells [51]. However, these levels of folic acid support endothelial cells growth when methionine is also present, which means that they are sufficient for DNA synthesis. Supplementation of endothelial cell cultures with folic acid redirects Hcy to the transmethylation pathway, which results in lower synthesis of Hcy-thiolactone and greater synthesis of methionine. The synthesis of Hcy-thiolactone in endothelial cell cultures is also inhibited by the supplementation with high-density lipoprotein (HDL) [51], which carries PON1 protein exhibiting Hcy-thiolactone hydrolyzing activity [57; 58; 59; 60].

Hcy-Thiolactone is Elevated in Hyperhomocysteinemic Humans and Mice

The findings that cultured human cells, including vascular endothelial cells, have the ability to metabolize Hcy to Hcy-thiolactone suggest that Hcy-thiolactone is likely to be synthesized *in vivo* in humans and animals. With the recent developments of highly selective and sensitive HPLC-based assays [53; 67], the demonstration of the *in vivo* relevance of Hcy-thiolactone became possible. In particular, the Hcy-thiolactone hypothesis [36] predicts that Hcy-thiolactone will be elevated under conditions predisposing to vascular disease, such as hyperhomocysteinemia. As described in the following sections, this prediction has recently been confirmed *in vivo* in humans and mice.

Human Genetic Hyperhomocysteinemia

It is well established that genetic deficiencies in the *CBS* or *MTHFR* gene lead to great elevation of plasma tHcy levels in humans and mice [16]. However, it was not known whether these genetic deficiencies affect Hcy-thiolactone levels. To answer this question we studied 14 patients with homocystinuria due to homozygous mutations in the CBS gene, 4 patients with hyperhomocysteinemia due to a homozygous mutation in the *MTHFR* gene, 6 unaffected siblings heterozygous for the *MTHFR* mutation, and 9 healthy unrelated subjects. We found that the CBS deficiency in humans leads to elevation of Hcy-thiolactone levels: mean plasma Hcy-thiolactone concentration in CBS deficient patients (14.4 nM) was 72-fold higher than in normal subjects [49]. This finding is consistent with my previous *ex vivo* observations that cultured human CBS-deficient fibroblasts synthesize more Hcy-thiolactone than normal fibroblasts [50].

We also found that 5-methyltetrahydofolate deficiency, caused by the MTHFR mutation leads to elevation of Hcy-thiolactone levels in humans: plasma Hcy-thiolactone in MTHFR-deficient patients (11.8 nM) was 24- or 59-fold higher than in MTHFR heterozygous or normal individuals, respectively [49]. This *in vivo* finding is consistent with our previous *ex vivo* observations that limiting availability of folic acid greatly enhances Hcy-thiolactone synthesis in human fibroblasts [50] and vascular endothelial cells [51]. It should be noted that, because MTHFR-deficient patients, like CBS-deficient patients, were on Hcy-lowering therapy, their Hcy-thiolactone concentrations represent minimal values. In one patient for whom samples were obtained before therapy, the therapy resulted in lowering plasma Hcy-thiolactone from 47.3 nM to 16.6 nM (tHcy was lowered from 208 μM before therapy to 66.2 μM after therapy) [49].

Mouse Dietary Hyperhomocysteinemia

Feeding a high methionine diet over extended periods of time is often used as a useful model of experimental hyperhomocysteinemia and atherosclerosis [14; 25; 26]. We found that plasma and urinary Hcy-thiolactone levels in mice fed a normal diet have a mean value of 3.7 nM and 140 nM, respectively [49]. We also found that a high methionine diet causes 3.7-fold and 25-fold increases in plasma and urinary Hcy-thiolactone, respectively, in mice. The distributions of Hcy-thiolactone between plasma and urine in mice fed a normal diet and humans are similar: much higher Hcy-thiolactone concentrations accumulate in urine than in plasma (urinary/plasma Hcy-thiolactone is 37 in mice [49] and 100 in humans [54]). This shows that urinary clearances of Hcy-thiolactone in mice and humans are similar, and that in mice, like in humans [54], >95% of the filtered Hcy-thiolactone is excreted in the urine. Furthermore, significantly higher urinary/plasma Hcy-thiolactone ratios are found in mice fed hyperhomocysteinemic diets than in the animals fed a normal diet. This finding suggests that urinary clearance of Hcy-thiolactone is much more efficient in hyperhomocysteinemic mice, compared to animals with normal tHcy levels.

Protein Lysine Residues are Targets for the Modification by Hcy-Thiolactone

Hcy-thiolactone is a novel Hcy metabolite, discovered in living organisms in the 1990's. Thus, although its propensity to react with primary amino groups has been recognized shortly after its chemical synthesis in the 1930's, the reactions of Hcy-thiolactone with proteins remained virtually unexplored, until the end of 1990's [46].

The discovery that Hcy-thiolactone and proteins containing N-linked Hcy (*N*-Hcy-protein) are formed by cultured mammalian, including human, cells has led to a hypothesis that the chemical reactivity of Hcy-thiolactone may underlie the involvement of Hcy in the pathology of human vascular disease [50]. This in turn prompted detailed studies of the reactions of Hcy-thiolactone with proteins [35; 36; 38; 46; 50; 70; 71; 82].

Initial studies have established that [^{35}S]Hcy-thiolactone added to human or animal serum disappears with a half-life of is from 0.25-1.5 hours, depending on the source of serum. I found that the disappearance of Hcy-thiolactone in serum is due to two major reactions: the formation of an *N*-Hcy-protein adduct, in which Hcy is attached *via* an isopeptide bond to the ε-amino group of a protein lysine residue (Equation 2) [38; 50], and enzymatic hydrolysis by serum paraoxonase/Hcy-thiolactonase to Hcy, which then forms a mixed protein-S-S-Hcy disulfide, mostly with the Cys34 of serum albumin (Figure 1) [38; 57; 58; 71; 82]. In the presence of [^{35}S]Hcy-thiolactone, each individual human or rabbit serum protein becomes *N*-homocysteinylated in proportion to its abundance in serum [38].

Hcy-thiolactone has a propensity to modify amino groups of free amino acids, albeit less efficiently than free lysine [50]. However, only the side chain amino groups of lysine residues in proteins, but not any other amino acid residues, are modified by Hcy-thioalctone [38; 71; 82]. In particular, Hcy-thiolactone does not appreciably react with the side chains of arginine, histidine, serine, or thereonine. Moreover, the N-terminal α-amino group in human serum albumin, hemoglobin, cytochrome *c*, or fibrinogen does not appear to react with Hcy-thiolactone. Using proteomic approaches only internal lysine residues were identified as targets for Hcy-thiolactone modification [42; 83; 84].

Second order rate constants for reactions of Hcy-thiolactone with individual purified proteins indicate that *N*-homocysteinylation is relatively robust and goes to completion within a few hours at physiological conditions of pH and temperature. A major determinant of the reactivity of most proteins with Hcy-thiolactone is their lysine content. For proteins that vary in size from 104 to 698 amino acid residues there is a very good correlation (r = 0.97) between protein's lysine content and its reactivity with Hcy-thiolactone. Larger proteins, such as fibrinogen (3588 amino acid residues) and low-density lipoproteins (LDL) (~5,000 amino acid residues), react with Hcy-thiolactone ~6-fold less efficiently than expected from their lysine contents. Of many lysine residues present in a protein only a few are predominant sites for the modification by Hcy-thiolactone, as has been shown for albumin [83], hemoglobin (H. Jakubowski, unpublished data), fibrinogen [42], and cytochrome c [84].

Protein *N*-Linked Hcy is a By-Product of Human Hcy Metabolism

Evidence from Tissue Culture Studies

The first indication that protein N-linked Hcy is likely to be an important component of Hcy metabolism in humans came from studies of Hcy-thiolactone metabolism in human tissue cultures [50]. Proteins from normal and CBS-deficient fibroblasts and breast cancer cells have been shown to contain small amounts of protein N-linked Hcy (0.4 to 2.4% relative to protein methionine). When metabolic conversion of Hcy to methionine was inhibited by the anti-folate drug aminopterin, the amounts of Hcy, Hcy-thiolactone, *and* protein N-linked Hcy increased [50].

Further experiments with cultured human umbilical vein endothelial cells provide evidence that the formation protein N-linked Hcy is likely to be important in human vascular tissues [51]. These experiments show that the formation of protein N-linked Hcy occurs concomitantly with the synthesis of Hcy-thiolactone in the presence of physiological concentrations of Hcy, methionine, and folic acid. Like the levels of Hcy-thiolactone, levels of protein N-linked Hcy are directly proportional to Hcy, and inversely proportional to methionine concentrations. Supplementation of endothelial cell cultures with folic acid inhibits the synthesis of extracellular and intracellular protein N-linked Hcy by facilitating the conversion of Hcy to methionine, thereby indirectly preventing synthesis of Hcy-thiolactone by methionyl-tRNA synthetase. The formation of extracellular, but not intracellular, protein N-linked Hcy in endothelial cell cultures is inhibited by supplementation with HDL [51], which carries an Hcy-thiolactone-hydrolyzing enzyme, paraoxonase 1 [57; 58; 59; 60].

The mode of Hcy incorporation into endothelial cell protein has been established by using Edman degradation, a classic protein chemistry procedure which releases from proteins amino acids having free α-amino group. About half of total Hcy incorporated into protein was found to be sensitive to Edman degradation [45; 51], suggesting that Hcy incorporation is due to reactions of Hcy-thiolactone with protein lysine residues (Equation 2) [38; 50]. The presence of a fraction of N-Hcy-protein that is resistant to Edman degradation suggests that translational, S-$nitroso$-Hcy-mediated, incorporation of Hcy into protein [65] also occurs in endothelial cell cultures.

Protein N-Linked Hcy is Present in Humans

To examine a possibility that N-Hcy-protein is relevant *in vivo* in the human body, I developed a highly selective and sensitive HPLC-based methods for the determination of protein N-linked Hcy [61] [61a]. The initial sample workup removes free and disulfide-linked Hcy by extensive treatments with the reducing agent dithiothreitol. The method is based on a quantitative conversion of protein N-linked Hcy to Hcy-thiolactone, which is achieved by acid hydrolysis under reducing conditions (in the presence of dithiothreitol). Hcy-thiolactone is then purified and quantified by HPLC on a cation exchange column direct UV detection (at A_{240}) [61] or fluorescence detection after post-column derivatization with orthophtaldialdehyde [61a].

That protein N-linked Hcy is present in human plasma proteins was first described in 2000 [82]. Subsequent studies have shown that protein N-linked Hcy occurs in all purified individual proteins examined so far [61]. The highest amounts of protein N-linked Hcy, 50 mol%, are present in human and equine ferritins [61a]. In human blood, 0.36-0.6 mol% of protein N-linked Hcy is present in hemoglobin, serum albumin, and γ-globulins, respectively. Other human serum proteins, such as fibrinogen, LDL, HDL, transferrin, and antitrypsin contain from 0.04 to 0.1 % of protein N-linked Hcy. N-Hcy-hemoglobin, present in normal blood at a concentration of 12.7 μM, constitutes a major Hcy pool in the human blood [61]. Interestingly, rodents have more N-linked Hcy in their blood proteins that humans [61a].

Although the levels of protein N-linked Hcy in individual human blood proteins correlate with the reactivity of these proteins toward Hcy-thiolactone [61], protein N-linked Hcy may also arise by *S-nitroso*-Hcy-mediated translational mechanism, in which Hcy substitutes a protein methionine residue [45]. However, the presence of protein N-linked Hcy in pig albumin [61], which does not contain methionine, strongly suggests that Hcy-thiolactone-mediated mechanism is responsible for Hcy incorporation.

Protein N-Linked Hcy is Elevated in Hyperhomocysteinemia and is Associated with Coronary Artery Disease (CAD) in Humans

The Hcy-thiolactone hypothesis [36] predicts that protein N-homocysteinylation will be elevated under conditions conducive to atherosclerosis, such as hyperhomocysteinemia. The verification of this prediction became possible with the development of sensitive chemical [61] and immunological assays [85] for protein N-linked Hcy in humans. Indeed, as predicted by the Hcy-thiolactone hypothesis, protein N-linked Hcy is elevated in subjects with genetic hyperhomocysteinemia [45; 61; 71; 82].

I found that human plasma contains from 0.1 to 13 μM protein N-linked Hcy, which represents up to 25% of plasma total Hcy [61]. Plasma concentrations of protein N-linked Hcy correlate positively with tHcy, suggesting that plasma tHcy level is a determinant of protein N-linked Hcy level. Interestingly, in some subjects, plasma levels of protein N-linked Hcy are lower than expected from their tHcy content; this suggests that factors other than tHcy can affect plasma protein N-linked Hcy levels [61]. A likely candidate for a determinant of plasma protein N-linked Hcy levels, is Hcy-thiolactonase activity [57; 59; 60], which has been shown to affect the formation of protein N-linked Hcy in HUVEC cultures [51] and in human serum *in vitro* [58].

We found that plasma protein N-linked Hcy levels are significantly elevated in CBS- or MTHFR-deficient patients and that CBS-deficient patients have significantly elevated levels of pro-thrombotic *N*-Hcy-fibrinogen [130]. These findings provide an explanation for increased atherothrombosis observed in CBS-deficient patients. Furthermore, plasma protein N-linked Hcy is elevated 10-fold in mice fed a pro-atherogenic high-methionine diet [131]. Inactivation of *Cbs*, *Mthfr*, or the proton coupled folate transporter (*Pcft*) gene in mice results in 19- to 30-fold increase in plasma protein N-linked Hcy levels [131]. These finding provide evidence that protein N-linked Hcy is an important metabolite associated with Hcy pathophysiology in humans and mice.

Other investigators have studied protein N-homocysteinylation in uremic patients [86; 87] to explain a link between hyperhomocysteinemia and higher cardiovascular risk and mortality observed in these patients [88]. Significantly higher protein N-linked Hcy levels were found in hyperhomocysteinemic uremic patients on hemodialysis than in control subjects [86; 87]. Interestingly, protein N-linked Hcy comprises less tHcy in hemodialysis patients than in control subjects [86; 87]. Similarly, protein N-linked Hcy comprises less tHcy in patients with higher plasma tHcy (50-120 μM) than in patients with lower plasma tHcy (5-40 μM) [61]. The lower protein N-linked Hcy/tHcy ratios suggest that the Hcy-thiolactone clearance is more effective at higher tHcy levels. This suggestion is supported by a finding that in mice fed a hyperhomocysteinemic high Met or Hcy diet urinary/plasma Hcy-thiolactone is 7-fold or 4-fold higher, respectively, compared to mice fed a normal diet [49].

Hyperhomocysteinemia in CAD patients is linked with increased mortality in these patients [23]. In one clinical study which examined a relationship between Hcy and coronary heart disease, plasma protein N-linked Hcy levels, like tHcy levels, were significantly higher in coronary heart disease patients than in controls [85]. Furthermore, there was a weak but significant positive correlation between protein N-linked Hcy level and the number of diseased coronary arteries: the higher protein N-linked Hcy level the greater the number of afflicted arteries.

Using polyclonal rabbit anti-*N*-Hcy-protein IgG antibodies [89], we have demonstrated that *N*-Hcy-protein is present in human cardiac tissues [90]. For example, we observed positive immunohistochemical staining of myocardium and aorta samples from cardiac surgery patients. Control experiments have demonstrated that the staining was specific for *N*-Hcy-protein. No immunostaining was observed with rabbit preimmune IgG, with iodoacetamide-treated tissues (which destroys the *Nε*-Hcy-Lys epitope), or with the antibody pre-adsorbed with *N*-Hcy-albumin [90]. Further support for a role of *N*-Hcy-protein in atherogenesis is provided by our finding of increased immunohistochemical staining for *N*-Hcy-protein in aortic lesions from ApoE-/- mice with hyperhomocysteinemia induced by a high methionine diet, relative to the mice fed a control chow diet [90].

Modification by Hcy-Thiolactone Causes Protein Damage

In proteins that were studied thus far, usually a few lysine residues are predominant targets for the modification by Hcy-thiolactone. For example, Lys525 [83] is a predominant site of albumin N-homocysteinylation *in vitro* and *in vivo*. Four lysine residues of cytochrome c (Lys8 or 13, Lys 86 or 87, Lys 99, and Lys 100) are susceptible to N-homocysteinylation [84]. Twelve lysine residues of fibrinogen (7 in Aα chain, 2 in Bβ chain and 3 in γ chain) were found to be susceptible to the modification by Hcy-thiolactone [42]. Four lysine residues (Lys16, Lys56 in α chain and Lys59, Lys95 in β chain) are predominant sites of N-homocysteinylation in hemoglobin (H. Jakubowski, unpublished).

The acylation of a basic ε-amino group of a protein lysine residue (pK=10.5) by Hcy-thiolactone generates an *Nε*-Hcy-Lys residue containing a much less basic amino group (pK~7) and a free thiol group (*Eq.* 1). This substitution is expected to significantly alter protein structure and function. Indeed, hemoglobin, albumin [83], and cytochrome c [38] are sensitive to *N*-homocysteinylation; incorporation of one Hcy/mol protein induces gross structural alterations in these proteins. For instance, *N*-Hcy-cytochrome c becomes resistant to proteolytic degradation (by trypsin, chymotrypsin, and pronase) [84] and susceptible to aggregation due to intermolecular disulfide bond formation [38], which also interferes with the red-ox state of the heme iron by rendering it reduced [84]. *N*-Hcy-hemoglobin, in contrast to unmodified hemoglobin, is susceptible to further irreversible damage by oxidation. Of the two physiological forms of human albumin, albumin-Cys34-S-S-Cys (containing cysteine in a disulfide linkage with Cys34 of albumin) is modified by Hcy-thiolactone faster than mercaptoalbumin (containing a free thiol at Cys34). Hcy-thiolactone-modified and unmodified forms of albumin exhibit different susceptibilities to proteolytic degradation by trypsin, chymotrypsin, or elastase [83].

Other proteins are inactivated only by incorporation of multiple Hcy residues. For example, complete loss of enzymatic activity occurs after N-homocysteinylation of eight lysine residues in MetRS (33% of total lysine residues) or eleven lysine residues in trypsin (88% of total lysine residues) [38]. Furthermore, extensively N-homocysteinylated proteins, such as fibrinogen, transferin, globulins, myoglobin, RNase A, and trypsin are prone to multimerization and undergo gross structural changes that lead to their denaturation and precipitation [38]. Chicken egg lysozyme is also denatured by extensive N-homocysteinylation [91].

N-Hcy-LDL, in which 10% or 25% lysine residues have been modified (i. e., containing 36 and 89 mol Hcy/mol LDL), is taken up and degraded by human monocyte-derived macrophages significantly faster than native LDL [92]. However, N-Hcy-LDL containing eight molecules of Hcy/mol LDL is taken up and degraded by leukemic L2C guinea pig lymphocytes to the same extent as native LDL via the high affinity LDL-specific receptor pathway [93].

Hcy-thiolactone may also inactivate enzymes by other mechanisms. For example, lysine oxidase, an important enzyme responsible for post-translational collagen modification essential for the biogenesis of connective tissue matrices, is inactivated by micromolar concentrations of Hcy-thiolactone, which derivatizes the active site tyrosinequinone cofactor with a half-life of 4 min [94].

Chronic Treatments with Hcy-Thiolactone are Harmful

As predicted by the Hcy-thiolactone hypothesis [36] [37a, 37b], chronic treatments of animals with Hcy-thiolactone cause pathophysiological changes similar to those observed in human genetic hyperhomocysteinemia. For example, Hcy-thiolactone infusions in baboons [95] or Hcy-thiolactone-supplemented diet in rats [96] produce atherosclerosis. Treatments with Hcy-thiolactone cause developmental abnormalities in chick embryos [97], including optic lens dislocation [98], a characteristic diagnostic feature present in the CBS-deficient human patients [16; 17; 18]. However, rabbits, which have the highest levels of serum Hcy-thiolactonase/PON1, and thus efficiently detoxify Hcy-thiolactone [57; 58; 71], are resistant to detrimental effects of Hcy-thiolactone infusions [99; 100].

Immunogenic Properties of Hcy-Thiolactone-Modified Proteins

Hcy-thiolactone-mediated incorporation of Hcy into protein (*Equation* 2) can impact cellular physiology through many routes. Protein modification by Hcy-thiolactone can disrupt protein folding, and create altered proteins with newly acquired interactions, or can lead to induction of autoimmune responses. During the folding process, proteins form their globular native states in a manner determined by their primary amino acid sequence [101; 102]. Thus, small changes in amino acid sequence caused by Hcy incorporation have the potential to create misfolded protein aggregates. Indeed, N-Hcy-proteins have a propensity to form protein aggregates [38]. Furthermore, the appearance of misfolded/aggregated proteins in the endoplasmic reticulum (ER) activates an unfolded protein response (UPR) signaling pathway, that, when overwhelmed, leads to cell death *via* apoptosis. Protein aggregates are known to be inherently toxic [103]. The toxicity of N-Hcy-LDL, which in contrast to native LDL, has the propensity to aggregate [92] and induces cell death in cultured human endothelial cells [40], is consistent with this concept. These pathways can be induced in cultured human endothelial cells and in mice by elevating Hcy [104; 105; 106; 107], which also elevates Hcy-thiolactone [49; 51]. Moreover, treatments with Hcy-thiolactone induce ER stress and UPR in retinal epithelial cells [108], as well as apoptotic death in cultured human vascular endothelial cells [39; 41]. In this scenario the formation of N-Hcy-proteins leads to the UPR and induction of the apoptotic pathway. Proteolytic degradation of N-Hcy-proteins can generate potentially antigenic peptides, which can be displayed on cell surface and induce adaptive immune response.

Atherosclerosis is now widely recognized as a chronic inflammatory disease that involves innate and adaptive immunity [7; 10; 11]. That inflammation is important is supported by studies showing that increased plasma concentration of markers of inflammation, such as C-reactive protein, interleukin-1, serum amyloid A, and soluble adhesion molecules are independent predictors of vascular events [9]. Autoantibodies against modified LDL were found to be elevated in vascular disease patients in some, but not all studies [12; 13]. Lipid peroxidation is thought to play a central role in the initiation of both cellular and humoral responses. Reactive aldehydes resulting from phospholipid peroxidation, such as malondialdehyde, 4-hydroxynonenal, and 1-palmitoyl-2-(5-oxovaleroyl)-*sn*-glycero-3-phosphocholine can modify lysine residues in LDL and in other proteins. The resulting oxidized lipids-protein adducts, e.g., malondialdehyde-LDL, carry neo-self epitopes which are recognized by specific innate and adaptive immune responses. As will be discussed in the following sections of this chapter, protein N-homocysteinylation by Hcy-thiolactone [35; 36] also appears to play an important role.

N-Hcy-Proteins are Immunogenic

By generating structurally altered proteins, the modification by Hcy-thiolactone, like other chemical modifications, such as glycation, acetylation, methylation, ethylation, carbamylation [7], can render proteins particularly immunogenic. Indeed, intradermal inoculations of rabbits with N-Hcy-LDL induces the synthesis of anti-N-Hcy-LDL antibodies in these animals [109]. Furthermore, immunization of rabbits with Hcy-thiolactone-modified keyhole limpet hemocyanin (KHL) leads to generation of antibodies that bind to N-Hcy-LDL [89; 110]. Of considerable interest are the observations that antisera from such immunizations bound not only to the N-Hcy-LDL but to a variety of other human proteins on which the N-linked Hcy epitope was present, such as N-Hcy-albumin, N-Hcy-hemoglobin, N-Hcy-transferrin, N-Hcy-antitrypsin, but not to native unmodified proteins. $N\varepsilon$-Hcy-$N\alpha$-acetyl-Lys, but not $N\varepsilon$-acetyl-$N\alpha$-Hcy-Lys, prevented the rabbit antibodies from binding to human N-Hcy-hemoglobin. This shows that the rabbit IgG specifically recognizes Hcy linked by isopeptide bond to ε-amino group of protein lysine residue; Hcy linked by peptide bond to α-amino group is not recognized. The rabbit antibodies bind short peptides containing the $N\varepsilon$-Hcy-Lys epitop. Hcy, Hcy-thiolactone, lysine, or unmodified lysine derivatives not are bound by the rabbit anti-N-Hcy-protein antibodies [110]. Furthermore, pre-immune rabbit serum exhibits significant titers of autoantibodies against N-Hcy-albumin [H. Jakubowski unpublished], which suggests that endogenous N-Hcy-proteins present in rabbit blood [61] are autoantigenic. Taken together, these data suggest that autoantibodies, once formed *in vivo* in response to N-Hcy-LDL would be capable of binding to endogenous N-Hcy-proteins.

An Auto-Immune Response to *N*-Hcy-Proteins in Humans

To determine whether N-Hcy-proteins are autoimmunogenic in humans, human sera were assayed for the presence of antibodies binding to N-Hcy-hemoglobin as an antigen. We found that each human serum tested showed some titer of IgG [110; 111; 112] and IgM (H. Jakubowski, unpublished a) auto-antibodies against N-Hcy-hemoglobin or N-Hcy-albumin.

The plasma levels of anti-N-Hcy-protein autoantibodies [89; 110; 111; 112] and protein N-linked Hcy [45; 61; 82; 83] vary considerably among individuals and are strongly correlated with plasma Hcy, but not with Cys or Met [110]. Such correlations can be explained by the Hcy-thiolactone hypothesis [36]: elevation in Hcy leads to inadvertent elevation in Hcy-thiolactone, observed *ex vivo* in human fibroblasts [50] and endothelial cells [51; 53], and *in vivo* in humans [49; 53; 54; 67] and mice [36; 49]. Hcy-Thiolactone mediates Hcy incorporation into proteins and the formation of neo-self antigens, $N\varepsilon$-Hcy-Lys-protein (**Eq. 1**). Raising levels of neo-self $N\varepsilon$-Hcy-Lys epitopes on proteins trigger an autoimmune response. The presence of IgM and IgG autoantibodies against N-Hcy-proteins in human blood [35; 36] suggest that Hcy incorporation into proteins triggers both innate and an adaptive immune response in humans.

Antigen Specificity of the Human Anti-*N*-Hcy-Proteins Autoantibodies

The anti-N-Hcy-protein IgG autoantibodies specifically recognize an $N\varepsilon$-Hcy-Lys epitope on N-homocysteinylated human proteins, such as N-Hcy-hemoglobin, N-Hcy-albumin, N-Hcy-transferrin, and N-Hcy-antitrypsin. The thiol group of N-linked Hcy is important for binding and proteins containing the $N\varepsilon$-Hcy-Lys epitope with its thiol blocked by the thiol reagent iodoacetamide are not bound by these autoantibaodies. Small molecules, such as $N\varepsilon$-Hcy-Lys, $N\varepsilon$-Hcy-$N\alpha$-acetyl-Lys, and $N\varepsilon$-Hcy-$N\alpha$-acetyl-LysAla are also bound by these autoantibodies, as demonstrated by their effective competition for autoantibody binding to antigen-coated microtiter plate wells [110]. High specificity of these autoantibodies is further demonstrated by our finding that $N\varepsilon$-acetyl-$N\alpha$-Hcy-Lys, in which

Hcy is attached to the α-amino group of lysine instead of the ε-amino group, did not compete with the human IgG binding. Lysine, LysAla, $N\alpha$-acetyl-Lys, Hcy or Hcy-thiolactone also did not compete with the human IgG binding. Taken together, these data suggest that human IgG specifically recognizes $N\varepsilon$-Hcy-Lys epitope on an $N\varepsilon$-Hcy-Lys-protein and that the antigen specificity of the human anti-N-Hcy-protein autoantibodies is essentially identical to the specificity of the rabbit anti-N-Hcy-protein antibodies generated by inoculations with N-Hcy-LDL or N-Hcy-KLH [110].

Anti-*N*-Hcy-Protein Autoantibodies are Associated with Stroke

Innate and adaptive immune responses directed against modified LDL are known to modulate the progression of vascular disease and increased plasma levels of markers of these responses are independent predictors of coronary events [6]. Although plasma levels of autoantibodies against oxidized or glycated LDL are often associated with vascular disease [12; 13], the role of anti-N-Hcy-protein auto-antibodies was unknown. In a case-control study [110], we examined the relation between anti-N-Hcy-protein auto-antibodies and stroke.

Our cohorts of 54 stroke patients (63.4 years old) and 74 healthy controls (66.3 years old) did not differ with respect to triglycerides, total cholesterol and LDL cholesterol levels, whereas HDL cholesterol was lower in stroke patients than in controls. We found significant differences in levels of anti-N-Hcy-protein IgG autoantibodies between the group of 39 male patients with stroke and the group of 29 healthy subjects. Male stroke patients had higher serum anti-N-Hcy-protein IgG levels than healthy controls [110]. Male stroke patients had also higher plasma tHcy than controls, consistent with earlier studies. Thus, both plasma tHcy and anti-N-Hcy-protein IgGs are associated with stroke in male subjects. Plasma levels of tHcy and anti-N-Hcy-protein IgG autoantibody in a group of 17 female stroke patients were similar to corresponding levels in a group of 45 female controls, suggesting that stroke in the female patients may have been caused by factors other than elevated Hcy or cholesterol. Furthermore, we found no differences in plasma cysteine or methionine concentrations between stroke patients and controls both for males and females. Thus, the high levels of anti-N-Hcy-protein autoantibodies in male stroke patients reflect high Hcy levels in these patients.

Anti-*N*-Hcy-Protein Autoantibodies are Associated with CAD

To test a concept that anti-N-Hcy-protein autoantibodies are an important feature of atherosclerosis, we examined the relation between anti-N-Hcy-protein autoantibodies and CAD in male subjects [111]. Our cohort of 88 male patients (45 years old) with angiographically documented CAD had significantly higher plasma levels of triglycerides, total cholesterol and LDL cholesterol, and lower levels of HDL cholesterol, compared to a cohort of 100 healthy male controls (43.5 years old). Significant differences in mean levels of anti-N-Hcy-protein IgG autoantibodies were found between a group of CAD male patients and a group of age-matched controls. Male CAD patients had 47 % higher serum levels of anti-N-Hcy-protein IgG autoantibodies than healthy controls. Levels of anti-N-Hcy-protein IgG were not associated with traditional risk factors. However, there was a weak positive correlation between the autoantibodies and plasma tHcy. Male CAD patients had also higher levels of plasma tHcy than controls, consistent with earlier studies. Thus, the higher levels of anti-N-Hcy-protein autoantibodies that are present in CAD male patients, like in stroke patients, reflect the higher levels of Hcy in these patients.

An age-adjusted risk for CAD related to seropositivity for anti-N-Hcy-protein IgG autoantibodies is 9.87 (95% CI 4.50-21.59, $p<10^{-5}$). In multivariate logistic regression analysis, seropositivity to anti-N-Hcy-protein IgG autoantibodies (OR, 14.82; 95% CI, 4.47 to 49.19; p=0.00002), smoking (OR, 8.84; 95% CI, 2.46 to 31.72; p=0.001), hypertension (OR, 43.45; 95% I, 7.91 to 238.7; p=0.0001), and HDL cholesterol (OR, 0.015; 95% CI, 0.002 to 0.098; p=0.00002 for each unit increase) were independent predictors of early CAD in men <50 years old ($\chi^2=26.17$, $p<10^{-5}$ for the increment in goodness of fit as compared to a three variable model employing smoking, HDL cholesterol, and hypertension). These analyses show that elevated levels of anti-$N\varepsilon$-Hcy-Lys-protein autoantibodies significantly contribute to the risk of CAD in male patients.

Anti-N-Hcy-Protein Autoantibodies are Associated with Uremia

As discussed above, the levels of N-Hcy-protein are elevated in uremic patients on hemodialysis [86; 87]. These finding suggests that an autoimmune response against N-Hcy-protein might also be enhanced in these patients. This possibility was examined in a group of 43 patients (58.8 years old) who were on maintenance hemodialysis for an average of 50 months and an age and sex matched group of 31 apparently healthy individuals [113]. Significantly higher levels of anti-N-Hcy-protein IgG autoantibodies were found in the hemodiallysis patients, compared with controls. Like in our previous studies [110], the levels of anti-N-Hcy-protein IgG autoantibodies were strongly correlated with plasma total Hcy, both in hemodialysis patients and in controls. Among the hemodialysis patients, a subgroup of survivors of myocardial infarction (n=14) had significantly higher levels of anti-N-Hcy-protein IgG autoantibodies than a subgroup of hemodialysis patients without a history of CAD (n=29) [113]. Taken together, these data suggest that an autoimmune response against N-Hcy-proteins contributes to the development of CAD in hemodialysis patients.

Hyperhomocysteinemia, N-Hcy-Protein, and an Innate Immune Response

We also found that the levels of anti-N-Hcy-protein autoantibodies are weakly, but significantly, correlated with plasma CRP levels (r=0.24, p=0.002) [111]. This finding suggests that N-Hcy-protein can also elicit an innate immune response. Many investigators, but not all [114; 115; 116], have linked Hcy to immune responses. For example, a weak, but significant, association between plasma total Hcy and CRP was observed in the Framingham Heart Study [117] and in the Physician's Health Study [118]. Holven et al. reported that in humans hyperhomocysteinemia is associated with increased levels of both CRP and interleukin-6 [119]. A similar positive association between Hcy and interleukin-6 was reported in patients with diabetic nephropathy [120]. Importantly, in the Holven et al. study, elevated level of interleukin-6 is observed in hyperhomocysteinemic individuals in the absence of hypercholesterolemia. Plasma total Hcy was positively associated with soluble tumor necrosis factor receptor in the Nurses' Health Study [121]. A positive correlation is observed between plasma tHcy and neopterin (a marker of Th1 type immune response) in Parkinson's disease patients [122]. Elevated Hcy is associated with elevated monocyte chemotactic protein-1 and increased expression of vascular adhesion molecules in humans [123; 124] and rats [125; 126; 127; 128]. Plasma Hcy is a determinant of TNF-α in hypertensive patients [129]. Furthermore, in mice dietary hyperhomocysteinemia is known to trigger atherosclerosis and enhance vascular inflammation, manifested by increased activation of NF-κB in the aorta and kidney, enhanced expression of VCAM-1 and RAGE in the aorta and TNF-α in plasma [14].

How Hcy can trigger these innate inflammatory responses is unknown, However, given that hyperhomocysteinemia causes elevation of Hcy-thiolactone and N-Hcy-protein levels in humans and mice [49], these responses are likely to be caused by N-Hcy-protein, particularly by N-Hcy-LDL. Consistent with this suggestion are the observations that N-Hcy-LDL is highly immunogenic [109], is present in human blood [61], and is taken up by macrophages faster than unmodified LDL [92]. Further studies are needed to elucidate the mechanism of Hcy-induced innate immune responses.

Possible Roles of Anti-N-Hcy-Protein Autoantibodies in Atherosclerosis

Our findings that anti-N-Hcy-protein autoantibodies are elevated in stroke and CAD patients suggest that an autoimmune response against N-Hcy-proteins is an important feature of atherosclerosis [35]. In general, antibodies protect against exogenous pathogens and endogenous altered neo-self molecules to maintain homeostasis by neutralization and clearance. Like autoantibodies against oxidatively modified LDL [7], the anti-N-Hcy-protein autoantibodies can be beneficial or deleterious. For example, the clearing of N-Hcy-protein proteins from circulation by the autoantibodies would be beneficial. On the other hand, binding of the anti-N-Hcy-protein autoantibodies to N-Hcy-proteins [35; 89] in tissues may contribute to the deleterious effects of hyperhomocysteinemia on many organs [16; 17; 18]. For instance, if the neo-self Nε-Hcy-Lys epitopes were present on endothelial cell membrane proteins, anti-N-Hcy-protein autoantibodies would form antigen-antibody complexes on the surface of the vascular wall. Endothelial cells coated with anti-N-Hcy-protein autoantibodies would be taken up by the macrophage *via* the Fc receptor, resulting in injury to the vascular surface. Under chronic exposures to excess Hcy, the neo-self epitopes Nε-Hcy-Lys, which initiate the injury, are formed continuously, and the repeating attempts to repair the damaged vascular wall would lead to an atherosclerotic lesion [35; 36].

Hcy-Lowering Therapy and Anti-N-Hcy-Protein Autoantibodies

If anti-N-Hcy-protein autoantibodies reflect plasma tHcy levels and arise through the mechanisms postulated by the Hcy-thiolactone hypothesis [36], then lowering plasma tHcy by folic acid supplementation should also lower plasma levels of anti-N-Hcy-protein autoantibodies. This prediction was tested in groups of hyperhomocysteinemic (plasma tHcy>15 μM) male patients (n=12) with angiographically documented CAD and healthy men (n=20) [112]. At baseline, the two groups did not differ with respect to age, tHcy, folate, lipid profile, and CRP. As in our two previous studies [110; 111], the baseline levels of anti-N-Hcy-protein autoantibodies were significantly higher in CAD patients than in healthy subjects and plasma tHcy was positively correlated with anti-N-Hcy-protein autoantibodies in both groups (r=0.77 to 0.85, p<0.0001 to 0.002) [112]. Furthermore, folate levels measured prior to folic acid supplementation correlated negatively with anti-N-Hcy-protein autoantibodies in healthy subjects (r=-0.58, p0.008) and in CAD patients (r=-0.9, p<0.0001).

Folic acid supplementation for 3 months or 6 months resulted in significant lowering of plasma tHcy (by 30%) and increased plasma folate levels (by 230%) in our CAD patients and controls, consistent with other Hcy-lowering studies [27; 28; 29; 30]. In healthy subjects, plasma levels of anti-N-Hcy-protein autoantibodies fell significantly (p<0.001) following 3 months (by 38%), and remained at a lower level at 6 months (by 48%), of folic acid supplementation. However, in CAD patients, surprisingly, plasma levels of anti-N-Hcy-protein autoantibodies fell by only 8.5-12% at 3 or 6 months of folic acid supplementation, but this effect was not significant [112]. The effects of Hcy-lowering therapy on anti-N-Hcy-protein autoantibodies suggest that the neo-self N-Hcy-protein antigens respond relatively quickly to changes in Hcy levels and can be cleared in healthy subjects. In contrast, the neo-self N-Hcy-protein antigens appear to persist in CAD patients and not to respond to Hcy lowering therapy. Interestingly, in another study the levels of anti-N-Hcy-protein IgG autoantibodies were found to be similar in groups of uremic patients on hemodialysis who were taking (n=37) or not taking (n=6) folic acid supplementation [113]. These findings suggest that the immune activation caused by protein N-homocysteinylation in uremia and in CAD patients cannot be easily reversed.

Taken together, the effects of Hcy-lowering therapy on anti-N-Hcy-protein autoantibodies support the involvement of Hcy in the synthesis of these autoantibodies according to a mechanism postulated by the Hcy-thiolactone hypothesis [36] (Figure 5).

Furthermore, our findings that lowering plasma Hcy by folic acid supplementation lowers anti-N-Hcy-protein autoantibodies in control subjects, but not in patients with CAD, support the involvement of an autoimmune response in CAD [112]. These findings also suggest that, while primary Hcy-lowering intervention by vitamin supplementation is beneficial, secondary intervention may be ineffective, and may explain at least in part the failure of vitamin therapy to lower cardiovascular events in MI patients [29; 30].

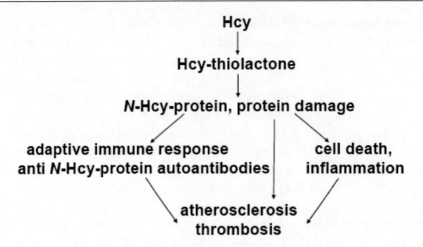

Figure 5. Hcy-thiolactone-mediated incorporation of Hcy into proteins leads to the induction of anti-N-Hcy-protein autoantibodies and is associated with atherosclerosis and thrombosis in humans.

Conclusion

Accumulating evidence suggests that elevated Hcy contributes to adaptive and innate immune responses in atherosclerosis in humans and experimental animals. In this chapter, I have discussed the evidence supporting a concept that the incorporation of Hcy into protein *via* isopetide linkages, causes alterations in the protein's structure and the formation of neo-self antigens that elicit anti-*N*-Hcy-protein autoantibodies, and emphasized their potential importance in vascular disease (Figure 5). Of many known natural Hcy metabolites, only the thioester Hcy-thiolactone can mediate the incorporation of Hcy into proteins *via* stable isopeptide bonds. Protein N-homocysteinylation creates altered proteins with newly acquired interactions, including immunogenic properties. Elevated levels of Hcy-thiolactone and protein N-linked Hcy are observed in genetic and dietary hyperhomocysteinemia in humans and mice. Levels of protein N-linked Hcy are also elevated in CAD patients. Protein N-homocysteinylation leads to the formation of neo-self protein N-linked Hcy epitopes, which cause an immune response in humans, manifested by the induction of anti-*N*-Hcy-protein autoantibodies. Levels of these autoantibodies correlate with plasma total Hcy, are elevated in stroke and CAD patients, and thus may play an important role in atherosclerosis. Primary Hcy-lowering vitamin therapy lowers the levels of anti-*N*-Hcy-protein autoantibodies in healthy subjects. In contrast, secondary vitamin intervention appears to be ineffective in reducing an autoimmune response: it lowers plasma tHcy, but not anti-*N*-Hcy-protein autoantibodies in CAD patients. These results support the Hcy-thiolactone hypothesis, which states that the metabolic conversion of Hcy to Hcy-thiolactone followed by the non-enzymatic protein modification by Hcy-thiolactone is an underlying mechanism that contributes to the pathophysiology of hyperhomocysteinemia. We are only beginning to understand pathophysiological consequences of *N*-Hcy-protein accumulation. Along with other aspects of protein N-homocysteinylation, identifying anti-*N*-Hcy-protein autoantibodies, and understanding their roles in health and disease are likely to yield an understanding of the basic mechanisms that evolved to deal with the consequences of Hcy-thiolactone formation.

References

[1]   E. Braunwald, Shattuck lecture--cardiovascular medicine at the turn of the millennium: triumphs, concerns, and opportunities. *N. Engl. J. Med.* 337 (1997) 1360-9.

[2]   J.T. Willerson, and P.M. Ridker, Inflammation as a cardiovascular risk factor. Circulation 109 (2004) II2-10.

[3]   P. Libby, The forgotten majority: unfinished business in cardiovascular risk reduction. *J. Am. Coll. Cardiol.* 46 (2005) 1225-8.

[4]   J.C. Tardif, T. Heinonen, D. Orloff, and P. Libby, Vascular biomarkers and surrogates in cardiovascular disease. *Circulation* 113 (2006) 2936-42.

[5]   A.J. Lusis, Atherosclerosis. *Nature* 407 (2000) 233-41.

[6]   C.J. Binder, M.K. Chang, P.X. Shaw, Y.I. Miller, K. Hartvigsen, A. Dewan, and J.L. Witztum, Innate and acquired immunity in atherogenesis. *Nat. Med.* 8 (2002) 1218-26.

[7]   C.J. Binder, P.X. Shaw, M.K. Chang, A. Boullier, K. Hartvigsen, S. Horkko, Y.I. Miller, D.A. Woelkers, M. Corr, and J.L. Witztum, The role of natural antibodies in atherogenesis. *J. Lipid. Res.* 46 (2005) 1353-63.

[8]   K. Croce, and P. Libby, Intertwining of thrombosis and inflammation in atherosclerosis. *Curr. Opin. Hematol.* 14 (2007) 55-61.

[9]   P. Libby, Inflammation in atherosclerosis. *Nature* 420 (2002) 868-74.

[10] P. Libby, and P.M. Ridker, Inflammation and atherothrombosis from population biology and bench research to clinical practice. *J. Am. Coll. Cardiol.* 48 (2006) A33-46.

[11] J.S. Forrester, and P. Libby, The inflammation hypothesis and its potential relevance to statin therapy. *Am. J. Cardiol.* 99 (2007) 732-8.

[12] G. Virella, and M.F. Lopes-Virella, Lipoprotein autoantibodies: measurement and significance. *Clin. Diagn. Lab. Immunol.* 10 (2003) 499-505.

[13] G. Virella, S.R. Thorpe, N.L. Alderson, M.B. Derrick, C. Chassereau, J.M. Rhett, and M.F. Lopes-Virella, Definition of the immunogenic forms of modified human LDL recognized by human autoantibodies and by rabbit hyperimmune antibodies. *J. Lipid. Res.* 45 (2004) 1859-67.

[14] M.A. Hofmann, E. Lalla, Y. Lu, M.R. Gleason, B.M. Wolf, N. Tanji, L.J. Ferran, Jr., B. Kohl, V. Rao, W. Kisiel, D.M. Stern, and A.M. Schmidt, Hyperhomocysteinemia enhances vascular inflammation and accelerates atherosclerosis in a murine model. *J. Clin. Invest.* 107 (2001) 675-83.

[15] H. Refsum, E. Nurk, A.D. Smith, P.M. Ueland, C.G. Gjesdal, I. Bjelland, A. Tverdal, G.S. Tell, O. Nygard, and S.E. Vollset, The Hordaland Homocysteine Study: a community-based study of homocysteine, its determinants, and associations with disease. *J. Nutr.* 136 (2006) 1731S-1740S.

[16] S.H. Mudd, H.L. Levy, and K. J.P., Disorders of transsulfuration. in: C.R. Scriver, A.L. Beaudet, W.S. Sly, and e. al, (Eds.), The metabolic and molecular bases of inherited disease, Mc Graw-Hill, New York, 2001, pp. 2007-2056.

[17] L.A. Kluijtmans, G.H. Boers, J.P. Kraus, L.P. van den Heuvel, J.R. Cruysberg, F.J. Trijbels, and H.J. Blom, The molecular basis of cystathionine beta-synthase deficiency in Dutch patients with homocystinuria: effect of CBS genotype on biochemical and clinical phenotype and on response to treatment. *Am. J. Hum. Genet.* 65 (1999) 59-67.

[18] S. Yap, G.H. Boers, B. Wilcken, D.E. Wilcken, D.P. Brenton, P.J. Lee, J.H. Walter, P.M. Howard, and E.R. Naughten, Vascular outcome in patients with homocystinuria due to cystathionine beta-synthase deficiency treated chronically: a multicenter observational study. *Arterioscler. Thromb. Vasc. Biol.* 21 (2001) 2080-5.

[19] K.S. McCully, Vascular pathology of homocysteinemia: implications for the pathogenesis of arteriosclerosis. *Am. J. Pathol.* 56 (1969) 111-28.

[20] D.S. Wald, M. Law, and J.K. Morris, Homocysteine and cardiovascular disease: evidence on causality from a meta-analysis. *Bmj* 325 (2002) 1202.

[21] S. Seshadri, Elevated plasma homocysteine levels: risk factor or risk marker for the development of dementia and Alzheimer's disease? *J. Alzheimers Dis.* 9 (2006) 393-8.

[22] S. Seshadri, A. Beiser, J. Selhub, P.F. Jacques, I.H. Rosenberg, R.B. D'Agostino, P.W. Wilson, and P.A. Wolf, Plasma homocysteine as a risk factor for dementia and Alzheimer's disease. *N. Engl. J. Med.* 346 (2002) 476-83.

[23] J.L. Anderson, J.B. Muhlestein, B.D. Horne, J.F. Carlquist, T.L. Bair, T.E. Madsen, and R.R. Pearson, Plasma homocysteine predicts mortality independently of traditional risk factors and C-reactive protein in patients with angiographically defined coronary artery disease. *Circulation* 102 (2000) 1227-32.

[24] K.A. Strauss, D.H. Morton, E.G. Puffenberger, C. Hendrickson, D.L. Robinson, C. Wagner, S.P. Stabler, R.H. Allen, G. Chwatko, H. Jakubowski, M.D. Niculescu, and S.H. Mudd, Prevention of brain disease from severe 5,10-methylenetetrahydrofolate reductase deficiency. *Mol. Genet. Metab.* 91 (2007) 165-75.

[25] A.B. Lawrence de Koning, G.H. Werstuck, J. Zhou, and R.C. Austin, Hyperhomocysteinemia and its role in the development of atherosclerosis. *Clin. Biochem.* 36 (2003) 431-41.

[26] S.R. Lentz, Mechanisms of homocysteine-induced atherothrombosis. *J. Thromb Haemost.* 3 (2005) 1646-54.

[27] J. Durga, M.P. van Boxtel, E.G. Schouten, F.J. Kok, J. Jolles, M.B. Katan, and P. Verhoef, Effect of 3-year folic acid supplementation on cognitive function in older adults in the FACIT trial: a randomised, double blind, controlled trial. *Lancet* 369 (2007) 208-16.

[28] J.D. Spence, H. Bang, L.E. Chambless, and M.J. Stampfer, Vitamin Intervention For Stroke Prevention trial: an efficacy analysis. *Stroke* 36 (2005) 2404-9.

[29] E. Lonn, S. Yusuf, M.J. Arnold, P. Sheridan, J. Pogue, M. Micks, M.J. McQueen, J. Probstfield, G. Fodor, C. Held, and J. Genest, Jr., Homocysteine lowering with folic acid and B vitamins in vascular disease. *N. Engl. J. Med.* 354 (2006) 1567-77.

[30] K.H. Bonaa, I. Njolstad, P.M. Ueland, H. Schirmer, A. Tverdal, T. Steigen, H. Wang, J.E. Nordrehaug, E. Arnesen, and K. Rasmussen, Homocysteine lowering and

cardiovascular events after acute myocardial infarction. *N. Engl. J. Med.* 354 (2006) 1578-88.

[31] R. Clarke, S. Lewington, P. Sherliker, and J. Armitage, Effects of B-vitamins on plasma homocysteine concentrations and on risk of cardiovascular disease and dementia. *Curr. Opin. Clin. Nutr. Metab. Care* 10 (2007) 32-9.

[32] D. Ingrosso, A. Cimmino, A.F. Perna, L. Masella, N.G. De Santo, M.L. De Bonis, M. Vacca, M. D'Esposito, M. D'Urso, P. Galletti, and V. Zappia, Folate treatment and unbalanced methylation and changes of allelic expression induced by hyperhomocysteinaemia in patients with uraemia. *Lancet* 361 (2003) 1693-9.

[33] S.J. James, S. Melnyk, M. Pogribna, I.P. Pogribny, and M.A. Caudill, Elevation in S-adenosylhomocysteine and DNA hypomethylation: potential epigenetic mechanism for homocysteine-related pathology. *J. Nutr.* 132 (2002) 2361S-2366S.

[34] D.W. Jacobsen, O. Catanescu, P.M. Dibello, and J.C. Barbato, Molecular targeting by homocysteine: a mechanism for vascular pathogenesis. *Clin. Chem. Lab. Med.* 43 (2005) 1076-83.

[35] H. Jakubowski, Anti-N-homocysteinylated protein autoantibodies and cardiovascular disease. *Clin. Chem. Lab. Med.* 43 (2005) 1011-4.

[36] H. Jakubowski, Pathophysiological consequences of homocysteine excess. *J. Nutr.* 136 (2006) 1741S-1749S.

[37] J. Perla-Kajan, T. Twardowski, and H. Jakubowski, Mechanisms of homocysteine toxicity in humans. *Amino Acids* 32 (2007) 561-72.
[37a] H. Jakubowski. The molecular basis of homocysteine thiolactone-mediated vascular disease. *Clin. Chem. Lab. Med.* 45 (2007) 1704-16.
[37b] H. Jakubowski. The pathophysiological hypothesis of homocysteine thiolactone-mediated vascular disease. *J Physiol Pharmacol.* 59 Suppl 9 (2008) 155-67.

[38] H. Jakubowski, Protein homocysteinylation: possible mechanism underlying pathological consequences of elevated homocysteine levels. *Faseb. J* 13 (1999) 2277-83.

[39] P. Mercie, O. Garnier, L. Lascoste, M. Renard, C. Closse, F. Durrieu, G. Marit, R.M. Boisseau, and F. Belloc, Homocysteine-thiolactone induces caspase-independent vascular endothelial cell death with apoptotic features. *Apoptosis* 5 (2000) 403-11.

[40] G. Ferretti, T. Bacchetti, C. Moroni, A. Vignini, L. Nanetti, and G. Curatola, Effect of homocysteinylation of low density lipoproteins on lipid peroxidation of human endothelial cells. *J. Cell Biochem.* 92 (2004) 351-60.

[41] M. Kerkeni, M. Tnani, L. Chuniaud, A. Miled, K. Maaroufi, and F. Trivin, Comparative study on in vitro effects of homocysteine thiolactone and homocysteine on HUVEC cells: evidence for a stronger proapoptotic and proinflammative homocysteine thiolactone. *Mol. Cell Biochem.* 291 (2006) 119-26.

[42] D.L. Sauls, E. Lockhart, M.E. Warren, A. Lenkowski, S.E. Wilhelm, and M. Hoffman, Modification of fibrinogen by homocysteine thiolactone increases resistance to fibrinolysis: a potential mechanism of the thrombotic tendency in hyperhomocysteinemia. *Biochemistry* 45 (2006) 2480-7.

[43] A. Undas, J. Brozek, M. Jankowski, Z. Siudak, A. Szczeklik, and H. Jakubowski, Plasma homocysteine affects fibrin clot permeability and resistance to lysis in human subjects. *Arterioscler. Thromb. Vasc. Biol.* 26 (2006) 1397-404.

[44] H. Jakubowski, and E. Goldman, Editing of errors in selection of amino acids for protein synthesis. *Microbiol. Rev.* 56 (1992) 412-29.

[45] H. Jakubowski, Translational accuracy of aminoacyl-tRNA synthetases: implications for atherosclerosis. *J. Nutr*. 131 (2001) 2983S-7S.

[46] H. Jakubowski, Molecular basis of homocysteine toxicity in humans. *Cell Mol. Life Sci.* 61 (2004) 470-87.

[47] H. Jakubowski, tRNA synthetase editing of amino acids, Encyclopedia of Life Sciences, John Wiley and Sons, Ltd, Chichester, UK, 2005, pp. http://www.els.net /doi:10.1038 /npg.els.0003933.

[48] H. Jakubowski, Accuracy of Aminoacyl-tRNA Synthetases: Proofreading of Amino Acids. in: M. Ibba, C. Francklyn, and S. Cusack, (Eds.), The Aminoacyl-tRNA Synthetases, Landes Bioscience/Eurekah.com Georgetown, TX, 2005, pp. 384-396.

[49] G. Chwatko, G.H. Boers, K.A. Strauss, D.M. Shih, and H. Jakubowski, Mutations in methylenetetrahydrofolate reductase or cystathionine {beta}-syntase gene, or a high-methionine diet, increase homocysteine thiolactone levels in humans and mice. *Faseb. J.* 21(2007)1707-13.

[50] H. Jakubowski, Metabolism of homocysteine thiolactone in human cell cultures. Possible mechanism for pathological consequences of elevated homocysteine levels. *J. Biol. Chem.* 272 (1997) 1935-42.

[51] H. Jakubowski, L. Zhang, A. Bardeguez, and A. Aviv, Homocysteine thiolactone and protein homocysteinylation in human endothelial cells: implications for atherosclerosis. *Circ. Res.* 87 (2000) 45-51.

[52] H. Jakubowski, Proofreading in vivo: editing of homocysteine by methionyl-tRNA synthetase in the yeast Saccharomyces cerevisiae. *Embo. J.* 10 (1991) 593-8.

[53] H. Jakubowski, The determination of homocysteine-thiolactone in biological samples. *Anal. Biochem.* 308 (2002) 112-9.

[54] G. Chwatko, and H. Jakubowski, Urinary excretion of homocysteine-thiolactone in humans. *Clin. Chem.* 51 (2005) 408-15.

[55] H. Jakubowski, and E. Goldman, Synthesis of homocysteine thiolactone by methionyl-tRNA synthetase in cultured mammalian cells. *FEBS Lett.* 317 (1993) 237-40.

[56] J. Zimny, M. Sikora, A. Guranowski, and H. Jakubowski, Protective mechanisms against homocysteine toxicity: the role of bleomycin hydrolase. *J. Biol. Chem.* 281 (2006) 22485-92.

[57] H. Jakubowski, Calcium-dependent human serum homocysteine thiolactone hydrolase. A protective mechanism against protein N-homocysteinylation. *J. Biol. Chem.* 275 (2000) 3957-62.

[58] H. Jakubowski, W.T. Ambrosius, and J.H. Pratt, Genetic determinants of homocysteine thiolactonase activity in humans: implications for atherosclerosis. *FEBS Lett.* 491 (2001) 35-9.

[59] M. Lacinski, W. Skorupski, A. Cieslinski, J. Sokolowska, W.H. Trzeciak, and H. Jakubowski, Determinants of homocysteine-thiolactonase activity of the paraoxonase-1 (PON1) protein in humans. *Cell Mol. Biol.* (Noisy-le-grand) 50 (2004) 885-93.

[60] T.B. Domagała, M. Łacinski, W.H. Trzeciak, B. Mackness, M.I. Mackness, and H. Jakubowski, The correlation of homocysteine-thiolactonase activity of the paraoxonase (PON1) protein with coronary heart disease status. *Cell Mol. Biol.* (Noisy-le-grand) 52 (2006) 4-10.

[61] H. Jakubowski, Homocysteine is a protein amino acid in humans. Implications for homocysteine-linked disease. *J. Biol. Chem.* 277 (2002) 30425-8.

[61a] Jakubowski H. New method for the determination of protein N-linked homocysteine. *Anal. Biochem.* 380 (2008) 257-61.

[62] S.H. Mudd, J.D. Finkelstein, H. Refsum, P.M. Ueland, M.R. Malinow, S.R. Lentz, D.W. Jacobsen, L. Brattstrom, B. Wilcken, D.E. Wilcken, H.J. Blom, S.P. Stabler, R.H. Allen, J. Selhub, and I.H. Rosenberg, Homocysteine and its disulfide derivatives: a suggested consensus terminology. *Arterioscler. Thromb. Vasc. Biol.* 20 (2000) 1704-6.

[63] H. Jakubowski, Mechanism of the condensation of homocysteine thiolactone with aldehydes. *Chemistry* 12 (2006) 8039-43.

[64] D.M. Reuben, and T.C. Bruice, Reaction of thiol anions with benzene oxide and malachite green. *J. Am. Chem .Soc.* 98 (1976) 114-121.

[65] H. Jakubowski, Translational incorporation of S-nitrosohomocysteine into protein. *J. Biol. Chem.* 275 (2000) 21813-6.

[66] H. Jakubowski, and A.R. Fersht, Alternative pathways for editing non-cognate amino acids by aminoacyl-tRNA synthetases. *Nucleic Acids Res.* 9 (1981) 3105-17.

[67] G. Chwatko, and H. Jakubowski, The determination of homocysteine-thiolactone in human plasma. *Anal. Biochem.* 337 (2005) 271-7.

[68] H. Jakubowski, Energy cost of translational proofreading in vivo. The aminoacylation of transfer RNA in Escherichia coli. *Ann. N Y Acad. Sci.* 745 (1994) 4-20.

[69] H. Jakubowski, Synthesis of homocysteine thiolactone in normal and malignant cells. in: I.H. Rosenberg, I. Graham, P.M. Ueland, and H. Refsum, (Eds.), Homocysteine Metabolism: From Basic Science to Clinical Medicine, Kluwer Academic Publishers, Norwell, MA, 1997, pp. 157-165.

[70] H. Jakubowski, Protein N-homocysteinylation: implications for atherosclerosis. *Biomed. Pharmacother.* 55 (2001) 443-7.

[71] H. Jakubowski, Biosynthesis and reactions of homocysteine thiolactone. in: D. Jacobson, and R. Carmel, (Eds.), Homocysteine in Health and Disease, Cambridge University Press, Cambridge, UK, 2001, pp. 21-31.

[72] H. Jakubowski, Proofreading in vivo. Editing of homocysteine by aminoacyl-tRNA synthetases in Escherichia coli. *J. Biol. Chem.* 270 (1995) 17672-3.

[72a] Sikora M, Jakubowski H. Homocysteine editing and growth inhibition in *Escherichia coli. Microbiology.* 155 (2009) 1858-65.

[73] H. Jakubowski, Proofreading in vivo: editing of homocysteine by methionyl-tRNA synthetase in Escherichia coli. *Proc. Natl. Acad. Sci. U S A* 87 (1990) 4504-8.

[74] W. Gao, E. Goldman, and H. Jakubowski, Role of carboxy-terminal region in proofreading function of methionyl-tRNA synthetase in Escherichia coli. *Biochemistry* 33 (1994) 11528-35.

[75] B. Senger, L. Despons, P. Walter, H. Jakubowski, and F. Fasiolo, Yeast cytoplasmic and mitochondrial methionyl-tRNA synthetases: two structural frameworks for identical functions. *J. Mol. Biol.* 311 (2001) 205-16.

[76] H. Jakubowski, and A. Guranowski, Metabolism of homocysteine-thiolactone in plants. *J. Biol. Chem.* 278 (2003) 6765-70.

[77] H. Jakubowski, Proofreading in trans by an aminoacyl-tRNA synthetase: a model for single site editing by isoleucyl-tRNA synthetase. *Nucleic Acids Res.* 24 (1996) 2505-10.

[78] H.Y. Kim, G. Ghosh, L.H. Schulman, S. Brunie, and H. Jakubowski, The relationship between synthetic and editing functions of the active site of an aminoacyl-tRNA synthetase. *Proc. Natl. Acad. Sci. U S A* 90 (1993) 11553-7.

[79] H. Jakubowski, The synthetic/editing active site of an aminoacyl-tRNA synthetase: evidence for binding of thiols in the editing subsite. *Biochemistry* 35 (1996) 8252-9.

[80] L. Serre, G. Verdon, T. Choinowski, N. Hervouet, J.L. Risler, and C. Zelwer, How methionyl-tRNA synthetase creates its amino acid recognition pocket upon L-methionine binding. *J. Mol. Biol.* 306 (2001) 863-76.

[81] H. Jakubowski, Aminoacylation of coenzyme A and pantetheine by aminoacyl-tRNA synthetases: possible link between noncoded and coded peptide synthesis. *Biochemistry* 37 (1998) 5147-53.

[82] H. Jakubowski, Homocysteine thiolactone: metabolic origin and protein homocysteinylation in humans. *J. Nutr.* 130 (2000) 377S-381S.

[83] R. Glowacki, and H. Jakubowski, Cross-talk between Cys34 and lysine residues in human serum albumin revealed by N-homocysteinylation. *J. Biol. Chem.* 279 (2004) 10864-71.

[84] J. Perla-Kajan, L. Marczak, L. Kajan, P. Skowronek, T. Twardowski, and H. Jakubowski, Modification by Homocysteine Thiolactone Affects Redox Status of Cytochrome c. *Biochemistry* 46 (2007) 6225-31.

[85] X. Yang, Y. Gao, J. Zhou, Y. Zhen, Y. Yang, J. Wang, L. Song, Y. Liu, H. Xu, Z. Chen, and R. Hui, Plasma homocysteine thiolactone adducts associated with risk of coronary heart disease. *Clin .Chim .Acta.* 364 (2006) 230-4.

[86] Y. Uji, Y. Motomiya, N. Hanyu, F. Ukaji, and H. Okabe, Protein-bound homocystamide measured in human plasma by HPLC. *Clin. Chem.* 48 (2002) 941-4.

[87] A.F. Perna, E. Satta, F. Acanfora, C. Lombardi, D. Ingrosso, and N.G. De Santo, Increased plasma protein homocysteinylation in hemodialysis patients. *Kidney Int.* 69 (2006) 869-76.

[88] F. Mallamaci, C. Zoccali, G. Tripepi, I. Fermo, F.A. Benedetto, A. Cataliotti, I. Bellanuova, L.S. Malatino, and A. Soldarini, Hyperhomocysteinemia predicts cardiovascular outcomes in hemodialysis patients. *Kidney Int.* 61 (2002) 609-14.

[89] J. Perla, A. Undas, T. Twardowski, and H. Jakubowski, Purification of antibodies against N-homocysteinylated proteins by affinity chromatography on Nomega-

homocysteinyl-aminohexyl-Agarose. *J. Chromatogr. B Analyt. Technol. Biomed. Life Sci.* 807 (2004) 257-61.

[90] Perła-Kaján J, Stanger O, Luczak M, Ziółkowska A, Malendowicz LK, Twardowski T, Lhotak S, Austin RC, Jakubowski H. Immunohistochemical detection of N-homocysteinylated proteins in humans and mice. *Biomed. Pharmacother.* 62 (2008) 473-9.

[91] C.E. Hop, and R. Bakhtiar, Homocysteine thiolactone and protein homocysteinylation: mechanistic studies with model peptides and proteins. *Rapid Commun. Mass Spectrom* 16 (2002) 1049-53.

[92] M. Naruszewicz, E. Mirkiewicz, A.J. Olszewski, and K.S. McCully, Thiolation of low density lipoproteins by homocysteine thiolactone causes increased aggregation and altered interaction with cultured macrophages. *Nutr. Metab. Cardiovasc. Dis.* 4 (1991) 70-77.

[93] M. Vidal, J. Sainte-Marie, J. Philippot, and A. Bienvenue, Thiolation of low-density lipoproteins and their interaction with L2C leukemic lymphocytes. *Biochimie* 68 (1986) 723-30.

[94] G. Liu, K. Nellaiappan, and H.M. Kagan, Irreversible inhibition of lysyl oxidase by homocysteine thiolactone and its selenium and oxygen analogues. Implications for homocystinuria. *J. Biol. Chem.* 272 (1997) 32370-7.

[95] L.A. Harker, S.J. Slichter, C.R. Scott, and R. Ross, Homocystinemia. Vascular injury and arterial thrombosis. *N. Engl. J. Med.* 291 (1974) 537-43.

[96] N. Endo, K. Nishiyama, A. Otsuka, H. Kanouchi, M. Taga, and T. Oka, Antioxidant activity of vitamin B6 delays homocysteine-induced atherosclerosis in rats. *Br. J. Nutr.* 95 (2006) 1088-93.

[97] T.H. Rosenquist, S.A. Ratashak, and J. Selhub, Homocysteine induces congenital defects of the heart and neural tube: effect of folic acid. *Proc. Natl. Acad .Sci. USA* 93 (1996) 15227-32.

[98] C. Maestro de las Casas, M. Epeldegui, C. Tudela, G. Varela-Moreiras, and J. Perez-Miguelsanz, High exogenous homocysteine modifies eye development in early chick embryos. *Birth Defects Res. A Clin. .Mol. Teratol.* 67 (2003) 35-40.

[99] S. Donahue, J.A. Struman, and G. Gaull, Arteriosclerosis due to homocyst (e) inemia. Failure to reproduce the model in weanling rabbits. *Am. J. Pathol.* 77 (1974) 167-3.

[100] A.N. Makheja, A.T. Bombard, R.L. Randazzo, and J.M. Bailey, Anti-inflammatory drugs in experimental atherosclerosis. Part 3. Evaluation of the atherogenicity of homocystine in rabbits. *Atherosclerosis* 29 (1978) 105-12.

[101] C.B. Anfinsen, Principles that govern the folding of protein chains. *Science* 181 (1973) 223-30.

[102] A. Fersht, Structure and mechansim in protein science, WH Freeman and Company, New York, 2000.

[103] M. Stefani, Protein misfolding and aggregation: new examples in medicine and biology of the dark side of the protein world. *Biochim. Biophys. Acta* 1739 (2004) 5-25.

[104] G.H. Werstuck, S.R. Lentz, S. Dayal, G.S. Hossain, S.K. Sood, Y.Y. Shi, J. Zhou, N. Maeda, S.K. Krisans, M.R. Malinow, and R.C. Austin, Homocysteine-induced

endoplasmic reticulum stress causes dysregulation of the cholesterol and triglyceride biosynthetic pathways. *J. Clin. Invest.* 107 (2001) 1263-73.

[105] C. Zhang, Y. Cai, M.T. Adachi, S. Oshiro, T. Aso, R.J. Kaufman, and S. Kitajima, Homocysteine induces programmed cell death in human vascular endothelial cells through activation of the unfolded protein response. *J. Biol. Chem.* 276 (2001) 35867-74.

[106] J. Zhou, J. Moller, C.C. Danielsen, J. Bentzon, H.B. Ravn, R.C. Austin, and E. Falk, Dietary supplementation with methionine and homocysteine promotes early atherosclerosis but not plaque rupture in ApoE-deficient mice. *Arterioscler. Thromb Vasc. Biol.* 21 (2001) 1470-6.

[107] G.S. Hossain, J.V. van Thienen, G.H. Werstuck, J. Zhou, S.K. Sood, J.G. Dickhout, A.B. de Koning, D. Tang, D. Wu, E. Falk, R. Poddar, D.W. Jacobsen, K. Zhang, R.J. Kaufman, and R.C. Austin, TDAG51 is induced by homocysteine, promotes detachment-mediated programmed cell death, and contributes to the cevelopment of atherosclerosis in hyperhomocysteinemia. *J. Biol. Chem.* 278 (2003) 30317-27.

[108] C.N. Roybal, S. Yang, C.W. Sun, D. Hurtado, D.L. Vander Jagt, T.M. Townes, and S.F. Abcouwer, Homocysteine increases the expression of vascular endothelial growth factor by a mechanism involving endoplasmic reticulum stress and transcription factor ATF4. *J. Biol. Chem.* 279 (2004) 14844-52.

[109] E. Ferguson, S. Parthasarathy, J. Joseph, and B. Kalyanaraman, Generation and initial characterization of a novel polyclonal antibody directed against homocysteine thiolactone-modified low density lipoprotein. *J. Lipid. Res.* 39 (1998) 925-33.

[110] A. Undas, J. Perla, M. Lacinski, W. Trzeciak, R. Kazmierski, and H. Jakubowski, Autoantibodies against N-homocysteinylated proteins in humans: implications for atherosclerosis. *Stroke* 35 (2004) 1299-304.

[111] A. Undas, M. Jankowski, M. Twardowska, A. Padjas, H. Jakubowski, and A. Szczeklik, Antibodies to N-homocysteinylated albumin as a marker for early-onset coronary artery disease in men. *Thromb Haemost.* 93 (2005) 346-50.

[112] A. Undas, E. Stepien, R. Glowacki, J. Tisonczyk, W. Tracz, and H. Jakubowski, Folic acid administration and antibodies against homocysteinylated proteins in subjects with hyperhomocysteinemia. *Thromb Haemost.* 96 (2006) 342-7.

[113] A. Undas, M. Kolarz, G. Kopec, R. Glowacki, E. Placzkiewicz-Jankowska, and W. Tracz, Autoantibodies against N-homocysteinylated proteins in patients on long-term haemodialysis. *Nephrol. Dial.Transplant.* 22 (2007) 1685-9.

[114] A.R. Folsom, M. Desvarieux, F.J. Nieto, L.L. Boland, C.M. Ballantyne, and L.E. Chambless, B vitamin status and inflammatory markers. *Atherosclerosis* 169 (2003) 169-74.

[115] G. Ravaglia, P. Forti, F. Maioli, L. Servadei, M. Martelli, G. Arnone, T. Talerico, M. Zoli, and E. Mariani, Plasma homocysteine and inflammation in elderly patients with cardiovascular disease and dementia. *Exp. Gerontol.* 39 (2004) 443-50.

[116] A.C. Peeters, B.E. van Aken, H.J. Blom, P.H. Reitsma, and M. den Heijer, The effect of homocysteine reduction by B-vitamin supplementation on inflammatory markers. *Clin. Chem. Lab. Med.* 45 (2007) 54-8.

[117] S. Friso, P.F. Jacques, P.W. Wilson, I.H. Rosenberg, and J. Selhub, Low circulating vitamin B(6) is associated with elevation of the inflammation marker C-reactive protein independently of plasma homocysteine levels. *Circulation* 103 (2001) 2788-91.

[118] L.E. Rohde, C.H. Hennekens, and P.M. Ridker, Survey of C-reactive protein and cardiovascular risk factors in apparently healthy men. *Am. J. Cardiol.* 84 (1999) 1018-22.

[119] K.B. Holven, P. Aukrust, K. Retterstol, T.A. Hagve, L. Morkrid, L. Ose, and M.S. Nenseter, Increased levels of C-reactive protein and interleukin-6 in hyperhomocysteinemic subjects. *Scand. J. Clin. Lab. Invest.* 66 (2006) 45-54.

[120] Y. Aso, N. Yoshida, K. Okumura, S. Wakabayashi, R. Matsutomo, K. Takebayashi, and T. Inukai, Coagulation and inflammation in overt diabetic nephropathy: association with hyperhomocysteinemia. *Clin. Chim. Acta* 348 (2004) 139-45.

[121] I. Shai, M.J. Stampfer, J. Ma, J.E. Manson, S.E. Hankinson, C. Cannuscio, J. Selhub, G. Curhan, and E.B. Rimm, Homocysteine as a risk factor for coronary heart diseases and its association with inflammatory biomarkers, lipids and dietary factors. *Atherosclerosis* 177 (2004) 375-81.

[122] B. Widner, F. Leblhuber, B. Frick, A. Laich, E. Artner-Dworzak, and D. Fuchs, Moderate hyperhomocysteinaemia and immune activation in Parkinson's disease. *J. Neural Transm.* 109 (2002) 1445-52.

[123] K.B. Holven, H. Scholz, B. Halvorsen, P. Aukrust, L. Ose, and M.S. Nenseter, Hyperhomocysteinemic subjects have enhanced expression of lectin-like oxidized LDL receptor-1 in mononuclear cells. *J. Nutr.* 133 (2003) 3588-91.

[124] R.W. Powers, A.K. Majors, S.L. Cerula, H.A. Huber, B.P. Schmidt, and J.M. Roberts, Changes in markers of vascular injury in response to transient hyperhomocysteinemia. *Metabolism* 52 (2003) 501-7.

[125] G. Wang, C.W. Woo, F.L. Sung, Y.L. Siow, and K. O, Increased monocyte adhesion to aortic endothelium in rats with hyperhomocysteinemia: role of chemokine and adhesion molecules. *Arterioscler. Thromb. Vasc. Biol.* 22 (2002) 1777-83.

[126] R. Zhang, J. Ma, M. Xia, H. Zhu, and W. Ling, Mild hyperhomocysteinemia induced by feeding rats diets rich in methionine or deficient in folate promotes early atherosclerotic inflammatory processes. *J. Nutr.* 134 (2004) 825-30.

[127] H. Lee, H.J. Kim, J.M. Kim, and N. Chang, Effects of dietary folic acid supplementation on cerebrovascular endothelial dysfunction in rats with induced hyperhomocysteinemia. *Brain Res.* 996 (2004) 139-47.

[128] H. Lee, J.M. Kim, H.J. Kim, I. Lee, and N. Chang, Folic acid supplementation can reduce the endothelial damage in rat brain microvasculature due to hyperhomocysteinemia. *J. Nutr.* 135 (2005) 544-8.

[129] Bogdanski P, Pupek-Musialik D, Dytfeld J, Lacinski M, Jablecka A, Jakubowski H. Plasma homocysteine is a determinant of tissue necrosis factor-alpha in hypertensive patients. *Biomed. Pharmacother.* 62 (2008) 360-5.

[130] Jakubowski H, Boers GH, Strauss KA. Mutations in cystathionine beta-synthase or methylenetetrahydrofolate reductase gene increase N-homocysteinylated protein levels in humans. *FASEB J* 22 (2008) 4071-6.

[131] Jakubowski H, Perla-Kajan J, Finnell RH, Cabrera RM, Wang H, Gupta S, Kruger WD, Kraus JP, Shih DM. Genetic or nutritional disorders in homocysteine or folate metabolism increase protein N-homocysteinylation in mice. *FASEB J.* 23 (2009) 1721-7.

In: Handbook of Cardiovascular Research
Editors: Jorgen Brataas and Viggo Nanstveit

ISBN 978-1-60741-792-7
© 2009 Nova Science Publishers, Inc.

Chapter V

Comorbidity in Systemic Lupus Erythematosus: Aspects of Cardiovascular Disease, Osteoporosis and Infections[*]

Irene E. M. Bultink[†], Ben A. C. Dijkmans
and Alexandre E. Voskuyl
Department of Rheumatology, VU University Medical Center,
Amsterdam, The Netherlands

Abstract

Over the last decades, the survival of patients with systemic lupus erythematosus (SLE) has improved dramatically. Having improved treatment for active lupus disease, the challenge is now to understand and prevent the long-term complications of the disease, which may be due to the disease itself or the therapies used. To date, long-term complications of SLE are now considered to be important, including cardiovascular disease, osteoporosis and infections.

Cardiovascular disease in patients with SLE, including coronary artery disease, ischemic cerebrovascular disease, and peripheral vascular disease, is the result of premature atherosclerosis. Besides the traditional risk factors (like hypertension, hypercholesterolaemia and smoking), renal insufficiency, raised homocysteine levels, and the presence of anti-phospholipid, antibodies have been recognized as additional risk factors for cardiovascular disease in SLE. Recent studies have demonstrated that the nitric oxide pathway and its endogenous inhibitor asymmetric dimethylarginine may also

---

[*] A version of this chapter was also published in *Progress in Systemic Lupus Erythematosus Research,* edited by Tomas I. Seward published by Nova Science Publishers, Inc. It was submitted for appropriate modifications in an effort to encourage wider dissemination of research.

[†] VU University Medical Center, Room 4A49, PO box 7057, 1007 MB Amsterdam. Tel: +31-20-4443432; Fax: +31-20-4442138.

be involved in the pathogenesis of cardiovascular organ damage in SLE. The metabolic syndrome and insulin resistance in SLE patients are current topics of research in this field.

Several studies have demonstrated a high prevalence of low bone mineral density in patients with SLE, especially in females. In the last few years, more attention is paid to osteoporotic fractures, one of the items of the organ damage index for SLE, and likely the most preventable form of musculoskeletal organ damage in SLE patients. Recent studies have demonstrated an increased frequency of symptomatic vertebral and nonvertebral fractures in patients with SLE. Moreover, a high prevalence of mostly asymptomatic vertebral fractures in patients with SLE was detected. These vertebral fractures were associated with previous use of intravenous methylprednisolone. The importance of identifying vertebral fractures in SLE patients is illustrated by the observed association between prevalent vertebral fractures and reduced quality of life as well as an increased risk of future vertebral and nonvertebral fractures in the general population.

Infection imposes a serious burden on patients with SLE. In case series, infectious complications were found in 25% to 45% of SLE patients, and infection as primary cause of death has been demonstrated in up to 50% of SLE patients. Defects of immune defence and treatment with corticosteroids and other immunosuppressive agents are supposed to play a role in the pathogenesis of infections in SLE. Recently, research has focused on the role of the lectin pathway of complement activation in the occurrence of infections in SLE.

In this review the results of recent studies on cardiovascular disease, osteoporosis and infectious complications in SLE will be discussed.

Introduction

Systemic lupus erythematosus (SLE) is a chronic autoimmune disorder that usually affects multiple organ systems and may be associated with considerable morbidity and mortality.

Over the last 3 decades, the survival of patients with SLE has improved dramatically. A 60% decrease in the standardized all-cause mortality rate (SMR) from 1970-1979 (SMR 4.9) to 1990-2001 (SMR 2.0) has been demonstrated in a large international multicenter study [1]. The improved health outcome in patients with SLE has been attributed to earlier and better diagnostic methods as well as better immunosuppressive treatment strategies. Despite the improved survival, mortality rates in patients with SLE are still significantly higher than those in the general population, across countries, and throughout the course of the disease, up to 20 years disease duration [1]. The most important causes of death in patients with SLE are disease activity (complicated by organ system involvement), treatment related complications such as infections, and long-term disease complications (particularly cardiovascular disease). From 1970 to 2001, a change in death causes in SLE patients has been observed [1-3]. In this period of time, a decrease in the rate of death primarily due to disease activity has occurred [1, 4], while death due to cardiovascular disease remained unchanged [4] or slightly increased, [1] and cardiovascular death is currently probably the commonest cause of death in lupus patients in the Western world [1, 4]. Despite improvements in immunosuppressive treatment strategies for active disease, infections are still an important cause of death in SLE patients, both early and late in the disease course [1-3, 5-7].

Apart from mortality, prognosis in SLE has also aspects with regard to morbidity. The prolonged survival of patients with SLE is also associated with considerable morbidity due to long-term complications of the disease. These long-term complications in SLE patients may be due to the disease itself, the therapies used, or comorbid diseases, and are associated with functional limitations and a reduced quality of life.

In this review, recent research in the field of three important long-term complications in patients with SLE will be discussed. First atherosclerotic cardiovascular disease, which is the major cause of cardiovascular, neuropsychiatric, and peripheral vascular organ damage in SLE patients, as assessed with the Systemic Lupus International Collaborating Clinics/American College of Rheumatology (SLICC/ACR) damage index score [8]. Secondly, osteoporosis and fractures, which contribute to damage in the most frequently involved system in SLE patients: the musculoskeletal system. In the third item, results of recent research on infectious complications in SLE will be highlighted.

Cardiovascular Disease in SLE

Over the last decades, accelerated atherosclerosis and premature cardiovascular disease (CVD), including coronary heart disease [9], ischaemic cerebrovascular disease [10], and peripheral vascular disease [11] has been identified as a major contributor to the morbidity and mortality of patients with SLE. In female SLE patients, the risk of myocardial infarction is 10-fold increased [12], the risk of stroke 8 to 10-fold [12, 13] and the risk of heart failure may be increased as much as 13-fold [13] as compared to age- and sex-matched healthy controls. Atherosclerotic events also tend to occur at younger ages in patients with SLE. In patients with SLE, the first myocardial infarction occurs at a mean age of 49 years as compared to 65 to 74 years in the general population, which illustrates the premature occurrence of CVD in SLE [9].

In addition, several studies have demonstrated a high prevalence of subclinical atherosclerosis in 17% to 40% of SLE patients, as measured by myocardial perfusion scans, presence of atherosclerotic plaques in the carotid artery and assessment of coronary artery calcifications by computer tomography [14-16]. Endothelial dysfunction, as defined by impaireded flow-mediated dilatation of the brachial artery, was present in 55% of SLE patients as compared to 26% of healthy persons in a recent study [17]. Data from an autopsy study performed in patients with SLE demonstrated that 52% of patients had moderate to severe atherosclerosis at the time of death, regardless of the cause of death [2].

Risk factors for CVD in SLE

The mechanisms underlying the accelerated atherosclerosis in SLE are not fully understood, but endothelial dysfunction and/or atherosclerosis in combination with prothrombotic factors are supposed to be important contributors to this process [18] . In recent years, both traditional and non-traditional risk factors have been identified, which play a role in the pathogenesis of CVD in SLE.

1. Traditional Risk Factors

Patients with SLE have an increased prevalence of several traditional risk factors for atherosclerosis, such as hypertension [12, 19, 20], diabetes mellitus [19], obesity [19, 20], inactivity [19-21], hypercholesterolaemia [20] and hypertriglyceridaemia [19] and these risk factors are, also in SLE patients, associated with an increased risk for CVD. However, even after adjustment for the presence of the traditional Framingham risk factors, the risk for cardiovascular events in patients with SLE is still 7 to 17-fold increased [12, 22]. Therefore, additional metabolic, inflammatory, medication related and lifestyle factors are suggested to contribute to the development of atherosclerosis and vascular disease in SLE.

2. Antiphospholipid Antibodies

The occurrence of a secondary antiphospholipid antibody syndrome in SLE patients is common and is characterized by both arterial and venous thrombosis [23].

The presence of lupus anticoagulant has been recognized as an independent risk factor for myocardial infarction [24] and cerebral arterial occlusion [25] in SLE patients. These findings support the idea that thrombosis plays a role in the increased risk of CVD in SLE. Studies of the relationship between the presence of lupus anticoagulant and atherosclerosis in SLE demonstrate conflicting results. In a Swedish study, the presence of lupus anticoagulant was associated with an increased intima-media thickness of the carotid artery [26], but in a recent study in the USA the presence of lupus anticoagulant or anticardiolipin (aCL) antibodies was not associated with coronary or carotid atherosclerosis [27].

The role of aCL and anti-ß2-glycoprotein 1 (ß2GP1) antibodies in the development of CVD in SLE is not completely clear. In the general population, the presence of aCL antibodies has been associated with an increased risk for future myocardial infarction [28, 29], but this finding has not been confirmed in SLE yet. In the study of Svenungsson and colleagues, both aCL antibodies and anti-ß2GP1 antibodies tended to be associated with arterial disease in lupus patients, but these associations were not statistically significant [26].

However, several other studies have suggested that aCL and anti-ß2GP1 antibodies might play a role in the atherosclerotic process in SLE [30-33]. The low-density lipoprotein (LDL) particle is susceptible to oxidative modification, which accounts for its atherogenic properties. Oxidized LDL (ox-LDL) contributes to the formation of foam cells in atherosclerotic lesions [30]. Ox-LDL can bind anti-ß2GP1, which results in ß2GP1-ox-LDL complexes [31]. Antibodies against these complexes are supposed to increase LDL uptake by macrophages, which contributes to foam cell formation, a process considered important in atherosclerotic plaque formation [33]. Moreover, it was demonstrated that binding of these antibodies to ß2GP1 on endothelial cells induces expression of adhesion molecules, which further enhances leukocyte adhesion to the endothelium [32]. The role of antibodies to ox-LDL in the pathogenesis of atherosclerosis in SLE is still under debate. The occurrence and high titres of these antibodies have been associated with the extent of atherosclerosis and CVD in reports, but other studies suggested that antibodies to ox-LDL play a protective role in the atherosclerotic process [33, 34]. Future research might provide more insight in the subtle interplay between thrombogenesis and atherogenesis and in the role of antiphospholipid antibodies in the pathogenesis of CVD in lupus.

3. SLE Related Risk Factors

Several diseases related factors have been recognized as independent risk factors for CVD in SLE.

In SLE patients, longer disease duration [9, 20, 21] and premature menopause [19] have been associated with an increased risk of CVD.

In addition, renal disease is an important contributor to CVD in lupus. Nephritis is a highly frequent complication in SLE and may cause proteinuria and renal failure. Nephrotic syndrome and proteinuria are associated with un unfavourable lipid profile [35] and atherosclerosis in SLE [36, 37]. Moreover, an elevated serum creatinine or history of renal disease are associated with atherosclerosis [38, 39].

Dyslipidaemia in SLE is characterized by a reduced high-density lipoprotein (HDL) cholesterol as well as an increased LDL cholesterol, VLDL cholesterol, triglycerides [40] and increased lipoprotein a (Lp(a)) [26, 41]. Dyslipidaemia occurs especially in active disease [40] and is associated with atherosclerosis and cardiovascular events [19, 26, 36]. The mechanisms underlying the dyslipidaemia in SLE are not well known, but tumor necrosis factor-α (TNF-α) induced de novo hepatic lipogenesis and inhibition of LDL are two possible mechanisms [18]. This hypothesis is supported by the strong associations found between elevated circulating levels of TNF-α, high triglycerides and low HDL levels in SLE patients [42]. Recently, the presence of anti-lipoprotein lipase antibodies (anti-LPL) in association with dyslipidaemia and increased inflammatory parameters have been demonstrated in patients with SLE [43]. Further research is necessary to unravel the role of these antibodies in the pathogenesis of atherosclerosis in lupus.

The role of antibodies against endothelial cells (aEC) in the development of CVD in SLE is not clear. These antibodies have been associated with vasculitis and disease activity [44] and direct stimulation of endothelial cells in SLE [45], but no correlation between aEC antibodies and CVD was found in one study [46].

Atherosclerosis can be considered to have an important inflammatory component and several inflammatory factors are supposed to promote atherosclerosis in SLE. In the general population, raised serum concentrations of C-reactive protein (CRP) are a strong predictor of future coronary events [47]. In line with this finding, raised serum levels of CRP were associated with subclinical atherosclerosis [39] and cardiovascular arterial events in SLE patients [48]. Moreover, serum levels of complement increase in response to inflammation and studies in the general population have demonstrated associations between high complement C3 levels and traditional cardiovascular risk factors and coronary heart disease [49, 50]. In lupus patients, increased complement C3 levels were correlated with increased vascular stiffness of the aorta [39] and with coronary calcifications in SLE [36]. Furthermore, we found an association between high C3 levels and metabolic syndrome score in female lupus patients [51]. This finding is in line with the results of a study by Chung et al, demonstrating an association between higher levels of inflammation and prevalence of the metabolic syndrome in patients with SLE [52]. In lupus, the systemic inflammatory response is accompanied by systemic complement activation and immune complex deposition in specific tissues. Complement activation induces endothelial cell activation, the release of monocyte chemoattractant protein-1 (MCP-1), and the release of IL-6 from vascular smooth muscle cells, which promote recruitment of leukocytes and atherosclerosis [53, 54]. Recently, Asanuma and colleagues found increased concentrations of IL-6 and MCP-1 in lupus patients and these cytokines were associated with inflammation, disease activity, body mass index and low HDL levels [14]. Moreover, IL-6 concentrations were correlated with coronary calcification [14]. Inflammation in SLE might also contribute to the dyslipidaemia associated with lupus by IL-6 mediated inhibition of lipoprotein lipase (LPL), the key enzyme in the metabolism of LDL and VLDL [15]. Reduced LPL activity has been demonstrated in lupus patients and was strongly associated with high triglyceride levels [55].

Recently, decreased binding of annexin V to endothelial cells has been proposed as a possible mechanism contributing to atherosclerosis in SLE [56]. Annexin V has anti-thrombotic properties and decreased binding of this plasma protein to endothelial cells, caused by antiphospholipid antibodies, might promote atherosclerosis. Associations between annexin V binding and carotid intima media thickness in lupus patients with a history of CVD have been demonstrated [56]. Further research is necessary to elucidate the role of annexin V and other inflammatory factors in the atherosclerotic process in lupus.

4. Oxidative Stress

Several studies have demonstrated increased oxidative stress in patients with SLE [57, 58]. In lupus patients with a history of cardiovascular events, raised plasma levels of ox-LDL have been demonstrated [26]. The contribution of ox-LDL to foam cell formation in atherosclerotic plaques has been debated. However, ox-LDL levels have also been associated with renal manifestations in SLE, and it is well known that nephritis and renal failure are risk factors for CVD. Therefore, the exact role of ox-LDL in the atherosclerotic process in SLE is still under debate and will be subject of more research.

The hypothesis that oxidative stress contributes to the atherosclerotic process in SLE is supported by a study demonstrating reduced activity of the antioxidant enzyme paraoxanase in SLE [59].

Recently, the role of the nitric oxide pathway and its endogenous inhibitor asymmetric dimethylarginine (ADMA) has been investigated in SLE. In the general population, high plasma ADMA levels are associated with endothelial dysfunction [60]. Moreover, high ADMA levels are a predictor of acute coronary events [61] and a risk factor for cardiovascular events and mortality in patients with end stage renal disease [62]. In patients with SLE, AMDA levels were significantly higher in patients with a history of cardiovascular events than in patients without a CVD history [63]. Moreover, high ADMA levels in SLE were associated with disease activity, high titers of anti-dsDNA antibodies [63, 64] and with coronary calcification [64]. The observed association between high ADMA levels and high titers of anti-dsDNA antibodies is in line with results from in vitro studies. Anti-dsDNA antibodies were shown to be reactive with the arginine-glycine-rich domains in recombinant heterogeneous nuclear ribonucleoprotein A2 (hnRNP A2) [65]. These domains are also preferred sites for the methylation of arginine to ADMA by type 1 protein arginine methyltransferase (PRMT1) [66]. In the presence of anti-dsDNA, methylation of hnRNP A2 by PRMT1 was increased to 3.5 times that of the control level. Therefore, anti-dsDNA antibodies might be a trigger for increased ADMA production by up regulating methylation of arginine residues by PRMT1. Furthermore, anti-dsDNA monoclonal antibodies were demonstrated to augment the inflammatory reaction by the release of proinflammatory cytokines from mononuclear cells [67]. These studies suggest that anti-dsDNA antibodies might play a role in the development of CVD in SLE by enhancing ADMA production and by enhancing the inflammatory reaction. However, a prospective study is required to answer definitively the question of whether high ADMA levels are an independent risk factor for future cardiovascular events in SLE.

5. Metabolic Risk Factors

In a prospective study in 337 patients with SLE from the Hopkins lupus cohort, raised plasma homocysteine levels were found in 15% of the patients and high homocysteine levels were an independent risk factor for stroke and arterial thrombosis [68]. This finding was confirmed by a Dutch study, reporting an increased risk for arterial thrombosis in SLE patients with high homocysteine levels [69].

The metabolic syndrome is a condition characterized by the clustering of cardiovascular risk factors, including hypertension, obesity, insulin resistance and dyslipidaemia, and is associated with an increased risk of diabetes mellitus and cardiovascular mortality in the general population, especially in women [70, 71]. Recently, research has focused on insulin resistance and the associated metabolic syndrome in SLE. In patients with SLE, an increased prevalence of insulin resistance was demonstrated [72, 73]. A study in the United Kingdom reported that 18% of female SLE patients, as compared with 2.5% of healthy female controls, fulfilled the criteria of the National Cholesterol Education Program (NCEP) metabolic syndrome [72]. A study by Chung et al in the United States reported that the metabolic syndrome was present in 29.4% of male and female SLE patients and 19.8% of healthy controls, using the NCEP definition [52]. In a recent study in 141 Dutch female SLE patients, the prevalence of the metabolic syndrome was 16% and a high metabolic syndrome score was associated with previous treatment with intravenous methylprednisolone, renal insufficiency, older age, higher erythrocyte sedimentation rate and higher C3 levels [51]. Moreover, the mean metabolic syndrome score was significantly higher in SLE patients with a history of cardiovascular events than in those without a previous cardiovascular event [51]. In both the Dutch and the USA study, associations were found between the metabolic syndrome and high levels of inflammation. Therefore, the metabolic syndrome might provide a link between inflammation and the increased vascular risk in SLE. A prospective study is necessary to investigate whether the metabolic syndrome is a predictor of cardiovascular events and mortality in patients with SLE.

6. The Role of Anti-Rheumatic Drugs

The role of corticosteroid treatment in the development of CVD in SLE has been investigated in many studies. Corticosteroids have a negative effect on blood pressure, glucose metabolism and body fat distribution. On the other hand, corticosteroids have an anti-inflammatory effect, which might be beneficial with respect to the atherosclerotic process. The evaluation of the effect of corticosteroids on CVD in SLE is complicated, since corticosteroids are usually prescribed in patients with more active disease. Therefore, a history of corticosteroid treatment might reflect a higher inflammatory disease state, which is supposed to be an important risk factor for CVD per se [47]. Associations between increased exposure to corticosteroids and atherosclerosis and cardiovascular events have been reported in patients with SLE [9, 20, 38], but other studies failed to find such an association [16, 74]. The benefit or harm of corticosteroids might be dose-dependent. In SLE patients, a daily dose of < 10 mg corticosteroids did not have an adverse effect on lipid levels [75], but a dose of > 10 mg daily was associated with increased cholesterol and triglyceride levels [75, 76]. The conflicting results of the studies on this subject illustrate the dual role of corticosteroid therapy with respect to the development of CVD in SLE.

Antimalarial drugs reduce the atherosclerotic risk in SLE by several mechanisms. First, antimalarials have an anti-inflammatory effect in mild to moderate disease activity. Secondly, a beneficial effect of antimalarials on the dyslipidaemia in SLE, especially in case of concomitant treatment with corticosteroids, has been reported in several studies [77-80]. In the third place, antimalarials may have a beneficial effect on insulin sensitivity, because these drugs prolong the half-life of the active insulin-receptor complex through the inhibition of insulin dissociation from its receptor [81]. However, the effect of antimalarials on insulin resistance has not been investigated in SLE patients yet.

Despite the great number of studies performed in the context of CVD and its risk factors in SLE, little is known about the role of other antirheumatic drugs. However, a negative association between previous cyclophosphamide use and the prevalence of carotid plaque was demonstrated in one study [16], suggesting that tight control of disease activity might be beneficial in the prevention of atherosclerosis in SLE.

Prevention and Treatment of CVD in SLE

Traditional risk factors, disease-related factors and the associated metabolic changes, immunologic factors, anti-phospholipid antibodies, lifestyle factors and use of antirheumatic drugs all contribute to the accelerated atherosclerosis and premature CVD in subgroups of patients with SLE. Prospective studies in large patient groups are necessary to evaluate the relative influence of each of these factors. In the meantime, physicians should use a proactive approach to suppress disease activity and other modifiable risk factors for atherosclerosis in these high-risk patients. Screening for risk factors in SLE patients is very important for several reasons. First, in patients with SLE, a high prevalence of multiple risk factors has been demonstrated [19, 20]. Secondly, a recent quality improvement study in Canada has demonstrated that hypertension and especially hypercholesterolaemia are not managed adequately in the majority of SLE patients [82]. In the third place, many of the risk factors mentioned may be relatively easily recognized and managed in clinical practice by lifestyle advices (stop smoking, physical activity, weight reduction) or medication (anti-hypertensive treatment, lipid lowering agents, anti-diabetic medication, anticoagulants, supplementation with folic acid and vitamin B12 in case of increased homocysteine levels). It was suggested by Bruce, that the diagnosis of SLE can be regarded as a risk factor for CVD itself, like diabetes, which has implications for the ideal targets for blood pressure, lipid levels and glucose levels in SLE patients [15].

The identification of biological markers of disease activity associated with atherosclerosis might be a tool to improve therapy and prevent cardiovascular complications in SLE.

In addition, physicians eagerly await the definitive results of current large-scale prospective studies evaluating the effect of different intervention strategies to reduce the risk for CVD in SLE. The preliminary results of a Canadian intervention study are promising [83].

Osteoporosis and Fractures in SLE

In recent years, osteoporosis and fractures have been recognized as important disease complications in patients with SLE. The growing interest in these unfortunate disease complications is justified for several reasons. First, in studies from 1990 to 2007, a high prevalence of low bone mineral density (BMD) in patients with SLE has been demonstrated, especially in female patients [84-101]. Secondly, osteoporotic fractures are an item of the SLICC/ACR organ damage index for SLE. In the third place, it was demonstrated in studies in the general population, that osteoporotic fractures are associated with a reduced quality of life [102], an increased risk of future fractures [103, 104], and an increased mortality rate [103].

Osteoporosis in SLE

A reduced BMD, as measured by Dual Energy X-ray absorptiometry (DEXA), is highly frequent in patients with SLE. Osteopenia is reported in 25-74% of SLE patients [93, 95, 101] and osteoporosis, defined as a T score less than -2.5 SD, is reported in 1-23% [84, 96, 98, 100]. The great majority of studies of BMD performed in patients with SLE had a cross-sectional study design [84, 86, 88-95, 97-100, 105-112]. Only a few longitudinal studies have been published [85, 113-116]. The prevalence of osteopenia and osteoporosis reported in studies in lupus patients differs widely as a consequence of differences between study populations with respect to size, mean age, ethnic background, menstrual status, disease severity and treatments used. The aetiology of bone loss in SLE is supposed to be multifactorial, involving both non-disease related and disease related factors.

Non-Disease Related Risk Factors for Osteoporosis in SLE

Higher age [84, 90, 93, 96, 101], low body-mass index [84, 86, 93], postmenopausal status [84, 86, 93, 94, 101], and non-Afro-Caribbean race [101] have been recognized as significant non-disease related risk factors for reduced BMD in patients with SLE. Two small studies in men demonstrated no increased prevalence of osteoporosis in male SLE patients [106, 109]. Several studies have evaluated the effects of smoking and alcohol use, but no significant associations with low BMD in patients with SLE have been reported [86, 90, 93,

101, 112, 113]. Data on other possible risk factors for low BMD (e.g. family history of osteoporosis and reduced mobility) are generally not available.

Disease Related Risk Factors for Osteoporosis in SLE

Disease duration, inflammation, renal failure, deficiency of 25(OH) vitamin D, reduced physical activity, hormonal factors and medication related factors have been suggested to play a role in the development of osteoporosis in SLE.

In contrast to two studies [98, 105] reporting an association between disease duration and BMD in SLE patients, most studies did not find such an association [84, 86, 88, 90, 94, 108, 112].

Disease activity is supposed to play a role in the development of osteoporosis in SLE [117]. Serum levels of pro-inflammatory cytokines, such as TNF-α, IL-1 and IL-6, are increased in patients with SLE [118] and production of bone-resorbing lymphokines by B-cells in SLE patients has been described [119]. These findings suggest that disease activity might be a risk factor for osteoporosis in SLE. Indeed, Petri and colleagues reported that disease activity, as measured by low serum C4 levels, was an independent predictor of low BMD in the lumbar spine [120]. However, no association between disease activity and BMD was found in all recent studies, including studies using cumulative measures for disease activity over time [86, 90, 94-96, 98, 100, 105, 106, 109, 115].

The relationship between BMD and organ damage in patients with SLE has been investigated in several studies, with conflicting results. In four studies [94, 98, 105, 111], higher organ damage score was significantly associated with low BMD in patients with SLE, but in four other studies [86, 90, 91, 93] no association between BMD and organ damage score in SLE patients was found. The reasons for this discrepancy are unclear.

Renal failure might contribute to the development of low BMD in patients with SLE through several mechanisms. Renal damage due to SLE may result in an impairment of vitamin D 1-hydroxylation by the kidneys, secondary hyperparathyroidism and increased osteoclastic bone resorption. However, no significant association between renal function and BMD was reported in recent studies [86, 90, 94], which might be explained by the relatively small number of patients with renal failure included in most recent studies and exclusion of patients with renal failure in several other studies [88, 92, 95, 98, 100, 106, 109, 110, 112].

Deficiency of 25(OH) vitamin D might be regarded as a non-disease related as well as a disease related risk factor for osteoporosis in SLE. However, the increased prevalence of 25(OH) vitamin D deficiency reported in patients with SLE, as compared to healthy controls [121] is usually ascribed to the disease related conscious avoidance of exposure to sunlight and/or the use of sunscreens [99, 105, 106, 121]. In a study in 107 Dutch SLE patients, deficiency of 25(OH) vitamin D was significantly associated with low BMD in the lumbar spine, but not at the hip [86].

Reduced physical activity is considered an important risk factor for the development of osteoporosis in several rheumatic disorders [117]. Bhattoa et al [84] reported a significant negative association between Steinbrocker functional classification and lumbar spine and hip

BMD in SLE patients, but other studies failed to demonstrate an association between physical activity and BMD in SLE patients [86, 90, 91, 115].

Several hormonal factors may be involved in the pathogenesis of low BMD in lupus. SLE is characterized by enhanced hydroxylation of estradiol, increased oxidation of testosterone and relatively low plasma levels of androgens, such as dehydroepiandrosterone sulphate (DHEAS). In addition, hyperprolactinaemia has been reported in patients with SLE, which may further decrease serum levels of estradiol and androgens [122]. In a study in 37 premenopausal SLE patients, a significant positive relationship between serum DHEAS levels and BMD was demonstrated [89]. In a small study in 20 male SLE patients, no association between hyperprolactinemia and low BMD was found [109]. Premature ovarian dysfunction as a result of active disease or caused by medication, is common in female SLE patients and contributes to bone loss by a reduction of overall estrogen exposure. In a study by Gordon et al [91], significantly decreased BMD values in SLE patients with a disordered menstrual history were found. These findings support the viewpoint that hormonal factors contribute to the development of low BMD in SLE.

The role of corticosteroids in the development of osteoporosis in SLE is still under debate. Various studies reported a relationship between corticosteroid use and low BMD [84, 85, 90, 91, 93, 94, 98, 100, 110], but several other studies did not find a significant relationship between corticosteroid treatment and BMD in SLE patients [86-89, 92, 96, 105, 106, 108, 109, 111-113]. The reasons for this discrepancy are unclear, but may be related to differences in patient populations in size, mean age and menstrual status, as well as differences between centers in treatment strategies for osteoporosis and use of corticosteroids. Moreover, corticosteroids might play a dual role with respect to the development of osteoporosis in SLE. On the one hand corticosteroid therapy may induce bone loss, but on the other hand corticosteroids might have a beneficial effect on bone mass by suppressing inflammation. Bone loss in patients with SLE might also be induced by other drugs which are commonly used in these patients. Cyclophosphamide may induce osteoporosis by induction of premature ovarian failure. In addition, long-term exposure to oral anticoagulation, and to a lesser extent, low-molecular-weight heparin, has been associated with increased bone loss in the general population [123], but this has not been investigated in patients with SLE.

Fractures in SLE

In contrast to the large number of studies on BMD, only a few studies on osteoporotic fractures in SLE have been published. In 4 studies, symptomatic vertebral and peripheral fractures occurring since disease onset were reported in 9-16.5% of SLE patients [84, 91, 93, 124]. The incidence of symptomatic vertebral and peripheral fractures was demonstrated to be 5 times higher in female SLE patients as compared to age-matched healthy women, and higher age and prolonged use of corticosteroids were identified as the most important risk factors for fractures [124]. In this large study, 10% of the symptomatic fractures were reported to be vertebral fractures.

Only two studies on prevalent vertebral fractures in SLE patients, using a standardized method to assess vertebral fractures, have been performed and in these studies at least 1 vertebral fracture was detected in 20-21% of the patients [86, 107]. In both studies, vertebral fractures were defined as a reduction of ≥ 20% of the vertebral body height. The frequency of vertebral fractures (20%) in 90 Dutch SLE patients with mean age 41 years, was high in comparison to the 12% prevalence of vertebral fractures in the general population of Europe with an age between 65 and 69 years [125]. Interestingly, in both studies on prevalent vertebral fractures in SLE, no association between oral corticosteroid use and vertebral fractures was found, but in the Dutch study, previous use of intravenous methylprenisolone was associated with prevalent vertebral fractures [86]. In both studies, BMD was not different between SLE patients with and without prevalent vertebral fractures [86, 107]. This finding is in line with results of a previous study in the general population, which reported that the proportion of fractures attributable to osteoporosis is modest, ranging from 10% to 44% [126]. These data suggest that bone quality contributes more to bone strength than bone quantity and point to the limited value of BMD measurement by DEXA in the assessment of future fracture risk. The high frequency of both peripheral and vertebral fractures demonstrated in SLE patients highlights the need to develop better strategies for the prevention and treatment of osteoporosis and fractures as important disease complications in lupus patients. The need for better prevention and treatment strategies is also illustrated by the relative high frequency of undertreatment of SLE patients with manifest osteoporosis or at high risk of the development of osteoporosis, as demonstrated in the Dutch study [86].

Prevention and Treatment of Osteoporosis in SLE

Prevention strategies directed toward SLE patients at risk for osteoporosis and fractures include advice for maintaining a normal body weight and daily performance of weight-baring physical activity. In addition, physicians should encourage a healthy diet and strongly advice against smoking. Moreover, adequate calcium and vitamin D supplementation should be prescribed. We advocate to perform BMD measurement by DEXA in SLE patients treated with corticosteroids and/or in postmenopausal patients with SLE. Moreover, as a consequence of the high prevalence of vertebral fractures demonstrated in SLE patients, physicians should consider to perform spine X-rays (analyzed using a standardized method for assessing vertebral deformities) next to BMD measurement of the spine and hip in the assessment of osteoporosis and future fracture risk. Postmenopausal women with osteoporosis and/or fractures and women on corticosteroids should be treated with appropriate antiosteoporosis medication, eg bisphosphonates. Results of a recent study in postmenopausal women in the general population have demonstrated a significant beneficial effect on BMD and a significantly reduced risk for symptomatic vertebral fractures (but not for other fractures) in patients continuing bisphosphonate therapy for 10 years as compared to patients who discontinued bisphosphonates after 5 years [127]. Moreover, the safety of long-term treatment with bisphosphonates up to 10 years was demonstrated in this study [127]. Bisphosphonates are contraindicated in patients with renal failure and in premenopausal lupus women planning pregnancy. Bisphosphonates are maintained in bone for a long period of time even after discontinuation of therapy, and fetal abnormalities due to bisphosphonates were demonstrated in animal studies [128]. Hormonal replacement therapy may be useful in postmenopausal women without an increased risk of thrombosis.

Infections in SLE

Importance of Infections in SLE

Infections are an important cause of morbidity and mortality in patients with SLE. Infections occur in 25% to 50% of SLE patients in case series [129-132] and a third of the infections in SLE patients were demonstrated to be major infections for which hospital admission is required [129, 130, 133]. Infection as primary cause of death has been reported in up to 50% of patients with SLE [5, 7].

Spectrum of Infections in SLE

SLE patients suffer from a broad spectrum of infections caused predominantly by community-acquired bacteria [129-131, 133], but also opportunistic infections are reported [5]. Among Indian SLE patients, tuberculosis was demonstrated to be the commonest infection [134]. Moreover, a high incidence (up to 21%) of Herpes zoster infection was found in several studies in SLE patients [129, 130, 135-139].

Risk Factors for Infections in SLE

Treatment with corticosteroids and immunosuppressive agents and defects in immune function (which may result from the disease itself and its therapy) are supposed to play a role in the pathogenesis [5], but also disease activity [7, 133, 140-142], disease duration [129, 143], active nephritis [135, 144] and decreased renal function [142] have been linked to an increased risk of infection in lupus patients.

The role of corticosteroid use as an independent risk factor for infections in SLE was demonstrated in several studies [130-132, 135, 145], but other studies failed to find such an association [129, 133, 140-142]. The impact of immunosuppressive drugs, such as cyclophosphamide, azathioprine and methotrexate, on the immune system is well established. Use of immunosuppressive drugs was identified as an independent risk factor for infections in some studies in SLE [131, 132, 142, 145], but not in other studies in patients with SLE [7, 86, 133, 140]. Some studies failed to demonstrate an additive effect of cytotoxic drugs in increasing the overall infection rate, but showed an increased incidence of Herpes zoster infections in patients using cyclophosphamide [136, 146] or azathioprine [135]. Since corticosteroids and immunosuppressive drugs are used mostly in patients with more severe disease, it is likely that both disease activity and drug therapy contribute to the increased infection risk in SLE. In a recent study, a strong negative association between hydroxychloroquine use and the occurrence of major infections was demonstrated [129]. This finding might be explained by the frequent use of hydroxychloroquine in the treatment of patients with mild lupus disease activity. Another explanation might be protection against infections due to the antimicrobial properties of hydroxychloroquine. However, antimalarials act against pathogenic organisms that are very uncommon in Western European countries [129].

Defects in the Complement System and Infections in SLE

Several defects in both humoral and cellular immunity have been described in lupus patients, which might contribute to an inadequate immune defence [5]. The potential role of macrophage defects, polymorphonuclear cell defects, defects in number and function of natural killer cells, T cells and B cells, immunoglobulin defects and dysfunction of the reticuloendothelial system in the pathogenesis of infections in SLE has been extensively described by Iliopoulos and Tsokos [5]. This chapter is restricted to the results of recent research on the contribution of the complement system to the increased infection risk in SLE.

The complement system plays an important role in host defence against microorganisms and the increased infection rate in SLE patients has been attributed in part to defects in the complement system [5]. A strong association between genetic deficiencies of early components of the classical pathway of complement activation and the development of SLE has been demonstrated [147]. In particular, deficiency of C1q is a major risk factor for the development of SLE. Moreover, deficiency of C1q might play a role in the susceptibility to infections in SLE, since C1q plays a role in the recognition and clearance of apoptotic material [148] and binds predominantly to antibodies and protein structures on bacteria and viruses, resulting in complement activation. The consumption of complement proteins by circulating and tissue-fixed immune complexes might also limit the amount of complement that is available for host defence against invading pathogens.

Deficiency of Mannose-Binding Lectin and Infections in SLE

Recently, the lectin pathway of complement activation has also been suggested to play a role in the pathogenesis of SLE [149] and in the occurrence of infections in SLE patients [150-152]. Mannose-binding lectin (MBL) is a serum protein that shares many features with C1q [153]. In contrast to C1q, which is a recognition molecule in the classical pathway of complement activation, MBL serves as one of the recognition molecules in the lectin pathway of complement activation [154]. MBL may activate complement through the lectin pathway by interacting with MBL-associated serine proteases (MASP). In addition, MBL can directly opsonise pathogenic microorganisms and enhance the activity of phagocytes [154].

In a meta-analysis of all available case-control studies, homozygosity for variant MBL alleles was demonstrated to be a minor risk factor for the presence of SLE [155]. A significant association between MBL codon 54 variant B and SLE was reported in that study.

In two Danish studies [150, 151] and a Japanese study [152], SLE patients homozygous for MBL variant alleles were at an increased risk for serious infections in comparison with patients who were heterozygous or homozygous for the normal allele. In contrast, in a study in Dutch SLE patients, no association between the biological activity of MBL and the occurrence of infections was found [129]. In this study, functional MBL activity was determined using three different assays: 1) an assay measuring functional MBL serum levels which is dependent only on the amount of functional protein, 2) an assay measuring activity of the MBL/MASP complex by assessing MBL-induced C4 deposition and 3) an assay measuring the complete MBL pathway activity in serum, which is sensitive to defects in all components of the MBL pathway. None of these assays demonstrated an association between deficient MBL activity and the occurrence of infections or major infections in patients with SLE [129]. There are two possible explanations for the discrepancy between the results of the genetic and the phenotypic studies. First, functional activity of MBL in serum not only is determined by mutations in the gene encoding MBL, but is also dependent on promoter polymorphisms, MASP activity, serum levels of other complement factors, and environmental factors [156, 157]. Therefore, measurement of functional MBL activity is supposed to be a better estimation of the in vivo situation than assessment of MBL genotypes when evaluating the association between the MBL pathway of complement activation and the occurrence of infections in SLE. Secondly, the discrepancy between the genotypic and phenotypic data could be explained by unidentified linkages between mutations or polymorphisms in the MBL gene with mutations or polymorphisms in other genes, which might influence the genetic approach. The results of this study suggest that deficiency of functional MBL activity does not play a role in the susceptibility to infections or major infections in SLE. However, this does not exclude an influence of defects in the complement system on the occurrence of infections in SLE. Therefore, future research will be focused on the role of defects of other complement factors and complement inhibitors in the pathogenesis of infections in SLE.

Diagnostic and Therapeutic Considerations

It is often difficult to distinguish infection from disease flare in febrile patients with SLE. As a consequence of an inadequate inflammatory response, signs and symptoms of infection may be subtle or absent, especially in patients treated with immunosuppressive drugs. On the other hand, clinical symptoms of lupus activity may simulate infection. Physicians should be aware that false-positive serological tests for several infections (e.g. Lyme disease, toxoplasmosis, syphilis), which are caused by polyclonal hypergammaglobulinaemia, are often found in SLE patients [5]. In addition, skin tests may be false-negative in case of corticosteroid use [5]. Chills and leukocytosis are markers favouring infection. Moreover, in a study in SLE patients, high C-reactive protein levels were associated with infection, in the absence of serositis [158]. Another study demonstrated increased serum procalcitonine levels in lupus patients with bacterial or fungal infections as compared to patients with viral infections or with lupus flare [159]. The presence of low complement levels and high serum anti-DNA antibody titers suggests lupus flare.

Strategies to reduce the morbidity and mortality related to infections in SLE include hygienic measures, prophylactic use of antimicrobial agents and immunisations.

Prophylaxis against *Pneumocystis carinii,* using a regimen of low-dose trimethoprim/ sulfamethoxazole or inhaled pentamidine should be considered in selected SLE patients being treated with immunosuppressive agents [160]. Moreover, prophylaxis with isoniazide is recommended in SLE patients with positive tuberculin skin test requiring high dose corticosteroids [161].

Although initial reports suggested that pneumococcal vaccinations in patients with SLE might induce disease exacerbations [162], recent studies demonstrated that vaccinations against influenza en pneumococcus are safe in this patient group [163, 164], although influenza vaccination was less effective in SLE patients than in controls [163].

Early diagnosis and treatment of infections in patients with SLE remains a difficult challenge for physicians. More research is necessary to develop laboratory tests that will improve differentiating between infections and disease exacerbations in patients with SLE.

Conclusion

The importance of CVD, osteoporosis, and infections as long-term complications in patients with SLE, can not be over emphasized. The aetiology of these complications in SLE is supposed to be multifactorial, including risk factors that also apply to the general population, disease-related and treatment-related risk factors. The relative contributions of these risk factors are not fully understood. Ongoing research should attempt to further unravel the pathogenic mechanisms, applying especially to SLE patients. Physicians treating patients with SLE should be aware of the long-term complications that might develop in their patients. In addition, SLE patients themselves need to understand how to modify lifestyle factors that increase the risk of premature atherosclerosis, osteoporosis, fractures and infectious complications. Treatment regimens will benefit from the results of large scale prospective studies evaluating the effect of different intervention strategies to reduce the risk of CVD, osteoporosis and infections in patients with SLE.

References

[1]   Bernatsky S, Boivin JF, Joseph L, Manzi S, Ginzler E, Gladman DD et al. Mortality in systemic lupus erythematosus. *Arthritis Rheum.* 2006;54(8):2550-7.

[2]   Abu-Shakra M, Urowitz MB, Gladman DD, Gough J. Mortality studies in systemic lupus erythematosus. Results from a single center. I. Causes of death. *J. Rheumatol.* 1995;22(7):1259-64.

[3]   Urowitz MB, Gladman DD. How to improve morbidity and mortality in systemic lupus erythematosus. *Rheumatology (Oxford)* 2000;39(3):238-44.

[4]   Bjornadal L, Yin L, Granath F, Klareskog L, Ekbom A. Cardiovascular disease a hazard despite improved prognosis in patients with systemic lupus erythematosus: results from a Swedish population based study 1964-95. *J. Rheumatol.* 2004;31(4):713-9.

[5]   Iliopoulos AG, Tsokos GC. Immunopathogenesis and spectrum of infections in systemic lupus erythematosus. *Semin Arthritis Rheum.* 1996;25(5):318-36.

[6]   Moss KE, Ioannou Y, Sultan SM, Haq I, Isenberg DA. Outcome of a cohort of 300 patients with systemic lupus erythematosus attending a dedicated clinic for over two decades. *Ann. Rheum Dis.* 2002;61(5):409-13.

[7]   Nossent JC. Course and prognostic value of Systemic Lupus Erythematosus Disease Activity Index in black Caribbean patients. *Semin. Arthritis Rheum.* 1993;23(1):16-21.

[8]   Gladman D, Ginzler E, Goldsmith C, Fortin P, Liang M, Urowitz M et al. The development and initial validation of the Systemic Lupus International Collaborating Clinics/American College of Rheumatology damage index for systemic lupus erythematosus. *Arthritis Rheum.* 1996;39(3):363-9.

[9]   Manzi S, Meilahn EN, Rairie JE, Conte CG, Medsger TA, Jr., Jansen-McWilliams L et al. Age-specific incidence rates of myocardial infarction and angina in women with systemic lupus erythematosus: comparison with the Framingham Study. *Am. J. Epidemiol.* 1997;145(5):408-15.

[10]   Kitagawa Y, Gotoh F, Koto A, Okayasu H. Stroke in systemic lupus erythematosus. *Stroke* 1990;21(11):1533-9.

[11]   McDonald J, Stewart J, Urowitz MB, Gladman DD. Peripheral vascular disease in patients with systemic lupus erythematosus. *Ann. Rheum Dis.* 1992;51(1):56-60.

[12]   Esdaile JM, Abrahamowicz M, Grodzicky T, Li Y, Panaritis C, du Berger R et al. Traditional Framingham risk factors fail to fully account for accelerated atherosclerosis in systemic lupus erythematosus. *Arthritis Rheum.* 2001;44(10):2331-7.

[13]   Ward MM. Premature morbidity from cardiovascular and cerebrovascular diseases in women with systemic lupus erythematosus. *Arthritis Rheum.* 1999;42(2):338-46.

[14]   Asanuma Y, Chung CP, Oeser A, Shintani A, Stanley E, Raggi P et al. Increased concentration of proatherogenic inflammatory cytokines in systemic lupus erythematosus: relationship to cardiovascular risk factors. *J. Rheumatol.* 2006; 33(3): 539-45.

[15]   Bruce IN. 'Not only...but also': factors that contribute to accelerated atherosclerosis and premature coronary heart disease in systemic lupus erythematosus. *Rheumatology (Oxford)* 2005;44(12):1492-502.

[16]   Roman MJ, Shanker BA, Davis A, Lockshin MD, Sammaritano L, Simantov R et al. Prevalence and correlates of accelerated atherosclerosis in systemic lupus erythematosus. *N. Engl. J. Med.* 2003;349(25):2399-406.

[17]   El-Magadmi M, Bodill H, Ahmad Y, Durrington PN, Mackness M, Walker M et al. Systemic lupus erythematosus: an independent risk factor for endothelial dysfunction in women. *Circulation* 2004;110(4):399-404.

[18]   Frostegard J. SLE, atherosclerosis and cardiovascular disease. *J. Intern. Med.* 2005;257(6):485-95.

[19]   Bruce IN, Urowitz MB, Gladman DD, Ibanez D, Steiner G. Risk factors for coronary heart disease in women with systemic lupus erythematosus: the Toronto Risk Factor Study. *Arthritis Rheum.* 2003;48(11):3159-67.

[20]   Petri M, Perez-Gutthann S, Spence D, Hochberg MC. Risk factors for coronary artery disease in patients with systemic lupus erythematosus. *Am. J. Med.* 1992;93(5):513-9.

[21] Manzi S, Selzer F, Sutton-Tyrrell K, Fitzgerald SG, Rairie JE, Tracy RP et al. Prevalence and risk factors of carotid plaque in women with systemic lupus erythematosus. *Arthritis Rheum.* 1999;42(1):51-60.

[22] Bessant R, Hingorani A, Patel L, MacGregor A, Isenberg DA, Rahman A. Risk of coronary heart disease and stroke in a large British cohort of patients with systemic lupus erythematosus. *Rheumatology (Oxford)* 2004;43(7):924-9.

[23] Harris EN, Gharavi AE, Boey ML, Patel BM, Mackworth-Young CG, Loizou S et al. Anticardiolipin antibodies: detection by radioimmunoassay and association with thrombosis in systemic lupus erythematosus. *Lancet* 1983;2(8361):1211-4.

[24] Petri M. The lupus anticoagulant is a risk factor for myocardial infarction (but not atherosclerosis): Hopkins Lupus Cohort. *Thromb. Res.* 2004;114(5-6):593-5.

[25] Jouhikainen T, Stephansson E, Leirisalo-Repo M. Lupus anticoagulant as a prognostic marker in systemic lupus erythematosus. *Br. J. Rheumatol.* 1993;32(7):568-73.

[26] Svenungsson E, Jensen-Urstad K, Heimburger M, Silveira A, Hamsten A, de Faire U et al. Risk factors for cardiovascular disease in systemic lupus erythematosus. *Circulation* 2001;104(16):1887-93.

[27] Farzaneh-Far A, Roman MJ, Lockshin MD, Devereux RB, Paget SA, Crow MK et al. Relationship of antiphospholipid antibodies to cardiovascular manifestations of systemic lupus erythematosus. *Arthritis Rheum.* 2006;54(12):3918-25.

[28] Vaarala O, Manttari M, Manninen V, Tenkanen L, Puurunen M, Aho K et al. Anti-cardiolipin antibodies and risk of myocardial infarction in a prospective cohort of middle-aged men. *Circulation* 1995;91(1):23-7.

[29] Wu R, Nityanand S, Berglund L, Lithell H, Holm G, Lefvert AK. Antibodies against cardiolipin and oxidatively modified LDL in 50-year-old men predict myocardial infarction. *Arterioscler. Thromb. Vasc. Biol.* 1997;17(11):3159-63.

[30] Haberland ME, Olch CL, Folgelman AM. Role of lysines in mediating interaction of modified low density lipoproteins with the scavenger receptor of human monocyte macrophages. *J. Biol. Chem.* 1984;259(18):11305-11.

[31] Kobayashi K, Kishi M, Atsumi T, Bertolaccini ML, Makino H, Sakairi N et al. Circulating oxidized LDL forms complexes with beta2-glycoprotein I: implication as an atherogenic autoantigen. *J. Lipid Res.* 2003;44(4):716-26.

[32] Matsuura E, Koike T. Accelerated atheroma and anti-beta2-glycoprotein I antibodies. *Lupus* 2000;9(3):210-6.

[33] van Leuven SI, Kastelein JJ, D'Cruz DP, Hughes GR, Stroes ES. Atherogenesis in rheumatology. *Lupus* 2006;15(3):117-21.

[34] Shoenfeld Y, Wu R, Dearing LD, Matsuura E. Are anti-oxidized low-density lipoprotein antibodies pathogenic or protective? *Circulation* 2004;110(17):2552-8.

[35] Leong KH, Koh ET, Feng PH, Boey ML. Lipid profiles in patients with systemic lupus erythematosus. *J. Rheumatol.* 1994;21(7):1264-7.

[36] Manger K, Kusus M, Forster C, Ropers D, Daniel WG, Kalden JR et al. Factors associated with coronary artery calcification in young female patients with SLE. *Ann. Rheum. Dis.* 2003;62(9):846-50.

[37] Theodoridou A, Bento L, D'Cruz DP, Khamashta MA, Hughes GR. Prevalence and associations of an abnormal ankle-brachial index in systemic lupus erythematosus: a pilot study. *Ann. Rheum. Dis.* 2003;62(12):1199-203.

[38] Doria A, Shoenfeld Y, Wu R, Gambari PF, Puato M, Ghirardello A et al. Risk factors for subclinical atherosclerosis in a prospective cohort of patients with systemic lupus erythematosus. *Ann. Rheum. Dis.* 2003;62(11):1071-7.

[39] Selzer F, Sutton-Tyrrell K, Fitzgerald SG, Pratt JE, Tracy RP, Kuller LH et al. Comparison of risk factors for vascular disease in the carotid artery and aorta in women with systemic lupus erythematosus. *Arthritis Rheum.* 2004;50(1):151-9.

[40] Borba EF, Bonfa E. Dyslipoproteinemias in systemic lupus erythematosus: influence of disease, activity, and anticardiolipin antibodies. *Lupus* 1997;6(6):533-9.

[41] Borba EF, Santos RD, Bonfa E, Vinagre CG, Pileggi FJ, Cossermelli W et al. Lipoprotein(a) levels in systemic lupus erythematosus. *J. Rheumatol.* 1994;21(2):220-3.

[42] Svenungsson E, Gunnarsson I, Fei GZ, Lundberg IE, Klareskog L, Frostegard J. Elevated triglycerides and low levels of high-density lipoprotein as markers of disease activity in association with up-regulation of the tumor necrosis factor alpha/tumor necrosis factor receptor system in systemic lupus erythematosus. *Arthritis Rheum.* 2003;48(9):2533-40.

[43] de Carvalho JF, Borba EF, Viana VS, Bueno C, Leon EP, Bonfa E. Anti-lipoprotein lipase antibodies: a new player in the complex atherosclerotic process in systemic lupus erythematosus? *Arthritis Rheum.* 2004;50(11):3610-5.

[44] D'Cruz DP, Houssiau FA, Ramirez G, Baguley E, McCutcheon J, Vianna J et al. Antibodies to endothelial cells in systemic lupus erythematosus: a potential marker for nephritis and vasculitis. *Clin. Exp. Immunol.* 1991;85(2):254-61.

[45] Carvalho D, Savage CO, Isenberg D, Pearson JD. IgG anti-endothelial cell autoantibodies from patients with systemic lupus erythematosus or systemic vasculitis stimulate the release of two endothelial cell-derived mediators, which enhance adhesion molecule expression and leukocyte adhesion in an autocrine manner. *Arthritis Rheum.* 1999;42(4):631-40.

[46] Cederholm A, Svenungsson E, Stengel D, Fei GZ, Pockley AG, Ninio E et al. Platelet-activating factor-acetylhydrolase and other novel risk and protective factors for cardiovascular disease in systemic lupus erythematosus. *Arthritis Rheum.* 2004;50(9): 2869-76.

[47] Ridker PM, Hennekens CH, Buring JE, Rifai N. C-reactive protein and other markers of inflammation in the prediction of cardiovascular disease in women. *N. Engl. J. Med.* 2000;342(12):836-43.

[48] Toloza SM, Uribe AG, McGwin G, Jr., Alarcon GS, Fessler BJ, Bastian HM et al. Systemic lupus erythematosus in a multiethnic US cohort (LUMINA). XXIII. Baseline predictors of vascular events. *Arthritis Rheum.* 2004;50(12):3947-57.

[49] Muscari A, Bastagli L, Poggiopollini G, Tomassetti V, Massarelli G, Cappelletti O et al. Different associations of C-reactive protein, fibrinogen and C3 with traditional risk factors in middle-aged men. *Int. J. Cardiol.* 2002;83(1):63-71.

[50] Onat A, Uzunlar B, Hergenc G, Yazici M, Sari I, Uyarel H et al. Cross-sectional study of complement C3 as a coronary risk factor among men and women. *Clin. Sci. (Lond)* 2005;108(2):129-35.

[51] Bultink IEM, Turkstra F, Diamant M, Dijkmans BAC, Voskuyl AE. Metabolic syndrome in women with systemic lupus erythematosus: Prevalence and association of metabolic syndrome score with disease characteristics and cardiovascular events. *Arthritis Rheum.* 2006;54(9):S270.

[52] Chung CP, Avalos I, Oeser A, Gebretsadik T, Shintani A, Raggi P et al. High prevalence of the metabolic syndrome in patients with systemic lupus erythematosus: association with disease characteristics and cardiovascular risk factors. *Ann. Rheum. Dis.* 2007;66(2):208-14.

[53] de Lemos JA, Morrow DA, Sabatine MS, Murphy SA, Gibson CM, Antman EM et al. Association between plasma levels of monocyte chemoattractant protein-1 and long-term clinical outcomes in patients with acute coronary syndromes. *Circulation* 2003; 107(5):690-5.

[54] Schieffer B, Selle T, Hilfiker A, Hilfiker-Kleiner D, Grote K, Tietge UJ et al. Impact of interleukin-6 on plaque development and morphology in experimental atherosclerosis. *Circulation* 2004;110(22):3493-500.

[55] Reichlin M, Fesmire J, Quintero-Del-Rio AI, Wolfson-Reichlin M. Autoantibodies to lipoprotein lipase and dyslipidemia in systemic lupus erythematosus. *Arthritis Rheum.* 2002; 46(11):2957-63.

[56] Cederholm A, Svenungsson E, Jensen-Urstad K, Trollmo C, Ulfgren AK, Swedenborg J et al. Decreased binding of annexin v to endothelial cells: a potential mechanism in atherothrombosis of patients with systemic lupus erythematosus. *Arterioscler. Thromb. Vasc. Biol.* 2005;25(1):198-203.

[57] Ames PR, Alves J, Murat I, Isenberg DA, Nourooz-Zadeh J. Oxidative stress in systemic lupus erythematosus and allied conditions with vascular involvement. *Rheumatology (Oxford)* 1999;38(6):529-34.

[58] Nuttall SL, Heaton S, Piper MK, Martin U, Gordon C. Cardiovascular risk in systemic lupus erythematosus--evidence of increased oxidative stress and dyslipidaemia. *Rheumatology (Oxford)* 2003;42(6):758-62.

[59] Delgado AJ, Ames PR, Donohue S, Stanyer L, Nourooz-Zadeh J, Ravirajan C et al. Antibodies to high-density lipoprotein and beta2-glycoprotein I are inversely correlated with paraoxonase activity in systemic lupus erythematosus and primary antiphospholipid syndrome. *Arthritis Rheum.* 2002;46(10):2686-94.

[60] Boger RH, Bode-Boger SM, Szuba A, Tsao PS, Chan JR, Tangphao O et al. Asymmetric dimethylarginine (ADMA): a novel risk factor for endothelial dysfunction: its role in hypercholesterolemia. *Circulation* 1998;98(18):1842-7.

[61] Valkonen VP, Paiva H, Salonen JT, Lakka TA, Lehtimaki T, Laakso J et al. Risk of acute coronary events and serum concentration of asymmetrical dimethylarginine. *Lancet* 2001;358(9299):2127-8.

[62] Zoccali C, Bode-Boger S, Mallamaci F, Benedetto F, Tripepi G, Malatino L et al. Plasma concentration of asymmetrical dimethylarginine and mortality in patients with end-stage renal disease: a prospective study. *Lancet* 2001;358(9299):2113-7.

[63] Bultink IE, Teerlink T, Heijst JA, Dijkmans BA, Voskuyl AE. Raised plasma levels of asymmetric dimethylarginine are associated with cardiovascular events, disease activity, and organ damage in patients with systemic lupus erythematosus. *Ann. Rheum. Dis.* 2005;64(9):1362-5.

[64] Kiani AN, Post W, Mahoney JA, Petri M. ADMA in SLE is associated with serologic activity, cardiovascular risk factors, and coronary calcium. *Arthritis Rheum.* 2005;52(9):S603.

[65] Sun KH, Tang SJ, Wang YS, Lin WJ, You RI. Autoantibodies to dsDNA cross-react with the arginine-glycine-rich domain of heterogeneous nuclear ribonucleoprotein A2 (hnRNP A2) and promote methylation of hnRNP A2. *Rheumatology (Oxford)* 2003;42(1):154-61.

[66] Gary JD, Clarke S. RNA and protein interactions modulated by protein arginine methylation. *Prog. Nucleic. Acid. Res. Mol. Biol* .1998;61:65-131.

[67] Sun KH, Yu CL, Tang SJ, Sun GH. Monoclonal anti-double-stranded DNA autoantibody stimulates the expression and release of IL-1beta, IL-6, IL-8, IL-10 and TNF-alpha from normal human mononuclear cells involving in the lupus pathogenesis. *Immunology* 2000;99(3):352-60.

[68] Petri M, Roubenoff R, Dallal GE, Nadeau MR, Selhub J, Rosenberg IH. Plasma homocysteine as a risk factor for atherothrombotic events in systemic lupus erythematosus. *Lancet* 1996;348(9035):1120-4.

[69] Fijnheer R, Roest M, Haas FJ, De Groot PG, Derksen RH. Homocysteine, methylenetetrahydrofolate reductase polymorphism, antiphospholipid antibodies, and thromboembolic events in systemic lupus erythematosus: a retrospective cohort study. *J. Rheumatol.* 1998;25(9):1737-42.

[70] Hanson RL, Imperatore G, Bennett PH, Knowler WC. Components of the "metabolic syndrome" and incidence of type 2 diabetes. *Diabetes* 2002;51(10):3120-7.

[71] Wilson PW, Kannel WB, Silbershatz H, D'Agostino RB. Clustering of metabolic factors and coronary heart disease. *Arch. Intern. Med* .1999;159(10):1104-9.

[72] El Magadmi M, Ahmad Y, Turkie W, Yates AP, Sheikh N, Bernstein RM et al. Hyperinsulinemia, insulin resistance, and circulating oxidized low density lipoprotein in women with systemic lupus erythematosus. *J. Rheumatol.* 2006;33(1):50-6.

[73] Sada KE, Yamasaki Y, Maruyama M, Sugiyama H, Yamamura M, Maeshima Y et al. Altered levels of adipocytokines in association with insulin resistance in patients with systemic lupus erythematosus. *J. Rheumatol.* 2006;33(8):1545-52.

[74] Asanuma Y, Oeser A, Shintani AK, Turner E, Olsen N, Fazio S et al. Premature coronary-artery atherosclerosis in systemic lupus erythematosus. *N. Engl. J. Med.* 2003; 349(25):2407-15.

[75] MacGregor AJ, Dhillon VB, Binder A, Forte CA, Knight BC, Betteridge DJ et al. Fasting lipids and anticardiolipin antibodies as risk factors for vascular disease in systemic lupus erythematosus. *Ann. Rheum. Dis.* 1992;51(2):152-5.

[76] Petri M, Spence D, Bone LR, Hochberg MC. Coronary artery disease risk factors in the Johns Hopkins Lupus Cohort: prevalence, recognition by patients, and preventive practices. *Medicine (Baltimore)* 1992;71(5):291-302.

[77] Borba EF, Bonfa E. Longterm beneficial effect of chloroquine diphosphate on lipoprotein profile in lupus patients with and without steroid therapy. *J. Rheumatol.* 2001;28(4):780-5.

[78] Petri M, Lakatta C, Magder L, Goldman D. Effect of prednisone and hydroxychloroquine on coronary artery disease risk factors in systemic lupus erythematosus: a longitudinal data analysis. *Am. J. Med.* 1994;96(3):254-9.

[79] Rahman P, Gladman DD, Urowitz MB, Yuen K, Hallett D, Bruce IN. The cholesterol lowering effect of antimalarial drugs is enhanced in patients with lupus taking corticosteroid drugs. *J. Rheumatol.* 1999;26(2):325-30.

[80] Wallace DJ, Metzger AL, Stecher VJ, Turnbull BA, Kern PA. Cholesterol-lowering effect of hydroxychloroquine in patients with rheumatic disease: reversal of deleterious effects of steroids on lipids. *Am. J. Med.* 1990;89(3):322-6.

[81] Bevan AP, Krook A, Tikerpae J, Seabright PJ, Siddle K, Smith GD. Chloroquine extends the lifetime of the activated insulin receptor complex in endosomes. *J. Biol. Chem.* 1997;272(43):26833-40.

[82] Urowitz MB, Gladman DD, Ibanez D, Berliner Y. Modification of hypertension and hypercholesterolaemia in patients with systemic lupus erythematosus: a quality improvement study. *Ann. Rheum. Dis.* 2006;65(1):115-7.

[83] Fortin PR, Abahamowicz M, Cymet A, Neville C, Harvey P, Su J et al. The health improvement and prevention program (HIPP) in systemic lupus erythematosus (SLE) shows preliminary benefits in reducing the estimated 8-year risk of cardiovascular disease. *Arthritis Rheum.* 2006;54(9):S791.

[84] Bhattoa HP, Bettembuk P, Balogh A, Szegedi G, Kiss E. Bone mineral density in women with systemic lupus erythematosus. *Clin. Rheumatol.* 2002;21(2):135-41.

[85] Boyanov M, Robeva R, Popivanov P. Bone mineral density changes in women with systemic lupus erythematosus. *Clin. Rheumatol.* 2003;22(4-5):318-23.

[86] Bultink IE, Lems WF, Kostense PJ, Dijkmans BA, Voskuyl AE. Prevalence of and risk factors for low bone mineral density and vertebral fractures in patients with systemic lupus erythematosus. *Arthritis Rheum.* 2005;52(7):2044-50.

[87] Chong HC, Chee SS, Goh EM, Chow SK, Yeap SS. Dietary calcium and bone mineral density in premenopausal women with systemic lupus erythematosus. *Clin. Rheumatol.* 2007;26(2):182-5.

[88] Formiga F, Moga I, Nolla JM, Pac M, Mitjavila F, Roig-Escofet D. Loss of bone mineral density in premenopausal women with systemic lupus erythematosus. *Ann. Rheum. Dis.* 1995;54(4):274-6.

[89] Formiga F, Moga I, Nolla JM, Navarro MA, Bonnin R, Roig-Escofet D. The association of dehydroepiandrosterone sulphate levels with bone mineral density in systemic lupus erythematosus. *Clin. Exp. Rheumatol.* 1997;15(4):387-92.

[90] Gilboe IM, Kvien TK, Haugeberg G, Husby G. Bone mineral density in systemic lupus erythematosus: comparison with rheumatoid arthritis and healthy controls. *Ann. Rheum. Dis.* 2000;59(2):110-5.

[91] Gordon C. Long-term complications of systemic lupus erythematosus. *Rheumatology (Oxford)* 2002;41(10):1095-100.

[92] Kalla AA, Fataar AB, Jessop SJ, Bewerunge L. Loss of trabecular bone mineral density in systemic lupus erythematosus. *Arthritis Rheum.* 1993;36(12):1726-34.

[93] Kipen Y, Buchbinder R, Forbes A, Strauss B, Littlejohn G, Morand E. Prevalence of reduced bone mineral density in systemic lupus erythematosus and the role of steroids. *J. Rheumatol.* 1997;24(10):1922-9.

[94] Lakshminarayanan S, Walsh S, Mohanraj M, Rothfield N. Factors associated with low bone mineral density in female patients with systemic lupus erythematosus. *J. Rheumatol.* 2001;28(1):102-8.

[95] Mok CC, Mak A, Ma KM. Bone mineral density in postmenopausal Chinese patients with systemic lupus erythematosus. *Lupus* 2005;14(2):106-12.

[96] Pineau CA, Urowitz MB, Fortin PJ, Ibanez D, Gladman DD. Osteoporosis in systemic lupus erythematosus: factors associated with referral for bone mineral density studies, prevalence of osteoporosis and factors associated with reduced bone density. *Lupus* 2004;13(6):436-41.

[97] Redlich K, Ziegler S, Kiener HP, Spitzauer S, Stohlawetz P, Bernecker P et al. Bone mineral density and biochemical parameters of bone metabolism in female patients with systemic lupus erythematosus. *Ann. Rheum. Dis.* 2000;59(4):308-10.

[98] Sinigaglia L, Varenna M, Binelli L, Zucchi F, Ghiringhella D, Gallazzi M et al. Determinants of bone mass in systemic lupus erythematosus: a cross sectional study on premenopausal women. *J. Rheumatol.* 1999;26(6):1280-4.

[99] Teichmann J, Lange U, Stracke H, Federlin K, Bretzel RG. Bone metabolism and bone mineral density of systemic lupus erythematosus at the time of diagnosis. *Rheumatol. Int.* 1999;18(4):137-40.

[100] Uaratanawong S, Deesomchoke U, Lertmaharit S, Uaratanawong S. Bone mineral density in premenopausal women with systemic lupus erythematosus. *J. Rheumatol* 2003;30(11):2365-8.

[101] Yee CS, Crabtree N, Skan J, Amft N, Bowman S, Situnayake D et al. Prevalence and predictors of fragility fractures in systemic lupus erythematosus. *Ann. Rheum. Dis.* 2005;64(1):111-3.

[102] Oleksik A, Lips P, Dawson A, Minshall ME, Shen W, Cooper C et al. Health-related quality of life in postmenopausal women with low BMD with or without prevalent vertebral fractures. *J. Bone Miner Res.* 2000;15(7):1384-92.

[103] Hasserius R, Karlsson MK, Nilsson BE, Redlund-Johnell I, Johnell O. Prevalent vertebral deformities predict increased mortality and increased fracture rate in both men and women: a 10-year population-based study of 598 individuals from the Swedish cohort in the European Vertebral Osteoporosis Study. *Osteoporos Int.* 2003;14(1):61-8.

[104] Klotzbuecher CM, Ross PD, Landsman PB, Abbott TA, III, Berger M. Patients with prior fractures have an increased risk of future fractures: a summary of the literature and statistical synthesis. *J. Bone Miner Res.* 2000;15(4):721-39.

[105] Becker A, Fischer R, Scherbaum WA, Schneider M. Osteoporosis screening in systemic lupus erythematosus: impact of disease duration and organ damage. *Lupus* 2001;10(11):809-14.

[106] Bhattoa HP, Kiss E, Bettembuk P, Balogh A. Bone mineral density, biochemical markers of bone turnover, and hormonal status in men with systemic lupus erythematosus. *Rheumatol Int.* 2001;21(3):97-102.

[107] Borba VZ, Matos PG, da Silva Viana PR, Fernandes A, Sato EI, Lazaretti-Castro M. High prevalence of vertebral deformity in premenopausal systemic lupus erythematosus patients. *Lupus* 2005;14(7):529-33.

[108] Dhillon VB, Davies MC, Hall ML, Round JM, Ell PJ, Jacobs HS et al. Assessment of the effect of oral corticosteroids on bone mineral density in systemic lupus erythematosus: a preliminary study with dual energy x ray absorptiometry. *Ann. Rheum. Dis* 1990;49(8):624-6.

[109] Formiga F, Nolla JM, Mitjavila F, Bonnin R, Navarro MA, Moga I. Bone mineral density and hormonal status in men with systemic lupus erythematosus. *Lupus* 1996; 5(6):623-6.

[110] Houssiau FA, Lefebvre C, Depresseux G, Lambert M, Devogelaer JP, Nagant de DC. Trabecular and cortical bone loss in systemic lupus erythematosus. *Br. J. Rheumatol.* 1996; 35(3):244-7.

[111] Lee C, Almagor O, Dunlop DD, Manzi S, Spies S, Chadha AB et al. Disease damage and low bone mineral density: an analysis of women with systemic lupus erythematosus ever and never receiving corticosteroids. *Rheumatology (Oxford)* 2006; 45(1):53-60.

[112] Li EK, Tam LS, Young RP, Ko GT, Li M, Lau EM. Loss of bone mineral density in Chinese pre-menopausal women with systemic lupus erythematosus treated with corticosteroids. *Br. J. Rheumatol.* 1998;37(4):405-10.

[113] Hansen M, Halberg P, Kollerup G, Pedersen-Zbinden B, Horslev-Petersen K, Hyldstrup L et al. Bone metabolism in patients with systemic lupus erythematosus. Effect of disease activity and glucocorticoid treatment. *Scand. J. Rheumatol.* 1998; 27(3):197-206.

[114] Jardinet D, Lefebvre C, Depresseux G, Lambert M, Devogelaer JP, Houssiau FA. Longitudinal analysis of bone mineral density in pre-menopausal female systemic lupus erythematosus patients: deleterious role of glucocorticoid therapy at the lumbar spine. *Rheumatology (Oxford)* 2000;39(4):389-92.

[115] Kipen Y, Briganti E, Strauss B, Will R, Littlejohn G, Morand E. Three year followup of bone mineral density change in premenopausal women with systemic lupus erythematosus. *J. Rheumatol* 1999;26(2):310-7.

[116] Pons F, Peris P, Guanabens N, Font J, Huguet M, Espinosa G et al. The effect of systemic lupus erythematosus and long-term steroid therapy on bone mass in pre-menopausal women. *Br. J. Rheumatol.* 1995;34(8):742-6.

[117] Star VL, Hochberg MC. Osteoporosis in patients with rheumatic diseases. *Rheum. Dis. Clin. North Am.* 1994;20(3):561-76.

[118] Al-Janadi M, al-Balla S, al-Dalaan A, Raziuddin S. Cytokine profile in systemic lupus erythematosus, rheumatoid arthritis, and other rheumatic diseases. *J. Clin. Immunol.* 1993; 13(1):58-67.

[119] Tanaka Y, Watanabe K, Suzuki M, Saito K, Oda S, Suzuki H et al. Spontaneous production of bone-resorbing lymphokines by B cells in patients with systemic lupus erythematosus. *J. Clin. Immunol.* 1989;9(5):415-20.

[120] Petri M. Musculoskeletal complications of systemic lupus erythematosus in the Hopkins Lupus Cohort: an update. *Arthritis Care Res.* 1995; 8(3):137-45.

[121] Muller K, Kriegbaum NJ, Baslund B, Sorensen OH, Thymann M, Bentzen K. Vitamin D3 metabolism in patients with rheumatic diseases: low serum levels of 25-hydroxyvitamin D3 in patients with systemic lupus erythematosus. *Clin. Rheumatol.* 1995;14(4):397-400.

[122] Lukert BP, Raisz LG. Glucocorticoid-induced osteoporosis. *Rheum. Dis. Clin. North Am.* 1994;20(3):629-50.

[123] Resch H, Pietschmann P, Krexner E, Willvonseder R. Decreased peripheral bone mineral content in patients under anticoagulant therapy with phenprocoumon. *Eur. Heart J.* 1991;12(3):439-41.

[124] Ramsey-Goldman R, Dunn JE, Huang CF, Dunlop D, Rairie JE, Fitzgerald S et al. Frequency of fractures in women with systemic lupus erythematosus: comparison with United States population data. *Arthritis Rheum.* 1999;42(5):882-90.

[125] Lips P. Epidemiology and predictors of fractures associated with osteoporosis. *Am. J. Med.* 1997;103(2A):3S-8S.

[126] Stone KL, Seeley DG, Lui LY, Cauley JA, Ensrud K, Browner WS et al. BMD at multiple sites and risk of fracture of multiple types: long-term results from the Study of Osteoporotic Fractures. *J. Bone Miner Res.* 2003;18(11):1947-54.

[127] Black DM, Schwartz AV, Ensrud KE, Cauley JA, Levis S, Quandt SA et al. Effects of continuing or stopping alendronate after 5 years of treatment: the Fracture Intervention Trial Long-term Extension (FLEX): a randomized trial. *JAMA* 2006;296(24):2927-38.

[128] Patlas N, Golomb G, Yaffe P, Pinto T, Breuer E, Ornoy A. Transplacental effects of bisphosphonates on fetal skeletal ossification and mineralization in rats. *Teratology* 1999; 60(2):68-73.

[129] Bultink IE, Hamann D, Seelen MA, Hart MH, Dijkmans BA, Daha MR et al. Deficiency of functional mannose-binding lectin is not associated with infections in patients with systemic lupus erythematosus. *Arthritis Res. Ther.* 2006; 8(6):R183.

[130] Gladman DD, Hussain F, Ibanez D, Urowitz MB. The nature and outcome of infection in systemic lupus erythematosus. *Lupus* 2002;11(4):234-9.

[131] Noel V, Lortholary O, Casassus P, Cohen P, Genereau T, Andre MH et al. Risk factors and prognostic influence of infection in a single cohort of 87 adults with systemic lupus erythematosus. *Ann. Rheum. Dis.* 2001;60(12):1141-4.

[132] Pryor BD, Bologna SG, Kahl LE. Risk factors for serious infection during treatment with cyclophosphamide and high-dose corticosteroids for systemic lupus erythematosus. *Arthritis Rheum.* 1996;39(9):1475-82.

[133] Zonana-Nacach A, Camargo-Coronel A, Yanez P, Sanchez L, Jimenez-Balderas FJ, Fraga A. Infections in outpatients with systemic lupus erythematosus: a prospective study. *Lupus* 2001;10(7):505-10.

[134] Shyam C, Malaviya AN. Infection-related morbidity in systemic lupus erythematosus: a clinico-epidemiological study from northern India. *Rheumatol Int.* 1996;16(1):1-3.

[135] Ginzler E, Diamond H, Kaplan D, Weiner M, Schlesinger M, Seleznick M. Computer analysis of factors influencing frequency of infection in systemic lupus erythematosus. *Arthritis Rheum.* 1978;21(1):37-44.

[136] Kahl LE. Herpes zoster infections in systemic lupus erythematosus: risk factors and outcome. *J. Rheumatol.* 1994;21(1):84-6.

[137] Moutsopoulos HM, Gallagher JD, Decker JL, Steinberg AD. Herpes zoster in patients with systemic lupus erythematosus. *Arthritis Rheum.* 1978;21(7):789-802.

[138] Pope JE, Krizova A, Ouimet JM, Goodwin JL, Lankin M. Close association of herpes zoster reactivation and systemic lupus erythematosus (SLE) diagnosis: case-control study of patients with SLE or noninflammatory nusculoskeletal disorders. *J. Rheumatol.* 2004;31(2):274-9.

[139] Wong KL. Pattern of SLE in Hong Kong Chinese: a cohort study. *Scand. J. Rheumatol.* 1992;21(6):289-96.

[140] Duffy KN, Duffy CM, Gladman DD. Infection and disease activity in systemic lupus erythematosus: a review of hospitalized patients. *J. Rheumatol.* 1991;18(8):1180-4.

[141] Nived O, Sturfelt G, Wollheim F. Systemic lupus erythematosus and infection: a controlled and prospective study including an epidemiological group. *Q. J. Med.* 1985;55(218):271-87.

[142] Petri M, Genovese M. Incidence of and risk factors for hospitalizations in systemic lupus erythematosus: a prospective study of the Hopkins Lupus Cohort. *J. Rheumatol.* 1992;19(10):1559-65.

[143] Jonsson H, Nived O, Sturfelt G. Outcome in systemic lupus erythematosus: a prospective study of patients from a defined population. *Medicine (Baltimore)* 1989;68(3):141-50.

[144] Lee P, Urowitz MB, Bookman AA, Koehler BE, Smythe HA, Gordon DA et al. Systemic lupus erythematosus. A review of 110 cases with reference to nephritis, the nervous system, infections, aseptic necrosis and prognosis. *Q. J. Med.* 1977;46(181):1-32.

[145] Hellmann DB, Petri M, Whiting-O'Keefe Q. Fatal infections in systemic lupus erythematosus: the role of opportunistic organisms. *Medicine (Baltimore)* 1987; 66(5):341-8.

[146] Austin HA, III, Klippel JH, Balow JE, le Riche NG, Steinberg AD, Plotz PH et al. Therapy of lupus nephritis. Controlled trial of prednisone and cytotoxic drugs. *N. Engl. J.* 1986; Med 314(10):614-9.

[147] Reveille JD. The molecular genetics of systemic lupus erythematosus and Sjogren's syndrome. *Curr. Opin. Rheumatol.* 1991;3(5):722-30.

[148] Nauta AJ, Daha MR, van Kooten C, Roos A. Recognition and clearance of apoptotic cells: a role for complement and pentraxins. *Trends Immunol.* 2003;24(3):148-54.

[149] Davies EJ, Snowden N, Hillarby MC, Carthy D, Grennan DM, Thomson W et al. Mannose-binding protein gene polymorphism in systemic lupus erythematosus. *Arthritis Rheum.* 1995;38(1):110-4.

[150] Garred P, Madsen HO, Halberg P, Petersen J, Kronborg G, Svejgaard A et al. Mannose-binding lectin polymorphisms and susceptibility to infection in systemic lupus erythematosus. *Arthritis Rheum.* 1999;42(10):2145-52.

[151] Garred P, Voss A, Madsen HO, Junker P. Association of mannose-binding lectin gene variation with disease severity and infections in a population-based cohort of systemic lupus erythematosus patients. *Genes Immun.* 2001;2(8):442-50.

[152] Takahashi R, Tsutsumi A, Ohtani K, Muraki Y, Goto D, Matsumoto I et al. Association of mannose binding lectin (MBL) gene polymorphism and serum MBL concentration with characteristics and progression of systemic lupus erythematosus. *Ann. Rheum. Dis.* 2005;64(2):311-4.

[153] Turner MW. Mannose-binding lectin: the pluripotent molecule of the innate immune system. *Immunol. Today* 1996;17(11):532-40.

[154] Turner MW, Hamvas RM. Mannose-binding lectin: structure, function, genetics and disease associations. *Rev. Immunogenet.* 2000;2(3):305-22.

[155] Lee YH, Witte T, Momot T, Schmidt RE, Kaufman KM, Harley JB et al. The mannose-binding lectin gene polymorphisms and systemic lupus erythematosus: two case-control studies and a meta-analysis. *Arthritis Rheum.* 2005;52(12):3966-74.

[156] Crosdale DJ, Ollier WE, Thomson W, Dyer PA, Jensenious J, Johnson RW et al. Mannose binding lectin (MBL) genotype distributions with relation to serum levels in UK Caucasoids. *Eur. J. Immunogenet* 2000;27(3):111-7.

[157] Hansen TK, Thiel S, Dall R, Rosenfalck AM, Trainer P, Flyvbjerg A et al. GH strongly affects serum concentrations of mannan-binding lectin: evidence for a new IGF-I independent immunomodulatory effect of GH. *J. Clin. Endocrinol. Metab.* 2001; 86(11):5383-8.

[158] ter Borg EJ, Horst G, Limburg PC, van Rijswijk MH, Kallenberg CG. C-reactive protein levels during disease exacerbations and infections in systemic lupus erythematosus: a prospective longitudinal study. *J. Rheumatol.* 1990;17(12):1642-8.

[159] Shin KC, Lee YJ, Kang SW, Baek HJ, Lee EB, Kim HA et al. Serum procalcitonin measurement for detection of intercurrent infection in febrile patients with SLE. *Ann. Rheum. Dis.* 2001;60(10):988-9.

[160] Porges AJ, Beattie SL, Ritchlin C, Kimberly RP, Christian CL. Patients with systemic lupus erythematosus at risk for Pneumocystis carinii pneumonia. *J. Rheumatol.* 1992; 19(8):1191-4.

[161] Gilliland WR, Tsokos GC. Prophylactic use of antibiotics and immunisations in patients with SLE. *Ann. Rheum. Dis.* 2002;61(3):191-2.

[162] Croft SM, Schiffman G, Snyder E, Herrmann K, James K, Jarrett MP. Specific antibody response after in vivo antigenic stimulation in systemic lupus erythematosus. *J. Rheumatol.* 1984;11(2):141-6.

[163] Holvast A, Huckriede A, Wilschut J, Horst G, De Vries JJ, Benne CA et al. Safety and efficacy of influenza vaccination in systemic lupus erythematosus patients with quiescent disease. *Ann. Rheum. Dis.* 2006;65(7):913-8.

[164] McDonald E, Jarrett MP, Schiffman G, Grayzel AI. Persistence of pneumococcal antibodies after immunization in patients with systemic lupus erythematosus. *J. Rheumatol.* 1984;11(3):306-8.

In: Handbook of Cardiovascular Research
Editors: Jorgen Brataas and Viggo Nanstveit

ISBN 978-1-60741-792-7
© 2009 Nova Science Publishers, Inc.

Chapter VI

Effects of Passive Smoking on the Levels of Coronary Artery Disease Risk Factors and Non-Enzymatic Antioxidants[*]

Andrzej Sobczak[†,1,2]*, Izabela Szołtysek-Bołdys*[1]
and Dariusz Gołka[3]

1. Department of General and Analytical Chemistry,
Medical University of Silesia, Sosnowiec, Poland
2. Department of Chemical Hazard, Institute of Occupational Medicine and
Environmental Health, Sosnowiec, Poland
3. Department of Pathology, Victoria Hospital,
Blackpool, United Kingdom

Abstract

Studies on the risk of coronary heart disease in persons exposed to environmental tobacco smoke have been conducted since mid eighties of the last century. Their results were published in numerous articles, including seven meta-analyses. The majority of them show that the risk of coronary artery disease is increased in passive smokers by about 20-30% in comparison with non-smoking controls. The effect is more significant that one might expect comparing the amounts of toxic substances aspirated by passive versus active smokers. This may result from increased levels of atherogenous substances

---

[*] A version of this chapter was also published in *Passive Smoking and Health Research,* edited by Nivek A. Jeorgensen published by Nova Science Publishers, Inc. It was submitted for appropriate modifications in an effort to encourage wider dissemination of research.

[†] Correspondence: Dr Andrzej Sobczak, Department of General and Analytical Chemistry, Medical University of Silesia, 41-200 Sosnowiec, Jagiellonska 4, Poland, tel: +48 32 364 15 69; fax: +48 32 2667860; e-mail: andsobcz@poczta.onet.pl.

in plasma, e.g. homocysteine and asymmetric dimethylarginine (an endogenous inhibitor of nitric oxide synthase) and from the weakened body self-defense due to decreased non-enzymatic antioxidants levels.

The purpose of the present study was the evaluation of the effects of passive smoking on the concentration of substances involved in pathogenesis of cardiovascular diseases, namely homocysteine, cysteine, asymmetric dimethylarginine, symmetric dimethylarginine and non-enzymatic antioxidants (α-tocopherol, γ-tocopherol, retinol).

Seventy-two men (mean age 39.3±2.7) years, were selected to the study. Non-smokers group included persons with plasma cotinine level not exceeding 10 ng/ml (31 men). Passive smokers group consisted of men with plasma cotinine level between 10 and 30 ng/ml (41 men). Plasma biochemical parameters were assessed with use of high performance liquid chromatotography. Plasma total homocysteine in passive smokers was statistically signifficantly higher than in non-smokers (10.17 versus 8.57 μmol/L). There was a significant positive correlation between plasma total homocysteine level and cotinine levels in passive smokers as well in the entire population. (r = 0.331; P = 0.034 and r = 0.332; P = 0.008, respectively). Plasma α-tocopherol levels in passive smokers were signifficantly lower than in non-smokers (12.31 versus 14.12 μg/ml). Both in passive smokers as well in the entire study population a significant negative correlation between cotinine and α-tocopherol levels in plasma was found (-0.378; P = 0.036 and – 0.220; P = 0.046, respectively). The changes in concentration of the remaining biochemical parameters were insignificant and did not correlate with plasma cotinine level. The obtained results indicate that chronic exposure to environmental tobacco smoke may result in elevated total plasma homocysteine level and may affect the body anti-oxidative barrier by lowering plasma α-tocopherol level.

Keywords: passive smoking, ETS, cotinine, homocysteine, cysteine, ADMA, SDMA, alpha-tocopherol, gamma-tocopherol, retinol.

Abbreviations

ADMA   asymmetric dimethylarginine;
CVD   cardiovascular disease;
ETS   environmental tobacco smoke;
MS, mainstream smoke;
NO, nitric oxide;
NOS,   nitric oxide synthase;
SDMA,   symmetric dimethylarginine,
SS,   sidestream smoke;
tCys,   total cysteine;
tHcy,   total homocysteine;

1. Introduction

Numerous environmental factors, including toxic, carcinogenous, and mutageinc environmental pollutants affect the biological existence of a human being. Tobacco smoke makes one of the sources next to emission associated with various areas of human activity. Poland, despite a decrease in number of smokers observed for two decades, still belongs to those countries with very high tobacco consumption. By the end of the 90's of the last century, approximately 10 millions of people smoked cigarettes [Sobczak et al., 2005]. These persons called active smokers are mainly exposed to substances present in mainstream smoke (MS) formed during puff.

It is estimated, that similar number of people in Poland are exposed to Environmental Tobacco Smoke (ETS) originating from Sidestream Smoke (SS) which forms during smolder between puffs. Moreover, ETS makes smoke exhaled by active smokers. Persons exposed to ETS are called passive smokers or second hand smokers.

Chemical composition and the concentration of particular SS and MS components may vary due to characteristic features of the cigarette (length, presence and type of filter, type of paper), tobacco used to its production, as well as smoking "technique", inhalation depth and rate, number of puffs and the size of stub [Ahijevych and Gillespie, 1997; Eissenberg et al., 1999; Patterson et al., 2003; Wood et al., 2004; Hammond et al., 2005].

Despite MS contains the most of the toxic components, some of them are present in increased amounts in SS. For example, the amount of carbon monoxide in SS, depending on the cigarette brand and smoking habit may be up to 3 times higher than in MS. On the other hand, the concentration of potent carcinogenic nitrosamines in SS may be few to few dozen times higher than in MS [Haroun et al., 1999].

Recently, Shick and Glantz [2005] evaluated, confidential results of the studies on the toxic properties of the Sidestream Smoke performed by Phillip Morris Tobacco Company in 80' of the last century in their secret Institut für Biologische Forschung in Germany. It turned out that inhaled fresh SS is approximately four times more toxic per gram total particulate matter (TPM) than MS. Moreover, it turned out that sidestream condensate is appoximately three times more toxic per gram and two to six times more tumourigenic per gram than main stream condensate by dermal application.

On the other hand, some researchers put the negative effect of ETS on the organisms of non-smokers exposed to it in question [Enstrom and Kabat, 2003]. One should however suspect that this is an attempt of tobacco industry to influence the scientists' opinion [Thun, 2003; Bornhäuser et al., 2006].

The importance of problem of harmful properties of ETS is reflected by the special report published in a prestigious american journal Circulation [Barnoya and Glantz, 2005].The retrospective analysis presented in this article regarded studies conducted since the second half of 1985 and encompassed several dozens of papers, including six meta-analyzes. All of them showed that a relative risk of heart disease in passive smokers is by 20%-30% higher than in non-smokers. Moreover, it was found that passive smoking has much worse impact on cardiovascular system that it could be expected comparing the amounts of toxic substances entering the body of passive and active smokers. In average, changes in some of the factors that influence heart diseases may reach 80-90% of values observed in smokers.

The tobacco smoke components may act directly or indirectly together with numerous chemical compounds present in the body. Some of these substances are involved in the pathogenesis of cardiovascular disease (CVD). One of such compounds is homocysteine (see figure 1 for structures of compounds discussed here). Elevated plasma total homocysteine level (tHcy) (reduced, oxidized, and bound to protein) is an independent CVD risk factor [Nygård et al., 1997; Nygård et al., 1998]. A total cysteine (tCy) level (similar to total homocysteine, total cysteine is the concentration of total amounts all cysteine fractions in the body) is also, however in a different and to minor degree, associated with peripheral vascular, cerebrovascular and coronary heart disease [El-Khairy et al., 2001].

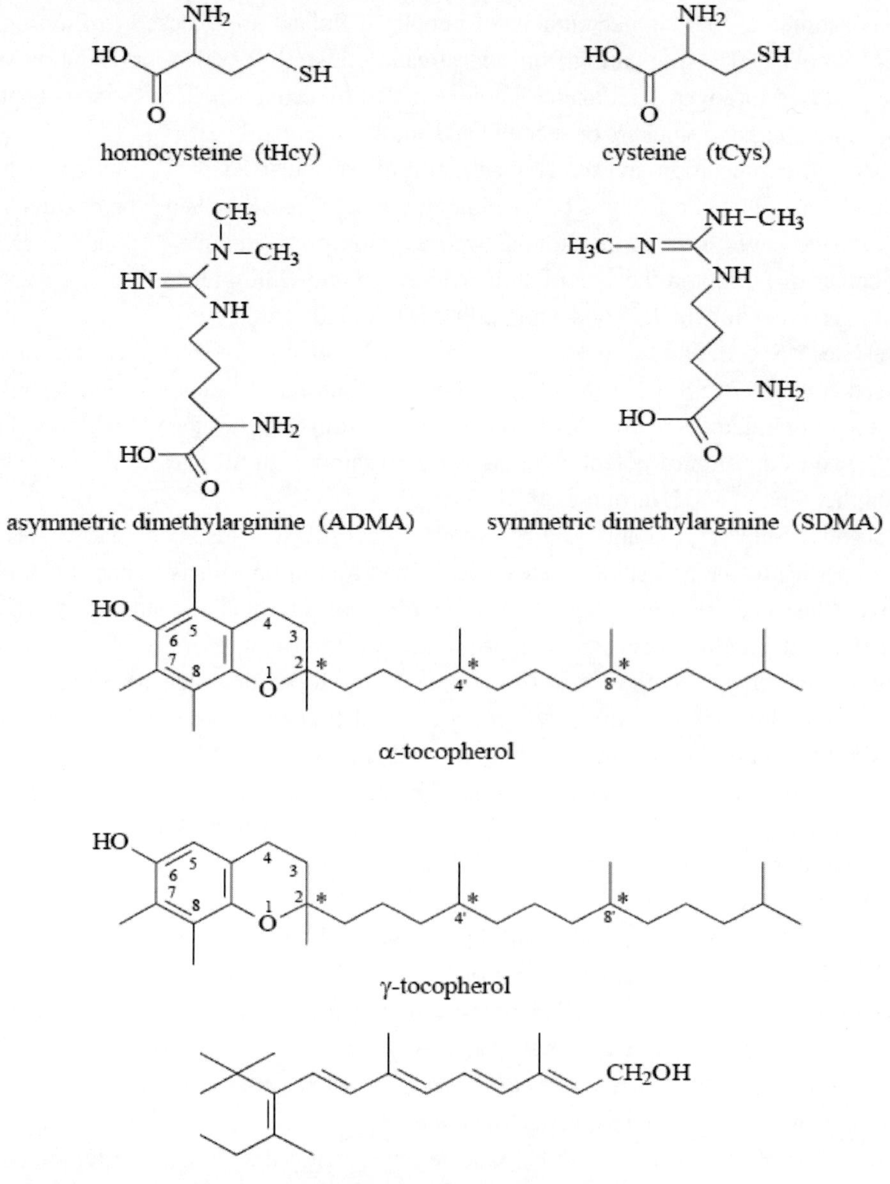

Figure 1. Structures of compounds discussed in this article

Recently, the number of publications regarding symmetric dimethylarginine (SDMA) and asymmetric dimethylarginine (ADMA) which are endogenous inhibitors of nitric oxide synthase (NOS) is rapidly growing. ADMA is believed to be a novel emerging risk factor in cardiovascular diseases [Böger et al., 2005; Böger, 2006].

Oxidative stress provoked by tobacco smoke causes redox instability and activation of body protective mechanisms. This results in some oxidants levels decrease. Concentrations of compounds involved in the neutralization of free radicals from tobacco smoke, e.g. antioxidative vitamins are useful, and frequently used, indicators in the evaluation of the body redox balance.

The purpose of the present study was to evaluate the effects of ETS on tHcy, tCys, ADMA, SDMA, retinol, γ-tocopherol and α- tocopherol.

2. Material and Methods

2.1. Study Subjects

The study group consisted of 72 volunteers (only men) aged 34- 45 (mean age 39.3± 2.7), ethnically homogenous, inhabitants of the same urban agglomeration (Katowice, Poland), with no history of coronary heart disease, diabetes and liver disease. These men did not suffered from arterial hypertension, 62 men presented normal lipid profile (total cholesterol level, LDL-cholesterol, HDL-cholesterol and triglycerides). Body mass index (BMI) was within normal range (18.5 – 24.9 kg/m^2) in 57 men and 15 were overweight (25.0 – 29.9 kg/m^2) according to the US National Institutes of Health classification [NIH, 1998].

All subjects declared in the questionnaire very similar nutritional habits, abstinence from alcohol consumption, did not actively exercise, and were drinking a maximum of one cup of coffee a day. The study subjects declared no vitamin intake three months before the study was done. The subjects were simultaneously qualified for the further study on tHcy,tCys, ADMA, SDMA, retinol, α- and γ-tocopherol levels.

Initially, the study subjects were classified into groups of non-smokers and passive smokers upon the questionnaire responses regarding the history of exposure, i.e. the time spent in rooms with smokers. The questionnaire data was verified by means of the plasma cotinine concentration measurements, and thereafter the study subjects were definitely included into the group of non-smokers and non-exposed to ETS and passive smokers (exposed to ETS). The arbitrary threshold values of cotinine concentration in plasma was <10 ng/ml for the group of nonsmokers, and 10≤ for passive smokers.

The nonsmokers group consisted of 31 men, the passive smokers group consisted of 41 men. Blood samples for the biochemical examinations were taken from the ulnar vein after a 12-hour period from the last meal.

The study protocol has been approved by the Bioethical Committee Medical University of Silesia.

2.2. Reagents

HPLC-grade acetonitrile, methanol and dichloromethane were purchased from Labscan (Dublin, Ireland). Ammonium 7-fluorobenzo-2-oxa-1,3-diazole-4-sulfonate (SBD-F) and phthaldialdehyde (OPA) were from Fluka (Buchs, Switzerland). Solid Phase Extraction (SPE) C_{18} columns were purchased from J.T. Baker (Deventer, Holland) and BondElut PRS SPE cartridges from Varian (Lake Forest, CA, USA). Standards: D,L-homocysteine, L-cysteine, ADMA, SDMA, α- and γ-tocopherol, retinol, cotinine, and internal standards: cysteamine, homoarginine, tocopherol acetate, ephedrine and other analytical grade chemicals were obtained from Sigma Chemical Co.(St. Louis, MO, USA) and from local commercial sources (POCh, Gliwice, Poland). Water was purified with Ropure and NANOpure systems (Barnstead, USA).

2.3. Equipment

Separations with high performance liquid chromatography (HPLC) method were performed with the use of a Merck Hitachi chromatograph consisting of the L-7100 pump, L-7400 UV detector, L-7485 fluorescence detector, and D-7000 interface. The system was controlled by HPLC System Manager (Merck Hitachi Model D-7000 Chromatography Data Station Software v. 4.1). Samples were injected using a Rheodyne Model 7125 injector with a 20 µl or 50 µl sample loop (Rheodyne, Cotati, USA). Before injection all samples were filtered through a GHP Acrodisc 13mm syringe filter, 0,45 µm (Pall, Ann Arbor, USA).

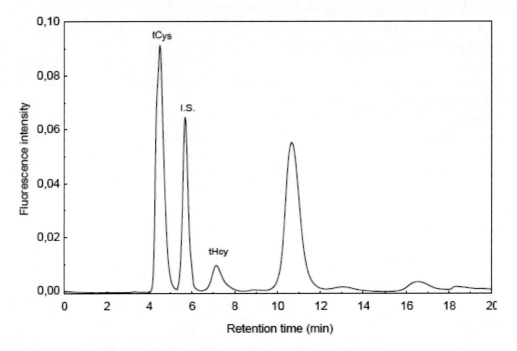

Figure 2. HPLC chromatogram of SBD-F derivatized plasma thiols sample. Peak identification: tCys, total cysteine; tHcy, total homocysteine; I.S., internal standard (cysteamine).

2.4. Biochemical Examinations

Total Homocysteine and Total Cysteine Measurement

Plasma tHcy and plasma tCys concentrations were determined simultaneously as described by Young at al. [1994]. Briefly, for analysis of plasma tHcy and tCys, EDTA treated blood samples were immediately placed on ice. The plasma was separated within 30 min. 50 μl of 10% (v/v) tri-n-butylphosphine in dimethylformamide was added to 200 μl of plasma and 50 μl of internal standard (cysteamine). The mixture incubated at 4°C for 30 minutes to release protein-bound homocysteine and cysteine. The solution was deproteinized with 250 μl of 10% (w/v) trichloroacetic acid containing 1 mmol/L EDTA under vigorous shaking, followed by centrifugation at 3000g for10 min. 100 μl of the supernatant was then mixed with 200 μl of 2.5 mol/L borate buffer (pH 9.5) containing 4 mmol/L EDTA and the mixture was derivatized with the thiol specific compound SBD-F. Finally, the mixture was incubated for 90 minutes at 60°C. A 20 μl aliquot was then used for HPLC analysis. The analysis was performed using a reversed-phase LiChrospher 100 RP 18 column (250 x 4.0 mm I.D., 5 μm particle size; E.Merck, Darmstadt, Germany) at room temperature. For chromatographic separation a binary gradient was used: phase A consistent of 0.1 mol/L acetate buffer (pH 4.0) containing 2 % methanol (v/v) and phase B of 0.1 mol/L phosphate buffer (pH 6.0) containing 5% methanol (v/v). A linear gradient from phase A to phase B over 20 minutes (0-100%) at a flow rate of 1 ml/min was used. The analytes were monitored by fluorescence detection at excitation wavelength 385 nm and emission wavelength 515 nm. Chromatogram of a plasma sample is shown in figure 2.

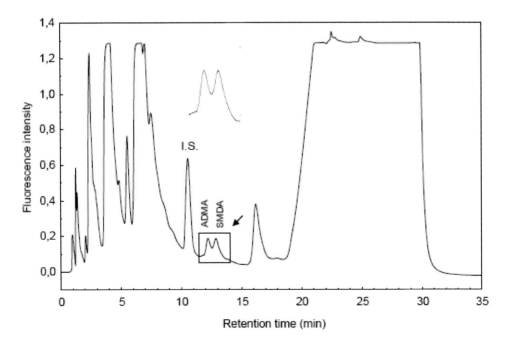

Figure 3. HPLC chromatogram of OPA derivatized ADMA and SDMA in plasma sample. Peak identification: ADMA, asymmetric dimethylarginine; SDMA, symmetric dimethylarginine; I.S., internal standard (homoarginine). Arrow indicates region where the Marquardt non-linear, least-square method was used to deconvolute ADMA and SDMA overlapping chromatogram peaks.

Asymmetric Dimethylarginine and Symmetric Dimethylarginine Measurement

ADMA and SDMA concentrations in plasma were determined simultaneously as described by Teerlink [2004]. 0.2 ml of plasma sample was mixed with 0.1 ml of internal standard (homoarginine) and 0.7 ml PBS. The Varian PRS SPE columns were used without preconditioning. After application of the samples, the columns were consecutively washed with 1.0 ml of 100 mM HCl and 1.0 ml methanol. Analytes were eluted in 3.0 ml tubes with 1.0 ml of concentrated ammonia:water:methanol (10:40:50). The solvent was removed by evaporation in vacuum. The residue was dissolved in 0.1 ml water and subsequently 0.1 ml of the OPA reagent was added and the mixture was shaken for 1 minute. Then 50 µl mixture was injected into the reverse-phase Supelcosil LC-DABS column (150 x 4.6 mm I.D., 3 µm particle size; Supelco, Bellefonte, PA, USA). Separation was performed under isocratic conditions with 100% mobile phase A (50 mM potassium phosphate buffer, pH 6.5, containing 8.7% acetonitrile) at a flow rate of 1.5 m,/min and room temperature. After elution of the last analyte, strongly retained compounds were quickly eluted by a 50% mobile phase B (acetonitrile:water = 50:50, v/v) from 20 to 27 min. Between 27 and 28 min the gradient returned to initial conditions and the column was equilibrated for an additional 7 min, resulting in a total run time of 35 min. Fluorecence was measured at excitation and emission wavelengths of 340 and 455 nm, respectively. The Marquardt non-linear, least-square method was used to deconvolute ADMA and SDMA overlapping chromatogram peaks and Exponential Modified Gaussian (EMG) function was used to model the chromatogram peaks. Chromatogram of a plasma sample is shown in figure 3.

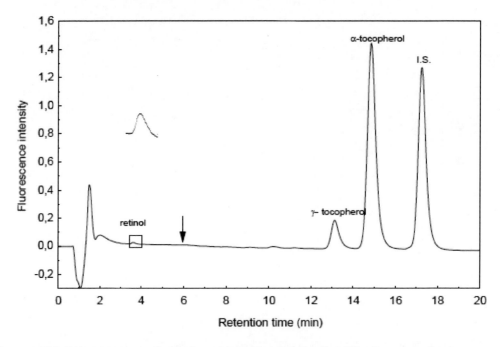

Figure 4. HPLC chromatogram of retinol, γ-tocopherol and α-tocopherol in plasma sample. Arrow indicates gain switch of the fluorescence detector. I.S, internal standard (tocopherol acetate).

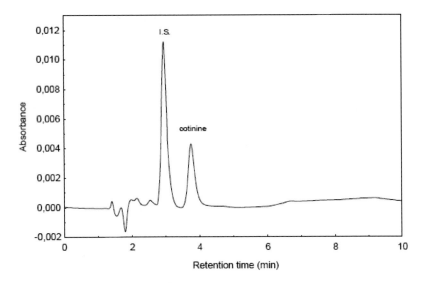

Figure 5. HPLC chromatogram of plasma cotinine sample. I.S., internal standard (ephedrine).

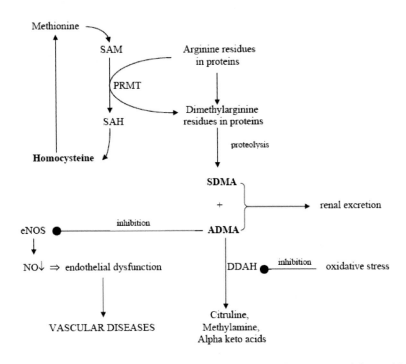

Figure 6. Metabolic interactions between homocysteine, ADMA and SDMA. Arginine residues in proteins are methylated by protein arginine methyltransferase (PRMT), which uses S-adenosylmethionine (SAM) as a methyl donor and produces S-adenosylhomocysteine (SAH). Homocysteine derived from the hydrolysis of SAH can be remethylated to methionine. ADMA and SDMA is derived from the proteolysis of proteins that contain methylated arginine residues. ADMA can cause endothelial dysfunction by inhibiting endothelial nitric oxide synthase (eNOS), whereas SDMA does not. The major pathway for metabolism of ADMA is via dimethylarginine dimethylaminohydrolase (DDAH), which produces citrulline, methylamine, and small amount of alpha keto acids. Dysregulation of DDAH by oxidative stress could be a potential reason for ADMA levels.

Retinol, γ-Tocopherol and α-Tocopherol Measurement

Both α– and γ-tocopherol and retinol were simultaneously measured with HPLC method [Sobczak et al., 1999]. Briefly, 50 μl of plasma was mixed with 50 μl of internal standard (tocopherol acetate) and 100 μl of ethanol were pipetted into Eppendorff test tubes wrapped with aluminum foil, and the mixture was shaken vigorously for 1 minute. Then 400 μl of butanol-ethyl acetate (1:1,v/v) mixture was added, and the tubes were shaken again for 1min. After adding 20 mg of anhydrous sodium sulphate, the tubes were shaken for 1 min and centrifuged for 10 min (3,000 g, 4°C). The supernatant was filtered through a GHP Acrodisc syringe filter. Then 20 μl of filtrate was injected into the reverse-phase LiChrospher 100 RP18 column (250 x 4.0 mm I.D., 5 μm particle size; E.Merck, Darmstadt, Germany). The separation was performed in isocratic system in reversed phase. For chromatographic separation, mobile phase acetonitryle-butanol (95:5, v/v) was used. The separation was conducted in room temperature. The fluorescence detector was used for retinol detection with 300 nm (excitation) and 480 nm (emission) wavelengths, and after 6 minute with 285 nm and 325 nm, respectively. Chromatogram of a plasma sample is shown in figure 4.

Cotinine Measurement

Cotinine was measured with HPLC method described by Picini et at [1992] with minor modifications. Briefly, 0.6 ml of the plasma was mixed with 0.1 ml of internal standard (ephedrine) was shaken with 1 ml of borate buffer pH10 for 10 minutes. The mixture was transferred to the SPE C_{18} column (J.T. Baker), which was preconditioned with 2 x 1 ml of methanol, 1 ml of water and finally with 1 ml of borate buffer, pH 9. The column was rinsed with 2 ml of water and the cotinine eluted with 2 x 250 μl of dichloromethane. The solution obtained was filtered through syringe filter. Then, 50μl of filtrate was placed upon the chromatographic column LiChrospher 100 RP 18 column (250 x 4.0 mm I.D., 5 μm particle size; E.Merck, Darmstadt, Germany). The separation was performed in isocratic system in reversed phase. The mobile phase was water-methanol-0.1 M sodium acetate-acetonitrile (63:23:6:8 v/v), adjusted to pH 4.3 with acetic acid. The separation was performed at room temperature. A UV detector was used for absorption at 254 nm. Chromatogram of a plasma sample is shown in figure 5.

2.5. Statistical Analysis

The results are expressed as mean ± standard deviation. Non-parametric statistical methods were chosen because of the limited number of observations. The Mann-Whitney U-test was used to examine whether there were differences between the groups. Pearson's correlation coefficients were calculated to evaluate relationships between different variables. For all significance calculations, P<0.05 was accepted as significant. The data were analyzed using STATISTICA (data analysis software system), v. 7.1. (StatSoft, Inc.2005).

3. Results

Volunteers included in the study, men only, were qualified into the study groups; non-smokers and not exposed to tobacco smoke (control group), and exposed to tobacco smoke (passive smokers) upon the plasma cotinine level. Selected physiological and biochemical parameters are shown in table 1.

The mean age in the non-smokers (control) group and passive smokers group was similar (38.5 and 41.0 years, respectively). Lipid profile parameters measured (total cholesterol, HDL cholesterol, LDL cholesterol and triglycerides) were within reference ranges used in laboratory diagnostics.

Table 1. Characteristics of subjects with respect to smoking status

Characteristics	Non-smokers n = 31	Passive smokers n = 41
Age (years)	38.5 ± 3.2	41.0 ± 2.3
BMI (kg/m^2)	22.9 ± 3.1	23.4 ± 2.9
Total cholesterol (mg/dL)	160.1 ± 37.4	165.7 ± 31.5
HDL cholesterol (mg/dL)	64.8 ± 12.0	55.5 ± 13.2
LDL cholesterol (mg/dL)	118.2 ± 24.9	120.6 ± 26.1
Triglycerides (mg/dL)	103.1 ± 33.5	100.1 ± 28.5

Table 2. The effect of ETS on the plasma levels of tHcy, tCys, ADMA, SDMA, retinol, γ-tocopherol, α-tocopherol and cotinine

Parameter	Non-smokers n = 31	Passive smokers n = 41	P-value
tHcy [μmol/L] min ÷ max	8.57 ± 2.52 $4,90 \div 15.77$	10.17 ± 2.96 $4.77 \div 17.72$	0.017
tCys [μmol/L] min ÷ max	196.8 ± 38.4 $137.8 \div 286.0$	219.7 ± 58.8 $124.8 \div 315.3$	0.130 (NS)
ADMA [μmol/L] min ÷ max	0.40 ± 0.17 $0.11 \div 0.77$	0.43 ± 0.17 $0.23 \div 0.91$	0.720 (NS)
SDMA [μmol/L] min ÷ max	0.39 ± 0.16 $0.18 \div 1.00$	0.39 ± 0.11 $0.24 \div 0.74$	0.592 (NS)
Retinol [μg/L] min ÷ max	0.65 ± 0.15 $0.42 \div 1.16$	0.60 ± 0.17 $0.28 \div 1.03$	0.192 (NS)
γ-Tocopherol [μg/L] min ÷ max	0.98 ± 0.42 $0.43 \div 2.02$	0.88 ± 0.23 $0.33 \div 1.29$	0.107 (NS)
α-Tocopherol [μg/L] min ÷ max	14.12 ± 4.19 $10.45 \div 26.51$	12.31 ± 2.44 $8.81 \div 18.47$	0.043
Cotinine [ng/ml] min ÷ max	4.14 ± 3.29 $0 \div 9.90$	18.93 ± 6.20 $10.66 \div 29.52$	<0.001

ETS, environmental tobacco smoke; tHcy, total homocysteine, tCys, total cysteine; ADMA, asymmetric dimethylarginine; SDMA, symmetric dimethylarginine; NS, non-significant.

Mean values, standard deviation as well as minimal and maximal values of studied parameter are presented in table 2. Thanks to arbitrary inclusion criteria, persons with plasma cotinine levels not exceeding 10 ng/ml were included into non-smokers group, and a mean cotinine level was established. It was 4.6 times lower than in passive smokers (4.14 ng/ml vs 18.93 ng/ml). Differences in plasma cotinine levels between non-smokers and passive smokers were statistically highly significant (p<0.001).

In terms of remaining parameters, statistically significant were differences plasma tHcy and α-tocopherol levels between non-smokers and passive smokers. The mean plasma tHcy level was by 18.7% higher in passive smokers in comparison with non-smokers. The mean plasma α-tocopherol level was, however, by 12.8% lower in passive smokers than in non-smokers.

Plasma levels of the remaining biochemical parameters, i.e. tCys, ADMA, SDMA, retinols and γ-tocopherol are statistically insignificant or even negligible (table 2).

Pearson's correlation coefficient for the relationships between plasma cotinine concentration and levels of the remaining parameters was used to assess the degree of tobacco smoke exposure (table 3). Such an analysis showed a statistical significance of the differences between plasma cotinine and α-tocopherol levels and between plasma cotinine and tHcy levels both in passive smokers group as well as among the entire population.

Passive smokers showed a positive and moderate (r= 0.331) correlation between plasma cotinine and tHcy levels. Pearson's correlation coefficient for the same value remained virtually unchanged among entire population. In both cases calculated correlation values were P =0.034 and P =0 .008, respectively.

There was an moderate negative correlation (r = - 0.378; P = 0.036) for the relationship between plasma cotinine and α-tocopherol levels in passive smokers. This relationship remained significant for the entire population (P=0.046) but the Pearson's correlation coefficient was -0.220, which places it within the range of minute correlation. Remaining plasma parameters studied showed a weak and insignificant correlation (table 3).

Table 3. The Pearson's correlation coefficient (r) for the relationships between plasma cotinine concentrations and plasma investigated biochemical parameters level

Cotinine versus	Passive smokers n = 41		All subject n = 72	
	r	P-value	r	P-value
tHcy	0.331	0.034	0.332	0.008
tCys	0.158	0.397 (NS)	0.262	0.140 (NS)
ADMA	0.156	0.403 (NS)	0.117	0.366 (NS)
SDMA	- 0.041	0.825 (NS)	- 0.029	0.820 (NS)
Retinol	0.218	0.240 (NS)	- 0.079	0.541 (NS)
γ-Tocopherol	0.317	0.083 (NS)	- 0.179	0.164 (NS)
α-Tocopherol	- 0.378	0.036	- 0.220	0.046

tHcy, total homocysteine, tCys, total cysteine; ADMA, asymmetric dimethylarginine; SDMA, symmetric dimethylarginine; NS, non-significant

Table 4. The Pearson's correlation coefficient (r) for the relationships between plasma tHcy concentrations and ADMA and SDMA

tHcy versus	Passive smokers n = 41		All subject n = 72	
	r	P-value	r	P-value
ADMA	0.332	0.032	0.249	0.041
SDMA	0.190	0.227 (NS)	0.174	0.176 (NS)

tHcy, total homocysteine, ADMA, asymmetric dimethylarginine; SDMA, symmetric dimethylarginine; NS, non-significant

Since homocysteine metabolism is associated with synthesis ADMA and SDMA, a correlation between tHcy and the plasma levels of both arginine derivates were assessed (table 4). Only in case of ADMA, a moderate, statistically significant relationship was found in the smokers' group (r = 0.332; P = 0.032) and a weak throughout the entire population (r = 0.249; P = 0.041).

4. Disccusion

The Assessment of the Tobacco Smoke Exposure

A questionnaire is the easiest and the most cost-effective way of gathering information regarding smoking habits. Data on the cigarette consumption in the past and at present and a number of cigarettes smoked a day let to distinguish following groups: non-smokers, former smokers (ex-smokers), and active smokers. Such a simple questionnaire is frequently used in studies requiring qualification of study persons into the groups of non-smokers, former smokers (ex-smokers), and active smokers.

The accuracy and reliability remains the most important issue associated with qualification of study persons into groups of non-smokers, passive smokers, and active smokers. Moreover, the exposure grading scale is not objective. The number of toxic substances present in the tobacco smoke is depends on so many factors that gathering appropriate information on questionnaire is virtually impossible. Studies show that the risk of second-hand smoke exposure (passive smoking) is in questionnaires underestimated [Whincup et al., 2004].

Tobacco smoke exposure assessment and thus the objective health risk assessment of passive and active tobacco smoking is possible with use of the laboratory quantitative measurements of markers and biomarkers of tobacco smoke exposure.

It is believed that nicotine and cotinine are the most selective and specific tobacco smoke biomarkers, whereby recently the examination of cotinine serum/plasma levels or urine concentration plays a major role [SRNT, 2002]. It is characterized by a longer half-life time (16-20 hours) than nicotine (1.5 hour). The measurements of cotinine may be performed both in physiological fluids (urine, plasma, serum, saliva, human milk, esophageal mucus) and also in hairs in persons exposed to tobacco smoke [Eliopoulos et al., 1994]. Numerous studies confirmed fact that cotinine is the best biomarker of smoking assessed in urine, serum or saliva with the sensitivity of 96-97% and specificity of 99-100% [Jarvis et al., 1987; Benowitz, 1996, Scherer and Richter, 1997; NCEH, 2003].

The selection of any biomarker of exposure of study persons to tobacco smoke results in the need of defining the cutoff points to distinguish non-smokers from passive smokers and active smokers.

Literature data regarding the cutoff cotinine values in plasma and in urine show a great variability (table 5). However, one should emphasize that the vast majority of authors classify study persons into smokers and non-smokers only. Occasionally, study persons are classified as non-smokers, passive smokers and active smokers.

Due to discrepant opinions on the selection of the most appropriate biomarker of tobacco smoke exposure, different threshold values and the questionable sufficiency of questionnaire in the assessment of tobacco smoke exposure, Society for Research on Nicotine and Tobacco (SRNT) appointed the team of experts lead by Professor Neal Benowitz. In 2002 the published a paper [SRNT, 2002], which recommends:

- cotinine as the most sensitive and specific biomarker of the tobacco smoke exposure;
- plasma/serum threshold cotinine levels of 15 ng/ml an urine concentration of 50 ng/ml to distinguish passive smokers from non-smokers.
- for studies on small populations, the assessment of tobacco smoke exposure by means of the measurements of biomarkers.

Considering the literature data presented in table 5, in our study we assumed a plasma cotinine level of 10 ng/ml as the cutoff point between non-smokers and passive smokers. One should however mention that food (potatoes, cauliflower, eggplant, tomatoes) may be a source of small amounts of nicotine [Benowitz, 1996; Karačonji, 2005]. Therefore, even persons not-exposed to ETS may show cotninie in their physiological fluids. Plasma cotinine levels of passive smokers range between 10 and 30 ng/ml. We think that the upper values may apply to persons smoking incidentally or smoking small number of cigarettes.

Table 5. Serum or plasma cotinine cutoff point in research

First author of references [year published]	Groups	Cutoff point [ng/ml]
Vartiainen [2002]; Bramer [2003]	non-smokers – smokers	10
Jarvis [1987]; Wagenknecht [1992]; Perez–Stable [1992]; Olivieri [2002]; Whincup [2004]	non-smokers – smokers	14
Cummings [1988]; Caraballo [2001]	non-smokers – smokers	13–15
Pirkle [1996]; Caraballo [1998]; Scott [2001a]	non-smokers – smokers	15
Lewis [2003]	non-smokers – smokers	20
Tangada [1997]; Quinn [1998]; Gunsolley [1998]	non-smokers – passive smokers – smokers	20–75

The Effects of Smoking on Total Homocysteine Level

A normal plasma tHcy in humans ranges between 5 and 15 μmol/l depending on sex and age, while a mean plasma level is higher in men than in women, and in older persons higher than in younger. In studies conducted by Ueland et al. [1993] in Western Europe, the mean plasma tHcy level in men was 13.0 μmol/l, and 10.0 μmol/l μmol/l in women. Similar values were found in epidemiological studies among Japanese population (12.6 versus 9.8 μmol/l) [Adachi et al., 2002]. Since age and sex are the strongest determinants of plasma tHcy level [El-Khairy et al., 1999; Jacques et al., 2001; Refsum at al., 2004] we decided to study only men aged between 34 and 45 years. The mean plasma tHcy level was 9.48 μmol/L.

Numerous publications suggest that tobacco smoking results in an increase of this amino acid in plasma. It is believed that the main cause of increased plasma tHcy level in smokers is deficiency of folic acid, vitamin B_6, and vitamin B_{12} that are involved in the homocysteine metabolism [Sobczak, 2003]. Recent studies show a synergistic effect of smoking and increased tHcy level on the development of coronary artery disease [Wilcken, 2002]. According to O'Callaghan et al. [2002], in smokers with a plasma tHcy level above 12 μmol/l, the risk of atherosclerosis is increased by 12 times in comparison with non-smokers with normal tHcy levels.

The vast majority studies on the effects of smoking on plasma tHcy levels compare active smokers with non-smokers. The literature data on plasma tHcy levels in passive smokers are very scanty. In the MEDLINE and EMBASE data bases since 1977 and 1989, respectively, till December 2005 there are just 5 quotations regarding passive smoking and homocyteine. Ganji and Kafai [2003] distinguish tobacco smoke exposure quartiles basing on the plasma cotinine levels. For the second quartile (plasma cotinine level between 0.087 ng/ml and 0.331) and third quartile (plasma cotinine level between 0.331 and 47.1 ng/ml) which one may consider a passive smoker' interval, the changes in tHcy in comparison with non-smokers are insignificant.

Bates et al. [2002] reported statistically highly significant (P = 0.006) differences in plasma tHcy levels in children aged between 7 and 10 years, whose mothers were active smokers in comparison to children whose mothers were non-smokers (5.95 μmol/l vs. 5.59 μmol/l), however the authors found these results unexpected and the effect of passive smoking on plasma tHcy level very unlikely.

Tröbs et al., observed a reverse situation [2002]. They found lower tHcy plasma content in non-smokers who lived with smokers in comparison with non-smokers not exposed to ETS (11.06 vs. 11.9 μmol/l). This relationship was, however, insignificant and the values correlated with sex only. The age range of the study population was 27 to 66 years which might have had affected the results.

In 2004, American Journal of Medicine published an article on the effects of passive smoking on inflammatory markers, including homocysteine, in men and women [Panagiotakos et al., 2004]. Men occasionally exposed to ETS (up to 3 times a week for at least 30 minutes) showed mean plasma tHcy level by 2.0 μmol/l (P>0.05) higher than the control group. The same difference in plasma tHcy levels was observed in persons exposed to smoke on regular basis (during more than three days a week) and here it was statistically significant (P<0.01).

At the same time, results of the study conducted in our center had been published [Sobczak et al., 2004]. They showed statistically significantly higher plasma tHcy levels in passive smokers in comparison with a control group (1.46 μmol/l, P<0.05). In this study, the passive smokers' group was qualified basing on urine cotinine concentration. Present results, which are based on plasma cotinine levels as a measure of tobacco smoke exposure, are similar to those presented in previous studies. Plasma tHcy level in passive smokers is by 1.6 μmol/l higher than in controls. However, in contrast to earlier studies, which did not show any correlation between urine cotinine concentration and plasma tHcy level, we found a statistically significant positive Pearson's correlation coefficient (r = 0.331, P<0.05) for the relationship between plasma cotinine and plasma tHcy levels.

The Effect of Passive Smoking on Total Cysteine

Cysteine is another amino acid containing a sulphhydryl group. Its chemical structure and physicochemical properties are similar to those of homocysteine. Plasma total homocysteine level in healthy individuals is about 20 times higher than tHcy level [Ueland et al., 1996]. Cysteine *in vivo* supports oxidative LDL modification, facilitates formation of foam cells [Parthasarathy, 1987], it forms adducts with NO, disturbs endothelial functions [Sheu et al., 2000], undergoes auto-oxidation which may lead to development of oxidative stress [Hogg, 1999]. Plasma tCys level is strongly associated with numerous factors (age, cholesterol level, diastolic blood pressure, coffee consumption) making a cardiovascular disease risk profile [El-Khairy et al., 1999].

Despite these, few reports of the studies on the relationship between plasma tCys levels and cardiovascular diseases have been published. The results of Europen Concerted Action Project published a few years ago show that similar to tHcy, also tCys level is associated, however to different and rather little degree, with coronary, cerebral and peripheral artery atherosclerosis [El-Khairy et al., 2001]. In contrast to tHcy, no relationship between tCys and the mortality or incidence of these disorders [El-Khairy et al., 2003]. Also, in contrary to tHcy, a tCys role as an independent atherosclerosis risk factor had not been confirmed [Van den Brandhof et al., 2001].

The mean plasma tCys level in men measured during European Concerted Action Project was 279.9 μmol/l [El-Khairy et al., 2001]. On the other hand, the its plasma level in men aged 40-42 years measured during Hordaland Homocysteine Study was 273.1 μmol/l and in men aged 43-64 years was 279.5 μmol/l [El-Khairy et al., 1999]. In the present study, the mean plasma tCys level in the entire study population (non-smokers and passive smokers) was 209.8 μmol/l.

Similar to homocysteine, tobacco smoking may affect plasma tCys level by means of decreaseing the level of vitamin B_6 being the cofactor of cystathionine β-synthase and cystathionine γ-lyase. The reaction of homocysteine trans-sulphuration to cysteine is inhibited. Consequently, the amounts of cysteine derived from homocysteine should reduce. The literature data on this subject are few and discrepant.

El-Khairy et al., [2001] showed a significant negative correlation between plasma tCys level and tobacco smoking. Similar conclusions were put forward by Brattstroom et al.,

[1994] who fund more than 8% decrease in plasma tCys (P<0.001) in smokers in comparison with non-smokers. The examination of plasma before and shortly after smoking one cigarette showed that 5 minutes after finishing smoking plasma tCys level decreased by 33% (P<0.001) but after 60 minutes its levels returns to the level measured before smoking [Tsuchiya et al., 2002].

On the other hand, a statistically significant but a weak negative correlation between plasma tCys level in non-smokers and smokers qualified into the groups of light, moderate and heavy smokers based upon the number of cigarettes smoked daily, was observed in Hordaland Homocysteine Study [El-Khairy et al., 1999]. However, one should emphasize that the highest tCy level was found in heavy smokers, lower in light smokers and the lowest in moderate smokers. Studies repeated six years later under the same program showed no significant relationship between the number of cigarettes smoked daily and the plasma tCys level [El-Khairy et al., 2003a].

Plasma tCys levels in passive smokers and in the control group in the present study do not let to draw unequivocal conclusions. Indeed, plasma tCys levels are by a dozen or so percent higher than in control group, but the differences were statistically insignificant. Neither in the smokers group, nor among the entire population, there was no statistically significant correlation between plasma cotinine and cysteine levels found. Similar results we obtained in the former studies in which we qualified study persons into study groups basing on the urine cotinine concentration [Sobczak et al., 2004]. Therfore, we suggest that tobacco smoke is not the main factor influencing plasma tCys level.

The Effects of Passive Smoking on the Asymmetric and Symmetric Dimethyloarginine

Homocysteine forms during methionine methylation with participation of S-adenozylomethionine (SAM). Increased biosynthesis of this amino-acid is associated with increased intensity of methyl group transfer reaction. Consequently, arginine ε-amin group methylation in proteins takes place, and subsequently the release of symmetric dimethyloarginine (SDMA) and a NOS inhibitor - asymmetric dimethyloarginine (ADMA) due to proteolysis (figure 6). This may in turn lead to, independently from other toxic tobacco smoke components, further NO level decrease leading to the development of mural thrombi and functional changes in the vascular wall [Cooke and Dzau, 1997; Diodati et al., 1988; Vallance et al., 1989]. At present, ADMA becomes an emerging important endothelial function risk factor [Lentz et al., 2003].

Only about 10% of ADMA is excreted from the body with urine. The remaining is metabolized by dimethlarginine dimethylaminohydrolase (DDAH) to citrulline, methylamine and small amounts of alpha keto acids. [Tran et al., 2003]. .

SDMA in turn, seems to be eliminated by renal excretion. SDMA does not affect the NOS activity to such extent as ADMA. It is, however, a potent competitor of L-arginine transport [Closs et al., 1997]. This suggests that SDMA may indirectly influence the NO synthesis in the body by means of limiting the arginine availability to NOS. Recently, Bode-Böger et al., [2006] found that SDMA might be a useful parameter for detecting patients in very early stages of chronic kidney disease and for determining their risk for developing cardiovascular disease.

In a number of reports it had been found that hyperhomocysteinemia is associated with elevated ADMA levels [Sydow et al., 2004; Dayal and Lentz 2005; Stühlinger and Stanger, 2005]. Therefore, smoking cigarettes may also cause an increase in plasma ADMA level in smokers by increasing plasma tHcy level. So far, only two reports compared plasma ADMA in non-smokers and active smokers. Eid et al. [2004] observed a statistically significant lower plasma ADMA levels in smokers than in non-smokers (- 7.7%, P = 0.037). Meanwhile, Wang et al. [2006] reported a significant increase in plasma ADMA levels in active smokers versus non-smokers (+9.3%, P =0.03). They did not find any differences in SDMA levels in both groups (0.37 μmol/L versus 0.38 μmol/L). In these studies, tHcy level was significantly higher in smokers group (by 23.8%).

The present study, for the first time presents the results of ADMA and SDMA measurements in the selected group of passive smokers. There was also a 7.5% difference in ADMA plasma levels between non-smokers and passive smokers, but it was statistically insignificant (P = 0.700). SDMA levels did not differ between both groups (0.39 μmol/L vs 0.39 μmol/L). However, there was a signifficant positive correlation between ADMA and tHcy levels in passive smokers as well as in the plasma of all men examined (r = 0.332, P = 0.032 and r = 0.249, P = 0.041, respectively). The obtained results are similar to those presented by Wang et al., [2006]. They calculated a Person's correlation coefficient for the relationship between plasma tHcy and ADMA levels in non-smokers and active smokers of 0.25, p<0.05 and 0.48, P<0.01 for SDMA.

The Effects of Passive Smoking on α-Tocopherol, γ-Tocopherol and Retinol

The intensive formation of reactive oxygen species observed in the ethiopathogenesis of atherosclerosis leads to oxidative modification of lipids, protein and nucleic acids. Their source may be endogenous (e.g. tiols auto-oxidation) as well as exogenous (e.g. tobacco smoke). This results in disturbed physiological redox balance in the body, thus resulting in depression of the anti-oxidative barrier by means. The proposed mechanisms include anti-oxidative enzymes inactivation and decreased levels of intra- and extracellular non-enzymatic anti-oxidants.

Vitamin E belongs to the most important non-enzymatic anti-oxidants, being the main lipid-soluble antioxidant of the biological membranes [Thakur and Srivastava, 1996].

The term "vitamin E" encompasses 8 natural hydrophobic compounds. All of them consist of 6-chromanol ring and side chain (phytyl chain) containing 16 carbon atoms (figure 1). Four of the substances discussed contain saturated side chain (group of tocopherols), while the remaining four have 3 double bounds (group of tocotrienols). Both tocopherols as well as tocotrienols are designated with first four letters of the Greek alphabet α, β, γ, δ. All tocopherol molecules contain chirality centres at the positions 2, 4' and 8', which make 8 optically active stereoisomers of each tocopherol. Among them 2R,4'R,8'R-α-tocopherol (shortly, R,R,R-α-tocopherol or simply α-tocopherol) is the most common substance and also the one showing the highest biological activity. If the relative α-tocopherol antioxidative activity in vitro (defined on the basis of the tocopherol reaction with fatty acids peroxyl radical) expressed in percentage is regarded as 100%, then the remaining values are 71% (β-tocopherol), 68% (γ-tocopherol), and 28% (δ-tocopherol), respectively [Schneider, 2005]. In the blood plasma, α-tocopherol makes circa 90% of the entire pool of substances known as vitamin E [Brigelius-Flohe and Traber, 1999]. Therefore, α-tocopherol is frequently identified with vitamin E. Second most common tocopherol form in plasma is γ-tocopherol. This is why these two forms raise the most interest.

Vitamin A is a traditional term including a series of compounds of animal origin. The biologically active Vitamin A forms include retinoids: retinol, retinal and retinoic acids. These are 20 carbon molecules containing a hexagonal ring with one double bond, 3 methyl groups, and a long-chain, branched substitute with a single hydroxyl, aldehyde, or carboxyl group, respectively. The main vitamin A form present in plasma (95%) is all-trans–retinol (figure 1). The most important Vitamin A functions include growth maintenance, reproduction, visual processes, epithelial differentiation, nerves myelinization and immune processes [Debier and Larondelle, 2005].

Table 6. Percentage differences between serum/plasma α-tocopherol, γ-tocopherol and retinol levels in nonsmokers, passive smokers, and active smokers

First author of references [year published]	Number of of study persons (sex)	Concentration changes in comparison with nonsmokers who are assumed as 100% [%]			
		Passive smokers	P_1-value	Active smokers	P_2-value
α-Tocopherol					
Takatsuka [1998]	124 (F/M)	- 17.3	<0.05	- 26.9	<0.05
Alberg [2000]	586 (F)	- 2.8	NS	- 1.1	NS
	560 (M)	- 5.2	NS	+ 0.5	NS
Wei [2001]	3901 (F)	- 3.6	NS	- 6.1	NS
	3972 (M)	- 1.1	NS	- 7.8	NS
Tröbs [2002]	1077 (F/M)	0.0 [1]	NS	- 6.7 [1]	<0.05
Dietrich [2003]	159 (F/M))	- 2.3	NS	- 1,0	NS
Sobczak [2004a]	117 (F/M)	- 5.7	<0.05	-9.2	<0.001
γ-Tocopherol					
Alberg [2000]	456 (F)	+ 3.7	NS	- 2.1	NS
	366 (M)	- 3.8	NS	- 3.0	NS
Dietrich [2003]	159 (F/M)	+ 30.0	<0.01	+ 31.6	0.032
Sobczak [2004a]	117 (F/M)	+1.1	NS	+3.2	NS
Retinol					
Dietrich [2003]	159 (F/M)	-5.1	NS	7.4	0.04

F – female; M – male; P_1 – statistical significance between passive smokers and nonsmokers; P_2 – statistical significance between active smokers and nonsmokers; NS – non-significant.

[1] α- and γ-tocopherol level expressed in (μmol/l) / cholesterol (mg/dl).

Tobacco smoke inducing oxidative stress causes a redox misbalance and triggers protective mechanisms. This results in decreased levels of some antioxidants. Anti-oxidant vitamins levels are useful and frequently applied indicators of the body redox balance. It is estimated that the blood levels of ascorbic acid, α-carotene, β-carotene and cryptoxanthin in active smokers are by more than 25% lower than in non-smokers [Alberg, 2002]. On the other hand, data on plasma α- and γ-tocopherols levels in persons exposed to tobacco smoke are discrepant [Sobczak and Gołka, 2006].

Studies, in which a questionnaire was the only inclusion criterion to study groups did not distinguished groups of passive smokers. Therefore, the number of articles devoted to the effects of tobacco smoke on the tocopherols levels in passive smokers is relatively low in comparison with analogous issue regarding active smokers. In the most of the analyzed reports plasma/serum α- and γ-tocopherol levels were lower in passive and active smokers in comparison with non-smokers. However, one should mention that some authors observed increased levels of these substances in smokers versus non-smokers [table 6].

In the present study, we observed a statistically significant decrease (by 12.8%) in α-tocopherol level in passive smokers as compared to non-smokers and significant and negative correlation between plasma α-tocopherol and cotinine levels both in passive smokers as well as among the entire population. The were no statistically significant changes in γ-tocopherol levels.

Lower plasma vitamin E levels in persons exposed to tobacco smoke may result from its different disintegration rates in smokers and non-smokers [Traber et al., 2001; Bruno et al., 2006]. In their experiment, Traber et al. [2001] supplemented smokers' and non-smokers' breakfasts with deuterium labeled vitamin E. They observed a more than 20% increase in vitamin E metabolism in smokers versus non-smokers. In vitro studies showed that in human plasma exposed to gaseous phase of the tobacco smoke, α-tocopherol level decreased faster than γ-tocopherol [Handelman et al.,1996]. This might explain decreased α-tocopherol levels and no change in γ-tocopherol levels in smokers in comparison with non-smokers.

The role of retinol in scavenge of reactive oxygen species and thus its role in the processes that maintain the oxidative-reduction balance in the body is lesser than the others non-enzymatic antioxidants. In a large retrospective analysis [Alberg, 2002] devoted to the effects of tobacco smoke on the non-enzymatic antioxidants there are no reports regarding retinol, but there are numerous articles on carotenoids, including vitamin A provitamin - β-carotene. Few articles on the effects of smoking on plasma retinol levels present similar results. Apart from few exceptions, the differences in plasma/serum retinol levels between smokers and non-smokers reach several percent and are insignificant [Marangon et al., 1998; Faure et al., 2006; Gabriel et al., 2006].

In the present study, the difference in plasma retinol level between persons exposed to tobacco smoke and control group was 7.7%, but it was statistically insignificant. There was also no correlation between plasma retinol and cotinine levels. Both literature data as well as our results indicate that retinol does not play any role in the formation of anti-oxidative barrier protecting against reactive oxygen species that enter the body with tobacco smoke.

5. Conclusion

Passive smoking does not affect plasma ADMA and SDMA levels. It seems that changes in plasma tHcy levels induced by ETS that might result in increased ADMA and SDMA levels are too little to affect levels of arginine derivates. In addition, no effect of passive smoking on tCys, γ-tocopherol and retinol levels was found.

It was showed that passive smoking increases plasma tHcy level. Increased tHcy level shows a positive correlation with plasma cotinine level in study persons. This confirms the relationship between the tobacco smoke exposure and homocyteine level. Moreover, exposure to ETS weakens the body anti-oxidative barrier by means of decrease in plasma α-tocopherol level. It seems that statistically significant changes in plasma tHcy and α-tocopherol levels although rather little, in a longer time interval may be one of the cardiovascular risk factors in passive smokers.

6. References

[1]   Adachi, H; Hirai, Y; Fujiura, Y; Matsuoka, H; Satoh, A; Imaizumi, T. Plasma homocysteine levels and atherosclerosis in Japan. Epidemiological study by use of carotid ultrasonography. *Stroke,* 2002, 33, 2177-2181.

[2]   Ahijevych, K; Gillespie, J. Nicotine dependence and smoking topography among black and white women. *Res. Nurs. Health.,* 1997, 20, 505-514.

[3]   Alberg, AJ. The influence of cigarette smoking on circulating concentrations of antioxidant micronutrients. *Toxicology,* 2002, 180, 121-137.

[4]   Alberg, AJ; Chen, JC; Zhao, H; Hoffman, SC; Comstock, GW; Helzlsouer, KJ; Houshold exposure to passive cigarette smoking and serum micronutrient concentrations. *Am. J. Clin. Nutr.,* 2000, 72, 1576-1582.

[5]   Barnoya, J; Glantz, SA. Cardiovascular effects of secondhand smoke. Nearly as large as smoking. *Circulation,* 2005, 111, 2684-2698.

[6]   Bates, CJ; Mansoor, MA; Gregory, J; Pentieva, K; Prentice, A; Correlates of plasma homocysteine, cysteine and cysteiny-glycine in respondents in the British National Diet and Nutrition Survey of Young People Aged 4-18 years, and a comparison with the Survey of People Aged 65 Years and Over. *Br. J. Nutr.,* 2002, 87, 71-79.

[7]   Benowitz, NL. Cotinine as a biomarker of environmental tobacco smoke exposure. *Epidemiol. Rev.,* 1996, 18, 188-204.

[8]   Bode-Böger, SM; Scalera, F; Kielstein, JT; Martens-Lobenhoffer, J; Breithardt, G; Fobker, M; Reinecke, H. Symmetrical dimethylarginine, a new combined parameter for renal function and extent of coronary artery disease. *J. Am. Soc. Nephrol.,* 2006, 17, 1128-1134.

[9]   Böger, RH; Cooke, JP; Vallance, P. ADMA, an emerging cardiovascular risk factor. *Vasc. Med.,* 2005, 10, S1-2.

[10]   Böger, RH. Asymmetric dimethylarginine (ADMA). A novel risk marker in cardiovascular medicine and beyond. *Ann. Med.,* 2006, 38, 126-136.

[11] Bornhäuser, A; McCarthy, J; Glantz, SA. German tobacco industry's successful efforts to maintain scientific and political respectability to prevent regulation of secondhand smoke. Tob. Control, 2006, 15, e1 (postprint available at, http//repositories.cdlib.org/ postprints/1143)

[12] Bramer, SL; Kallungal, BA. Clinical considerations in study designs that use cotinine as a biomarker. *Biomerkers*, 2003, 8, 187-203.

[13] Brattstrom, L; Lindgren, A; Israelsson, B; Andersson, A; Hultberg, B. Homocysteine and cysteine, determinants of plasma levels in middle-aged and elderly subjects. *J. Intern. Med.*, 1994, 236, 633-641.

[14] Brigelius-Flohe, R, Traber, MG. Vitamin E function and metabolism. *FASEB J.*, 1999, 13, 1145-1155.

[15] Bruno, RS; Leonard, SW; Atkinson, J; Montine, TJ; Ramakrishnan, R; Bray, TM; Traber, MG. Faster plasma vitamin E disappearance in smokers is normalized by vitamin C supplementation. *Free Radic. Biol. Med.*, 2006, 40, 689-697.

[16] Caraballo, RS; Giovino, GA; Pechacek, TF; Mowery, PD; Richter, PA; Strauss, WJ; Sharp, DJ; Eriksen, MP; Pirkle, JL; Maurer, KR. Racial and ethnic differences in serum cotinine levels of cigarette smokers, Third National Health and Nutrition Examination Survey, 1988-1991. *JAMA*, 1998, 280, 135 – 139.

[17] Caraballo, RS; Giovino, GA; Pechacek, TF; Mowery, PD. Factors associated with discrepancies between self-reports on cigarette smoking and measured serum cotinine levels among persons aged 17 years or older. Third National Health and Nutrition Examination Survey, 1988-1994. *Am. J. Epidemiol.*, 2001, 153, 807-814.

[18] Closs, EI; Basha, FZ; Habermeier, A; Forstermann, U. Interference of L-arginine analogues with L-arginine transport mediated by the y+ carrier hCAT-2B. *Nitric Oxide*, 1997, 1, 65-73.

[19] Cooke, JP; Dzau, VJ. Derangements of the nitric oxide synthase pathway, L-arginine and cardiovascular diseases. *Circulation*, 1997, 96, 379-382.

[20] Cummings, SR; Richard, RJ; Optimum cutoff points for biochemical validation of smoking status. *Am. J. Public Health*, 1988, 78, 574-575.

[21] Dayal, S; Lentz, SR. ADMA and hyperhomocysteinemia. *Vasc. Med.*, 2005, 10, S27-33.

[22] Debier, C; Larondelle, Y. Vitamins A and E, metabolism, roles and transfer to offspring. *Br. J. Nutr.*, 2005, 93, 153-174.

[23] Dietrich, M; Block, G; Norkus, EP; Hudes, M; Traber, MG; Cross, C.E; Packer, L. Smoking and exposure to environmental tobacco smoke decrease some plasma antioxidants and increase γ-tocopherol in vivo after adjustment for dietary antioxidant intakes. *Am. J. Clin. Nutr.*, 2003, 77, 160-166.

[24] Diodati, JG; Dakak, N; Gilligan, DM; Quyyumi, AA. Effect of atherosclerosis on endothelium-dependent inhibition of platelet activation in humans. *Circulation*, 1998, 98, 17-24.

[25] Eid, HA; Arnesen, H; Hjerkinn, EM; Lyberg, T; Seljeflot, I. Relationship between obesity, smoking, and the endogenous nitric oxide synthase inhibitor, asymmetric dimethylarginine. *Metabolism*, 2004, 53, 1574-1579.

[26] Eissenberg, T; Adams, C; Riggins, EC3rd, Likness, M. Smokers' sex and the effects of tobacco cigarettes, subject-rated and physiological measures. *Nicotine Tob. Res.*, 1999, 1, 317-324.

[27] Eliopoulos, C; Klein, J; Phan, MK; Knie, B; Greenwald, M; Chitayat, D; Koren, G. Hair concentrations of nicotine and cotinine in women and their newborn infants. *JAMA*, 1994, 271, 621-623.

[28] El-Khairy, L; Ueland, P.M; Nygård, O; Refsum, H; Vollset, S.E; Lifestyle and cardiovascular disease risk factors as determinants of total cysteine in plasma, the Hordaland Homocysteine Study. *Am. J. Clin. Nutr.*, 1999, 70, 1016-1024.

[29] El-Khairy, L; Ueland, PM; Refsum, H; Graham, IM; Vollset, SE; Plasma total cysteine as risk factor for vascular disease. The European Concerted Action Project. *Circulation*, 2001, 103, 2544-2549.

[30] El-Khairy, L; Vollset, SE; Refsum, H; Ueland, PM. Plasma total cysteine, mortality, and cardiovascular disease hospitalizations, the Hordaland Homocysteine Study. *Clin. Chem.*, 2003, 49, 895-900.

[31] El-Khairy, L; Vollset, SE; Refsum, H; Ueland, PM. Predictors of change in plasma total cysteine, longitudinal findings from the Hordaland Homocysteine Study. *Clin. Chem.*, 2003a, 49, 113-120.

[32] Enstrom, JE; Kabat, GC. Environmental tobacco smoke and tobacco related mortality in a prospective study of Californians, 1960-98. *BMJ*, 2003, 326, 1057-1066.

[33] Faure, H; Preziosi, P; Roussel, AM; Bertrais, S; Galan, P; Hercberg, S; Favier, A. Factors influencing blood concentration of retinol, α-tocopherol, vitamin C, and β-carotene in the French participants of the SU.VI.MAX trial. *Eur. J. Clin. Nutr.*, 2006, 60, 706-17.

[34] Gabriel, HE; Liu, Z; Crott, JW; Choi, SW; Song, BC; Mason, JB; Johnson, EJ. A comparison of carotenoids, retinoids, and tocopherols in the serum and buccal mucosa of chronic cigarette smokers versus nonsmokers. *Cancer Epidemiol. Biomarkers Prev.*, 2006, 15, 993-999.

[35] Ganji, V; Kafai, MR. Demographic, health, lifestyle, and blood vitamin determinants of serum total homocysteine concentrations in the third National Health and Nutrition Examination Survey, 1988-1994. *Am. J. Clin. Nutr.*, 2003, 77, 826-833.

[36] Gunsolley, JC; Quinn, SM; Tew, J; Gooss, CM; Brooks, CN; Schenkein, HA. The effect of smoking on individuals with minimal periodontal destruction. *J. Periodontol.*, 1998, 69, 165-170.

[37] Hammond, D; Fong, GT; Cummings, M; Hyland, A. Smoking topography, brand switching, and nicotine delivery, results from an in vivo study. *Cancer Epidemiol. Biomarkers Prev.*, 2005, 14, 1370-1375.

[38] Handelman, GJ; Packer, L; Cross, CE. Destruction of tocopherols, carotenoids, and retinol in human plasma by cigarette smoke. *Am. J. Clin. Nutr.*, 1996, 63, 559-565.

[39] Haroun, L, Dunn, AJ, Ting, D. Exposure Measurement and Prevalence. [In] Health Effects of Exposure to Environmental Tobacco Smoke. The Report of the California Environmental Protection Agency. [Ed.] Zeise L; Bethesda, MD, National Institutes of Health 1999.

[40] Hogg, N. The effect of cyst(e)ine on the auto-oxidation of homocysteine. *Free Radic. Biol. Med.,* 1999, 27, 28-33.

[41] Jacques, PF; Bostom, AG; Wilson, PWF; Rich, S; Rosenberg, IH; Selhub, J. Determinants of plasma total homocysteine concentration in the Framingham Offspring cohort. *Am. J. Clin. Nutr.,* 2001, 73,613-621.

[42] Jarvis, MJ; Tunstall-Pedoe, H; Feyerabend, C; Vesey, C; Saloojee, Y. Comparison of tests used to distinguish smokers from nonsmokers. *Am. J. Public. Health,* 1987, 77, 1435-1438.

[43] Karačonji, I.B. Facts about nicotine toxicity. *Arh. Hig. Rada Toksikol.,* 2005, 56, 363-371.

[44] Lentz, SR; Rodionov, RN; Dayal, S. Hyperhomocysteinemia, endothelial dysfunction, and cardiovascular risk, the potential role of ADMA. *Atherosclerosis,* 2003, Suppl. 4, 61-65.

[45] Lewis, SJ; Cherry, NM; McL Niven, R; Barber, PV; Wilde, K; Povey, AC. Cotinine levels and self-reported smoking status in patients attending a bronchoscopy clinic. *Biomarkers,* 2003, 8, 218-228.

[46] Marangon, K; Herbeth, B; Lecomte, E; Paul-Dauphin, A; Grolier, P; Chancerelle, Y; Artur, Y; Siest, G. Diet, antioxidant status, and smoking habits in French men. *Am. J. Clin. Nutr.,* 1998, 67, 231-239.

[47] NCEH (National Center for Environmental Health), Division of Laboratory Sciences. Second national report on human exposure to environmental chemicals. Atlanta, Georgia, 2003 NCEH Pub. No. 02-0716

[48] NIH (National Institutes of Health). Clinical guidelines on the identification and treatment of overweight and obesity in adults. The Evidence Report. 1998 NIH Pub. No. 98-4083

[49] Nygård, O; Refsum, H; Ueland, PM; Vollset, SE. Major life style determinants of plasma total homocysteine distribution, the Hordaland Homocysteine Study. *Am. J. Clin. Nutr.,* 1998, 67, 263-270.

[50] Nygård, O; Nordrehaug, JE; Refsum, H; Ueland, PM; Farstad, M; Vollset, SE. Plasma homocysteine levels and mortality in patients with coronary artery disease. *N. Engl. J. Med.,* 1997, 337, 230-236.

[51] O'Callaghan, R; Meleady, R; Fitzgerald, T; Graham, I; and the European COMAC group. Smoking and plasma homocysteine. *Eur. Heart J.,* 2002, 23,1580-1586.

[52] Olivieri, M; Poli, A; Zuccaro, P; Ferrari, M; Lampronti, G; De Marco, R; Lo Cascio, V; Pacifici, R. Tobacco smoke exposure and serum cotinine in a random sample of adults living in Verona, Italy. *Arch. Environ. Health,* 2002, 57, 355-359.

[53] Panagiotakos D.B; Pitsavos C; Chrysohoou C; Skoumas J; Masoura C; Toutouzas P; Stefanadis C; Effect of exposure to secondhand smoke on markers of inflammation, the ATTICA Study. *Am. J. Med.* 2004, 116, 145-150.

[54] Parthasarathy, S. Oxidation of low-density lipoprotein by thiol compounds leads to its recognition by the acetyl LDL receptor. *Biochim. Biophys. Acta,* 1987, 917, 337-340.

[55] Patterson, F; Benowitz, N; Shields, P; Kaufmann, V; Jepson, C; Wileyto, P; Kucharski, S; Lerman, C. Individual differences in nicotine intake per cigarette. *Cancer Epidemiol. Biomarkers Prev.,* 2003, 12, 468-461.

[56] Perez-Stable, EJ; Marin, G; Marin, BV. Benowitz, NL. Misclassification of smoking status by self-reported cigarette consumption. *Am. Rev. Respir. Dis.,* 1992, 145, 53-57.

[57] Pichini, S; Altieri, I; Pacifici, R; Rosa, M; Ottaviani, G; Zuccaro, P. Simultaneous determination of cotinine and trans-3'-hydroxycotinine in human serum by high-performance liquid chromatography. *J. Chromatogr.,* 1992, 577, 358-361.

[58] Pirkle, JL; Flegal, KM; Bernert, JT; Brody, DJ; Etzel, RA; Maurer, KR. Exposure of the US population to environmental tobacco smoke, the Third National Health and Nutrition Examination Survey, 1988 to 1991. *JAMA,* 1996, 275, 1233-1240.

[59] Quinn, SM; Zhang, JB; Gunsolley, JC; Schenkein, HA; Tew, JG. The influence of smoking and race on adult periodontitis and serum IgG2 levels. *J. Periodontol.,* 1998, 69, 171-177.

[60] Refsum, H; Smith, AD; Ueland, PM; Nexo, E; Clarke, R; McPartlin, J; Johnston, C; Engbaek, F; Schneede, J; McPartlin, C; Scott, JM. Facts and recommendations about total homocysteine determinations: an expert opinion. *Clin. Chem.,* 2004, 50, 3-32.

[61] Scherer, G; Jarczyk, L; Heller, WD; Biber, A; Neurath, GB; Adlkofer, F. Pharmacokinetics of nicotine, cotinine and 3'-hydroxycotyninie in cigarette smokers. *Klin. Wochenschr.,* 1988, 66, 5-11.

[62] Scherer, G; Richter, E. Biomonitoring exposure to environmental tobacco smoke (ETS), a critical reappraisal. *Hum. Exp. Toxicol.,* 1997, 16, 449-459.

[63] Schick, S; Glantz, SA. Philip Morris toxicological experiments with fresh sidestream smoke, more toxic than mainstream smoke. *Tob. Control,* 2005, 14, 396-404.

[64] Schneider, C. Chemistry and biology of vitamin E. *Mol. Nutr. Food Res.,* 2005, 49, 7-30.

[65] Scott, DA; Palmer, RM; Stapleton, JA. Dose-years as an improved index of cumulative tobacco smoke exposure. *Med. Hypotheses,* 2001, 56, 735-736.

[66] Sheu, FS; Zhu, W; Fung, PC. Direct observation of trapping and release of nitric oxide by glutathione and cysteine with electron paramagnetic resonance spectroscopy. *Biophys. J.,* 2000, 78, 1216-1226.

[67] Sobczak, A; Gołka, D; Szołtysek-Bołdys, I. The effects of tobacco smoke on plasma alpha- and gamma-tocopherol levels in passive and active cigarette smokers. *Toxicol. Lett.* 2004a, 151, 429-437.

[68] Sobczak, A; Gołka, D. The effects of cigarette smoking on the human plasma tocopherols levels. [In] Focus on Vitamin E Research [Ed.] M. Braunstein, New York, Nova Science Publishers, 2006 (in press)

[69] Sobczak, A; Skop, B; Kula, B. Simultaneous determination of serum retinol and α- and γ- tocopherol levels in type II diabetic patients using high-performance liquid chromatography with fluorescence detection. *J. Chromatogr. B. Biomed. Sci Appl.,* 1999, 730, 265-271.

[70] Sobczak, A; Wardas, W; Zielińska –Danch, W; Pawlicki, K. The influence of smoking on plasma homocysteine and cysteine levels in passive and active smokers. *Clin. Chem. Lab. Med.,* 2004, 42, 408-414.

[71] Sobczak, A; Wardas, W; Zielińska-Danch, W; Szołtysek-Bołdys, I. Biomarkers of tobacco smoke.[in polish]. *Przegl. Lek.,* 2005, 62, 1192-1199.

[72] Sobczak, A. The effects of tobacco smoke on the homocysteine level – a risk factor of atherosclerosis. *Addict. Biol.,* 2003, 8, 147-158.

[73] SRNT (Society for Research on Nicotine and Tobacco), Subcommitee on Biochemical Verification. Biochemical verification of tobacco use and cessation. *Nicotine Tob. Res.,* 2002, 4, 149-159.

[74] Stühlinger, MC; Stanger, O. Asymmetric dimethyl-L-arginine (ADMA), a possible link between homocyst(e)ine and endothelial dysfunction. *Curr. Drug. Metab.,* 2005, 6, 3-14.

[75] Sydow, K; Hornig, B; Arakawa, N; Bode-Böger, SM; Tsikas, D; Münzel, T; Böger, RH. Endothelial dysfunction in patients with peripheral arterial disease and chronic hyperhomocysteinemia, potential role of ADMA. *Vasc. Med.,* 2004, 9, 93-101.

[76] Takatsuka, N; Kawakami, N; Ito Y; Kabuto, M; Shimizu, H. Effects of passive smoking on serum levels of carotenoids and α-tocopherol. *J. Epidemiol.,* 1998, 8, 146-151.

[77] Tangada, SD; Califano, JV; Nakashima, K; Quinn, SM; Zhang, JB; Gunsolley, JC; Schenkein, HA; Tew, JG. The effect of smoking on serum IgG2 reactive with Actinobacillus actinomycetemcomitans in early-onset periodontitis patients. *J. Periodontol.,* 1997, 68, 842-850.

[78] Teerlink, T. Determination of the endogenous nitric oxide synthase inhibitor asymmetric dimethylarginine in biological samples by HPLC. *Methods Mol. Med.,* 2004, 108, 263-274.

[79] Thakur, M.L; Srivastava, US. Vitamin E metabolism and its application. *Nutr. Res.,* 1996, 16, 1767-1809.

[80] Thun, MJ. More misleading science from the tobacco industry. Delaying clean air laws through disinformation. *BMJ USA,* 2003, 3, 352.

[81] Traber, MG; Winklhofer-Roob, BM; Robb, JM; Khoschsorur, G; Aigner, R; Cross, C; Ramakrishnan, R; Brigelius-Flohe, R. Vitamin E kinetics in smokers and nonsmokers. *Free Radic. Biol. Med.,* 2001, 31, 1368-1374.

[82] Tran, CTL; Leiper, JM; Vallance, P; The DDAH/ADMA/NOS pathway. *Atherosclerosis,* 2003, Suppl. 4, 33-40.

[83] Tröbs, M; Renner, T; Scherer, G; Heller, WD; Geiss, HC; Wolfram, G; Haas, GM; Schwandt, P. Nutrition, antioxidants, and risk factor profile of nonsmokers, passive smokers and smokers of the Prevention Education Program (PEP) in Nuremberg, Germany. *Prev. Med.,* 2002, 34, 600-607.

[84] Tsuchiya, M; Asada, A; Kasahara, E; Sato, EF; Shindo, M; Inoue, M. Smoking a single cigarette rapidly reduces combined concentrations of nitrate and nitrite and concentrations of antioxidants in plasma. *Circulation,* 2002, 105, 1155-1157

[85] Ueland, PM; Mansoor, MA; Guttormsen, AB; Müller, F; Aukrust, P; Refsum, H; Svardal, AM. Reduced, oxidized and protein-bound forms of homocysteine and other aminothiols in plasma comprise the redox thiol status – a possible element of the extracellular antioxidant defense system. *J. Nutr.,* 1996, 126, 1281S-1284S.

[86] Ueland, PM; Refsum, H; Stabler, SP; Malinow, MR; Anderson, A; Allen, RH. Total homocysteine in plasma and serum, methods and clinical applications. *Clin. Chem.,* 1993, 39, 1764-1779.

[87] Vallance, P; Collier, J; Moncada, S. Effects of endothelium derived nitric oxide on peripheral arteriolar tone in man. *Lancet,* 1989, 334, 997-1000.

[88] Van den Brandhof, WE; Haks, K; Schouten, EG; Verhoef, P. The relation between plasma cysteine, plasma homocysteine and coronary atherosclerosis. *Atherosclerosis,* 2001, 157, 403-409.

[89] Vartiainen, E; Seppälä, T; Lillsunde, P; Puska, P. Validation of self reported smoking by serum cotinine measurement in a community-based study. *J. Epidemiol. Community Health,* 2002, 56, 167-170.

[90] Wagenknecht, LE; Burke, GL; Perkins, LL. Haley, NJ; Friedman, GD. Misclassification of smoking status in the CARDIA study, a comparison of self-report with serum cotinine levels. *Am. J. Public Health,* 1992, 82, 33-36.

[91] Wang, J; Sim, AS; Wang, XL; Salonikas, C; Naidoo, D; Wilcken, DEL. Relations between plasma asymmetric dimethylarginine (ADMA) and risk factors for coronary disease. *Atherosclerosis,* 2006, 184, 383-388.

[92] Wei, W; Kim, Y; Boudreau, N. Association of smoking with serum and dietary levels of antioxidants in adults, NHANES III, 1988-1994. *Am. J. Public Health,* 2001, 91, 258-264.

[93] Whincup, PH; Gilg, JA; Emberson, JR; Jarvis, MJ; Feyerabend, C; Bryant, A; Walker, M; Cook, DG. Passive smoking and risk of coronary heart disease and stroke, prospective study with cotinine measurement. *BMJ,* 2004, 329, 200-205.

[94] Wilcken, DEL. Homocysteine, smoking and vascular disease. *Eur. Heart J.,* 2002, 23,1559-1560.

[95] Wood, T; Wewers, ME; Groner, J; Ahijevych, K. Smoke constituent exposure and smoking topography of aldolescent daily cigarette smokers. *Nicotine Tob. Res.,* 2004, 6, 853-862.

[96] Young, PB; Molloy, AM; Scott, JM; Kennedy, DG. A rapid high performance liquid chromatographic method for determination of homocysteine in porcine tissue. *J. Liq. Chromatogr.,* 1994, 17, 3553-3561.

In: Handbook of Cardiovascular Research
Editors: Jorgen Brataas and Viggo Nanstveit

ISBN 978-1-60741-792-7
© 2009 Nova Science Publishers, Inc.

Chapter VII

Effects of Melatonin on Cardiovascular System

Ewa Sewerynek[*]

Department of Bone Metabolism, Endocrinology and Metabolic Diseases,
The Medical University of Łódź, Poland

Abstract

The evidence obtained during more than last 10 years suggests that melatonin exerts some effects on the cardiovascular system. It is especially important in the case of elderly people, because of the increased incidence of both, acute and chronic heart diseases. In the course of aging concentrations of some of the hormones decrease, e.g., melatonin, dehydroepiandrosterone, eostrogensoestrogen, etc. It has been shown that melatonin concentration in serum and the level of its main metabolite 6-sulphatoxymelatonin in urine are lower in older people compared to younger population. The melatoninergic receptors demonstrated in vascular system are functionally associated with either vasoconstrictory, vasoconstrictory or vasodilatory effects of this pineal indoleamine. In the 90ties of the last century melatonin was established as a potent antioxidant. In the pathogenesis of some age-related diseases the generation of free radicals play an important role. Melatonin contributes to the general cardioprotection in rat models of oxidative stress induced by myocardial ischemia-reperfusion or adriamycin-induced cardiotoxicity. It has been shown that patients with coronary heart disease have a low melatonin production rate, especially those with the higher risk of cardiac infarction and/or of the sudden death. The suprachiasmatic nucleus and, possibly, the melatoninergic system may modulate cardiovascular rhythmicity. It has been shown, that melatonin may influence other age-related problems including hypercholesterolemia and hypertension. People with high levels of LDL-cholesterol and also those with

[*] Ewa Sewerynek Department of Bone Metabolism, Chair of Endocrinology and Metabolic Diseases, The Medical University of Łódź, 91-425 Łódź, Dr Sterling Str Nr 5, Poland, Phone/Fax: (48) (42) 632 25 94,E-mail: ewa.sewerynek@wp.pl; ewa@tyreo.am.lodz.pl.

hypertension have lower levels of melatonin compared to the population without lipid disturbance and with the normal blood pressure. It has been shown that melatonin suppresses the formation of cholesterol, reduces LDL oxidation and accumulation in the vascular system. The administration of melatonin decreases blood pressure to the normal levels.

It has been observed, that melatonin replacement therapy may decrease the incidence of sudden cardiac deaths, especially in elderly patients with deficiency of its endogenous level. This review summarises up-to-date knowledge about correlation between the cardiovascular system and melatonin.

Keywords: melatonin, cardiovascular system, hypertension, hypercholesterolemia, ischemia-reperfusion

Introduction

Cardiovascular diseases in many countries pose a serious problem, and they are frequently the cause of disability and/or mortality. There are many options of treatment leading to reduction of cardiac damage, such as non-invasive or cardio-surgical procedures. In elderly subjects, the incidence of heart diseases, both acute and chronic, systematically increases. The evidence indicates that melatonin influences the cardiovascular system (Sewerynek, 2002; Reiter and Tan, 2003).

It is well-known that melatonin in serum plays an important role in the regulation of various neural and endocrine processes that are synchronized with the daily change of the photoperiod (Reiter, 1992). The half-life of serum melatonin in humans is approximately 41 min (Fourtillan et al., 2000). Most of the circulating melatonin is metabolised in the liver to 6-hydroxymelatonin and subsequently to 6-sulfatoxymelatonin (6-hydroxymelatonin sulfate) which is excreted into the urine. It has been shown that concentrations of serum melatonin and urinary levels of 6-sulphatoxymelatonin, decrease in the course of ageing both in humans and animals (Karasek and Reiter, 2002). It has also been found that in old mice serum melatonin levels were reduced by 80% in 27-month old mice relative to 12 month (Lahiri et al., 2004). Levels of the melatonin metabolite, 6-hydroxymelatonin sulfate were significantly higher than free melatonin in all examined tissues (liver, kidney, cerebral cortex, heart); the highest being in the cerebral cortex. In 12-month old animals this metabolite concentration was 1000-fold greater than that of melatonin in the cerebral cortex compared to only 3-fold greater in serum. Any age-related decline of tissue melatonin was reversed by supplementation with dietary melatonin.

However, it has been reported that during childhood and adolescence the absolute melatonin production remainesremains constant. The authors suggest that the observed decreased melatonin levels in plasma in young population is mainly related to the increase in body size rather than to the decrease of melatonin secretion (Griefahn et al., 2003).

Rhythms of Cardiac Events

Similarly to other organs and systems, the cardiovascular system exhibits a diurnal rhythm, e.g. heart rate, blood pressure and vascular tone decrease at night (Panza et al., 1991; Burgess et al., 1997). Daily variations in the incidence of cardiac events have also been observed. Coca (1994) demonstrated that blood pressure falls during the night. Nicolau et al. (1991) suggested that cardiac mortality rate has its peaks early in the morning, coinciding with the peaks in systolic and diastolic blood pressure.

It has been shown that cardiovascular system has also seasonal rhythms. It has been observed that: 1) heart rate variability is the lowest in winter (Kristal-Boneh et al., 2000), 2) the incidence of cardiac arrest is the highest in winter (Peckowa et al., 1999), and 3) blood pressure values are higher in winter than in summer (Kristal-Boneh et al., 1997). There is some information about seasonal variations in the incidence of cardiac events, e.g.: 1) seasonal variations of acute myocardial infarction show winter peaks and summer drops (Sayer et al., 1997), 2) cardiac mortality rate has its peak in July and also from December to February (Nicolau et al., 1991), 3) cardiac output of rats has low values in spring and summer and high in autumn and winter (Back and Strubelt, 1975).

Epidemiological studies have shown that cardiological events occur most frequently in the morning between 6.00 a.m. and 12.00 a.m. (Muller et al., 1987). Additionally, it has been observed that the incidence of cardiac arrests is the highest in the morning (from 8.00 to 11.00 a.m.) and in the afternoon (from 4.00 to 7.00 p.m.) (Peckowa et al., 1998; 1999).

It is well known that an acute heart attack has a daily, seasonal and, perhaps, ultradian rhythm; on the other side, cardiological events, such as angina pectoris and sudden death, display circadian rhythms (Tarquini et al., 1993). Also, a number of known cardiovascular risk factors, such as hormones, metabolic parameters, lifestyle, blood pressure, fibrinogenesis, as well as fibrinolytic activity demonstrate periodical oscillations.

The suprachiasmatic nucleus and, possibly, the melatoninergic system can modulate the cardiovascular rhythm. During the night, when the level of melatonin is highest, the heart rate decreases, the cardiac output is higher, the blood pressure drops, the level of cholesterol declines and the activity of calcium pump increases.

Autonomic Nerve System

It has been reported that there is a close correlation between autonomic nerve system and melatonin release. Cardiovascular blunting during the night is at least partially linked to the autonomic activity and increased risk of cardiac events (Huikuri et al., 1992; Verdecchia et al., 1993). In animals, the data obtained indicates that the cardiovascular response to melatonin may be mediated to some extend, by reducing noradrenergic activity (Visvanathan et al., 1986; Chuang et al., 1993). In men, melatonin administration may exert suppressive effects on the sympathetic tone (Nishiyama et al., 2001). Oral administration of melatonin increases cardiac vagal tone, decreases blood pressure and vascular reactivity and norepinephrine level (Cagnacci et al., 1998; Arangino et al., 1999; Nishiyama et al., 2001). The findings of Ray (2003) indicate that in humans, a high concentration of melatonin can attenuate the reflex sympathetic increases that occur in response to orthostatic stress. These alterations appear to be mediated by melatonin-induced changes to the baroreflexes.

The fact of seasonal variations in blood pressure of patients treated with beta-adrenergic receptor blockers (Lemmer, 1989) and the fact that the circadian rhythm of the heart rate was maintained in patients after heart transplantation (Wenting et al., 1987), indicate that seasonal and daily variations in the sympathetic tone may not be the only controlling factors. This suggests an involvement of some other mechanisms.

In patients with coronary artery disease a decreased melatonin level in serum has been observed (Sakotnik et al., 1999). The possible use of β-adrenoceptor blockers, which reduce melatonin synthesis, may be an important factor responsible for low melatonin levels in these patients. Stoschitzky et al. (1999) have shown that β-blockers decrease melatonin release via a specific inhibition of β_1-receptors. Nathan et al. (1997) have demonstrated a dose-dependent relationship between β_1-receptor blockade and the suppression of nocturnal plasma melatonin in humans. On the other hand, Girotti et al. (2000) did not observe any significant difference in the levels of 6-sulphatoxymelatonin excretion in patients, either treated or not treated with β-adrenoceptor blockers.

Lower nocturnal melatonin levels may induce sleep disturbances which are well-known side effects of β-adrenergic antagonists. Several studies indicate that sleep disorders occur more frequently in coronary patients than in non-coronary or normal subjects. Since low melatonin levels can be associated with sleep disturbances, at least, in elderly patients, low melatonin secretion, reported in coronary patients, could play a causal role in this respect.

Melatonin Receptors in Cardiovascular System

The presence of vascular melatoninergic receptors has been demonstrated, together with their functional associations with vasoconstrictor or vasodilatory effects of melatonin. The receptors for melatonin have been detected in walls of cerebral and caudal arteries of rats (Capsoni et al., 1994; Visvanathan et al., 1990; Masana et al., 2002), in myoblasts, and coronary arteries of chick (Pang et al., 2002), as well as in walls of cerebral arteries of subhuman primates (Stankow et al., 1993). The expression of the MT_1 receptor in human coronary arteries, derived from healthy heart donors, has been described (Ekmekcioglu et al., 2001). It has been suggested that MT_2 melatonin receptors, expressed in vascular smooth muscles, mediate vasodilation, in contrast to vascular MT_1 receptors mediating vasoconstriction (Masana et al., 2002). Direct actions of melatonin on blood vessels have also been reported (Satake et al., 1991; Weekley, 1993).

Ageing and gonadal steroids influence the expression of vascular melatonin receptors in animals (Vanecek et al., 1990; Seltzer et al., 1992). Doolen et al. (1999) attempted to determine whether estrogenoestrogen modulates the function of vascular melatonin receptors. They reported that estradiol enhanced MT_2 melatonin receptor function in the thermoregulatory caudal artery of female rat, resulting in an increased vasodilatation in response to melatonin. In that experimental model, as mention above, MT_1 receptors mediated melatonin-induced vasoconstriction, while MT_2 receptors mediated melatonin-induced vasodilatation (Dooden et al., 1998).

Melatonin Levels in Heart Diseases

A decrease in nocturnal serum melatonin levels has been observed in patients with coronary artery disease (Yaprak et al., 2003). Despite large individual variations into each group found in this study, patients with coronary artery disease secreted less melatonin at 02:00 a.m., 04:00 a.m. and 08:00 a.m. when compared to healthy people. Also decreased nocturnal melatonin levels were observed during acute myocardial infarction (Dominquez-Rodriguez et al., 2002). Urinary 6-sulphatoxymelatonin excretion was significantly lower in patients with unstable angina, compared to healthy subjects or patients with stable angina (Girotti et al., 2000). Additionally, the authors observed that the concentrations of 6-sulphatoxymelatonin correlated negatively with the age in healthy subjects, but not in coronary patients. Brugger et al. (1995) have shown that serum melatonin concentrations at night were more than five times lower in patients with coronary heart disease than in those in controls. The authors have suggested that melatonin reduces sympathetic activity, which is higher during the day. This effect is important for humans in order to relax during the night. In the morning, the opposite effect can be observed – melatonin concentrations decrease and the sympathetic activity is regained. The results of Harris et al. (2001) indicate that melatonin is unlikely to drive the previously observed pre-sleep increase in cardiac parasympathetic activity.

As previously mentioned, it has been observed that patients with coronary heart disease have a low melatonin production rate, which correlates with the stage of the disease, e.g., deeper decreases are observed in patients with higher risk of cardiac infarction and/or sudden death. Several studies suggest that some immunological factors can play an important role in the pathogenesis of coronary diseases, such as the reactive C protein or cytokines. By activation of cytokine receptors in the endothelium of cerebral vessels, increased serum cytokine levels augment the synthesis of hypothalamic corticotropin-releasing hormone (CRH) and suppress the activity of the pituitary-adrenal axis (Kakucska et al., 1993; Licino and Li, 1997). The data indicates that increased circulating CRH levels suppress melatonin secretion (Kellner et al., 1997) or 6-sulphatoxymelatonin excretion with urine in humans (Girotti et al., 2000).

Lipid Metabolism

Hypercholesterolemia is one of the most serious problems related to age. It has been shown that chronic melatonin administration decreases serum total cholesterol levels (Aoyama et al., 1988; Chan and Tang, 1995). Hoyos et al. (2000) have shown that melatonin diminishes total cholesterol and LDL-cholesterol levels, while increasing high-density lipoprotein (HDL)-cholesterol in diet-induced hypercholesterolemia in rats. The results of that study confirm that melatonin participates in the regulation of cholesterol metabolism and in the prevention of oxidative damage to membranes. Pita et al. (2002) have shown that oral melatonin administration modifies fatty acid composition of rat plasma and liver lipids in rats fed with high-cholesterol diet for 3 months. In this long-term experiment, the analysis of lipid fractions revealed that only cholesterol ester fraction was affected by melatonin.

Additionally, they found that melatonin reduced arterial fatty infiltration, induced by cholesterol feeding. Although the authors suggest that these effects may partially be related to antioxidative properties of melatonin, a possible modulation of the activity of some hepatic enzymes can be suggested (e.g., delta-9desaturase, lecithin-cholesterol acyltransferase).

Also, other authors have shown that melatonin can inhibit LDL oxidation (Pieri et al., 1996; Kelly and Loo, 1997; Bonnefort-Rousselot et al., 2002). Furthermore, Seegar et al. (1997) have demonstrated that, although melatonin itself appears to have little anti-atherogenic activity during LDL oxidation, melatonin precursors and breakdown products inhibit LDL oxidation, as compared to vitamin E. In contrast, Abyja et al. (1997) have reported that melatonin cannot prevent LDL lipid peroxidation. Wakatsuki et al. (2000) found that melatonin treatment reduced LDL susceptibility to oxidative modification in normolipidemic post-menopausal women. Thus, the oxidised form of LDL-cholesterol (ox-LDL) plays a principal role in the development of atherosclerosis. The findings of Okatani et al. (2000) suggest that ox-LDL potentiates the vascular tension in human umbilical artery, probably by suppressing the endothelial synthesis of nitric oxide (NO). In that experiment, melatonin significantly suppressed the vasospastic effect of ox-LDL, possibly because it generally scavenges that hydroxyl radical induced by this lipid fraction.

People with high levels of low-density lipoprotein (LDL)-cholesterol have low levels of melatonin. It has been shown that melatonin suppresses the formation of cholesterol by 38% and reduces LDL accumulation by 42% in freshly isolated human mononuclear leukocytes (Muller-Wieland et al., 1994). Cohen (1995) observed a 10%-20% reduction cholesterol in women, using the B-oval pill. It is a very significant fact in context of the Angier's suggestion (1995), that even 10%-15% depletion in blood cholesterol results in a 20% to 30% reduction of the risk of coronary heart disease. On the other hand, no changes have been shown in total cholesterol, HDL-cholesterol, and triglycerydestriglycerides concentration after 6 months of melatonin administration in insomniac patients (Siegrist et al., 2001) and in women in age 64-80 (Pawlikowski et al., 2002).

Hypertension

The administration of melatonin reduces blood pressure in normal (Chuang et al., 1993), pinealectomized (Holmes and Sugden, 1976), and spontaneously hypertensive rats (Kawashima et al., 1987), whereas hypertension is induced by pinealectomy in rats (Karppanen et al., 1973; Holmes and Sugden, 1976). Laflamme et al. (1998) have suggested that melatonin may act as the main antihypertensive agent by stimulating the central inhibitory adrenergic pathways, thereby diminishing the basal tone of the peripheral sympathetic nervous system. The hypotensive action of melatonin appears to be, at least partly, associated with the inhibition of basal sympathoadrenal tone and, finally, it could be mediated by blocking the postsynaptic α_1-adrenergic receptor-induced inositol phosphate formation. On the other hand, the hypotensive effect of melatonin in rats is not mediated neither by melatonin receptors nor α-adrenoreceptors (Wu et al., 1998). The antioxidative effect of melatonin may be important in hypertensive rats, which either demonstrate a lower content of endogenous antioxidants or a greater sensitivity to free radicals of the vascular tissue.

One of the mechanisms that might be responsible for hypertension-induced myocardial dysfunction in an increase of oxidative stress observed both in humans (Higashi et al., 2002) and animals (De Nigris et al., 2001). It has been shown that long-term antioxidant intervention e.g. vitamin E or C) improves myocardial microvascular function in experimental hypertension (Rodriguez-Porcel et al., 2004). Melatonin's antihypertensive effects may be due to reduction of oxidative stress, decrease of NF-κβ activation and depletion of intestinal renal inflammation (Nava et al., 2003).

People with hypertension demonstrate lower melatonin levels than those with normal blood pressure. The administration of the melatonin declines blood pressure to the normal range. It has been shown that exogenous melatonin taken at bedtime reduces blood pressure of both normo- (Cagnacci et al., 1997;1998; Arangino et al., 1999; Lusardi et al., 1997) and hypertensive persons (Birau et al., 1981). Additionally, melatonin influences the resistance of large arteries to blood flow in both men (Arangino et al., 1999) and young women (Cagnacci et al., 1998).

Cagnacci et al. (1998) examined the influence of melatonin administration in a dose of 1 mg on the circulation of young, healthy women. They found that melatonin greatly influences artery blood flow, decreases blood pressure, and blunts noradrenergic activation. Likewise, Arangino et al. (1999) observed that melatonin, in a dose 1 mg, reduces blood pressure and decreases catecholamine level after 90 min in human subjects. A decrease of even 5mm to 10 mm Hg in blood pressure plays a very important role. Rich-Edwards et al. (1995) suggested that, in hypertensive subjects, a similar decrease in diastolic blood pressure is associated with a 20% reduction of cardiovascular mortality. Arangino et al. (1999) indicated that endogenous melatonin contributes to the nocturnal decrease in blood pressure and of catecholamine levels.

Arterial hypertension is frequently associated with type 1 diabetes. Cavallo et al. (2004a) showed that administration of 5 mg melatonin at bedtime amplifies the nocturnal drop in diastolic blood pressure in normotensive adolescents with type 1 diabetes. In the next paper, the authors suggested that the cardiovascular effect of melatonin is dose-dependent. Higher dose of melatonin (10 mg/day) was more effective in lowering both the systolic and the diastolic blood pressure during sleep (Cavallo et al., 2004b).

The Role on Nitric Oxide

Nitric oxide (NO) was originally identified as a principal endothelium-derived vascular relaxation factor. In 1998, the Nobel Prize in Physiology and Medicine has been awarded for the discovery that NO can be a signalling molecule in the cardiovascular system.

In the meantime, it has been shown that the main pineal hormone - melatonin may influence NO production (Pozo et al., 1994, 1997). Cagnacci et al. (2000) examined the effect of melatonin on the vascular reactivity in postmenopausal women, who were or were not subjected to hormone replacement therapy (HRT). They found that the circulatory response to melatonin is preserved in postmenopausal women on HRT but not in untreated postmenopausal women. In their subsequent paper, Cagnacci et al. (2001) found that melatonin increases nitric oxide (NO) levels only in HRT-treated but not in unnot treated postmenopausal women. These results indicate that melatonin may amplify the reported estrogenoestrogen capacity to increase a nitric oxide synthase (NOS). The authors suggested that, because a normal night-time decline of blood pressure protects women from cardiovascular accidents (Verdecchia et al., 1993), estradiol capability to maintain the circulatory response to melatonin may represent one of the mechanisms mediating the reduction of the cardiovascular risk in postmenopausal women.

Weekley (1991) found that melatonin relaxes the aorta smooth muscle lining in rats. The vascular endothelium may contribute to the regulation of vascular smooth muscle tone by producing such vasoconstrictors as endothelin-1 (Yanagisawa et al., 1988) and tromboxane (Svensson et al., 1977), as well as vasodilators, such as prostacyclin (Weksler et al., 1997) and NO (Fuechgott and Vanhoutte, 1988). Okatani et al. (1997) demonstrated that pre-treatment with a NOS inhibitor (L-N^G-monomethyl arginine), suppressed the potential effect of hydrogen peroxide (H_2O_2) on the vascular tension in umbilical artery segments, suggesting that H_2O_2 may exert its vasospastic effect by inhibiting NOS in the endothelium. Melatonin modulates NOS activity and, therefore, influences NO production (Pozo et al., 1994; 1997). Cuzzocrea et al. (2000) demonstrate that melatonin treatment in a model of shock by splanchnic artery occlusion exerts a protective effect due to inhibition of the expression of adhesion molecule and peroxynitrite-related pathways and subsequent reduction of neutrophil-mediated cellular injury. The results of the study of Wakatsuki et al. (2000) indicate that H_2O_2 may impair NO synthesis in the endothelium of human umbilical arteries. Melatonin significantly suppresses the H_2O_2-induced inhibition effect of NO production, most probably through its ability to scavenge hydroxyl radicals.

Calcium Metabolism

Calcium (Ca^{+2}) plays an important role in physiology of the heart. Melatonin may participate in the regulation of myocardial Ca^{+2} homeostasis. It has been shown that this indoleamine enhances the activity of the membrane calcium pump and regulates calmodulin (Chen et al., 1993; Benitez-King et al., 1996; Anton-Tay et al., 1998). Melatonin may regulate intracellular calcium levels by preventing calcium from overloading. The results of Mei et al. (Mei et al., 2001) suggest a specific melatonin receptor-mediated action on the calcium channel of the chick myocytes. The increase of high-voltage calcium current induced by melatonin may enhance myocyte contractility and cardiac output.

Antioxidative Effect of Melatonin

As mentioned above, the results of many publications suggest an impending decrease in circulating melatonin concentrations at different stages of the coronary disease. The results of epidemiological studies have demonstrated a lower incidence of coronary artery disease and mortality rate in persons who consume larger quantities of antioxidants, like vitamin E, beta-carotene, and vitamin C in their diet (Marchioli, 1999). The antioxidants, including melatonin, can play a beneficial role in reducing the incidence of coronary events. The antioxidative property of melatonin has been demonstrated for more than 12 years (Tan et al., 1993; Reiter et al., 1995; Stasica et al., 1998). Our results have shown protective effect of melatonin against oxidative stress induced by many xenobiotics or carcinogens, e.g.: lipopolysaccharide, hydrogen peroxide, iron, iodide, thyrotoxicosis, potassium bromate, delta-aminolevulinic acid, cadmium and liver ischemia-reperfusion (Karbownik et al., 2001a,b; Karbownik and Reiter, 2002; Karbownik et al., 2005; Sewerynek et al., 1995a,b,c; Sewerynek et al., 1999; Swierczynska-Machura et al., 2004; Wiktorska et al., 2005). Tan et al. (1998) observed that melatonin protected against arrhythmia induced by ischemia-reperfusion in isolated rat hearts. Sahna et al. (2002a,b) suggested that physiological melatonin concentrations are important to reduce the ischemia-reperfusion arrhythmias, myocyte damage and mortality, while pharmacological concentrations of this hormone did not increase its beneficial effect. In the following paper they showed (Sahna et al., 2005) that melatonin administration exerts a mitigating effect on infarct size. As suggested Castagnino et al. (2002) significant cytoprotective effect of melatonin is especially demonstrable in an early phase of myocardial infarction in rats.

One or more brief periods of ischemia, followed reperfusion, increase the tolerance of the heart to subsequent prolonged ischemia. This phenomenon is known as ischemic preconditioning (Murry et al., 1986). Andreadou et al. (2004) in rabbits showed that melatonin did not prevent the beneficial effect of ischemic after two cycles of preconditioning on infarct size despite its antioxidant effect against oxidative stress. Authors suggested that there are some limitations of their findings because the results could be quite different if only one cycle of preconditioning had been used in the presence of melatonin.

The cardioprotective activity of melatonin may be mediated by its antioxidative property and its capacity for neutrophil inhibition in myocardial ischemia-reperfusion (Lee et al., 2002). Melatonin reduces the damage induced by chemical hypoxia and reoxygenation in rat cardiomyocytes (Salie et al., 2001). Melatonin alone or in combination with hGH decreased the injured area after cardiac infarction by 86%-87% and reduced the number of cardiac lesions by 75%-80% (Abyja et al., 1997). Isoproterenol is a β-adrenergic agonist which may produce acute myocardial necrosis in high dosages. Some of the mechanisms explain isoproterenol-induced myocardial injury including hypoxia, calcium overload and excessive production of free radicals resulting from oxidative metabolism of catecholamines (Acikel et al., 2003). It has been examined that melatonin protected against isoproterenol-induced myocardial damage.

Antracycline antibiotics are widely used in antineoplastic treatment of haemopoietic or solid tumours. Cardiotoxicity is one of the most serious side effects of these drugs (Wojtacki et al., 2000). Morishima et al. (1999) reported that melatonin protected against adriamycin (doxorubicin hydrochloride)-induced cardiomyopathy, the pathogenesis of which may involve free radical and lipid peroxidation. In that study, melatonin was shown to affect zinc turnover, which acts as an antioxidant. Similar results were obtained by others; melatonin was an effective antioxidant against cardiotoxicity of myocardium generated by adriamycin (Agapito et al., 2001; Xu et al., 2001a,b; 2002; Dziegiel et al., 2002a). The protective effect of melatonin can partly depend on stimulation of catalase activity in cardiomyocytes subjected to the action of doxorubicin (Dziegiel et al., 2003). Idarubicin is an antracycline antibiotics used in the treatment of acute leukaemia and other malignancies. Amifostine is well-known cell protector and similarly to melatonin involves free radical scavenging. It has been shown that amifostine reduces apoptosis and DNA damage in normal cells (lymphocytes) and cancer cells (leukemic K562 and HeLa cells). Melatonin protected both normal and cancerian cells against genotoxic effect and apoptosis induced by idarubicin. The authors concluded that despite its recognized potential as an antioxidant, melatonin should be administered with caution when it is used in combination with cancer chemiotherapy agents, especially in the case of leukemias (Majsterek et al., 2004). Additionally, it has been examined the cytostatic effectiveness of daunorubicin applied in parallel with melatonin in rats with transplanted Morris hepatoma (Dziegiel et al., 2002b). On one side, melatonin protects cardiomyocytes by decreasing the intensity of daunorubicin-induced apoptosis, but on the other side it weakens the cytostatic activity of this drug, as it was demonstrated by the less frequent necrosis and apoptosis in cells of the transplantable Morris hepatoma.

Melatonin also suppresses the iron-induced lipid peroxidation in many tissues, including the heart (Sewerynek et al., 1995b; Tang et al., 1997; Karbownik et al., 2001b). Arteaga et al. (2000) compared the antioxidative effect of a few antioxidants. They showed that the antioxidant potency of estradiol in vitro was 10-100 times higher than that of α- and γ-tocopherol and melatonin in protection against the oxidation of LDL-cholesterol from postmenopausal women. Benot et al. (1999) suggests that the antioxidative mechanism of melatonin plays a very important role in blood pressure reduction and in the protection against atherosclerosis.

Clinical data concerning the relation between antioxidative effect of melatonin on cardiovascular system in humans is very scarce. Dominguez-Rodriguez et al. (2002) examined serum levels of melatonin and some parameters of oxidative stress (glutathione peroxidase and lipid peroxidation levels) in light/dark period in patients with acute myocardial infarction. They showed that acute myocardial infarction is associated with a nocturnal melatonin deficit in serum and increases oxidative stress. They suggested that melatonin, at least in part, is depleted during night to reduce the free radicals formed in acute myocardial infarction.

An additional problem is connected with cardiac surgery. The number of patients who undergo cardiac surgery especially cardiopulmonary bypass increases every year. The generation of free radical and fluidity of cellular membrane increasing after surgery may induce post-operative complications and mortality in these patients. Together with the fact that melatonin synthesis decreases in patients with coronary artery disease (Sakotnik et al., 1999) become an argument for the use of melatonin for prevention and therapeutic strategy during surgery (Ochoa et al., 2003).

Summing up, melatonin may exert its effect on circulation by: 1) interference with autonomic nervous system; 2) via specific receptors; 3) by a direct effect on the hypothalamus; 4) as an antioxidant; 5) by relaxing aorta smooth muscles.

Concluding up-to-date knowledge about relationship between cardiovascular system and pineal hormone, it may be suggested that especially in old patients with decreased concentrations of melatonin and higher risk of many cardiological diseases, melatonin replacement therapy might to be taken into consideration. The aim of such supplementation with melatonin could be a decrease in the incidence of sudden cardiac deaths during acute myocardial infarction diseases and hypertension.

References

Abyja, PM, Liebmann, P, Hayn, M et al. Antioxidant role of melatonin in lipid peroxidation of human LDL. *FEBS Lett*, 1997, 413, 289-293.

Acikel, M, Buyukokuroglu, ME, Aksoy, H et al. Protective effects of melatonin against myocardial injury induced by isoproterenol in rats. *J. Pineal Res*, 2003, 35, 75-79.

Agapito, MT, Antoli, Y, del Brio, MT et al. Protective effect of melatonin against adriamycin toxicity in the rat. *J. Pineal Res,* 2001, 31, 23-30.

Andreadou, I, Iliodromitis, EK, Mikros, E et al. Melatonin does not prevent the protection of ischemic preconditioning in vivo despite its antioxidant effect against oxidative stress. *Free Rad. Biol. Med*, 2004, 37, 500-510.

Angier, N. Health Benefits from Soy Protein. New York Times. 1995, Aug. 3, p. A1

Anton-Tay, F, Mortiney, R, Tovar, R et al. Modulation of subcellular distribution of calmodulin by melatonin in MDCK cell. *J. Pineal Res*, 1998, 24, 35-42.

Aoyama, H, Mori, N, Mori, W. Effects of melatonin on genetic hypercholesterolemia in rats. *Atherosclerosis*, 1988, 69, 269-272.

Arangino, S, Cagnacci, A, Angiolucci, M et al. Effects of melatonin on vascular reactivity, catecholamine levels, and blood pressure in healthy men. *Am. J. Cardiol*, 1999, 83, 1417-1419.

Arteaga, E, Rojas, A, Villaseca, P et al. The effect of 17β-estradiol and α-tocopherol on the oxidation of LDL cholesterol from postmenopausal women and the minor effect of γ-tocopherol and melatonin. *Menopause,* 2000, 7, 112-116.

Back, G, Strubelt, O. Seasonal variations of cardiac output in rats. *Experientia*, 1975, 15, 1304-1306.

Benitez-King, G, Rios, A, Martinez, A et al. In vitro inhibition of Ca2+/calmodulin-dependent kinase II activity by melatonin. *Biochim Biophys Acta,* 1996, 1290, 191-196.

Benot, S, Goberna, R, Reiter, RJ et al Physiological levels of melatonin contribute to the total antioxidative capacity of human serum. *J. Pineal Res,* 1999, 27, 59-64.

Birau, N, Peterssen, U, Meyer, C et al. Hypotensive effect of melatonin in essential hypertension. *IRSC Med. Sci,* 1981, 9, 906-909.

Bonnefort-Rousselot, D, Cheve, G, Gozzo, A et al. Melatonin related compounds inhibit lipid peroxidation during copper or free radical-induced LDL oxidation. *J. Pineal Res,* 2002, 33, 109-117.

Brugger, P, Marktl, W, Herold, M. Impaired nocturnal secretion of melatonin in coronary heart disease. *Lancet,* 1995, 345, 1408-1412.

Burgess, HJ, Trinder, J, Kim, Y et al. Sleep and circadian influences on cardiac autonomic nervous system activity. *Am. J. Physiol,* 1998, 274, H1761-H1768.

Cagnacci, A, Arangino, S, Angiolucci, M et al. Influence of melatonin administration on the circulation of women. *Am.. J. Physiol,* 1998, 274, R335-R338.

Cagnacci, A, Arangino, S, Angiolucci, M et al. Effect of exogenous melatonin on vascular reactivity and nitric oxide in postmenopausal women: role of hormone replacement therapy. *Clin. Endocrinol,* 2001, 54, 261-266.

Cagnacci, A, Sodani, R, Yen, SSC. Melatonin enhances cortisol levels in aged women: reversible by estrogens. *J. Pineal Res,* 1997, 22, 81-85.

Cagnacci, A, Zanni, AL, Veneri, MG et al. Influence of exogenous melatonin on catecholamine levels of postmenopausal women prior and during oestradiol replacement. *Clin. Endocrinol,* 2000, 53, 367-377.

Capsoni, SM, Viswanathan, M, De Oliveira, AM et al. Characterization of melatonin receptors and signal transduction system in rat arteries forming the circle of Willis. *Endocrinology,* 1994, 135, 373-378.

Castagnino, HE, Lago, N, Centrella, JM et al. Cytoprotection by melatonin and growth hormone in early rat myocardial infarction as revealed by Feulgen DNA staining. *Neuroendocrinol. Lett,* 2002, 23, 391-395.

Cavallo, A, Daniels, SR, Dolan, LM et al. Blood pressure response to melatonin in type 1 diabetes. *Ped. Diabetes,* 2004a, 5, 26-31.

Cavallo, A, Daniels, SR, Dolan, LM et al. Blood pressure-lowering effect of melatonin in type 1 diabetes. *J. Pineal Res,* 2004b, 36, 262-266.

Chan, TY, Tang, PL. Effect of melatonin on the maintenance of cholesterol homeostasis in the rat. *Endocr. Res,* 1995, 21, 681-696.

Chen, LD, Tan, DX, Reiter, RJ et al. In vivo and in vitro effects of the pineal gland and melatonin on $[Ca^{2+} + Mg^{2+}]$-dependent ATPase in cardiac sarcolemna. *J. Pineal Res,* 1993, 14, 178-183.

Chuang, JI, Chen, SS, Lin, MT. Melatonin decreases brain serotonin release, arterial pressure and heart rate in rats. *Pharmacology,* 1993, 47, 91-97.

Coca, A. Circadian rhythm and blood pressure control: physiological and pathophysiological factors. *J. Hypertens Suppl,* 1994, 12, S13-21.

Cohen, M, Josimovich, J, Brzezinski, A. *Melatonin: From Contraception to Breast Cancer Prevention.* Potomac, Maryland: Sheba Press. 1995, p.76

Cuzzoorea, S, Constantino, G, Mazzon, E et al. Beneficial effects of melatonin in a rat model of splanchnic artery occlusion and reperfusion. *J. Pineal Res,* 2000, 28, 52-63.

Dominquez-Rodriguez, A, Abreu-Gonzalez, P, Garcia, MJ et al. Decreased nocturnal melatonin levels during acute myocardial infarction. *J Pineal Res,* 2002, 33, 248-252.

Doolen, S, Krause, DN, Dobocovich, M et al. Melatonin mediates two distinct responses in vascular smooth muscle. *Eur. J. Pharmacol,* 1998, 345, 67-69.

Doolen, S, Krause, DN, Duckles, SP. Estradiol modulates vascular response to melatonin in rat caudal artery. *Am. J. Physiol,* 1999, 276, H1281-H1288.

Dziegiel, P, Jethon, Z, Suder, E et al. M. Role of exogenous melatonin in reducing the cardiotoxic effect of daunorubicin and doxorubicin in the rat. *Exp. Toxicol. Pathol,* 2002a, 53, 433-439.

Dziegiel, P, Murawska-Cialowicz, E, Jethon, Z et al. Melatonin stimulates the activity of protective antioxidative enzymes in myocardial cells of rats in course of doxorubicin intoxication. *J. Pineal Res,* 2003, 35, 183-187.

Dziegiel, P, Surowiak, P, Rabczynski, J et al. Effect of melatonin on cytostatic effects of daunorubicin on myocardium and on transplantable Morris hepatoma in rats. *Pol. J. Pathol,* 2002b, 53, 201-204.

Ekmekcioglu, C, Haslmayer, P, Philipp, C et al. 24h varations in the expression of the mt1 melatonin receptor subtype in coronary arteries derived from patients with coronary heart disease. *J. Recept Signal Transduct Res*, 2001, 21, 85-91.

Fourtillan, JB, Brisson, AM, Gobin, P et al. Bioavailability of melatonin in humans after day-time administration of D(7) melatonin. *Biopharm. Drug Dispos*, 2000, 21, 15-22.

Fuechgott, RF, Vanhoutte, PM. Endothelium-derived relaxing and contracting factors. *FASEB J*, 1988, 3, 2007-2018.

Girotti, L, Lago, M, Ianavsky, O et al. Low urinary 6-sulphatoxymelatonin levels in patients with coronary artery disease. *J. Pineal Res*, 2000, 29, 138-142.

Griefahn, B, Brode, P, Blaszkewicz, M et al. Melatonin production during childhood and adolescence: a longitudinal study on the excretion of urinary 6-hydroxymelatonin sulfate. *J. Pineal Res*, 2003, 34, 26-31.

Harris, AS, Burgess, HJ, Dawson, D. The effect of day-time exogenous melatonin administration on cardiac autonomic activity. *J. Pineal Res,* 2001, 31, 199-205.

Higashi, Y, Sasaki, S, Nakagawa, K et al. Endothelial function and oxidative stress in renovascular hypertension. *N. Engl. J. Med*, 2002, 346, 1954-1962.

Holmes, SW and Sugden, D. The effect of melatonin on pinealectomy-induced hypertension in the rat. *Br. J. Pharmacol,* 1976, 56, 360-361.

Hoyos, M, Guerrero, JM, Perez-Cano, R et al. Serum cholesterol and lipid peroxidation are decreased by melatonin in diet-induced hypercholesterolemic rats. *J. Pineal Res*, 2000, 28, 150-155.

Huikuri, HV, Linnaluoto, MK, Seppanen, T et al. Circadian rhythm of heart rate variability in survivors of cardiac arrest. *Am. J. Cardiol,* 1992, 70, 610-615.

Kakucska, I, Qi, Y, Clark, BD et al. Endotoxin-induced corticotropin-releasing hormone gene expression in the hypothalamic paraventricular nucleus is mediated centrally by interleukin-1. *Endocrinology*, 1993, 133, 815-821.

Karasek, M, Reiter, RJ. Melatonin and aging. *Neuroendocrinol Lett,* 2002, 23(suppl 1), 14-16.

Karbownik, M, Gitto, E, Lewinski, A et al. Induction of lipid peroxidation in hamster organs by the carcinogen cadmium: melioration by melatonin. *Cell Biol. Toxicol*, 2001a, 17, 33-40.

Karbownik, M, Gitto, E, Lewinski, A et al. Relative efficacies of indole antioxidants in reducing autoxidation and iron-induced lipid peroxidation in hamster testes. *J. Cell Biochem,* 2001b, 81, 693-699.

Karbownik, M, Reiter, RJ. Melatonin protects against oxidative stress caused by delta-aminolevulinic acid: implications for cancer reduction. *Cancer Invest,* 2002, 20, 276-286.

Karbownik, M, Stasiak, M, Zasada, K et al. Comparison of potential protective effects of melatonin, indole-3-propionic acid, and propylthiouracil against lipid peroxidation caused by potassium bromate in the thyroid gland. *J. Cell Biochem*, 2005, 95, 131-138.

Karppanen, H, Airaksinen, MM, Sarkimaki, I. Effects in rats of pinealectomy and oxypertine on spontaneous locomotor activity and blood pressure during various light schedules. *Ann. Med. Exp. Biol. Fenn,* 1973, 51, 93-103.

Kawashima, K, Miwa, Y, Fujimoto, K et al. Antihypertensive action of melatonin in the spontaneously hypertensive rat. *Clin. Exp. Theo Pract,* 1987, A9, 1121-1131.

Kellner, M, Yassauridis, A, Manz, B et al. Corticotropin-releasing hormone inhibits melatonin secretion in healthy volunteers - A potential link to low-melatonin syndrome in depression? *Neuroendocrinology,* 1997, 65, 284-290.

Kelly, MR and Loo, G. Melatonin inhibits oxidative modification of human low-density lipoprotein. *J. Pineal Res,* 1997, 22, 203-209.

Kristal-Boneh, E, Froom, P, Harari, G et al. Summer-winter differences in 24h variability of heart rate. *J. Cardiovasc. Risk,* 2000, 7, 141-146.

Kristal-Boneh, E, Harari, G, Green, MS. Seasonal change in 24-hour blood pressure and heart rate is greater among smokers than nonsmokers. *Hypertension,* 1997, 30, 436-441.

Laflamme, KA, Wu, L, Foucart, S et al. Impaired basal sympathetic tone and alpha 1-adrenergic responses in association with the hypotensive effect of melatonin in spontaneously hypertensive rats. *Am. J. Hypertens,* 1998, 11, 219-229.

Lahiri, DK, Ge, Y-W, Sharman, EH et al. Age-related changes in serum melatonin in mice: higher levels of combined melatonin and 6-hydroxymelatonin surfate in the cerebral cortex than in serum, heart, liver and kidney tissues. *J. Pineal Res,* 2004, 36, 217-223.

Lee, Y-M, Chen, H-R, Hsiao, G et al. Protective effects of melatonin on cardial ischemia-reperfusion injury in vivo. *J. Pineal Res,* 2002, 33, 72-80.

Lemmer, B. Circadian rhythms in the cardiovascular system. In: Arendt J, Minors DS, Waterhouse JM, editors. *Biological Rhythms in Clinical Practice,* Boston: Butterworths; 1989. p. 51-70.

Licino, J and Li, W. Pathways and mechanisms for cytokine signaling of the central nervous system. *J. Clin. Invest,* 1997, 100, 2941-2947.

Lusardi, P, Preti, P, Savino, S et al. Effect of bedtime melatonin ingestion on blood pressure of normotensive subjects. *Blood Pressure Monitor,* 1997, 2, 99-103.

Majsterek, I, Gloc, E, Blasiak, J et al. A comparison of the action of amifostine and melatonin on DNA-damaging effects and apoptosis induced by idarubicin in normal and cancer cells. *J. Pineal Res,* 2005, 38, 254-263.

Marchioli, R. Antioxidant vitamins and prevention of cardiovascular disease: laboratory, epidemiological and clinical trial data. *Pharmacol. Res,* 1999, 40, 227-238.

Masana, MI, Doolen, S, Ersahin, C et al. MT_2 melatonin receptors are present and functional in rat caudal artery. *J Pharmacol Exp Ther,* 2002, 302, 1295-1302.

Mei, YA, Lee, PPN, Wie, H. Melatonin and ist analogs potentiate the nifedipine-sensitive high-voltage-activated calcium current in chick embryonic heart cells. *J. Pineal Res,* 2001, 30, 13-21.

Morishima, I, Okumura, K, Matsui, H et al. Zinc accumulation in adriamycin-induced cardiomyopathy in rats: Effects of melatonin, a cardioprotective antioxidant. *J. Pineal Res,* 1999, 26, 204-210.

Muller, JE, Ludmer, PL, Willich, SN et al. Circadian varations in the frequency of sudden cardiac death. *Circulation,* 1987, 75, 131-138.

Muller-Wieland, D, Behnke, B, Koopmann, K et al. Melatonin inhibits LDL receptor activity and cholesterol synthesis in freshly isolated human mononuclear leukocytes. *BBRC*, 1994, 203, 416-421.

Murry, CE, Jennings, RB, Reimer, KA. Preconditioning with ischemia: a delay of lethal cell injury in ischemia myocardium. *Circulation*, 1986, 74, 1124-1136.

Nathan, PJ, Maguire, KP, Burrows, GD et al. The effect of atenolol, a β1-adrenergic antagonist, on nocturnal plasma melatonin secretion: Evidence for a dose-response relationship in humans. *J. Pineal Res,* 1997, 23, 131-135.

Nava, M, Quiroz, Y, Vaziri, N et al. Melatonin reduces renal interstinal inflammation and improves hypertension in spontaneously hypertensive rats. *Am. J. Physiol. Renal. Physiol*, 2003, 284, F447-F454.

De Nigris, F, Lerman, LO, Condorelli, M et al. Oxidation-sensitive transcription factors and molecular mechanisms in the arterial wall. *Antioxid. Redox. Signal,* 2001, 3, 1119-1130.

Nicolau, GY, Haus, E, Popescu, M et al. Circadian, weekly, and seasonal variations in cardiac mortality, blood pressure, and catecholamine excretion. *Chronobiol. Int*, 1991, 8, 149-159.

Nishiyama, K, Yasue, H, Moriyama, Y et al. Acute effects of melatonin administration on cardiovascular autonomic regulation in healthy men. *Am. Heart J,* 2001, 141, E9.

Ochoa, JJ, Vilchez, MJ, Palacios, MA et al. Melatonin protects against lipid peroxidation and membrane rigidity in erythrocytes from patients undergoing cardiopulmonary bypass surgery. *J. Pineal Res*, 2003, 35, 104-108.

Okatani, Y, Wakatsuki, A, Watanabe, K et al. Melatonin inhibits vasospastic action of oxidized low-density lipoprotein in human umbilical arteries. *J. Pineal Res*, 2000, 29, 74-80.

Okatani, Y, Watanabe, K, Sagara, Y. Effect of nitric oxide, prostacyclin, and tromboxane on the vasospastic action of hydrogen peroxide on human umbilical artery. *Acta Obstet Gynecol. Scand*, 1997, 76, 515-520.

Pang, CS, Xi, AC, Brown, GM et al. [125I] Iodomelatonin binding and interaction with B-adrenergic signalling in chick heart/coronary artery physiology. *J. Pineal Res*, 2002, 32, 243-252.

Panza, JA, Epstein, SE, Quyyumi, AA. Circadian variation in vascular tone and ist relation to α-sympathetic vasoconstrictor activity. *N. Engl. J. Med,* 1991, 325, 986-990.

Pawlikowski, M, Kolomecka, M, Wojtczak, A et al. Effects of six months melatonin treatment on sleep quality and serum concentrations of estradiol, cortisol, dehydroepiandrosterone sulfate, and somatostatuin C in erderly women. *Neuroendocrinol. Lett*, 2002, 23, 17-19.

Peckova, M, Fahrenbruch, CE, Cobb, LA et al. Circadian variations in the occurrence of cardiac arrests: initial and repeat episodes. *Circulation*, 1998, 98, 31-39.

Peckowa, M, Fahrenbruch, CE, Cobb, LA et al. Weekly and seasonal variation in the incidence of cardiac arrests. *Am. Heart J*, 1999, 137, 384.

Pieri, C, Marra, M, Gaspar, R et al. Melatonin protects LDL from oxidation but dose not orevent the apolipoprotein derivatization. *Biochem. Biophys. Res. Commun*, 1996, 222, 256-260.

Pita, ML, Hoyos, M, Martin-Lacave, I et al. Long-term melatonin administration increases polyunsaturated fatty acid percentage in plasma lipids of hypercholesterolemic rats. *J. Pineal Res,* 2002, 32, 179-186.

Pozo, D, Reiter, RJ, Calvo, JP et al. Physiological concentrations of melatonin inhibit nitric oxide synthase in rat cerebellum. *Life Sci,* 1994, 55, PL455-PL460.

Pozo, D, Reiter, RJ, Calvo, JR et al. Inhibition of cerebellar nitric oxide synthase and cyclic GMP production by melatonin via complex formation with calmodulin. *J. Cell Biochem,* 1997, 65, 430-442.

Ray, ChA. Melatonin attenuates the sympathetic nerve responses to orthostatic stress in humans. *J. Physiol,* 2003, 551, 1043-1048.

Reiter, RJ. The ageing pineal gland and its physiological consequences. *BioEssays,* 1992, 14, 169-175.

Reiter, RJ, Melchiorri, D, Sewerynek, E et al. A review of the evidence supporting melatonin's role as an antioxidant. *J. Pineal Res,* 1995, 18, 1-11.

Reiter, RJ, Tan, D-X. Melatonin: a novel protective agent against oxidative injury of the ischemic/reperfused heart. *Cardiovascular Res,* 2003, 58, 10-19.

Rich-Edwards, JW, Manson, JE, Hennekens, CH et al. The primary prevention of coronary heart disease in women. *N. Engl. J. Med,* 1995, 332, 1758-1766.

Rodrigez-Porcel, M, Herrman, J, Chade, AR et al. Long-term antioxidant intervention improves myocardial microvascular function in experimental hypertension. *Hypertension,* 2004, 43, 493-498.

Sahna, E, Acet, A, Kaya Ozer, M et al. Myocardial ischemia-reperfusion in rats: reduction of infarct size by either supplemental physiological or pharmacological doses of melatonin. *J. Pineal Res,* 2002a, 33, 234-238.

Sahna, E, Olmez, E, Acet, A. Effects of physiological and pharmacological concentrations of melatonin on ischemia-reperfusion arrhythmias in rats: can the incidence of sudden cardiac death be reduced? *J. Pineal Res,* 2002b, 32, 194-198.

Sahna, E, Parlakpinar, H, Turkoz, Y et al. Protective effects of melatonin on myocardial ischemia-reperfusion induced infarct size and oxidative changes. *Physiol. Res,* 2005, 54, 491-495.

Sakotnik, A, Liebmann, PM, Stoschitzky, K et al. Decreased melatonin synthesis in patients with coronary artery disease. *Eur. Heart J,* 1999, 20, 1314-1317.

Salie, R, Harper, I, Cillie, Ch et al. Melatonin protects against ischaemic-reperfusion myocardial damage. *J. Mol. Cell Cardiol,* 2001, 33, 343-357.

Satake, N, Oe, H, Sawada, T et al. Vasorelaxing action of melatonin in rat isolated aorta: possible endothelium dependent relaxation. *Gen. Pharmacol,* 1991, 22, 1127-1133.

Sayer, JW, Wilkinson, P, Ranjadajalan, K et al. Attenuation or absence of circadian and seasonal rhythms of acute myocardial infarction. *Heart* 1997, 77, 325-329.

Seegar, H, Mueck, AO, Lippert, TH. Effect of melatonin and metabolities on copper-mediated oxidation of low density lipoprotein. *Br. J. Clin. Pharmacol,* 1997, 44, 283-284.

Seltzer, A, Viswanathan, M, Saavedra, JM. Melatonin-binding sites in brain and caudal arteries of the female rat during the estrous cycle and after estrogen administration. *Endocrinology,* 1992, 130, 1896-1902.

Sewerynek, E, Melchiorri, D, Chen, LD et al. Melatonin reduces both basal and bacterial lipopolysaccharide-induced lipid peroxidation in vitro. *Free Rad. Biol. Med*, 1995a, 19, 903-909.

Sewerynek, E, Poeggeler, B, Melchiorri, D et al. H_2O_2-induced lipid peroxidation in rat brain homogenates is greatly reduced by melatonin. *Neurosci Lett*, 1995b, 195, 203-205.

Sewerynek, E, Reiter, RJ, Melchiorri, D et al. Oxidative damage in the liver induced by ischemia-reperfusion: Protection by melatonin. *Hepatogastroenterology*, 1995c, 43, 898-905.

Sewerynek, E, Wiktorska, J, Lewinski, A. Effects of melatonin on the oxidative stress induced by thyrotoxicosis in rats. *Neuroendocrinol. Lett*, 1999, 20, 157-163.

Sewerynek, E. Melatonin and cardiovascular system. *Neuroendocrinol. Lett*, 2002, 23 (suppl 1), 79-83.

Siegrist, C, Benedetti, Orlando A. Lack of changes in serum prolactin, FSH, TSH, and estradiol after melatonin treatment in doses that improve sleep and reduce benzodoazepine consumption in sleep-disturbed, middle-aged, and erderly patients. *J. Pineal Res*, 2001, 30, 34-42.

Stankow, B, Fraschini, F. High Affinity melatonin binding sites in the vertebral brain. *Neuroendocrinol. Lett*, 1993, 15, 149-164.

Stasica, P, Ulanski, P, Rosiak, JM. Melatonin as a hydroxyl radical scavenger. *J. Pineal Res*, 1998, 25, 65-66.

Stoschitzky, K, Sakotnik, A, Lercher, P et al. Influence of beta-blockers on melatonin release. *Eur. J. Clin. Pharmacol*, 1999, 55, 111-115.

Swierczynska-Machura, D, Lewinski, A, Sewerynek, E. Melatonin effects on Schiff's base levels induced by iodide administration in rats. *Neuroendocrinol. Lett*, 2004, 25, 70-74.

Svensson, J, Strandberg, K, Tuvemo, T et al. Thromboxane A2: Effects of airway and vascular smooth muscle. *Prostaglandins*, 1977, 74, 425-236.

Tan, DX, Chen, LD, Poeggeler, B et al. Melatonin, A potent, endogenous hydroxyl radical scavenger. *Endocrine Reg*, 1993, 1, 57-60.

Tan, DX, Manchester, LC, Reiter, RJ et al. Ischemia/reperfusion-induced arrhythmias in the isolated rat heart: Prevention by melatonin. *J. Pineal Res*, 1998, 25, 184-191.

Tang, PL, Xu, MF, Qian, ZM. Different behaviour of cell membranes towards iron-induced oxidative damage and the effects of melatonin. *Biol. Signals*, 1997, 6, 291-300.

Tarquini, B, Tarquini, R, Perfetto, F et al. Chronobiology in epidemiology and preventive medicine. *Ann. Ist Super Sanita*, 1993, 29, 559-67.

Vanecek, J, Kosar, E, Vorlicek, J. Daily changes in melatonin binding sites and the effect of castration. *Mol. Cell Endocrinol*, 1990, 73, 161-170.

Verdecchia, P, Schillaci, G, Gatteschi, C et al. Blunted nocturnal fall in blood pressure in hypertensive women with future cardiovascular morbid events. *Circulation*, 1993, 88, 986-992.

Visvanathan, M, Hissa, R, George, JC. Suppression of sympathetic nervous system by short photoperiod and melatonin in the Syrian hamster. *Life Sci*, 1986, 38, 73-79.

Visvanathan, M, Laitinen, JT, Saaveda, JM. Expression of melatonin receptors in arteries involved in thermoregulation. *Proc. Natl. Acad. Sci. USA*, 1990, 87, 6200-6203.

Wakatsuki, A, Okatani, Y, Ikenoue, N et al. Melatonin inhibits oxidative modification of low-density lipoprotein particles in normolipidemic post-menopausal women. *J. Pineal Res*, 2000, 28, 136-142.

Wakatsuki, A, Okatani, Y. Melatonin protects against the free radical-induced impairment of nitric oxide production in the human umbilical artery. *J. Pineal Res*, 2000, 28, 172-178.

Weekley, LB. Melatonin-induced relaxation of rat aorta: Interaction with adrenergic agonists. *J. Pineal Res*, 1991,11, 28-34.

Weekley, LB. Effects of melatonin on isolated pulmonary artery and vein: role of vascular endothelium. *Pulm Pharmacol*, 1993, 6, 149-154.

Weksler, B, Marcus, A, Jaffe, E. Synthesis of prostaglandin I2 (prostacyclin) by cultured human and bovine endothelial cells. *Proc. Natl. Acad. Sci. USA,* 1997, 74, 3922-3926.

Wenting, DJ, Meiracker, VD, Simoons, AH et al. Circadian variation of heart rate but not of blood pressure after heart transplantation. *Transplant Proc*, 1987, 19, 2554-2555.

Wiktorska, JA, Lewinski, A, Sewerynek, E. Effects of different antioxidants on lipid peroxidation in brain homogenates induced by thyrotoxicosis in rats. *Neuroendocrinol. Lett*, 2005, 26, 269-274.

Wojtacki, J, Lewicka-Nowak, E, Leśniewski-Kmak, K. Anthracycline-induced cardiotoxicity: clinical course, risk factors, pathogenesis, detection and prevention – review of the literature. *Med. Sci. Monitor,* 2000, 6, 411-420.

Wu, L, Wang, R, de Champlain, J. Enhanced inhibition by melatonin of α-adrenoceptor-induced aortic contraction and inositol phosphate production in vascular smooth muscle cells from spontaneously hypertensive rats. *J. Hypertens,* 1998, 16, 339-347.

Xu, M, Ashraf, M. Melatonin protection against lethal myocyte injury induced by doxorubicin as reflected by effects on mitochondrial membrane potential. *J. Mol. Cell Cardiol,* 2002, 34, 75-79.

Xu, MF, Ho, S, Qian, ZM et al. Melatonin protects against cardiac toxicity of doxorubicin in rat. *J. Pineal Res*, 2001a, 31, 301-307.

Xu, MF, Tang, PL, Qian, ZM et al. Effects by doxorubicin on the myocardium are mediated by oxygen free radicals. *Life Sci,* 2001b, 68, 889-901.

Yanagisawa, M, Kurihara, H, Kimura, S et al. A novel potent vasoconstrictor peptide produced by vascular endothelial cells. *Nature*, 1988, 332, 411-415.

Yaprak, M, Altun, A, Vardar, A et al. Decreased nocturnal synthesis of melatonin in patients with coronary artery disease. *Internat. J. Cardiology*, 2003, 89, 103-107.

In: Handbook of Cardiovascular Research   ISBN 978-1-60741-792-7
Editors: Jorgen Brataas and Viggo Nanstveit   © 2009 Nova Science Publishers, Inc.

Chapter VIII

Plasma Serotonin and Platelet Serotonin Transporter: Molecular and Cellular Aspects in Cardiovascular Research

Fusun Kilic[*]*, *Endrit Ziu and Samuel Freyaldenhoven*

University of Arkansas for Medical Sciences, Little Rock, AR, USA

Abstract

The serotonin transporter (SERT) on the surface membrane of platelets is a primary and saturable mechanism for serotonin uptake from plasma. After the uptake of 5-hydroxytryptamine (5HT) by SERT, 5HT is stored in dense granules that are released following stimulation of platelet and other intravascular events. 5HT is a monoamine neurotransmitter that also functions as a vasoconstrictor during blood vessel injury and as a mitogen during early embryogenesis. Alterations in 5HT levels in the nervous system or blood plasma are associated with a number of neuropsychiatric disorders and cardiovascular disease.

The 5HT uptake capacity of platelets depends on the number of SERT molecules on the plasma membrane, which exhibits a biphasic relationship to plasma 5HT concentration. Specifically, the density of SERT molecules on the platelet surface is down-regulated when plasma 5HT is elevated, *in vitro* or *in vivo,* to a level that was observed during hypertension. Thus, high 5HT at high levels appears to limit its own uptake into platelets by down-regulating SERT, and results in a "platelet to plasma shift" in 5HT distribution.

In exploring the factors involved in the intracellular movement of SERT, we focused on the associations between platelet SERT, Rab4, and vimentin. Mechanistically, our studies investigate the link between elevated plasma 5HT and the intracellular tethering

---

[*]Address correspondence to: kilicfusun@uams.edu, Department of Biochemistry and Molecular Biology, College of Medicine, University of Arkansas for Medical Sciences, 4301 West Markham Street, #516, Little Rock, AR 72205

of SERT by Rab4, and the 5HT-mediated phosphorylation of vimentin that arrests SERT recycling on a paralyzed vimentin network. These novel findings support the hypothesis that high plasma 5HT leads to abnormalities in the platelet trafficking of SERT, which reduces the density of SERT molecules on the plasma membrane to deplete 5HT content.

Overall, we provide the first detailed information on the 5HT-mediated biochemical pathways that regulate the number of functional SERT molecules on the platelet surface. The importance of understanding the structure, function, and regulation of SERT is underscored by the observations that plasma 5HT may be elevated in the plasma, either locally or globally, during atherosclerosis, hypertension, stroke, and other cardiovascular diseases.

5HT in Plasma and Platelet

Platelets store and secrete 5-Hydroxytryptamine (5HT), also known as serotonin, which is an intermediate product of tryptophan metabolism. 5HT is primarily located in the enterochromaffin cells of the intestine, serotonergic neurons of the brain, and platelets of the blood. 5HT is well established as a neurotransmitter in the central nervous system (1-3), but it also plays diverse roles in cardiovascular function. The involvement of elevated plasma 5HT in cardiovascular diseases including coronary artery diseases, atherothrombosis, cerebrovascular ischemia, and myocardial infarction has been implicated (4-7). The plasma 5HT level is important, and it should be kept at a steady level. However, once elevated, plasma 5HT must be taken up by platelets in order to bring it back to the physiological level.

Serotonin transporter (SERT), on the plasma membrane of platelet, is responsible for the accumulation of 5HT by peripheral cells (Fig. 1) (8). After 5HT is taken up by SERT into the cytoplasm of platelet, it is either sequestered in the dense granules by vesicular monoamine transporters (VMAT) or degraded by monoamine oxidase. Although, there is always some unbound, free 5HT in the platelet cytoplasm and dense granules, cardiovascular diseases have been linked to elevated plasma 5HT levels (9-16).

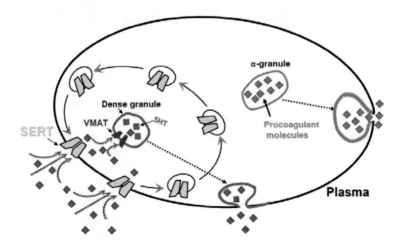

Figure 1. A schematic diagram of platelet organelles and SERT. After uptake, 5HT is stored in dense granules which can be recycled to the plasma membrane. Additionally, platelets contain α-granules that store procoagulant molecules.

Knock-out of the SERT gene in rat (17) and mouse (18) models has helped to elucidate the relationship between platelet SERT expression, circulating 5HT levels in plasma, and the contribution of these influences to platelet physiology. For example, these studies demonstrated that platelets were almost completely depleted of 5HT in *SERT* knockout (-/-) rodent models. These findings confirmed the role of platelet SERT in clearing plasma 5HT.

The source of the initial elevation in plasma 5HT levels remains controversial but may originate from an increase rate of 5HT synthesis or secretion from the enterochromaffin cells of the intestine due to the initial stage of a disease. Studies in the platelets of mice lacking the gene for tryptophan hydroxylase (TPH), which is the rate-limiting enzyme in the synthesis of 5HT in peripheral cells, demonstrated a requirement for intracellular 5HT together with Ca^{2+} for the release of granules during platelet activation (19, 20). These studies in isolated platelets indicated that 5HT-stimulation accelerated the exocytosis of granules, which secrete their contents, 5HT, ADP, and procoagulant molecules, such as fibrinolytic regulators, growth factors, chemokines, immunologic modulators, P-selectin, von Willebrand factor, thrombospondin, fibrinogen, and fibronectin (19, 20). Therefore, these data demonstrate that the rate of exocytosis of platelet granules and the 5HT uptake rates of platelets are manipulated with the plasma 5HT in a concentration-dependent manner. Motivated by these findings, we started our investigation on the type of relationship between plasma 5HT and the platelet SERT (21).

To correlate hypertension and the impact of plasma 5HT on platelet SERT, we obtained blood samples from 25 adult men between the ages of 45 and 50 years presenting to the emergency department with high blood pressure only due to leading trauma or stress (episodic hypertension). The blood samples were collected from these subjects during the episode and after the hypertension had subsided. Through this study, we had access to samples that provided superb "treated" and "control" samples that were unaffected by ongoing treatment that might confound study outcomes. We compared the biochemical and biogenesis characteristics of platelet SERT during hypertension and after hypertension subsided (21).

The major difference between hypertensive and normotensive plasma was the 5HT concentration. While the 5HT concentration of hypertensive plasma was as high as 2 nM, it decreased to 0.7-1.0 nM after hypertension subsided. We then compared the 5HT uptake rates of hypertensive and normotensive platelets. 5HT uptake rates of hypertensive platelets were lower than the normotensive ones due to a decrease in V_{max} with a similar K_m; also, the decrease in V_{max} was primarily due to a decrease in the density of SERT on the platelet membrane, with no change in whole cell expression. Additionally, while the platelet 5HT content decreased 33%, the plasma 5HT content increased 33%.

Furthermore, we tested these *in vivo* findings on isolated platelets following 5HT pretreatment. Our *in vitro* studies agreed with the *in vivo* data by showing the level of SERT proteins on the plasma membrane and the 5HT uptake rates of platelets initially rise as plasma 5HT levels are increased, but then fall below normal as the plasma 5HT level continues to rise (21). These findings clearly indicated a biphasic relationship between plasma 5HT-level and the platelet SERT density on the plasma membrane, more specifically, down-regulation of platelet SERT in the presence of high level of 5HT in plasma. Therefore, we hypothesized that in a hypertensive state, the elevated plasma 5HT levels induces a loss in

5HT uptake function in platelets via a decrease in the density of SERT molecules on the plasma membrane. Through the feedback effect of this proposed mechanism, plasma 5HT controls its own concentration levels by modulating the uptake properties of platelet SERT (Fig. 2).

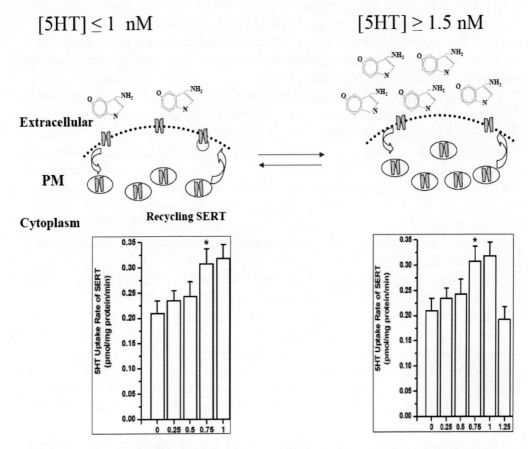

Figure 2. Model for 5HT-dependent plasma membrane density of platelet SERT. Based on our earlier studies, we propose that the density of SERT molecules on the plasma membrane, which defines the 5HT uptake rate of platelets, exhibits a biphasic relationship to plasma 5HT concentration. An initial increase in the plasma 5HT concentration (≤ 1 nM) up-regulates platelet SERT. However, further increase in plasma 5HT concentration (≥ 1 nM, as found in the plasma samples of hypertensive subjects) down-regulates platelet SERT. Indeed, our in vivo and in vitro studies confirm a dynamic relationship between extracellular 5HT elevation, loss of surface SERT, and depletion of platelet 5HT.

While the regulatory roles of substrates and inhibitors on their transporters are well established, the mechanism by which 5HT regulates SERT, specifically in platelet, has remained elusive. The substrates of the γ-aminobutyric acid transporter (GAT) (22, 23), DAT (24), and the excitatory amino acid transporter (EAAT1) have been shown to up-regulate the expression of the transporter on the cell membrane, i.e., glutamate increases the surface expression of EAAT1 (25). SERT is an important target for many therapeutic agents that enhance serotonergic signaling (e.g., for treatment of affective neuropsychiatric disorders) and is involved in the mechanism of some drugs of abuse [e.g., cocaine and MDMA (ectasy)]

(26, 27). These compounds affect recycling and internalization and thereby the density of SERT on the plasma membrane (28).

Activation of protein kinase C (PKC) decreases the number of SERT molecules on the plasma membrane; however, this effect of PKC is blocked in the presence of 5HT at high levels (28). Importantly, Whitworth *et al.*, (2003) demonstrated that 5HT-mediated signals have a role in regulating the number of transporters at or near the synapse by changing the subcellular redistribution of SERT in neurons and glia (29). These studies confirm that the functional efficiency of SERT is regulated by its membrane trafficking pathways, i.e., internalization and recycling of the transporter (30-32).

In order to evaluate our findings with the down-regulation of platelet SERT in the presence of high level plasma 5HT, we first studied the known impacts of plasma 5HT on platelet biology. Our literature search brought two independent pathways which are altered in plasma 5HT-dependent manner: Rab4 and vimentin.

Plasma 5HT and Platelet Rab4

In platelets, plasma 5HT at high levels appears to be closely related to regulated exocytosis in which Rho and Rab4 are implicated (20, 33, 34). The Rab protein family of Ras-related small GTP-binding proteins (GTPase) regulates vesicular traffic (20, 33, 35). There are more than 60 Rab protein family members in mammalian cells, and individual Rab proteins are localized to the cytoplasmic leaflet of distinct compartments in both the endocytotic and exocytotic pathways (36). These proteins, with a molecular mass between 20 kDa and 30 kDa, are highly homologous to the yeast YPT1 and SEC4 proteins, which play a crucial role in endocytosis and exocytosis. Rab4 is associated with early endosomes and regulates membrane recycling (36-38). Rab4 also regulates exocytic events from other post-Golgi compartments in cells with specialized functions (36). In adipocytes, Rab4 controls recycling of the insulin-regulated glucose transporter GLUT4 (39), and recombinant Rab4 stimulates α–granule secretion in platelets *in vitro* (19). All Rab proteins contain highly conserved domains required for guanine nucleotide binding, GTP/GDP exchange, and GTP hydrolysis that are essential for their proper targeting and function (34).

Importantly with regard to our studies, elevations of 5HT in the blood plasma activate Rab4 in platelets via modification of 5HT, which is known as serotonylation or transamidation (Fig. 3A-D) (20). Platelets contain high levels of transglutaminase (TGase) that catalyze the transamidation reaction between 5HT and small GTP-binding proteins, including Rab4 (19, 20). In response to elevation in plasma 5HT, the platelet phosphatidylinositol pathway is activated, resulting in increased intracellular Ca^{2+}. The subsequent activation of Ca^{2+}-dependent TGase covalently modifies Rab4 at its phosphate binding domain with intracellular, free 5HT (20, 40). Bacterial TGase transamidates the Gln residue of the DTAGQE sequence within the GTP hydrolysis domain of Rho which produces constitutively active Rho (40). The DTAGQE signature is conserved in all Rab proteins. However, it has not been established whether the Rab4 effector network involved in actin-myosin dynamics and membrane trafficking is regulated through the transamidation to a constitutively active form of Rab4 (20).

Plasma 5HT and Platelet Vimentin

Studies of axon growth cones and wound healing have demonstrated that signals created by 5HT result in rearrangements of the myosin-actin cytoskeleton and other actin-binding protein bundles (41-43). In addition to the actin cytoskeleton, the intermediate filament network also regulates the trafficking of proteins between cytoplasmic compartments and surface membrane (41-43).

Vimentin is the major structural component of the intermediate filaments in cells of mesenchymal origin including platelets (44). In muscle cells, it was shown that 5HT-stimulation activates p21 activating kinase (PAK), which in turn phosphorylates vimentin on the serine residue at position 56 (Fig. 3E-G) (45). Following phosphorylation, the curved filamentous structure of vimentin undergoes reorganization and straightens (46).

In exploring the communication between plasma 5HT and platelet SERT, we studied whether SERT associates with vimentin and Rab4 during translocation from/to plasma membrane, and whether these associations are impaired in a plasma 5HT-dependent manner.

SERT

SERT is a member of a larger family of Na^+- dependent transporters in prokaryotes and animals, which is designated the SLC6 or NSS family. The biogenic amine transporter family, which also includes the dopamine transporter (DAT) and the norepinephrine transporter (NET), shares about 60% amino acid identity overall (47-50). Hydropathy analysis predicts that SERT contains 12 transmembrane domains and that both the amino (N) and carboxyl (C) terminus are exposed to the cytoplasm.

The termini domains of monoamine transporter proteins have garnered significant attention for their importance in transport function and localization. Significant work has been accomplished in identifying the importance of the C-terminal region of DAT and NET in transporter function, expression, and localization (51-54). Syntaxin 1A (55, 56) and secretory carrier membrane protein 2 (57) interacts with the N-terminus of SERT. Hic-5 (58) and α-synuclein (59) are identified in a complex with SERT. Several proteins have been identified in association with the C-terminus of SERT such as PICK1 (60-62), the actin cytoskeleton (63), neuronal nitric oxide synthase, Sec23A, Sec24C (60), and fibrinogen, an activator of integrin αIIbβ3 (64).

Additionally, the interaction with MacMARCKS has been shown to modulate 5HT uptake, endocytosis, and phosphorylation of SERT via activating protein kinase C (PKC) (65). Studies have also shown that PKC-dependent modulation of SERT is correlated with extracellular 5HT levels (58, 66). More specifically, it has been suggested that the final 20 amino acids of the C-terminal of SERT are critical for the functional expression of the transporter (67, 68). While the protein-protein interactions plays a significant role in the processing of the newly biosynthesized proteins to their final destiny, their post-translational glycosyl modification are important in that processing as well (69), but in platelet this is at a negligible level.

Like the other membrane proteins, SERT is packed in a secretory vesicle and enters into the membrane trafficking pathway. Depending on the plasma 5HT level, once the platelets are separated from megakaryocytes, SERT-carrying small vesicles either stay in the cytoplasm or are moved to the plasma membrane of platelet. The number of available transporters on the plasma membrane defines the 5HT uptake capacity of platelets. Upon clearance of 5HT from the extracellular matrix into the cytoplasm of the cell, SERT moves from plasma membrane and is sequestered in the small vesicle to recycle in cytoplasm. In platelets, the biosynthesis of proteins is minimal and is much lower than the rate of their degradation. Consequently, some of the factors which may play a role in the membrane trafficking of transporter are not there anymore. Therefore, platelet provides an excellent model to study the plasma 5HT level-dependent membrane trafficking of SERT as well as the cellular steps and factors that regulate the translocation of SERT to/from plasma membrane.

While the regulatory roles of substrates and inhibitors on receptors and transporters are accepted, the mechanism by which plasma 5HT alters the recycling dynamic of SERT in the platelet, specifically in a concentration-dependent manner, has remained elusive. Our studies with hypertensive and normotensive blood samples demonstrated that in response to elevation in the plasma 5HT level, the number of SERT molecules on the plasma membrane is down-regulated in platelet. However, the mechanism by which 5HT accomplishes this task remains to be explored.

In general, translocation of proteins from/to the plasma membrane is mediated by their association with other proteins that facilitate their movement between the surface membrane and intracellular compartments. The molecular pathways that alter platelet SERT trafficking in response to elevated plasma 5HT were unknown before our studies (68, 70). In these recently published studies, we explored two independent pathways that control the translocation of SERT from/to platelet plasma membrane and are altered in response to elevated plasma 5HT via activating Rab4 and PAK to phosphorylate vimentin (68, 70).

5HT Transamidates Rab4 and Facilitates its Binding to SERT

The 5HT uptake capacity of SERT is related to the density of transporter molecules on the plasma membrane, which is regulated by membrane trafficking, internalization, and recycling of the transporter (21, 68-70). At physiological levels, the numbers of SERT molecules should be stoichiometrically balanced between the plasma membrane and intracellular pools. The signaling mechanisms regulating the translocation of SERT between the plasma membrane and intracellular locations have not yet been described.

In a recent study we investigated the mechanism by which high concentrations of plasma 5HT alter the redistribution of SERT. Specifically, in 2 nM 5HT stimulated-platelets the 5HT uptake rates and the surface expression of SERT become much lower than the untreated counterparts (21). Using two Rab4 mutants, Rab4Q67L, which is a constitutively active form of Rab4 (71), and Rab4N121I, which is an empty form of Rab4 that cannot bind to nucleotides (72), we demonstrated that Rab4 must be in the active GTP-form to bind to SERT (68). A functional interaction between Rab4 and SERT is implied by the finding that co-expression of SERT and Rab4 resulted in very low 5HT uptake rates and a very low density of SERT on the plasma membrane. Although high level plasma 5HT is not the only factor to activate Rab4 to form Rab4-GTP, in the absence or at low concentrations of plasma 5HT, neither co-immunoprecipitation assays nor immunofluorescence microscopy analysis can determine an interaction between Rab4 and SERT. Therefore, our data strongly suggest that the SERT-Rab4 association occurs following the activation of Rab4 to Rab4-GTP. If Rab4 is not transamidated as in the Rab4N121I mutant, then it cannot associate with SERT. However, Rab4Q67L cannot be transamidated but can associate with SERT regardless of 5HT-concentration (68).

Furthermore, we monitored the cellular distribution of SERT in response to plasma 5HT at low and high concentrations by comparing them with an untreated condition. At elevated plasma 5HT levels, the 5HT uptake rates of cells became low due to a decrease in the density of SERT on the plasma membrane with an accumulation at intracellular locations in association with Rab4. Overall, in this study we clearly demonstrated an association between Rab4-GTP and SERT in a plasma 5HT level-dependent manner. These data give some insight into a possible mechanism through which plasma 5HT is involved in the plasma membrane density of SERT molecules. The role of Rab4 on translocation of intracellular SERT protein to the plasma membrane is further illustrated by locating the SERT-Rab4 association domain on the C-terminus of SERT which is responsible for the regulation of SERT and its effective delivery to the plasma membrane.

Based on our findings, we hypothesize that in the presence of plasma 5HT at high concentration, SERT on the platelet plasma membrane initially takes 5HT into platelets at a high rate. Free 5HT in platelets is transamidated on Rab4, and this leads intracellular SERT to recognize the 5HT bound to the GTP-GDP hydrolysis domain, thus placing Rab4 in an active GTP-form that associates with SERT. This association changes the distribution of transporters between intracellular locations versus those on the plasma membrane and modulates 5HT uptake. This may continue until plasma 5HT levels return to physiological levels where the concentration is no longer sufficient to transamidate Rab4 (68). Based on these findings we propose that plasma 5HT controls its own concentration through down-regulating the number of SERT molecules on the plasma membrane via enabling an association between Rab4 and SERT which retains SERT molecules intracellularly.

SERT uses Vimentin Network in Recycling Process

In the serum of prehypertensive subjects in which the plasma 5HT level was slightly higher than physiological levels, 5HT uptake rates and the density of SERT on the platelet plasma membrane were found to be significantly higher than those on platelets from normotensive states (21). However, in plasma of hypertensive subjects in which 5HT concentration was further elevated, the 5HT uptake rates of SERT was low due to a decrease in the number of the transporters on the platelet plasma membrane (21). We started to identify the mediators playing a role in 5HT-dependent regulation of SERT density on the plasma membrane. Following our report on the role of the C-terminus in the localization and trafficking of SERT via Rab4 a small GTPase in a plasma 5HT-dependent manner, we applied proteomic approaches to identify other platelet proteins interacting with the C-terminus of SERT (70). Our studies revealed vimentin was one of the proteins that bind to the C-terminus of SERT in the cytoplasm and on the plasma membrane of platelet.

It was reported that 5HT-stimulation of cells phosphorylates vimentin on the serine residue at position 56 via PAK (45). Following 5HT-dependent phosphorylation, the curved filamentous structure of vimentin undergoes disassembly and spatial reorganization and straightens (46).

Therefore, we next analyzed the role of plasma 5HT on the vimentin-SERT association in platelets, i.e., whether the disassembly and spatial reorganization of the vimentin network affects the translocation and, in turn, the cellular distribution of SERT molecules. Our data clearly demonstrated that in the presence of elevated plasma 5HT, association of SERT with phosphovimentin reduces the density of SERT on the plasma membrane (Fig. 3E-G).

Therefore, we hypothesize that plasma 5HT–mediated phosphovimentin-SERT association accelerates the internalization of SERT. In parallel, as we discussed above, translocation of SERT to plasma membrane is blocked by serotonylation of Rab4 which reduces the number of SERT on the platelet surface. Thus, the vimentin and Rab4 pathways act in concert to down-regulate SERT on the platelet plasma membrane under conditions in which plasma 5HT is above physiological levels. However, SERT on the platelet plasma membrane would be expected to continue clearing plasma 5HT, albeit at a lower Vmax, until plasma 5HT levels return to physiological levels (Fig. 4G-A).

Conclusion

The findings in these studies showed for the first time that elevated plasma 5HT dynamically interacts with distinct biochemical mechanisms in platelets to attenuate SERT expression on the plasma membrane, resulting in a loss of the primary mechanism for plasma 5HT uptake. Thus, our findings provided the first molecular elucidation of the physiological regulation by 5HT of SERT in platelets. Importantly, our early findings in isolated platelets suggested that their aggregation is enhanced under elevated 5HT conditions. Findings by others in TPH knockout mice strengthen our confidence in our hypothesis. These studies in TPH knockout mice showed that in the absence of 5HT, platelets showed a blunted secretion of granules and a reduced risk of thrombosis. Conversely, the exocytosis of α-granules was accelerated in 5HT-stimulated platelets (19, 20). Importantly, clinical studies also suggested that platelet activation is enhanced in the presence of elevated plasma 5HT levels (73-75).

Considering the role of 5HT in platelet aggregation, a loss of platelet SERT coupled with elevated plasma 5HT may play a significant role in the cluster of cardiovascular diseases including diabetes, metabolic syndrome, atherosclerosis, and peripheral arterial disease, which are thought to reflect a prothrombotic state susceptible to coagulation and thrombotic events. Numerous factors have been identified that confer susceptibility to thrombosis, including a loss of endothelial-derived nitric oxide, vascular smooth muscle cell hypertrophy, hyperinsulinemia and other metabolic abnormalities, obesity, and inflammation (20, 2, 6, 73-75). The development of possible antithrombotic therapies for patients with cardiovascular disease has focused on reducing these risk factors rather than on promoting endogenous mechanisms of anti-thrombosis. In this regard, therapies designed to promote the expression of SERT on the platelet surface may represent a novel approach to alleviating thrombotic events by taking advantage of an endogenous protective mechanism already in place to reduce plasma 5HT.

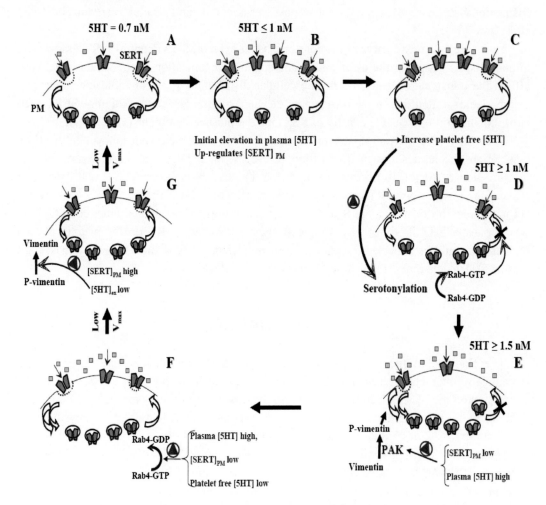

Figure 3. The biphasic effect of plasma 5HT on platelet SERT. Based on our data, we propose that plasma 5HT at a slightly high concentration ($0.7 \geq 5HT \leq 1.0$) causes an elevation in the density of SERT molecules on the plasma membrane (A-B). However, at a very high level as we found during the hypertension status ($1.0 \geq 5HT \leq 1.5$) leads to abnormalities in the platelet trafficking of SERT (C-F), which reduces the density of SERT molecules on the plasma membrane ([SERT]plasma membrane) (D-F). These events appear to promote platelet aggregation (E, F). However, even at the highest levels of plasma 5HT, there are always a number of SERT molecules on the plasma membrane that still continue to clear plasma 5HT, but at a lower rate (Vmax) (F-A), most likely until the plasma 5HT levels return to physiological levels.

Acknowledgements

We thank Ms. Shelly Lensing for critical review of the text. These works were supported by grants from the National Alliance for Research on Schizophrenia and Depression, American Heart Association (0660032) and the NICHD/National Institutes of Health (HD053477) (to F. K.).

References

[1] J. L.R. Rubenstein. Development of Serotonergic Neurons and Their Projections. *Biol Psychiatry* 1998. 44:145–150.

[2] Walther, D.J., and Bader, M. Serotonin synthesis in murine embryonic stem cells. *Molecular Brain Research* 1999. 68: 55–63.

[3] Hendricks, T., Francis, N., Fyodorov, D., and Deneris, ES. "The ETS Domain Factor Pet-1 Is an Early and Precise Marker of Central Serotonin Neurons and Interacts with a Conserved Element in Serotonergic Genes." *The J. of Neuroscience,* 1999. 19(23):10348–10356.

[4] William HS, Jesse AB, Stephen EK. Effect of antidepressants and their relative affinity for the serotonin transporter on the risk of myocardial infarction *Circulation.* 2003. (108):32-36.

[5] Fumeron F., Betoulle D, Nicaud V, Evans A, Kee F, Ruidavets JB, Arveiler D, Luc G, Cambien F. Serotonin transporter gene polymorphism and myocardial infarction. *Circulation* 2002 (105), 2943-2945.

[6] Coto E, Reguero JR, Alvarez V. 5-hydroxytryptamine 5-HT2A receptor and 5-hydroxytryptamine transporter polymorphisms in acute myocarial infarction. *Clin Sci. (Lond.)* 2003. (104), 241-245

[7] Jane RM, Rajender RA, Rebecca KB. Interaction between selective serotonin reuptake inhibitors and nonsteroidal anti-inflammatory drugs: Review of the literature. *Pharmacotherapy* 2006; 26(9): 1307-1313.

[8] Rudnick G. Active transport of 5-hydroxytryptamine by plasma membrane vesicles isolated from human blood platelets *J Biol Chem.* 1977. 252(7):2170-4.

[9] Vikenes K, Farstad M, Nordrehaug JE. Serotonin is associated with coronary artery disease and cardiac events. *Circulation.* 1999. 100(5):483-9.

[10] van den Berg EK, Schmitz JM, Benedict CR, Malloy CR, Willerson JT, Dehmer GJ. Transcardiac serotonin concentration is increased in selected patients with limiting angina and complex coronary lesion morphology. *Circulation.* 1989. 79(1):116-24

[11] Ni W, Watts SW. 5-hydroxytryptamine in the cardiovascular system: focus on the serotonin transporter (SERT). *Clin Exp Pharmacol Physiol.* 2006. 33(7):575-83.

[12] Pietraszek MH, Takada Y, Takada A, Fujita M, Watanabe I, Taminato A, Yoshimi T.Blood serotonergic mechanisms in type 2 (non-insulin-dependent) diabetes mellitus. *Thromb Res.*1992. 66(6):765-74.

[13] Kaumann AJ, Levy FO. 5-hydroxytryptamine receptors in the human cardiovascular system. *Pharmacol Ther.* 2006. 111(3):674-706. Review.

[14] Ban Y, Watanabe T, Miyazaki A, Nakano Y, Tobe T, Idei T, Iguchi T, Ban Y, Katagiri T. Impact of increased plasma serotonin levels and carotid atherosclerosis on vascular dementia. *Atherosclerosis*. 2007. 95(1):153-9.

[15] Nebigil CG, Choi DS, Dierich A, Hickel P, Le Meur M, Messaddeq N, Launay JM, Maroteaux L. Serotonin 2B receptor is required for heart development. *Proc Natl Acad Sci U S A*. 2000. 97(17):9508-13.

[16] Pino R, Cerbai E, Calamai G, Alajmo F, Borgioli A, Braconi L, Cassai M, Montesi GF, Mugelli A. Effect of 5-HT4 receptor stimulation on the pacemaker current I(f) in human isolated atrial myocytes. *Cardiovasc Res*. 1998. 40(3):516-22.

[17] Homberg JH, Mudde JM, Braam B, Ellenbroek B, Cuppen E. Blood pressure in mutant rats lacking the 5-hydroxytryptamine transporter. *Hypertension*. 2006. 48:e115-e116.

[18] Bengel D, Murphy DL, Andrews AM *et al.* Altered brain serotonin homeostasis and locomotor insensitivity to 3,4-methylenedioxymethamphetamine ('ecstasy') in serotonin transporter deficient mice. *Mol.Pharmacol*. 1998. 53: 649–55.

[19] Shirakawa, R., Yoshioka, A., Horiuchi, H., Nishioka, H., Tabuchi, A., and Kita, T. Small GTPase Rab4 regulates Ca^{2+}-induced α-granule secretion in platelets. J. Biol. Chem. 2000. 275:33844–33849.

[20] Walther DJ, Peter JU, Winter S, Holtje M, Paulmann N, Grohmann M, Vowinckel J, Alamo-Bethencourt V, Wilhelm CS, Ahnert-Hilger G, Bader M. Serotonylation of small GTPases is a signal transduction pathway that triggers platelet alpha-granule release. *Cell*. 2003. 26;115(7):851-62.

[21] Brenner, B., Harney, JT., Ahmed, BA., Jeffus, BC., Unal, R., Mehta J.L., and Kilic, F. Plasma serotonin level and the platelet serotonin transporter. *J. Neurochem*. 2007. 102(1):206-216.

[22] Wang D, Quick MW. Trafficking of the plasma membrane gamma-aminobutyric acid transporter GAT1. Size and rates of an acutely recycling pool. *J Biol Chem*. 2005. 13;280 (19):18703-9.

[23] Farhan H, Reiterer V, Korkhov VM, Schmid JA, Freissmuth M, Sitte HH. Concentrative export from the endoplasmic reticulum of the gamma-aminobutyric acid transporter 1 requires binding to SEC24D. *J Biol Chem*. 2007. 282(10):7679-89

[24] Holton KL, Loder MK, Melikian HE. Nonclassical, distinct endocytic signals dictate constitutive and PKC-regulated neurotransmitter transporter internalization. *Nat Neurosci*. 2005. 8(7):881-8.

[25] Duan S, Anderson CM, Stein BA, Swanson RA. Glutamate induces rapid upregulation of astrocyte glutamate transport and cell-surface expression of GLAST. *J Neurosci* 1999. 19:10193–10200.

[26] Kilic F., Murphy D., Rudnick G. A human serotonin transporter mutation causes constitutive activation of transport activity. *Mol. Pharm*. 2003. 64: 4-12.

[27] Murphy DL, Andrews AM, Wichems CH, Li Q, Tohda M, and Greenberg B. Brain serotonin neurotransmission: an overview and update with an emphasis on serotonin subsystem heterogeneity, multiple receptors, interactions with other neurotransmitter systems, and consequent implications for understanding the actions of serotonergic drugs. *J Clin Psychiatry*. 1998. 59 Suppl 15: 4–12.

[28] Ramamoorthy S, Blakely RD. Phosphorylation and sequestration of serotonin transporters differentially modulated by psychostimulants. *Science*. 1999. 285(5428):763-6.

[29] Whitworth TL, Herndon LC, Quick MW. Psychostimulants differentially regulate serotonin transporter expression in thalamocortical neurons. *J Neurosci*. 2003. 22(1):RC192.

[30] Ramamoorthy, S., Baumen, A.L., Moore, K.R., Han, H., Yang-Fen, T., Chang, A.S., Ganapathy, V., Blakely, R.D. Antidepressant- and cocaine-sensitive human serotonin transporter: molecular cloning, expression, and chromosomal localization. *Proc. Natl. Acad. Sci.* U.S.A. 1993. 90: 2542-2546.

[31] Wang X, Baumann MH, Xu H, Morales M, Rothman RB. (+/-)-3,4-Methylenedioxymethamphetamine administration to rats does not decrease levels of the serotonin transporter protein or alter its distribution between endosomes and the plasma membrane. *J Pharmacol Exp Ther*. 2005. 314(3):1002-12.

[32] Muller HK, Wiborg O, Haase J. Subcellular redistribution of the serotonin transporter by secretory carrier membrane protein 2. *J Biol Chem*. 2006. 281(39):28901-9.

[33] Symons M, and Rusk N. Control of vesicular trafficking by Rho GTPases. *Curr Biol*. 2003. 13;13(10):R409-18.

[34] Deneka M, Neeft M, van der Sluijs P. Regulation of membrane transport by rab GTPases. *Crit Rev Biochem Mol Biol*. 2003. 38(2):121-142.

[35] Chavrier P, Parton RG, Hauri HP, Simons K, Zerial M. Localization of low molecular weight GTP binding proteins to exocytic and endocytic compartments. *Cell* 1990. 62:317–329.

[36] Jones MC, Caswell PT, Norman JC. Endocytic recycling pathways: emerging regulators of cell migration. *Curr Opin Cell Biol*. 2006. 18(5):549-57.

[37] Mohrmann K, van der Sluijs P. Regulation of membrane transport through the endocytic pathway by rabGTPases. *Mol Membr Biol*. 1999. 16(1):81-7.

[38] Borner GH, Harbour M, Hester S, Lilley KS, Robinson MS. Comparative proteomics of clathrin-coated vesicles. *J Cell Biol*. 2006. 20;175(4):571-8.

[39] Cormont M, Bortoluzzi MN, Gautier N, Mari M, van Obberghen E, Le Marchand-Brustel Y. Potential role of Rab4 in the regulation of subcellular localization of Glut4 in adipocytes. *Mol Cell Biol*. 1996. 16(12):6879-86.

[40] Aktories K, Barbieri JT. Bacterial cytotoxins: targeting eukaryotic switches. *Nat Rev Microbiol*. 2005. 3(5):397-410.

[41] Zhou, F., and Cohan, CS. Growth Cone Collapse through Coincident Loss of Actin Bundles and Leading Edge Actin without Actin Depolymerization. *J. Cell Biol*. 2001. 153:1071–1083.

[42] Togo, T., and Steinhardt, RA. Nonmuscle Myosin IIA and IIB Have Distinct Functions in the Exocytosis-dependent Process of Cell Membrane Repair. *Molecular Biology of the Cell* 2004. 15:688–695.

[43] Musch, A., Cohen, D., and Rodriguez-Boulan, E. Myosin II is involved in the production of constitutive transport vesicles from the TGN. *J. Cell Biol*. 1997. 138, 291–306.

[44] McNicol A, Israels SJ. Platelet dense granules: structure, function and implications for haemostasis. *Thromb Res.* 1999. 95(1):1-18. Review.

[45] Tang DD, Bai Y, Gunst SJ. Silencing of p21-activated kinase attenuates vimentin phosphorylation on Ser-56 and reorientation of the vimentin network during stimulation of smooth muscle cells by 5-hydroxytryptamine. *Biochem J.* 2005. 388(Pt 3):773-83.

[46] Li QF, Spinelli AM, Wang R, Anfinogenova Y, Singer HA, Tang D.D. Critical role of vimentin phosphorylation at Ser-56 by p21-activated kinase in vimentin cytoskeleton signaling. *J Biol Chem.* 2006. 10;281(45):34716-24.

[47] Blakely, R.D., Ramamoorthy, A., Schroeter, S., Qian, Y., Apparsundaram, S., Galli, A., DeFelice, L.J. Regulated phosphorylation and trafficking of antidepressant-sensitive serotonin transporter proteins. *Biol. Psychiatry.* 1998. 44, 169-78.

[48] Rudnick, G., and Clark, J.From synapse to vesicle: the reuptake and storage of biogenic amine neurotransmitters. *Biochim. Biophys. Acta Rev. Bioenerg.* 1992. 1144:249–263.

[49] Blakely, R.D., Berson, H.E., Fremeau R.T. Jr., Caron, M.G., Peek, M.M., Prince, H.K., Bradley, C.C. Cloning and expression of a functional serotonin transporter from rat brain. Nature. 1991. 354, 66-70.

[50] Hoffman, B.J., Mezey, E., Brownstein, M.J. Cloning of a serotonin transporter affected by antidepressants. *Science.* 1991. 254, 579-80.

[51] Binda, F., Lute, B.J., Dipace, C., Blakely, R.D., Galli, A. The N-terminus of the norepinephrine transporter regulates the magnitude and selectivity of the transporter-associated leak current. *Neuropharmacology* 2006. 50, 354-61.

[52] Bjerggaard, C., Fog, J.U., Hastrup, H., Madsen, K., Loland, C.J., Javitch, J.A., Gether, U. Surface targeting of the dopamine transporter involves discrete epitopes in the distal C terminus but does not require canonical PDZ domain interactions. *J. Neurosci.* 2004. 24, 7024-36.

[53] Distelmaier, F., Wiedemann, P., Bruss, M., Bonisch, H. Functional importance of the C-terminus of the human norepinephrine transporter. *J. Neurochem.* 2004. 91, 537-46.

[54] Bauman, P.A. and Blakely, R.D. Determinants within the C-terminus of the human norepinephrine transporter dictate transporter trafficking, stability, and activity. *Arch. Biochem. Biophys.* 2002. 404, 80-91

[55] Quick MW. Role of syntaxin 1A on serotonin transporter expression in developing thalamocortical neurons. *Int J Dev Neurosci* 2002. 20:219–224.

[56] Quick MW Regulating the conducting states of a mammalian serotonin transporter. *Neuron.* 2003. 40:537–549.

[57] Muller HK, Wiborg O, Haase J Subcellular redistribution of the serotonin transporter by secretory carrier membrane protein 2. *J Biol Chem* 2006. 281:28901–28909.

[58] Carneiro AM, Blakely RD Serotonin-, protein kinase C-, and Hic-5-associated redistribution of the platelet serotonin transporter. *J Biol Chem.* 2006. 281:24769–24780.

[59] Wersinger C, Rusnak M, Sidhu A. Modulation of the trafficking of the human serotonin transporter by human alpha-synuclein. *Eur J Neurosci.* 2006. 24:55–64.

[60] Chanrion B, Mannoury la Cour C, Bertaso F, Lerner-Natoli M, Freissmuth M, Millan MJ, Bockaert J, Marin P. Physical interaction between the serotonin transporter and

neuronal nitric oxide synthase underlies reciprocal modulation of their activity. *Proc Natl Acad Sci U S A.* 2007. 104(19):8119-24.

[61]   Torres GE, Yao WD, Mohn AR, Quan H, Kim KM, Levey AI, Staudinger J, Caron MG. Functional interaction between monoamine plasma membrane transporters and the synaptic PDZ domain-containing protein PICK1. *Neuron.* 2001. 30:121–134.

[62]   Madsen KL, Eriksen J, Milan-Lobo L, Han DS, Niv MY, Ammendrup-Johnsen I, Henriksen U, Bhatia VK, Stamou D, Sitte HH, McMahon HT, Weinstein H, Gether U. Membrane Localization is Critical for Activation of the PICK1 BAR Domain. *Traffic.* 2008. 9(8):1327-43.

[63]   Mochizuki, H., Amano, T., Seki, T., Matsubayashi, H., Mitsuhata, C., Morita, K., Kitayama, S., Dohi, T., Mishima, H.K., Sakai, N. Role of C-terminal region in the functional regulation of rat serotonin transporter (SERT). *Neurochem. Int.* 2005. 46, 93-105.

[64]   Steiner JA, Carneiro AM, Blakely RD. Going with the Flow: Trafficking-Dependent and -Independent Regulation of Serotonin Transport. *Traffic* 2008. 9, 1393-402.

[65]   Jess U, El Far O, Kirsch J, Betz H. Interaction of the C-terminal region of the rat serotonin transporter with MacMARCKS modulates 5-HT uptake regulation by protein kinase C. *Biochem Biophys Res Commun.* 2002. 294, 272–279.

[66]   Qian, Y., Galli, A., Ramamoorthy, S., Risso, S., DeFelice, L. J., and Blakely, R. D. (1997). "Protein kinase C activation regulates human serotonin transporters in HEK-293 cells via altered cell surface expression." *J. Neurosci.* 17, 45–57

[67]   Larsen, M.B., Fjorback, A.W., Wiborg, O. The C-terminus is critical for the functional expression of the human serotonin transporter. *Biochemistry.* 2006. 45, 1331-7.

[68]   Ahmed, BA., Jeffus, BC., Harney, JT., Bukhari, SIA., Unal, R., Lupashin, VV., van der Sluijs, P., Kilic, F. Serotonin transamidates Rab4 and facilitates its binding to the C terminus of serotonin transporter. *J. Biol. Chem.* 2008. 283(14):9388-98.

[69]   Ozaslan, D., Wang, S., Ahmed, B., Bene, A., Kocabas, AM., and Kilic, F. Glycosyl Modification Facilitates Homo- and Hetero-Oligomerization of Serotonin Transporter. A Specific Role for the Sialic Acid Residues. *J. Biol. Chem.* 2003. 278: 43991-44000.

[70]   Ahmed, B., Bukhari, S.I.A.., Harney, J., Jeffus, B., Thyparambil, S., Fraer, M., Rusch, N.J., Zimniak, P., Lupashin, V., Tang, D., and Kilic, F. The translocation of serotonin transporter is impeded on serotonin-altered vimentin network: A mechanism by which serotonin dictates the cellular distribution of serotonin transporter. *PLoS ONE.* 2009. 4(3):e4730

[71]   Gerez L, Mohrmann K, van Raak M, Jongeneelen M, Zhou XZ, Lu KP, van Der Sluijs P. Accumulation of rab4GTP in the cytoplasm and association with the peptidyl-prolyl isomerase pin1 during mitosis. *Mol Biol Cell.* 2000.11(7):2201-11.

[72]   Lazzarino DA. Blier P. Mellman I. The monomeric guanosine triphosphatase rab4 controls an essential step on the pathway of receptor-mediated antigen processing in B cells. *J Exp Med.* 1998. 188(10):1769-74

[73]   Saxena PR, Villalón CM. Cardiovascular effects of serotonin agonists and antagonists. *J Cardiovasc Pharmacol.* 1990. 15 Suppl 7:S17-34. Review.

[74]   Watts SW. 5-HT in systemic hypertension: foe, friend or fantasy? *Clin Sci* (Lond). 2005 108(5):399-412. Review.

[75] Doggrell SA. The role of 5-HT on the cardiovascular and renal systems and the clinical potential of 5-HT modulation. *Expert Opin Investig Drugs.* 2003 May;12(5):805-23. Review.

In: Handbook of Cardiovascular Research
Editors: Jorgen Brataas and Viggo Nanstveit

ISBN 978-1-60741-792-7
© 2009 Nova Science Publishers, Inc.

Chapter IX

Methods for Handling Inter-Hospital Transfer in Acute Myocardial Infarction Research

John M. Westfall *

Department of Family Medicine, University of Colorado at
Denver Anschutz Medical Campus, Denver, CO, USA

Abstract

Context Patients are frequently transferred during their care for acute myocardial infarction. The clinical risks and benefits associated with inter-hospital transfer have not been fully evaluated.

Objective: To compare and contrast the analytic methods used to handle transferred patients in previous acute myocardial infarction research.

Design: Systematic review of acute myocardial infarction literature over the past 10 years.

Main Outcomes: Benefits and risks of various methods used for handling transferred patients in acute myocardial infarction research

Results: Seven major methods for dealing with inter-hospital transfer emerged: 1) Count each hospitalization as a separate event. 2) Delete transferred patients from analysis. 3) Link the data from different hospitals and produce a record of the "episode" of acute myocardial infarction. 4) Analyze data on transferred patients the same as on non-transferred patients. 5) Transfer patients are the specific population of interest. 6) Diagnosis, treatment, outcomes are attributed to the index hospital. 7) Control for transfer in logistic regression modeling. Several studies included a combination of these methods.

Conclussion: Inter-hospital transfer in the care of acute MI is common and increasing. From a clinical standpoint, determining the patient most likely to benefit from inter-hospital transfer will help guide clinicians faced with this difficult decision. From a

---

* Corresponding author: email address: jack.westfall@ucdenver.edu.

health services standpoint it is essential to understand the implications of using a particular method for handling transfer patients, the impact on data collection, the data lost, the appropriate analyses, and the generalizability of findings.

Background

Patients are frequently transferred during their care for acute myocardial infarction. The clinical risks and benefits associated with inter-hospital transfer have not been fully evaluated. Inter-hospital transfer, particularly out of rural regions also has serious implications for clinical care and health services research.[1] There has been a recent rise in medical publications, both clinical trials and editorials on whether inter-hospital transfer or local care is better. [2-6] A thorough understanding of the issues surrounding inter-hospital transfer will lead to a better understanding of its impact on patient outcomes from both a clinical and health services perspective. Numerous studies have analyzed patients with acute myocardial infarction and have dealt with patient transfers in various ways. The purpose of this paper is to review the published methods for handling inter-hospital transfers and discuss the benefits and risks of each method.

Definitions of Transfer

Patients suffering acute MI are frequently transferred into or out of a hospital for further medical care. Published literature on acute MI is the product of research studies; hence, we use the term "study hospital" to define a hospital involved in a research study. A "non-study hospital" is a hospital not involved in that specific research study. Figure 1 provides a graphic description of acute MI patient flow from the point of initial patient presentation through the potential locations for treatment and movement between locations.

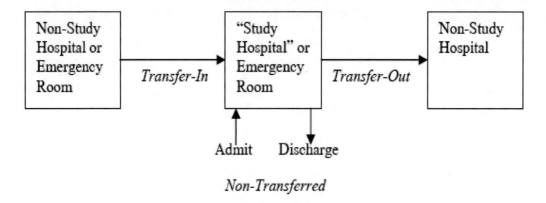

Figure 1. Transfer of Patients Into and Out of a "Study Hospital".

There are four groups of patients related to inter-hospital transfer in acute MI research. 1) *Non-transferred* patients are patients who receive all their care at one acute care hospital; from presentation, through treatment, to discharge. 2) *Transfer-in* patients are patients that are transferred into a study hospital. There is little or no data on the care they received prior to transfer into the study hospital. *Transfer-in* patients can be transferred in from another acute care facility or from an emergency department at another acute care facility. 3) *Transfer-out* patients are patients who are transferred out of a study hospital. *Transfer-out* patients can be initially admitted to the study hospital, receive care, and then transferred to another acute care facility, or can be transferred out directly from the emergency department. Subsequent non-study hospital care, procedures, discharge treatments, and outcomes are often not available for *transfer-out* patients. 4) There is a small group of patients admitted to a hospital, transferred only for a particular treatment (e.g. angiogram, angioplasty), immediately returned, and subsequently discharged from the index hospital.

The unit of analysis is an essential component of any research on acute MI. In acute MI research the unit of analysis may be; 1) the patient, 2) the treating physician, or 3) the hospital. The study objective should determine the unit of analysis. The unit of analysis should then help direct the decision of how to handle transferred patients. For example, if the clinical question is the incidence of acute MI the unit of analysis should be the patient. Choosing the patient as the unit of analysis then requires linking of the multiple hospitalizations to get an accurate incidence rate. If the clinical question is the use of reperfusion for acute MI in community hospitals then the unit of analysis may be the hospital. In this case the essential data is from the index hospital during the first 12 hours after the patient presents. For hospitals without angioplasty capabilities it may also be necessary to collect data on the number of patients transferred specifically for reperfusion with angioplasty or to obtain data from the second hospital. Because treatment for acute MI includes immediate treatment (first 2-6 hours) and later treatment (1-5 days), identifying the most appropriate manner for collecting patient specific data and for handling transferred patients is important for accurate results and conclusions. It may be more difficult to enroll patients from rural and smaller community hospitals into clinical trails due to small numbers and limited availability of research staff and resources.

Methods

We searched Medline using keywords; "acute myocardial infarction" *or* "myocardial ischemia" *and* "rural" *or* "transfer". We limited this set to human, English language and publication from 1995-2004. This provided 326 articles for initial review. We deleted 93 articles that related to *genetic transfer*. Because inter-hospital transfer was not the primary question in the vast majority of these articles, the Medline search did not adequately identify all research on acute MI that analyzed transferred patients. Therefore, we also culled the general literature on care and treatment of acute MI and obtained additional articles by reviewing the bibliography and endnotes of articles on care and treatment of acute MI. Rather than an exhaustive review of acute myocardial infarction, the purpose of this paper is to provide a thorough review of the wide range of methods for dealing with inter-hospital transfer in the published literature. While not including every article on acute MI, our final sample includes the major studies and numerous smaller studies on acute MI that dealt with transferred patients. Our final sample of articles which will be cited individually in the appropriate section includes examples from the Cooperative Cardiovascular Project (CCP), National Registry of Myocardial Infarction (NRMI), Pennsylvania Health Care Cost Containment Council (PH4C), California Health Outcomes Project (CHOP), the State Health Reports for Connecticut, Georgia, Washington, Colorado, the National Center for Health Statistics (NCHS), National Institute of Health Heart Lung and Blood Institute Chart book (NIH/NHLBI), Myocardial Infarct Triage and Intervention project (MITI), the Dartmouth Health Atlas of Medicare patients and numerous other individual studies on acute MI.

Results

Seven major methods for dealing with inter-hospital transfer emerged: 1) Count each hospitalization as a separate event. 2) Delete transferred patients from analysis. 3) Link the data from different hospitals and produce a record of the "episode" of acute myocardial infarction, regardless of how many hospitalizations occurred. 4) Analyze data on transferred patients the same as on non-transferred patients. 5) Transfer patients are the specific population of interest. 6) Diagnosis, treatment, outcomes are attributed to the index hospital. 7) Control for transfer in logistic regression modeling. Table 1 summarizes these methods and gives a brief overview of the benefits and risks for each.

Several other methods were used in individual smaller studies and reflect subtle differences from the major methods listed above. Many authors utilized a combination of methods to handle transferred patients. Figure 2 provides a graphic description of the major analytic methods on a theoretical sample of 200 acute MI patients.

1) *Count each hospitalization as a separate event.* Hospitalization is the unit of analysis in this method. This method provides a rough estimate of the incidence of acute MI and provides an accurate estimate of hospitalization for acute MI and the general utilization of health resources for acute MI. However, no linkage between hospitals is possible. Because each transferred patient accounts for 2 or more hospitalizations for acute MI, the true incidence of acute MI is less than the incidence of hospitalization for acute MI. The rate of inter-hospital transfers has increased rapidly over the last decade resulting in a growing discrepancy between hospitalization rate and incidence rate. [7] The discrepancy is particularly great in rural regions where a higher proportion of patients is transferred out for ongoing care of their acute MI. For studies on treatments and outcomes, counting each hospitalization will underestimate the treatment rates and mortality rates among the transferred patients.

Hospital discharge data does not include data on emergency department visits. Therefore, if a patient is transferred directly from the emergency department of one hospital to a second hospital they do not appear in the hospital discharge data from the first hospital.

Table 1. Benefits and Risks of Various Methods for Dealing with Transfer Patients in Health Services Research

Method for Handling Transferred Patients	Benefits	Risks	Citations of studies using this method
1) Count each hospitalization as a separate event.	• Can use large public administrative databases • Easy assignment of responsibility for treatment and outcomes	• Significantly overestimates incidence • Separates the treatment to 1 patient provided at 2 hospitals	7-16
2) Delete transferred patients from analysis.	• Avoids assignment of responsibility to individual hospital or physician • Allows for analysis when no data on subsequent hospital care available (transfer-out patients)	• Because transferred patients are different than non-transferred patients introduces significant bias into analysis	17-31
3) Link the data from multiple hospitals and produce a record of the "episode" of acute myocardial infarction.	• Provides complete description of all care provided and allows for analysis of the impact of specific treatment on outcome	• Difficult to get all the records from non-study hospitals • Time consuming and more expensive • Unable to assign responsibility to single institution or physician	32-37
4) Analyze data on transferred patients the same as on non-transferred patients.	• Easy to collect data and analyze • Common for individual hospital Quality Improvement projects • Able to compare *early* treatment between institutions and providers	• No mortality outcome data for transfer-out patients unless link to another database • No data on discharge medications, treatments	38, Numerous individual hospital QI reports
5) Transfer patients are the specific population of interest.	• Direct comparison between transfer and non-transfer patients • Able to study the impact of transfer on treatment and outcomes	• Expensive and time consuming to track patients between institutions • Need to plan a priori when designing study • Need to deal with multiple institutions, systems, and physicians	39-43
6) Diagnosis, treatment, outcomes are attributed to the index hospitalization.	• Index hospital gets "credit" for appropriate transfer of patients for specialized care • Recognizes the link between early care and outcomes	• Transfer-in hospitals do not get "credit" for improving the outcome of transferred patients • Assumes there is no intrinsic benefit to transfer	44-45
7) Control for transfer in logistic regression modeling.	• Can analyze retrospective data and secondary databases	• Many not fully account for the large differences between transferred and non-transferred patients	46-49

The National Center for Health Statistics (NCHS) [8], National Institute of Health Heart Lung and Blood Institute Chart book (NIH/NHLBI) [9], Dartmouth Health Atlas [10] of Medicare patients Dartmouth Health Atlas, and the state health reports for Connecticut [11], Georgia [12], Washington [13], Colorado [14] utilize this method and base their published rates for disease and acute myocardial infarction on the number of hospital discharges making no attempt to correct for inter-hospital transfer. Their estimates of acute myocardial infarction incidence are likely inflated by 10-20% and even more so for rural regions. Kostis et al. used this method to determine time trends in "occurrence and outcome" of acute MI in New Jersey between 1986 and 1996. [15] Their estimate on the incidence of acute MI is likely overestimated because the transferred patients were counted twice. Their finding of a decrease in in-hospital mortality is inaccurate because of the increasing number of transferred patients who show up in the denominator for calculations of in-hospital mortality. In contrast, Naylor et al. linked hospitalization using a matching algorithm specifically to obtain an accurate denominator for calculation of case-fatality rates. [16]

2) *Delete transferred patients/data from analysis.* There are four subsets within this major heading; a) delete all transferred patients, b) delete only transfer-in patients, c) delete only transfer-out patients. d) Transfer is an exclusion criterion for "ideal" candidate of therapy. Deleting transferred patients removes those patients from the study. If inter-hospital transfer were a random event, deleting transferred patients would have little impact on the study results. The published findings that transferred patients are more likely to be young, male, and have lower in-hospital mortality means that deleting transferred patients from the analysis introduces a major bias against hospitals with high transfer-out rates. [1,17]

Several CCP [18,19] and NRMI [20,21] publications deleted transferred patients from their analysis. Thiemann et al. reported from the CCP that mortality from acute myocardial infarction was higher in smaller and rural hospitals and in patients cared for by primary care physicians; however, they deleted 25% of their sample due to inter-hospital transfer. [22] Casale's report from the Pennsylvania data also found higher in-hospital mortality in rural hospitals and in patients cared for by primary care physicians. [23] Their study deleted over 9000 patients (23% of the total sample) due to inter-hospital transfer. Using the CCP data, Baldwin et al. reported specifically on rural patients with AMI. [24] They deleted patients transferred-in to the study hospitals. They found that patients transferred out of study hospitals were younger, less ill, and more likely to receive recommended treatments.

A method of patient identification that leads to inadvertent deletion of transfer-out patients is retrospective identification of acute MI patients from admission and discharge data. [25] Patients transferred from an emergency room to another hospital are not included because they do not appear in the transfer-out hospital discharge data. No information on the care provided in the first emergency room is available for analysis.

Deleting only transfer-in patients may be an attractive alternative because it still allows for analysis using large secondary and administrative datasets and decreases the risk of enriching the pool of patients in hospitals with high transfer-in rates. It may be appropriate for studying early treatment of MI. [26,27] However, it also removes them from the transfer-out hospital patient pool, specifically in terms of later hospital care and discharge medications and treatments.

Similarly, deleting transfer-out patients from analysis penalizes hospitals with high transfer-out rates. Krumholz et al. deleted transfer-out patients because they could not determine their ultimate discharge medications. [28] At the time of transfer, many patients are not receiving beta-blockers, ace-inhibitors, and have not undergone revascularization. These transferred patients may receive these treatments at the second hospital, but because they did not receive them in the index hospital prior to discharge, the index hospital appears to have lower rates for these treatments. [29]

Another method under this rubric is to include transferred patients but only include data from the index hospitalization. Transferred patients are identified by the "type of admission" code and hospital data on patients identified as transferred from another acute care facility are not included in analysis. This method is attractive as it allows for analysis of secondary databases and large administrative databases that include no way of linking multiple hospitalizations for a single patient. This method is effective for studying early treatment of acute MI and for studying the indications for inter-hospital transfer. However, because there is no data on subsequent hospitalizations in the transferred patients and no way to link hospitalizations, it is not possible to compare later treatments, discharge medications, and mortality. [30]

Transferred patients may be deleted from the group of "ideal" candidates for specific treatments. [31] This is another mechanism similar to deleting transferred patients. For example, a patient is seen in an ER, diagnosed with ST elevation acute MI, treated with thrombolytics and transferred to an urban hospital. Because they were transferred they are not considered an "ideal" candidate and are excluded from the data analysis. Conversely, if they did not receive lytic therapy even though he/she was a candidate for it, because of transfer the patient is erroneously considered not an "ideal" candidate for therapy. Transferred patients are younger and healthier, thus more likely to be "ideal" candidates for therapy. However, because they are deleted, the transfer-out hospital does not get credit for providing treatment or take responsibility for not providing treatment.

3) *Link the data from multiple hospitals and produce a record of the "episode" of acute myocardial infarction.* This linking should occur prospectively so that a complete record of presentation, treatment, discharge, and outcome is collected. However, for large retrospectively collected data it is possible to link multiple hospitalizations for a single patient using matching algorithms or patient identifiers. The downside of linking hospitalizations is the increased cost and time necessary to create reliable "episodes" for individual patients.

One recent article utilizing CCP data attempted to link patients transferred between two CCP hospitals, but also deleted all patients in whom their first hospitalization was a transfer from a non-CCP hospital. [32] The Connecticut substudy of the CCP linked transfers between hospitals to study the impact of on-site catheterization. [33] They linked data for 3 years and found little difference in cost and mortality between hospitals with and without on-site catheterization.

The CHOP and MITI studies linked hospital transfers to produce a complete continuous record for each episode. [34,35] The MITI also found that transferred patients were younger and had a lower mortality than patients who were not transferred. In contrast, the CHOP found higher rates of adverse outcomes among transferred patients. [36]

Vermeer et al. studied a comparison between thrombolysis and primary PTCA in patients presenting to a hospital without PTCA capabilities. [37] A random sample of patients were transferred to a hospital with PTCA capabilities and then transferred back to the index hospital immediately or within one day. The authors linked the data from the transfer, however, in this case, the transfer was short and for one specific reason, therefore it did not require an enormous amount of extra work. Because transfer simply for a procedure and then transfer back to the index hospital is rare in the United States, it is unlikely that this type of analysis will become common.

4) *Analyze data on transferred patients the same as on non-transferred patients.* This method analyzes all patients the same, whether they were transferred in or out. This is a simple method for an individual hospital to analyze the care it provides and is accurate for hospitals with low transfer-in and transfer-out rates. This method works well for individual hospital quality improvement projects. Patil et al. studied the admissions for AMI to one hospital to better understand their own population of patients. [38] Because there is no subsequent data on transfer-out patients, this method may underestimate the treatments of smoking cessation, aspirin and beta-blockers on discharge. Because transfer-in patients have little data from their index hospital it may underestimate reperfusion strategies such as thrombolytics or early transfer for angioplasty. There is no inter-hospital linkage even for patients transferred between 2 study hospitals so an individual patient may be counted twice.

5) *Transfer patients are the specific population of interest.* [39-41] This analysis studies the transferred patients as a separate group of specific interest. They may be compared to each other and to non-transferred patients. Comparisons between transferred and non-transferred patients should account for the demographic and clinical differences between these groups. Theroux et al. studied the impact of early treatment of acute MI in hospitals with high transfer-out rates. [42] While they reported differences in treatment and outcomes between transferred and non-transferred patients they caution that this comparison had "limited significance" due to the biased selection process inherent in non-randomized assignment of transfer. Madsen et al. conducted a randomized trial of transfer for PTCA with local conservative treatment. [43] They studied only patients with post infarction ischemia after the initial treatment for acute MI but prior to discharge. This randomized, controlled trial found improvement in clinical outcomes for patients undergoing the more invasive treatment.

6) *Subsequent care/procedures are attributed to the index hospitalization.* [44] This method requires linkage of data from multiple hospitalizations. It is attractive because the data from subsequent hospitalizations dealing with procedures, costs, and disposition can be obtained from administrative databases rather than requiring complete data from full chart abstraction from all hospitals involved in the care of the patient. However, this method focuses the unit of analysis on the index hospital and may overestimate the impact of early care. The index hospital gets credit for appropriately transferring patients for specialized care. The index hospital also gets "credit" for the care provided by subsequent hospitals/providers. [45] Hospitals with high transfer-in rates do not get adequate "credit" for the care they provide. Any subtle volume-outcome relationship will be lost because this method assumes that other than the major quality indicators, the care provided in all institutions is roughly equivalent.

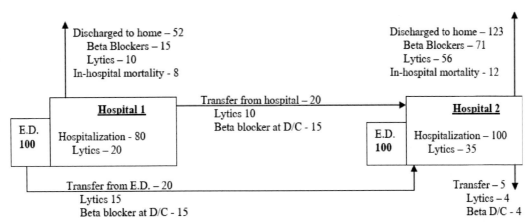

100 patients with acute myocardial infarction present to each hospital emergency department. Hospital 1 is a small community hospital that transfers 20 patients immediately from the emergency department to another hospital and 20 more patients later during their hospitalization. Hospital 2 is a larger urban tertiary care hospital that accepts many transfers and only transfers out occasional patients based on patient preference or insurance requirements. Both hospitals provide identical care to their patients for thrombolytics/reperfusion (35%), beta-blockers at discharge (50%), and both have 10% in-hospital mortality. The assumptions in this model are all based on published reports for treatments and the published findings that transferred patients are younger, have lower expected mortality, are more likely to receive lytic therapy and beta-blockers at discharge, and have lower in-hospital mortality.

Hospital 1 ends up with 52 patients discharged home, 40 patients transferred to hopsital 2 and 8 in-hospital deaths. Hospital 2 ends up with 123 patients discharged, 5 patients transferred and 12 in-hospital deaths. Below are the results for treatment and in-hospital mortality resutling from the various methods for handling transferred pateints. There is wide variation in the outcomes among the various methods for handling transferred patients. The gold-standard is to link data from all hospitals which provides the accurate finding that these 2 hospitals behave in the same manner. However, based on the method for handling transferred patients, the results can be quite different. For instance, when deleting all transferred patients, the results appears that Hospital 2 provided much better care than Hospital 1 (lytics 33% v 17%; beta-blockers 48% v 29%) and in-hospital mortality appears much lower (10.5% v 13%).

Figure 2. Theoretical treatment and outcomes of 200 patients with Acute MI depending on method of handling inter-hospital transfers.

7) *Control for transfer differences with logistic regression modeling.* Transferred and non-transferred patients are very different demographically and clinically. Logistic regression attempts to control for these differences. Giles et al. only used data from the index hospitalizations to compare race and gender differences in rates of invasive cardiac procedures. [46] They attempted to control for transfer in their analysis. However, because transfer may occur specifically to obtain invasive cardiac procedures and transferred patients are substantially different than non-transferred patients, bias was introduced into the analysis. Regression analysis may not fully control for significant differences between transferred patients and non-transferred patients. It does not adequately control for the subtle differences between transfer-in patients and transfer-out patients and variations in the types of hospitals with high transfer-in or high transfer-out rates, for example, presence of E.R. Physicians, telemetry technicians, cardiac trained nurses, and the presence of an ICU. The official report from the Pennsylvania Health Care Cost Containment Council (PHC4) developed two

regression models, one for patients admitted directly and one for transfer-in patients. [47,48] While partially sorting out the assignment of "credit" and "responsibility", because the transfer-in patients are younger and healthier, the PHC4 hospitals with high transfer-out rates are penalized by not including the transferred patients in their pool .[1]

Method 1. 220 discharges for acute MI – mortality 20/220 = 9%. True mortality is 20/200 = 10%		
Method 2a. Delete all transferred patients	Hospital 1	Hospital 2
Mortality	8/60 = 13.%	10/95 = 10.5%
Lytics	10/60 = 17%	31/95 = 33%
Beta blocker at D/C	15/52 = 29%	41/85 = 48%
Method 2b. Delete all transfer-in patients – no data from other hospital		
Mortality	10/100 = 10%	10/100 = 10%
Lytics	35/100 = 35%	35/100 = 35%
Beta blocker at D/C	15/92 = 16%	45/90 = 50%
Method 2c. Delete all transfer-out patients – no data from subsequent hospital		
Mortality	8/60 = 13.3%	12/135 = 8.9%
Lytics	10/60 = 17%	31/135 = 23%
Beta blocker at D/C	15/52 = 29%	45/123 = 37%
Method 2d. Transfer is an exclusion for "ideal" candidate of therapy.		
Mortality	8/60 = 13%	10/95 = 10.5%
Lytics	10/60 = 17%	31/95 = 33%
Beta blocker at D/C2	15/52 = 29%	41/85 = 48%
Method 3. Link data from hospitals -		
Mortality	10/100 = 10%	10/100 = 10%
Lytics	35/100 = 35%	35/100 = 35%
Beta blocker at D/C	45/90 = 50%	45/90 = 50%
Method 4. Analyze transferred and non-transferred patients the same.		
Mortality	8/100 = 8%	12/140 = 8.6%
Lytics	35/100 = 35%	35/140 = 25%
Beta blocker at D/C	15/92 = 16%	71/128 = 55%
Method 5.Transfer Patients are the specific population of interest.		
Mortality	3/45 = 6.7%	
Lytics	29/45 = 64%	
Beta blocker at D/C	34/45 = 76%	
Method 6. Subsequent Care and outcomes attributed to the index hospitalization		
Mortality	10/100 = 10%	10/100 = 10%
Lytics	35/100 = 35%	35/100 = 35%
Beta blocker at D/C	45/90 = 50%	45/90 = 50%
Method 7. Unable to conduct regression analysis for theoretical patient		

Several newer methods for controlling for differences have been recently proposed. Propensity score analysis uses a similar approach to logistic regression to control for differences in measured variables by replacing the multiple confounding covariates with one function of these covariates. [49] However, neither logistic regression nor propensity score analysis can control for unmeasured differences between patient populations.

Instrumental variable (IV) analysis attempts to control for the unmeasured patient differences often found in non-randomized retrospective and cross-sectional data. The goal of IV analysis is a post-hoc pseudo randomization of patients to better define the impact of a specific treatment. McClellan used IV analysis to determine the incremental benefit of angioplasty of elderly patients with acute MI. [50] Instrumental variable analysis is limited in application due to the difficulty identifying an appropriate instrumental variable and limited experience of health services researchers with this method.

Discussion

The inclusion, exclusion, or linkage of transferred patients in a study should be determined by the research question. Quality improvement studies may focus on the hospital admission as the unit of analysis, while studies on case-fatality or incidence should focus on the patient or episode of acute myocardial infarction. However, several large studies have utilized hospital discharges as a proxy measure for incidence of acute MI and inappropriate handling of transfers in other studies has lead to biased results.

Much of the problem has been due to uncertainty in whether transfer should be an independent variable or a dependent variable. That is, is transfer a treatment of acute myocardial infarction, an outcome of the treatment of acute myocardial infarction, or a neutral occurrence that has no relationship to treatment or outcomes? Many researchers have chosen to handle transfer as a neutral occurrence, but because transfer is so common and transferred patients are different than non-transferred patients have had difficulty adequately handling transfer status in their analysis.

Transfer Issues Related to Clinical Care

Ultimately, the goal of cardiac research is to improve patient care, decrease mortality, improve quality of life, and decrease unnecessary costs. The impact of inter-hospital transfer on clinical care is generally unknown. Only several studies were designed specifically to study transfer and these were looking at transfer for specific treatments, not transfer in general. Transfer muddies the waters of cardiac research and most research has dealt with transfer as a problem to be overcome rather than as an important component of care to be studied and understood. Overwhelmingly, the inferences made and conclusions published about transfer were done so based on studies not designated to answer any questions about transfer. Newer studies designed specifically to answer the question of whether immediate transfer for angioplasty is better than local care with intravenous thrombolysis promise to shed some light on this difficult decision. However, these trials need to include truly rural and remote communities in order to fully answer this important question. The impact of transfer for other acute MI care deserves further investigation.

Because transfer is increasingly common, understanding the risks and benefits is essential to providing the best care to patients suffering acute MI or acute coronary syndromes. The benefit of transfer to a hospital with a higher level of service seems intuitive. Certainly, patients who benefit from angioplasty, coronary artery bypass surgery, or invasive monitoring will, by definition, benefit from transfer to receive those services. The benefit to other groups is less clear. The volume/outcome relationship previously reported should be reinterpreted carefully due to the significant bias introduced into the analyses by deleting transferred patients. The potential downsides to transfer include; complications occurring during transport, delay in reperfusion therapy and other medical care, and separation of patients from their family and/or support group. Theroux et al. reported a higher rate of bleeding complications among the transferred patients in their study [34]. With the growing emphasis on the relationship between depression and acute MI mortality, the clinical impact of transferring a patient from their current social support network will also require further study. Additionally, the emerging interest in pay-for-performance provides additional impetus to clearly identify the care and outcomes associated with individual physicians and hospital. [51, 52] As seen in Figure 2, the method chosen for handling transferred patients can dramatically alter the reported performance outcomes of interest to payors.

Transfer Issues Related to Health Services Research

Health services researchers have spent considerable time evaluating the diagnosis and treatment of acute MI. As the number one cause of death in the U.S., even small changes in diagnostic accuracy and incremental improvement in outcome translates to hundreds if not thousands of patients with better outcomes each year.

Health services researchers have sought to determine the best physicians, hospitals, insurance programs, and delivery systems for acute MI care [27,39]. To do this requires the ability to determine the responsibility for the care patients receive. For patients cared for in 1 hospital by 1 physician this is simple. Add in a physician group, primary care v specialist care, co-insurance, and risk adjustment, and determining responsibility and/or credit becomes less clear. Move patients between hospitals and the relationship between care and outcomes becomes nearly impossible.

Commonly studied outcomes for acute MI include both intermediate outcomes (reperfusion therapy, use of aspirin, beta-blocker, ACE-Inhibitors, rehabilitation services, etc) and patient-oriented outcomes (mortality, quality of life, functional status). If there is a firm link between intermediate outcomes and final outcomes then measurement of intermediate outcomes may be appropriate. If there is no firm link between intermediate outcomes and final outcomes then it is important to measure final outcomes. For example, it is firmly established that aspirin is associated with a significant improvement in mortality for patients with acute MI. It is reasonable to measure aspirin use as an accepted measure of good care. The difference between reperfusion with lytics vs. angioplasty is less well established; therefore it is not adequate to simply measure the rate of angioplasty as a measure of good care. Transfer is an important unresolved issue in this sense. The link between transfer and outcomes has not yet been established; therefore it is essential to study inter-hospital transfer more rigorously. Many of these same issues have been identified in the area of trauma care; regionalization of trauma management, timing and method of patient transport [53, 54]. Unfortunately, no clear outcomes data or consensus has emerged from the trauma transfer literature.

The focus in much cardiac research has been on describing differences and assigning responsibility rather than identifying the best strategy of care for patients with acute MI (Cardiologist v noncardiologist, rural v urban, males v females). The crucial question that addresses both the clinical care of acute MI and the health services questions on acute MI should be; what is the best process of care for this patient? The answer may be different depending on where the patient lives, what hospital the patient presents to, the type of acute MI or acute coronary syndrome the patient is suffering, the availability of specialized cardiac services and cardiology consultants. Not all patients with acute MI will present in the first hour of chest pain to a tertiary hospital with a high volume angioplasty lab during the regular workday. For patients presenting to rural and frontier hospitals, or urban hospitals without angiography services, what is the best process of care for this patient? In the context of inter-hospital transfer, which patient will benefit from transfer?

Conclusion

Inter-hospital transfer in the care of acute MI is common and increasing. Transfer patients have been handled in numerous ways in health research; from full inclusion to complete deletion from the analysis. While this article has focused on the issues surrounding transfer in acute MI, many of the issues are similar for transfer patients with other medical conditions. From a health services standpoint it is important to understand the implications of using a particular method for handling transfer patients, the impact on data collection, the data lost, the appropriate analyses, the generalizability of the findings. From a clinical standpoint it is crucial to further study the issue of inter-hospital transfer and determine the risks and benefits to transfer in acute MI care.

Competing Interests

The authors declare that they have no competing interests.

Authors' Contributions

The author warrants that his submission to the article is original and that he has full power to enter into this agreement. A previous version of this article has appeared in Clinical Medicine: Cardiology 2008:2 1-12. Clinical Medicine: Cardiology is published under the Creative Commons Attribution by License and Dr. Westfall maintained full copyright. Dr.

Westfall conceived of the project, reviewed the literature, developed the conceptual models related to inter-hospital transfer and wrote the manuscript.

References

[1]   Jollis JG, Romano PS. Pennsylvania's Focus on Heart Attack--grading the scorecard. *N. Engl. J. Med*. 338;(14):983-7, 1998 Apr 2.

[2]   Bednar F, Widimsky P, Krupicka J, Groch L, Aschermann M, Zelizko M, et al. Interhospital transport for primary angioplasty improves the long-term outcome of acute myocardial infarction compared with immediate thrombolysis in the nearest hospital (one-year follow-up of the PRAGUE-1 study).[see comment]. *Can. J. Cardiol*. 1919; (10):1133-7, 2003 Sep.

[3]   Waters RE 2nd, Singh KP, Roe MT, Lotfi M, Sketch MH Jr, Mahaffey KW, et al. Rationale and strategies for implementing community-based transfer protocols for primary percutaneous coronary intervention for acute ST-segment elevation myocardial infarction. [Review] [26 refs]. *J. Am. Coll. Cardiol*. 1943;(12):2153-9, 2004 Jun 16.

[4]   Dalby M, Bouzamondo A, Lechat P, Montalescot G. Transfer for primary angioplasty versus immediate thrombolysis in acute myocardial infarction: a meta-analysis.[see comment]. *Circulation* 108;(15):1809-14, 2003 Oct 14.

[5]   Patel MR, Armstrong PW. To transfer or not to transfer: Acute myocardial infarction reperfusion. *Am. Heart J*. 2004 Apr;147(4):573-4.

[6]   Choi S. Is transfer for primary angioplasty better than on-site fibrinolytic therapy for acute myocardial infarction? *CMAJ Canadian Medical Association Journal* 169;(7): 695, 2003 Sep 30.

[7]   Westfall JM, McGloin J. Impact of double counting and transfer bias on estimated rates and outcomes of acute myocardial infarction. *Med. Care* 2001 May;39(5):459-68.

[8]   Lawrence L, Hall MJ. 1997 Summary: National Hospital Discharge Survey. Advance Data from Vital and Health Statistics; no. 308. Hyattsville, MD: National Center for Health Statistics, 1999.

[9]   National Institute of Health, National Heart, Lung, and Blood Institute, U.S. Department of Health and Human Services. Morbidity and Mortality: 1998 Chartbook on Cardiovascular, Lung and Blood Diseases. 1998.

[10] Dartmouth Medical School, Robert Wood Johnson Foundation. The Quality of Medical Care in the United States, A Report on the Medicare Program.AHA Press, 1999.

[11] State of Connecticut Office of Health Care Access. Hospital Discharge Data. Hartford, CT: 1998.

[12] Georgia Department of Human Resources, American Heart Association, Southeast Affiliate. 1999 Georgia State of the Heart Report: Statistics for Cardiovascular Diseases, including County-by County Mortality. 1999. Report No.: DPH99.3HW.

[13] Washington State Department of Health. The Health of Washington State: Coronary Heart Disease. Olympia, WA: 1996.

[14] Dusenbury LJ. Cardiovascular Disease Risk Factors: Morbidity and Mortality in Colorado Residents, 1989-1993. Denver, CO.: Colorado Department of Public Health and Environment, 1995.

[15] Kostis JB, Wilson AC, Lacy CR, Cosgrove NM, Ranjan R, Lawrence-Nelson J, et al. Time trends in the occurrence and outcome of acute myocardial infarction and coronary heart disease death between 1986 and 1996 (a New Jersey statewide study).[see comment]. *Am. J. Cardiol.* 1988; (8):837-41, 2001 Oct 15.

[16] Naylor CD, Chen E. Population-wide mortality trends among patients hospitalized for acute myocardial infarction: the Ontario experience, 1981 to 1991. *J. Am. Coll. Cardiol.* 1924;(6):1431-8, 1994 Nov 15.

[17] Mehta RH, Stalhandske EJ, McCargar PA, Ruane TJ, Eagle KA. Elderly patients at highest risk with acute myocardial infarction are more frequently transferred from community hospitals to tertiary centers: reality or myth? *Am. Heart J.* 138;(4 Pt 1):688-95, 1999 Oct.

[18] Chen J, Radford MJ, Wang Y, Marciniak TA, Krumholz HM. Do "America's Best Hospitals" perform better for acute myocardial infarction?[see comment]. *N. Engl. J. Med.* 340;(4):286-92, 1999 Jan 28.

[19] Allison JJ, Kiefe CI, Weissman NW, Person SD, Rousculp M, Canto JG, et al. Relationship of hospital teaching status with quality of care and mortality for Medicare patients with acute MI. *JAMA* 2000 Sep;284(10):1256-62.

[20] Magid DJ, Calonge BN, Rumsfeld JS, Canto JG, Frederick PD, Every NR, et al. Relation between hospital primary angioplasty volume and mortality for patients with acute MI treated with primary angioplasty vs thrombolytic therapy.[see comment]. *JAMA* 284;(24):3131-8, 2000 Dec 27.

[21] Every NR, Frederick PD, Robinson M, Sugarman J, Bowlby L, Barron HV. A comparison of the national registry of myocardial infarction 2 with the cooperative cardiovascular project. *J. Am. Coll. Cardiol.* 1933;(7):1886-94, 1999 Jun.

[22] Thiemann DR, Coresh J, Oetgen WJ, Powe NR. The association between hospital volume and survival after acute myocardial infarction in elderly patients. *N. Engl. J. Med.* 1999 May;340(21):1640-8.

[23] Casale PN, Jones JL, Wolf FE, Pei Y, Eby LM. Patients treated by cardiologists have a lower in-hospital mortality for acute myocardial infarction. *J. Am. Coll. Cardiol.* 1998 Oct;32(4):885-9.

[24] Baldwin LM, MacLehose RF, Hart LG, Beaver SK, Every N, Chan L. Quality of care for acute myocardial infarction in rural and urban US hospitals. *J. Rural Health* 1920; (2):99-108, 2004.

[25] Tu JV, Austin PC, Chan BT. Relationship between annual volume of patients treated by admitting physician and mortality after acute myocardial infarction.[see comment]. *JAMA* 285;(24):3116-22, 2001 Jun 27.

[26] Willison DJ, Soumerai SB, Palmer RH. Association of physician and hospital volume with use of aspirin and reperfusion therapy in acute myocardial infarction. *Med. Care* 1938; (11):1092-102, 2000 Nov.

[27] Krumholz HM, Murillo JE, Chen J, Vaccarino V, Radford MJ, Ellerbeck EF, et al. Thrombolytic therapy for eligible elderly patients with acute myocardial infarction.[see comment]. *JAMA* 277;(21):1683-8, 1997 Jun 4.

[28] Krumholz HM, Radford MJ, Wang Y, Chen J, Heiat A, Marciniak TA. National use and effectiveness of beta-blockers for the treatment of elderly patients after acute myocardial infarction: National Cooperative Cardiovascular Project.[erratum appears in *JAMA* 1999 Jan 6;281(1):37]. *JAMA* 280;(7):623-9, 1998 Aug 19.

[29] Frances CD, Go AS, Dauterman KW, Deosaransingh K, Jung DL, Gettner S, et al. Outcome following acute myocardial infarction: are differences among physician specialties the result of quality of care or case mix? *Arch Intern. Med.* 159;(13):1429-36, 1999 Jul 12.

[30] Nash IS, Corrato RR, Dlutowski MJ, O'Connor JP, Nash DB. Generalist versus specialist care for acute myocardial infarction. *Am. J. Cardiol.* 1983; (5):650-4, 1999 Mar 1.

[31] O'Connor GT, Quinton HB, Traven ND, Ramunno LD, Dodds TA, Marciniak TA, et al. Geographic variation in the treatment of acute myocardial infarction: the Cooperative Cardiovascular Project. *JAMA* 1999 Feb;281(7):627-33.

[32] Druss BG, Bradford DW, Rosenheck RA, Radford MJ, Krumholz HM. Mental disorders and use of cardiovascular procedures after myocardial infarction.[see comment]. *JAMA* 283;(4):506-11, 2000 Jan 26.

[33] Krumholz HM, Chen J, Murillo JE, Cohen DJ, Radford MJ. Admission to hospitals with on-site cardiac catheterization facilities :impact on long-term costs and outcomes. *Circulation* 1998;(19):2010-6, 1998 Nov 10.

[34] Romano PS, Luft HS, Rainwater JA, Zach AP. Report on Heart Attack 1991-1993, Volume 2: Technical Guide. Sacramento, CA: California Office of Statewide Health Planning and Development, 1997 Dec.

[35] Every NR, Parsons LS, Fihn SD, Larson EB, Maynard C, Hallstrom AP, et al. Long-term outcome in acute myocardial infarction patients admitted to hospitals with and without on-site cardiac catheterization facilities. MITI Investigators. Myocardial Infarction Triage and Intervention.[see comment]. *Circulation* 1996;(6):1770-5, 1997 Sep 16.

[36] Romano PS, Zach A, Luft HS, Rainwater J, Remy LL, Campa D. The California Hospital Outcomes Project: Using administrative data to compare hospital performance. *Jt. Comm. J. Qual. Improv.* 1995 Dec;21(12):668-82.

[37] Vermeer F, Oude Ophuis AJ, vd Berg EJ, Brunninkhuis LG, Werter CJ, Boehmer AG, et al. Prospective randomised comparison between thrombolysis, rescue PTCA, and primary PTCA in patients with extensive myocardial infarction admitted to a hospital without PTCA facilities: a safety and feasibility study. *Heart* 1982;(4):426-31, 1999 Oct.

[38] Patil SS, Joshi R, Gupta G, Reddy MV, Pai M, Kalantri SP. Risk factors for acute myocardial infarction in a rural population of central India: a hospital-based case-control study.[see comment]. *Natl. Med. J. India* 1917;(4):189-94, 2004 Jul-Aug.

[39] Widimsky P, Groch L, Zelizko M, Aschermann M, Bednar F, Suryapranata H. Multicentre randomized trial comparing transport to primary angioplasty vs immediate

thrombolysis vs combined strategy for patients with acute myocardial infarction presenting to a community hospital without a catheterization laboratory. The PRAGUE study.[see comment]. *Eur. Heart J.* 1921;(10):823-31, 2000 May.

[40] Feit F, Mueller HS, Braunwald E, Ross R, Hodges M, Herman MV, et al. Thrombolysis in Myocardial Infarction (TIMI) phase II trial: outcome comparison of a "conservative strategy" in community versus tertiary hospitals. The TIMI Research Group.[see comment]. *J. Am. Coll. Cardiol.* 1916;(7):1529-34, 1990 Dec.

[41] Leimbach WN Jr, Hagan AD, Vaughan HL, Sonnenschein RC, McCoy JD, Basta LL. Cost and efficacy of intravenous streptokinase plus PTCA for acute myocardial infarction when therapy is initiated in community hospitals. *Clin. Cardiol.* 1911;(11): 731-8, 1988 Nov.

[42] Theroux P, Alexander J Jr, Dupuis J, Pesant Y, Gervais P, Grandmont D, et al. Upstream use of tirofiban in patients admitted for an acute coronary syndrome in hospitals with or without facilities for invasive management. PRISM-PLUS Investigators. *Am. J. Cardiol.* 1987;(4):375-80, 2001 Feb 15.

[43] Madsen JK, Grande P, Saunamaki K, Thayssen P, Kassis E, Eriksen U, et al. Danish multicenter randomized study of invasive versus conservative treatment in patients with inducible ischemia after thrombolysis in acute myocardial infarction (DANAMI). DANish trial in Acute Myocardial Infarction.[see comment]. *Circulation* 1996;(3):748-55, 1997 Aug 5.

[44] Every NR, Larson EB, Litwin PE, Maynard C, Fihn SD, Eisenberg MS, et al. The association between on-site cardiac catheterization facilities and the use of coronary angiography after acute myocardial infarction. Myocardial Infarction Triage and Intervention Project Investigators.[see comment]. *N. Engl. J. Med.* 329; (8):546-51, 1993 Aug 19.

[45] Chen J, Radford MJ, Wang Y, Krumholz HM. Care and outcomes of elderly patients with acute myocardial infarction by physician specialty: the effects of comorbidity and functional limitations. *Am. J. Med.* 108;(6):460-9, 2000 Apr 15.

[46] Giles WH, Anda RF, Casper ML, Escobedo LG, Taylor HA. Race and sex differences in rates of invasive cardiac procedures in US hospitals. Data from the National Hospital Discharge Survey. *Arch Intern. Med.* 155;(3):318-24, 1995 Feb 13.

[47] Pennsylvania Health Care Cost Containment Council. Technical Report. Focus on Heart Attack in Pennsylvania: A 1993 Summary Report for Health Benefits Purchasers, Health Care Providers, Policy-makers, and Consumers. Part A. Harrisburg, PA, 1996.

[48] Pennsylvania Health Care Cost Containment Council. Technical Report. Focus on Heart Attack in Pennsylvania: A 1993 Summary Report for Health Benefits Purchasers, Health Care Providers, Policy-makers, and Consumers. Part B. Harrisburg, PA, 1996.

[49] Rubin DB. Estimating causal effects from large data sets using propensity scores. [Review] [31 refs]. *Ann. Intern. Med.* 127;(8 Pt 2):757-63, 1997 Oct 15.

[50] McClellan M, McNeil BJ, Newhouse JP. Does more intensive treatment of acute myocardial infarction in the elderly reduce mortality? Analysis using instrumental variables. *JAMA* 272;(11):859-66, 1994 Sep 21.

[51] Lindenauer PK, Remus D, Roman S, Rothberg MB, Benjamin EM, Ma A, et al. Public Reporting and Pay for Performance in Hospital Quality Improvement. *N. Engl. J. Med.* 2007 Feb;356(5):486-96.

[52] Rosenthal MB, Dudley RA. Pay-for-performance: will the latest payment trend improve care?. *JAMA.* 297(7):740-4, 2007 Feb 21.

[53] Rogers FB, Shackford SR, Osler TM, Vane DW, Davis JH. Rural trauma: the challenge for the next decade. *Journal of Trauma-Injury Infection and Critical Care* 1999 Oct; 47(4): 802-21, .

[54] Newgard CD, McConnell KJ, Hedges JR. - Variability of trauma transfer practices among non-tertiary care hospital emergency departments. *Acad. Emerg. Med.* 2006 Jul; 13(7):746-54.

In: Handbook of Cardiovascular Research   ISBN 978-1-60741-792-7
Editors: Jorgen Brataas and Viggo Nanstveit   © 2009 Nova Science Publishers, Inc.

Chapter X

In Vivo Tracking of the Cardially Delivered Stem Cells in Ischemic Heart Disease – Cell Fate, Proliferation and Migratory Itinerary

Mariann Gyöngyösi, Silvia Charwat, Jeronimo Blanco,
Terez Marian, Rayyan Hemetsberger, Noemi Pavo,
Aniko Posa, Aliasghar Khorsand, Imre J Pavo,
Örs Petnehazy, Zsolt Petrasi, Iván Horváth, Johann Wojta,
Kurt Huber, Dara L. Kraitchman, Gerald Maurer
and Dietmar Glogar

Department of Cardiology, Medical University of Vienna, Austria
Centro de Investigación Cardiovascular (CSIC-ICCC), CIBER-BBN, Barcelona, Spain
PET Centrum - Institute of Nuclear Medicine, The University of Debrecen, Hungary
Institute of Diagnostic Imaging and Radiation Oncology, University of Kaposvar,
Hungary
Downtown Animal Clinic, Budapest, Hungary
The Johns Hopkins University, School of Medicine,
Russell H. Morgan Department of Radiology and Radiological Science,
Baltimore, MD, USA
3rd Department of Medicine (Cardiology and Emergency Medicine),
Wilhelminenhospital, Vienna, Austria
Department of Cardiology, Medical University of Vienna, Pecs, Hungary

Abstract

Cardiac transplantation of stem cells (SCs) has been shown to improve regional
perfusion and systolic function of the failing heart after myocardial infarction (MI).

However, once delivered to the heart, unlabeled cells cannot be visualized or tracked *in vivo*. While iron oxide-labeled SCs can be detected by magnetic resonance imaging (MRI), this method is insensitive to a small number of cells, is hindered by the label dilution due to cell division and migration, and cannot distinguish live from dead cells.

The reporter gene approach is a promising method to track SC fate non-invasively.

Because the reporter probe is expressed only in living cells and is passed to daughter cells upon cell division without dilution, the sensitivity for *in vivo* detection is enhanced. Using a reporter system, multimodality (bioluminescence, fluorescence, and positron emission tomography (PET)) imaging permits longitudinal monitoring of the cell survival, homing, and proliferation, if the reporter gene is stably expressed.

We have adapted and validated the reporter gene method for *in vivo* monitoring of cardiac SC therapy in a large animal model of MI that would facilitate translational research.

Domestic pigs underwent a closed-chest, reperfused acute myocardial infarction (AMI), which mimics most human AMI, followed by percutaneous intramyocardial injections of autologous mesenchymal stem cell (MSC) transfected stably with a trifusion reporter gene containing the renilla luciferase (RL)-red fluoroscent protein (RFP)-herpes simplex truncated thymidine kinase (tTK, PET-reporter) (LV-RL-RFP-tTK).

The osteogenic, chondrogenic and adipogenic differentiation of the MSCs was not altered by transfection. Both cell viability and proliferation assays showed no significant difference between the nontransfected MSCs and LV-RL-RFP-tTK-MSCs. Serial PET imaging demonstrated focal [18F]-FHBG tracer uptake of the injured anterior myocardial wall accompanied by a pattern of intense tracer foci at the local injections of the LV-RL-RFP-tTK-MSCs when injected in 2 sites at 8 h post delivery. Ten days after LV-RL-RFP-tTK-MSC implantation, fluorescence confocal microscopy of the myocardium showed the presence of RFP+ cells in the area surrounding the intramyocardial injections. Analysis of luciferase enzyme activities revealed decreased level of expression of the RL gene in the myocardial injection sites, but increasing number of surviving cells in the remote organs at 8 days post-delivery. Fluorescence confocal microscopy confirmed the presence of RFP+ cells in a mediastinal lymph node, thereby validating the migration of the LV-RL-RFP-tTK-MSCs.

1. Introduction

1.1. Rational for in Vivo Tracking of the Implanted Stem Cells in Regenerative Medicine

In the last decade new medical and interventional options for patients with acute myocardial ischemia has dramatically decreased the early mortality of acute myocardial infarctions (AMI). Conversely, this has led an increase in the number of patients with heart failure due to moderately to severely impaired left ventricular function. Therefore, medical interest in cardiac regeneration therapy is growing to treat these patients, and research into gene- and cell-based therapies has become intense. Despite encouraging results of the cardiac cell therapy on global left ventricular function in a recent meta-analysis [1,2], the fate, the distribution, and potential side effects of bioengineered adult bone-marrow cells in remote organs has not yet been elucidated. Various non-invasive imaging, including positron emmision computer tomography (PET), single photon emission computer tomography

(SPECT) and magnet resonance imaging (MRI) have shown poor engraftment of administered stem cells at the site of tissue injury, raising doubts whether sufficient numbers of effector cells can be delivered to achieve the required biological effect and uncertainty about the cell fate. Furthermore, cells engineering to overexpress pro-survival factors, such as vascular endothelial growth factor (VEGF) or granulocyte colony stimulating factor (G-CSF), the cardiac transplanted cells might exhibit unwanted angiogenesis and tumorigenesis in the remote organs. Stable transfection of cells with therapeutic genes, e.g., VEGF, using viral vectors can promote angiogenesis in ischemic tissues, but also carries the risk for gene overexpression, and the potential hazard of undesirable vector shuttle [3]. Thus, tracking of the transplanted stem cells has the potential of increasing both the safety and efficacy of cell-based gene therapy in human regenerative medicine for ischemic or degenerative organ disorders.

1.2. Animal Models of Cell Tracking

Although experimental models can never replicate the complexity and unique nature of human cardiovascular disease, animal studies can yield useful information on logistic issues, such as optimum cell type, delivery method, and timing of cell therapy. Several methods to making the implanted cells visible have been studied in small animals models, offering a more cost-effective approach than the large animal models.

1.2.1. Small Animal Models

Small animal models have the inherent advantage of the feasibility of studying a large number of cohorts for high statistical power and high reproducibility especially in genetically modified models. Almost all reporter gene tracking methods employing different optical imaging (bioluminescence, fluorescence, micro-PET) were first evaluated in small animal models.

After peripheral intravenous injection in athymic rats, [111]Indium labelled endothelial and haematopoietic progenitor cells were shown to accumulate mainly in the liver and spleen. At 1 and 96 hours after injections approximately 71% of the whole body activity was detected in these organs [4,5]. Histological examination showed an accumulation of endothelial progenitor cells (EPCs) in the border zone of the infarction [4]. Due to the large size of bone marrow-derived MSCs, systemic delivery to rats after MI resulted in entrapment of the donor cells mainly in the lungs, with significantly smaller amounts in the liver, heart, and spleen [6]. Delivery by left ventricular cavity infusion resulted in drastically lower lung uptake, better uptake in the heart, and specifically higher uptake in infarcted compared with sham-MI hearts. Histological examination at 1 week after infusion identified labeled cells either in the infarcted or border zone but not in remote viable myocardium or sham-MI hearts. Labeled cells were also identified in the lung, liver, spleen, and bone marrow [6].

1.2.2. Large Animal Models

Successful in vivo imaging of the SCs requires imaging techniques that can be easily translated to the clinics. Many preclinical small animal studies of stem cell tracking are not readily adaptable to clinical practice. The main reasons are: 1) the lack of feasibility of using autologous stem cells; 2) the pretreatment of the animals before allogeneic or xenogenic stem cell transplantation might negatively influence the survival of the recipient animals and/or the cells themselves; 3) the delivery mode is vastly different; and 4) the number of cells in relation to the recipient organ is not readily scalable to human body mass index. On the other hand, large animal models of cell therapy allow the usage of a more similar ischemic event using closed-chest and reperfused techniques and standard clinically available PET, SPECT, and MR imaging scanners for ease of clinical translation.

In a large animal model of infarction, intravenous administration of [111]Indium-labelled mesenchymal stem cells showed accumulation in the lungs shortly after injection and redistributed to the liver, spleen and kidneys over time by SPECT imaging [7,8]. In a study by Hou et al., three stem cell administration techniques were compared in pigs [9]. Retrograde coronary sinus delivery was performed with a double-balloon catheter to minimize washout of delivered cells into the systemic circulation via distal, low-resistance venovenous anastomoses. Intracoronary delivery was performed with a normal angioplasty balloon inflated to low pressure [9]. Lastly, intramyocardial injections were given via an open chest approach to the anterior surface of the heart. Interestingly, the predominant activity (counted as the percentage of locally retained radioactivity in the different organs to total radioactivity) was detected in lungs one hour after delivery in all three methods. After intravenous injection 43.3%, after intracoronary delivery 47.1% and after intramyocardial injection 26.3% of the cells were found in the lungs. The heart showed a retention rate of 3.2%, 2.6% and 11.3% after retrograde coronary sinus, intracoronary and intramyocardial delivery, respectively, without reaching statistical significance between intravenous and intramyocardial injection [9]. In a study of Freyman et al., intracoronary (IC) and endocardial injection of MSCs post-MI resulted in increased engraftment within infarcted tissue when compared with intravenous (IV) infusion, and intracoronary was more efficient than endocardial [10]. However, intracoronary delivery was also associated with a higher incidence of decreased coronary blood flow. Endocardial delivery into acutely infarcted myocardial tissue was safe and well tolerated and was associated with decreased remote organ engraftment with compared with IC and IV deliveries [10]. In another large animal infarction model, $6.8 \pm 1.8\%$ of 18F-FDG-labeled mononuclear cells were found in the infarcted myocardium at one-hour post administration with the remaining activity found primarily in the liver and spleen. In the heart, mononuclear cells were detected predominantly in the border zone of the infarction, and the cell retention correlated very well with the infarct size [11].

The inference that can be derived from these large animal models of a variety of delivery techniques is that the majority of delivered cells are not retained in the heart. Another clinical implication of these findings is the potential that the stem cells could have unwanted effects in other organs to which they were not primarily targeted but to which they are distributed [9].

2. Tracking of Implanted Stem Cells in Humans

To date only few cardiac tracking studies have been performed in patients with a limited number of subjects. In one trial, three subjects early after coronary angioplasty received intravenous delivery of ^{18}F-FDG-labelled bone marrow mononuclear cells (BM-MNCs) [12]. No PET signal above background lung activity was seen. In this same study, intracoronary injection of unselected BM-MNCs led to 1-2% myocardial activity 75 minutes after administration. Enrichment with CD34 positive cells led to a significantly higher activity of 14-39% in the heart. In both patient groups of intracoronary injections, the activity was limited to the injected vascular territory. [12].

Penicka et al. injected 99mTc-labelled BM-MNCs into the LAD via using an over-the-wire balloon 9 days after AMI and stenting. The balloon was inflated for 3 minutes during BM-MNC injection and then deflated for 3 minutes to allow reflow [13]. This manoeuvre was repeated 5 times. Nuclear imaging studies were performed at 2 and 18 hours after transplantation and showed that the majority of transplanted cells accumulated in the spleen. The estimated radioactivity uptake by the heart was 5% of the injected dose at 2 hours and 1% at 18 hours after transplantation. PET imaging demonstrated that peak radioactivity in the heart marched from the LAD territory to the apex and surrounding segments, which was the region with reduced perfusion and viability [13].

3. Methods of In Vivo Tracking

There are many methods to label cells for tracking. Ideally, the tracking agent should demonstrate several characteristics. [14] The label should be biocompatible, safe and non-toxic even when metabolized. No change in protein expression, cell metabolism, or cell survival should occur. Ideally, one should be able to distinguish a single cell at any anatomic location and simultaneously determine cell numbers in a quantification manner. The tracking agent should not be diluted by cell division and remain detectable for months to years. Furthermore it should only be incorporated by stem cells and destroyed by cell death.

The most commonly used methods for in vivo tracking are the direct, non-specific labelling with contrast agents or specific labelling with reporter genes. Of these methods, direct labelling is the easiest method for cellular imaging and cell tracking.

3.1. Direct Non-Specific Labeling

3.1.1. MRI

The most widely used imaging for direct labelling is MRI. Two major groups of MRI contrast agents, the paramagnetic metal chelates such as Gadolinium (Gd) chelate and iron oxide particles are widely used. These contrast agents may be internalized into the cells intended to track by phagocytosis or magnetoelectroporation.

Gadolinium (Gd) chelates are effective contrast agents because of their 7 unpaired electrons. By shortening longitudinal relaxation rates (T1), a hyperintense contrast can be induced. To generate optimal signal for detection by a 1.5-T MRI, a currently clinical standard MRI, intracellular concentrations greater than 50 μmol/L are required [15,16]. One of the main problems with Gd chelates is that the concentration that is needed is high because of the restricted visibility of intracellular water. Because free gadolinium is highly toxic, gadolinium-based contrast agents are chelated. For cell labeling, another concern is that the gadolinium complex will become dechelated if the cell dies leading to toxic free gadolinium.

Another class of MRI contrast agenst is the superparamagnetic iron oxides. These particles vary in size from large superparamagnetic iron particles (SPIO), which have a diameter of >50 nm, to ultrasmall SPIO (USPIO), which are <50 nm to monocrystalline iron oxide nanoparticle (MION) agents [17]. The iron cores are coated with agents, such as dextran or siloxane in a polymer capsule to prevent aggregation [18]. These iron oxide nanoparticles create a large magnetic moment that leads to substantial disturbances in the local magnetic field and a rapid dephasing of protons in the vicinity of the nanoparticles. MR imaging techniques, such as gradient echo techniques, that do not compensate for dephasing are particularly sensitized to detecting these nanoparticles. Concentrations of iron in the pictogram range are sufficient to generate detectable hypointense signals on T2*-weighed images [19-21]. Because free iron from degraded labeled cells is recycled using into the normal iron pool, toxicity concerns compared to gadolinium chelates are greatly reduced. Since iron oxide particles create a negative signal, there may be problems distinguishing labeled cells from haemoglobin degradation products such as methaemoglobin and haemosiderin such as may occur with microvascular obstruction after an acute ischemic event.

Potential disadvantages of MRI labelling include the fact that the contrast agent is not linked to cell viability, so dead cells, macrophages that phagocytize the dying cells, or free particles can be imaged. After several cell divisions, the contrast agent per cell will be diminished and the daughter cells may no longer be visible [22,23]. Compared to PET scanning, the sensitivity of MR is much lower. On average, on the order of 10^5 must be present for detection for cardiovascular applications with conventional MRI scanners without any sequence modification. This threshold of detection can be lowered using high-field magnets (11.7-T) such that single cells containing a single iron particle can be detected and tracked [24]. Furthermore, MRI is contraindicated in patients with some cardiac devices, such as pacemakers and internal cardiac defibrillators (ICDs). Areas of ischemia, calcification, and haemorrhage may also appear as hypointensites and therefore are require specialized techniques to distinguish [20].

The advantage of the direct unspecific labelling with Gd or SPIOs is that these clinically approved agents have been used in clinical cell labeling trials for cardiac and non-cardiac applications [25-27]. In 2003, two research groups have published the first successful in vivo tracking of intracardially injected stem cells using MRI in large animal model of MI [28,29].

In contrast with PET or other nuclear techniques, MRI is a 3D technique with high spatial resolution and exquisite soft tissue detail for anatomical localization. In addition, information about global and regional function can be readily obtained without ionizing radiation, thereby lending the technique to serial imaging in the clinical setting.

3.1.2. Ultrasound

Because of its availability and low cost, echocardiography remains an attractive option for clinical trials of cardiac stem cell therapy [30]. A variety of contrast agents for echocardiography have been developed such as nanoparticles, liposome, or microbubbles. Technological advances in molecular imaging agents for echocardiography offer the potential to image in vivo cellular morphology and/or characterize pathophysiologic processes [31]. In addition, echocardiography has been reported to have the potential to detect a single cell loaded with a single unit of contrast. Limitations of ultrasound for in vivo cell tracking include lack of accuracy in cell quantification, spatial resolution, and lack of robust techniques for intracellular accumulation of the agent. Finally, as this imaging modality is a transthoracic, 2-dimensional–based technique, anatomical inaccessibility of certain cardiac structures could present an important limitation [15].

3.1.3. Radiolabelled Cells Tracked with Nuclear Imaging

Radiolabelling can be performed in animal and also in clinical studies using clinically approved tracers, such as ^{99m}Tc and ^{18}F-FDG. The cells are incubated with radioactive isotopes, such as ^{111}Indium oxide [32], ^{99m}Tc, or ^{18}F-FDG and then transplanted. The radiation of positron annihilation is detected with a gamma camera. The detectability of cells over time mainly depends on the physical half time of the tracers, which is for example 62.7 h for Indium. Hence, tracking beyond ~5-7 days is limited with the available substances [33], which is a clear disadvantage of the direct radiotracer cell labeling for in vivo tracking.

Further disadvantage of this method the relatively low radioactivity of single molecules. A typical patient dose of 10 to 20 mCi is equivalent to 3.5 to 7^{12} radioactive molecules. To detect a single stem cell, about 0.01% of the injected dose would have to be concentrated in/on the cell, which is a formidable technical challenge [14]. Additionally, nuclear labelling may impair the cell integrity as high concentrations of the radioisotope used.

Compared to MRI, nuclear imaging has a higher sensitivity for enhanced information on cell homing and perfusion with a lower background signal, but at a lower spatial resolution [34].

3.2. Reporter Gene Approach

For preclinical applications, the reporter gene approach is currently one of the best methods for monitoring the cell fate, proliferation and migration; its usefulness has been proven for small animals [35-37] and for large animals [38,39). This approach involves inserting a reporter gene(s) into stem cells for the purpose of creating a gene product expressed by the cell that can be used for tracking. To prevent loss of the reporter upon cell division, a stable transfection is required with extensive molecular manipulation. However, reporter genes are extremely useful in assessing survival status of the implanted cells because the reporter is expressed as long as the cells survive and is passed to daughter cells upon cell division [36-40].

Using this labelling technique, it is possible to characterize and quantify biologic processes on the cellular and subcellular level. Reporter genes of choice can be transferred to cell exogenously to detect the expressed protein with an injected reporter probe that accumulates only in the transduced cells after in vivo administration [35].

In cases of non-stable transfection using adenovirus or non-viral transfection methods (e.g., electroporation or nucleofection), a limited time (usually up to 2 weeks) is available for cell tracking. Non-stable transduction leads to episomal gene expression, because the reporter gene is not integrated into the chromatin of mother or daughter cells. This can be a severe limitation if the desired goal of noninvasive imaging is to track stem cell survival and proliferation longitudinally [41]. Using adenovirus for gene manipulation, the expression of immunogenic adenoviral proteins may occur, which could lead to host immune response against cells expressing the reporter gene [41]. In contrast with the viral vector, where the transfection efficacy may reach high level (from 28% to almost 100%), non-viral method has a much less transfection efficacy of about 5-20% [41]. On the other hand, stable constitutive expression of the reporter gene can be achieved by using lentivirus as a viral promoter with integration of the reporter gene into the chromatin.

A number of reporter genes have been developed for radionuclide imaging, generally divided into three different classes, using either receptors, transporters, or enzymes. In receptor-based reporters, the radioactive tracer binds to a gene-encoded protein, while enzyme-based systems use reporter gene production of a specific enzyme, such as herpes simplex virus type-1 thymidine kinase (HSV1-tk) [36] resulting in the accumulation of a radioactive metabolite of the tracer. The expression of HSV1-tk can be visualized using a radioactive PET or SPECT reporter probe. The HSV1-tk gene expresses a viral thymidine kinase. The HSV1-thymidine kinase protein (HSV1-TK) phosphorylates thymidine, resulting in monophosphates, which are converted by cellular enzymes to di- and triphosphates that are trapped inside the cells. By taking advantage of the high sensitivity of PET or SPECT imaging modalities, it is possible to administer the substrate for thymidine kinase that is labeled with a positron or single-photon emitting radioisotope for detection of HSV1-tk expression.

An important development is the multimodality bi- or tri-fusion reporter systems, which can be studied using both optical and radionuclide imaging [37,41,42]. The trifusion gene expresses red fluorescent protein, Renilla luciferase, and the HSV1-TK enzyme. Cellular fluorescence expression can be monitored using microscopic techniques, while *in vivo* monitoring can be performed using both optical and PET or SPECT methods. This fusion reporter offers the possibility of using the particular imaging technique that best suits the application; fluorescence for studying individual cells or for cell sorting, bioluminescence for high sensitivity *in vivo* imaging in small animals, and PET or SPECT when quantitative accuracy is important, or for the translation to humans [35]. Massoud et al. have reported micro-PET whole-body coronal images of a rat injected with 18-fluorodeoxyglucose (FDG) [43], which technique was associated with the development of the PET-reporter probes. The first in vivo tracking of the direct intramyocardial injections of adenovirus expressing wild-type HSV1-tk reporter genes in healthy, non-infarcted pigs with clinical PET scanner was reported by Myagawa et al. [38]. This study confirmed the feasibility of the *in vivo* visualization of PET reporters in large animal model but without a cell carrier [38]. Recently we have adapted the reporter gene method for in vivo tracking of the percutaneously, intramyocardially-delivered cells in the closed chest, reperfused AMI in large animal model

[39]. The clinical application of PET-based reporter gene imaging is anticipated to expand over the next several years [39]. Human reporter genes will play an increasingly more important role in this development, and it is likely that one or more reporter systems (human gene and complimentary radiopharmaceutical) will take leading roles.

Initial applications of reporter gene imaging in patients will be developed for gene therapy and adoptive cell-based therapies. These studies will benefit from the availability of efficient human reporter systems that can provide critical monitoring information for viral-based gene therapies, oncolytic bacterial and viral therapies, and adoptive cell-based therapies. Translational applications of noninvasive in vivo reporter gene imaging are likely to include: (a) quantitative monitoring of gene therapy vectors for targeting and transduction efficacy in clinical protocols by imaging the location, extent and duration of transgene expression; (b) monitoring of cell trafficking, targeting, replication and activation in adoptive T-cell and stem/progenitor cell therapies; (c) and assessments of endogenous molecular events using different inducible reporter gene imaging systems [44].

Another way to internalize the radiotracer is via active transporters such as the Sodium-Iodide-Symporter (NIS). This transmembrane glycoprotein physiologically transports many different ions like I^-, ClO_3^-, SCN^-, $TcO4^-$ and others into thyrocytes and to a lesser extend to gastric mucosa cells. Radioactive iodide ($^{123}I^-$, $^{124}I^-$ and $^{131}I^-$) and $^{99m}TcO_4^-$, which use this transporter are often used for cell imaging. [45-47]. They enter the cell with a Na^+ gradient established by a Na^+/K^+-ATPase pump. Internalization via the NIS features the advantage that this transporter is innate in humans and other laboratory animals so it should not induce an immune reaction and can be used in a preclinical and clinical setting. The human NIS gene ressembles the ones found in pigs, rats and mice by 80% [44]. Since the thyroid, stomach, and salivary glands express the NIS, these organs are not optimal targets for exogenous transduction of cells to produce the NIS. In addition, the amount of tracer within the cells will depends on the blood concentrations as falling plasma iodide leads to clearance from the cells.

Although the reporter gene strategy permits tracking and quantification of stem cells over the course of months, genetic manipulation of the stem cells is required. In addtion, an infrastructure for 18F chemistry, a PET scanner, and radiation exposure (albeit it intermittent) to the stem cells and subject is needed. This technique features the advantage that only viable cells that produce the translated protein are detected even after several cell divisions if the transfection is stable. We have shown that this can be a semiquantitative technique since there is a positive correlation between the reporter protein and the number of active cells [39].

A limitation of reporter gene labelling is the unresolved issue of reporter gene silencing. With gene silencing, genes are functionally and reversibly "knocked out" by the cell on the epigenetic level before transcription or thereafter. Transcriptional silencing comprises mechanisms such as DNA methylation where a methyl group is covalently linked to CpG dinucleotides (cytosine next to guanine separated by a phosphate) at the promoter region and thus inhibits bondage of transcription factors. In histone deacetylation, specific enzymes remove acetyl groups from an ε-N-acetyl lysine amino acid on a histone, which results in tighter packing of the DNA. A mechanism of post-transcriptional gene silencing is RNA interference where a short double stranded RNA guide strand destroys the messenger RNA.

For the therapeutic use of transplanted cells, gene silencing can be suppressed with methylation inhibitors and transcriptional activators. Among the substances named 5-azacytidine induces the highest activity of reporter protein confirmed by PCR in vitro and bioluminescence in vivo. Pharmacologic inhibitors of gene silencing could lead to the clinical applicability of this method [40].

Despite bearing a conceptual promise, the use of reporter gene imaging to monitor cell transplantation is still limited to animal model studies. In order to proceed from bench to bedside, further work is required to develop non-immunogenic probes, improved transfection stability, and reductions in the interference of transfection with the cell function and desired molecular effect. Additional work is necessary to establish a robust approach for cell visualization that is also practical for use in the clinical setting [34].

3.3. Optical Imaging

Fluorescent protein and luciferase are well-established reporter genes in biochemical and molecular investigations. Cooled charge-coupled devices (CCD) are used in small animal experiments to detect the emitted light. They are sensitive to the visible light spectrum and near-infrared light. Because of the sensitivity of liquid-cooled CCD cameras and the low background level of visible light emitted from tissues, bioluminescent imaging has great sensitivity.

3.3.1. Fluorescence

Fluorescence imaging uses organic (e.g., green fluorescent protein, small-molecule polymethines) or organic/inorganic hybrids (e.g., quantum dots) as exogenous contrast agents for in vivo imaging [14]. In many cases LacZ and green fluorescence protein (GFP) are used as targets [35]. The agent is excited by an external light source with a wavelength a little shorter than that of the emitted light. Attenuation of light causes a loss of signal with increasing tissue depth from the detector.

Today, the most favoured wavelength is near infrared (NIR, 700-1000 nm) because at that wavelength absorbance spectra for all biomolecules reaches a minima compared to visible wavelengths [400-750nm] [48]. In addition to the high tissue absorption, major disadvantages of NIR fluorescence are the dilution of the agent with each cell division and the possibility of uptake by non-stem cells after stem cell death [14].

3.3.2. Bioluminescence

Bioluminescence refers to the spontaneous emission of light by a living organism as the result of a chemical reaction during which chemical energy is converted to light energy and not to an externally induced process. Luciferase is the enzyme that oxidates luciferin to oxyluciferin, a reaction that requires adenosine-triphosphate (ATP) and produces CO_2, phosphate, and light. In the case of Fluc (a luciferase from the firefly Photinus pyralis) a portion of this chemical energy is released as visible light (blue to yellow-green in color) with an emission spectrum (490- to 620-nm wavelengths) that peaks at 560 nm. This type of light has a very high absorption in living tissue.

Unfortunately, luciferase genes and substrates described to date, which are associated with very high absorption and scatter in living tissue, generate only visible (400-700 nm) light. The need to take cell depth into account (when considering accuracy of detection) represents another important drawback. Also, xenogenous gene-expression and the injection of potentially immunogenic non-human substrates hamper the clinical applicability [35,49].

Fluorescent and bioluminescent imaging studies are simple, relatively inexpensive, and very user friendly. Another advantage, especially for bioluminescence imaging, is its high sensitivity to detect low levels of gene expression, due to the absence of background light emission caused by external illumination. Moreover, biologic hypotheses can be tested rapidly in living experimental models, because these methods have been widely used in many in vitro reporter gene assays. Biologic information regarding fluorescent protein expression from in vitro cell systems also easily translated to in vivo whole-body systems, such as movement of specific cells, monitoring promoter activity, or several cellular factors. In addition, optical imaging modalities are suitable for high-throughput screening due to ease of operation, short acquisition times (usually 10–60 s), and the capability for simultaneous measurement.

4. Multimodality Imaging for *In Vivo* Tracking of Percutaneously Intramyocardially Injected Stem Cells Transfected with Trifusion Reporter Genes in Pre-Clinical Experiment of Closed Chest/Reperfused AMI

We have adapted and validated the cell-based reporter gene method for *in vivo* monitoring of cardiac SC therapy in a large animal MI model that would facilitate translational research [39].

Domestic pigs underwent closed chest reperfused AMI (which condition is the most similar to human AMI and primary percutaneous coronary intervention), followed by intramyocardial injections of autologous mesenchymal stem cell transfected with the envelope plasmid pMD-G-VSVG, the packaging plasmid pCMV-DR8.2, and an expression plasmid construct containing the renilla luciferase (RL)-red fluoroscent protein (RFP)-herpes simplex truncated thymidine kinase (tTK, PET-reporter) (LV-RL-RFP-tTK).

In vitro assays showed, that the osteogenic, chondrogenic and adipogenic differentiation was not altered by transfecting of the MSCs. Both cell viability and proliferation assays showed no significant difference between the nontransfected MSCs and LV-RL-RFP-tTK-MSCs. Serial PET imaging demonstrated focal [18F]-FHBG tracer uptake of the anterior myocardial wall accompanied by a pattern of intense tracer foci at the local injections of the when injected in 2 sites at 8 h post delivery (Figure 1).

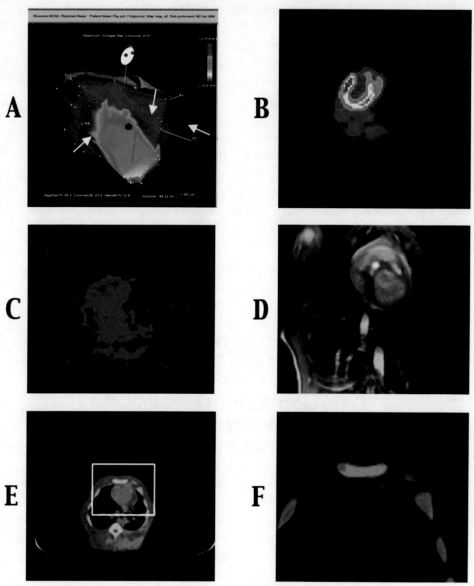

Gyöngyösi et al. Circulation: Cardiovascular Imaging 2008;1:94-103, with permission.

Figure 1. A. Endocardial mapping of a pig heart 16 days post-MI. Voltage map with the sites (black points) of the NOGA-guided intramyocardial injections of the LV-RL-RFP-tTK-MSC (white arrows at the border zone of infarction) and non-transfected MSCs (yellow arrow at the non-infarcted posterior wall). Normal viability is represented by blue and pink colors. Yellow and green color represents decreased viability in the mid-distal anterior wall and red non-viability at the heart apex. B. 13N-ammonia positron emission tomography (PET) with transmission scan of the pig heart (supine position) 16 days post-AMI indicating perfusion defect in the anterior wall and apex. C. [18F]-FHBG tracer uptake in the 2 injected points, representing the location of the LV-RL-RFP-tTK-MSC 8 hours after cell delivery into the myocardium (PET-transmission scan, pig in supine position). No activity in the posterior wall, where the non-transfected MSCs were injected. D. Fusion image of MRI (grayscale) and [18F]-FHBG-PET (hot scale) indicating tracer accumulation in the sites only where LV-RL-RFP-tTK-MSC were intramyocardially injected. E. [18F]-FHBG-PET-CT hybrid image for localization of the injected cells in the anterior wall. F. Magnification of the ROI of [18F]-FHBG-CT.

In the following experiments, we have injected the LV-RL-RFP-tTK-MSCs in 10-12 sites of the border zones of infarction, similarly to the human cardiac stem cell therapy. Autoradiography of the myocardium 3h after intravenous administration of 10 mCi (~0.33 mCi/kg) [18F]-FHBG confirmed the presence of radioactivity in the myocardium with LV-RL-RFP-tTK-MSCs, in contrast with the non-treated myocardium (Figure 2).

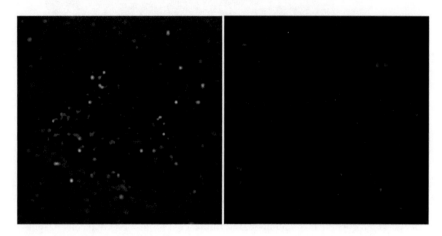

Figure 2. Autoradiographic localization of LV- RL-RFP-tTK-MSC in the injected area (left) but only background activity in the normal myocardium (right).

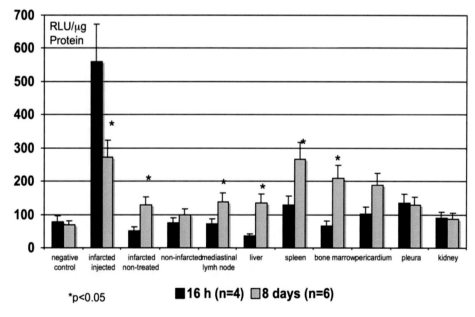

Figure 3. Luciferase assay 16h and 8 days after cardiac cell delivery. Decrease in the number of transplanted cells from 16h to 8 days, while increase of luciferase acivity in the remote organs.

Gyöngyösi et al. Circulation: Cardiovascular Imaging 2008;1:94-103, with permission.

Figure 4. Image of a mediastinal lymph node: red fluorescent protein positive cells in lymph node 10 days post cardiac delivery.

Luciferase activity was measured 16h and 8 days post-delivery in the homogenized tissues using components of the Dual-Luciferase Reporter Assay and expressed in relative light units (RLU) per µg protein. Luciferase activity decreased in the injected myocardial area from 16h to 8±1 days, while it increased significantly in the infarcted non-treated myocardium, and remained at the level of the negative control of the non-infarcted myocardium. Significantly increased luciferase activity was measured at 8±1 days in the mediastinal lymph nodes, liver, spleen and the bone marrow. The luciferase level was slightly elevated in the pericardium and pleura at 16h, which increased nonsignificantly at 8 days (Figure 3.).

Fluorescence confocal microscopy confirmed the presence of RFP+ cells in a mediastinal lymph node 10 days after intamyocardial cell delivery, confirming the migration of the LV-RL-RFP-tTK-MSCs (Figure 4).

References

[1]   Abdel-Latif A, Bolli R, Tleyjeh IM, Montori VM, Perin EC, Hornung CA, et al. Adult bone marrow-derived cells for cardiac repair: a systematic review and meta-analysis. *Arch Intern. Med.* 2007;167(10):989-97.

[2]   Zhou R, Acton PD, Ferrari VA. Imaging stem cells implanted in infarcted myocardium. *J. Am. Coll. Cardiol.* 2006;48(10):2094-106.

[3]   Blömer U, Gruh I, Witschel H, Haverich A, Martin U. Shuttle of lentiviral vectors via transplanted cells in vivo. *Gene Therapy.* 2005; 12:67-74.

[4]   Aicher A, Brenner W, Zuhayra M, Badorff C, Massoudi S, Assmus B, et al. Assessment of the tissue distribution of transplanted human endothelial progenitor cells by radioactive labeling. *Circulation* 2003;107(16):2134-9.

[5]   Brenner W, Aicher A, Eckey T, et al. 111In-labeled CD34+ hematopoietic progenitor cells in a rat myocardial infarction model. *J. Nucl. Med.* 2004;45(3):512-8.

[6]   Barbash IM, Chouraqui P, Baron J, Feinberg MS, Etzion S, Tessone A, et al. Systemic delivery of bone marrow-derived mesenchymal stem cells to the infarcted myocardium: feasibility, cell migration, and body distribution. *Circulation* 2003;108(7):863-8.

[7]   Chin BB, Nakamoto Y, Bulte JW, Pittenger MF, Wahl R, Kraitchman DL. 111In oxine labelled mesenchymal stem cell SPECT after intravenous administration in myocardial infarction. *Nucl. Med. Commun.* 2003;24(11):1149-54.

[8]   Kraitchman DL, Tatsumi M, Gilson WD, et al. Dynamic imaging of allogeneic mesenchymal stem cells trafficking to myocardial infarction. *Circulation* 2005;112(10): 1451-61.

[9]   Hou D, Youssef EA, Brinton TJ, Zhang P, Rogers P, Price ET, et al. Radiolabeled cell distribution after intramyocardial, intracoronary, and interstitial retrograde coronary venous delivery: implications for current clinical trials. *Circulation* 2005;112(9 Suppl): I150-6.

[10] Freyman T, Polin G, Osman H, Crary J, Lu MM, Cheng L, Palasis M, Wilensky RL. A quantitative, randomized study evaluating three methods of mesenchymal stem cell delivery following myocardial infarction. *Eur. Heart J.* 2006;27:1114–1122.

[11] Qian H, Yang Y, Huang J, Gao R, Dou K, Yang G, et al. Intracoronary delivery of autologous bone marrow mononuclear cells radiolabeled by 18F-fluoro-deoxy-glucose: tissue distribution and impact on post-infarct swine hearts. *J. Cell Biochem.* 2007; 102(1): 64-74.

[12] Hofmann M, Wollert KC, Meyer GP, Menke A, Arseniev L, Hertenstein B, et al. Monitoring of bone marrow cell homing into the infarcted human myocardium. *Circulation* 2005;111(17):2198-202.

[13] Penicka M, Widimsky P, Kobylka P, Kozak T, Lang O. Images in cardiovascular medicine. Early tissue distribution of bone marrow mononuclear cells after transcoronary transplantation in a patient with acute myocardial infarction. *Circulation* 2005;112(4):e63-5.

[14] Frangioni JV, Hajjar RJ. In vivo tracking of stem cells for clinical trials in cardiovascular disease. *Circulation* 2004;110(21):3378-83.

[15] Hoshino K, Ly HQ, Frangioni JV, Hajjar RJ. In vivo tracking in cardiac stem cell-based therapy. *Prog. Cardiovasc. Dis.* 2007;49(6):414-20.

[16] Modo M, Cash D, Mellodew K, Williams SC, Fraser SE, Meade TJ, et al. Tracking transplanted stem cell migration using bifunctional, contrast agent-enhanced, magnetic resonance imaging. *Neuroimage* 2002;17(2):803-11.

[17] Wang YX, Hussain SM, Krestin GP. Superparamagnetic iron oxide contrast agents: physicochemical characteristics and applications in MR imaging. *Eur. Radiol.* 2001; 11(11): 2319-31.

[18] Shen T, Weissleder R, Papisov M, Bogdanov A, Jr., Brady TJ. Monocrystalline iron oxide nanocompounds (MION): physicochemical properties. *Magn. Reson. Med.* 1993; 29(5):599-604.

[19] Jung CW. Surface properties of superparamagnetic iron oxide MR contrast agents: ferumoxides, ferumoxtran, ferumoxsil. *Magn. Reson. Imaging* 1995;13(5):675-91.

[20] Kustermann E, Roell W, Breitbach M, et al. Stem cell implantation in ischemic mouse heart: a high-resolution magnetic resonance imaging investigation. *NMR Biomed.* 2005; 18(6):362-70.

[21] Bulte JW, Kraitchman DL. Iron oxide MR contrast agents for molecular and cellular imaging. *NMR Biomed.* 2004;17(7):484-99.

[22] Penn MS. Cell-based gene therapy for the prevention and treatment of cardiac dysfunction. *Nat. Clin. Pract. Cardiovasc. Med.* 2007;4 Suppl 1:S83-8.

[23] Kraitchman DL, Bulte JWM. Imaging of stem cells using MRI. *Basic Res. Cardiol.* 2008; 103:105–113.

[24] Shapiro EM, Skrtic S, Sharer K, Hill JM, Dunbar CE, Koretsky AP. MRI detection of single particles for cellular imaging. *Proc. Natl. Acad. Sci. USA* 2004;101(30):10901-6.

[25] Amsalem Y, Mardor Y, Feinberg MS, Landa N, Miller L, Daniels D, et al. Iron-oxide labeling and outcome of transplanted mesenchymal stem cells in the infarcted myocardium. *Circulation* 2007;116(11 Suppl):I38-45.

[26] Zhu J, Zhou L, XingWu F. Tracking neural stem cells in patients with brain trauma. *N. Engl. J. Med.* 2006;355(22):2376-8.

[27] de Vries IJ, Lesterhuis WJ, Barentsz JO, et al. Magnetic resonance tracking of dendritic cells in melanoma patients for monitoring of cellular therapy. *Nat. Biotechnol.* 2005; 23(11):1407-13

[28] Kraitchman DL, Heldman AW, Atalar E, Amado LC, Martin BJ, Pittenger MF, Hare JM, Bulte JW. In vivo magnetic resonance imaging of mesenchymal stem cells in myocardial infarction. *Circulation* 2003;107:2290–2293

[29] Hill JM, Dick AJ, Raman VK, Thompson RB, Yu ZX, Hinds KA, Pessanha BS, Guttman MA, Varney TR, Martin BJ, Dunbar CE, McVeigh ER, Lederman RJ. Serial cardiac magnetic resonance imaging of injected mesenchymal stem cells. *Circulation* 2003;108:1009-1014

[30] Morawski AM, Lanza GA, Wickline SA: Targeted contrast agents for magnetic resonance imaging and ultrasound. *Curr. Opin. Biotechnol.* 2005;16:89-92

[31] Liang HD, Blomley MJ: The role of ultrasound in molecular imaging. *Br. J. Radiol.* 2003; 76 Spec No 2:S140-508 2003.

[32] Kofidis T, Lebl DR, Swijnenburg RJ, Greeve JM, Klima U, Robbins RC. Allopurinol/uricase and ibuprofen enhance engraftment of cardiomyocyte-enriched human embryonic stem cells and improve cardiac function following myocardial injury. *Eur. J. Cardiothorac. Surg.* 2006;29(1):50-5.

[33] Bengel FM. Nuclear imaging in cardiac cell therapy. *Heart Fail Rev.* 2006;11(4):325-32.

[34] Beeres SL, Bengel FM, Bartunek J, Atsma DE, Hill JM, Vanderheyden M, et al. Role of imaging in cardiac stem cell therapy. *J. Am. Coll. Cardiol.* 2007;49(11):1137-48.

[35] Acton PD, Zhou R. Imaging reporter genes for cell tracking with PET and SPECT. *Q. J. Nucl. Med. Mol. Imaging* 2005;49(4):349-60.

[36] Gambhir SS, Herschman HR, Cherry SR, et al. Imaging transgene expression with radionuclide imaging technologies. *Neoplasia* 2000;2:118-1388

[37] Ray P, Wu AM, Gambhir SS. Optical bioluminescence and positron emission tomography imaging of a novel fusion reporter gene in tumor xenografts of living mice. *Cancer Res.* 2003;63:1160-5.

[38] Miyagawa M, Anton M, Haubner R, Simoes MV, Städele C, Erhardt W, Reder S, Lehner T, Wagner B, Noll S, Noll B, Grote M, Gambhir SS, Gansbacher B, Schwaiger M, Bengel FM. PET of Cardiac Transgene Expression: Comparison of 2 Approaches Based on Herpesviral Thymidine Kinase Reporter Gene. *J. Nucl. Med.* 2004;45:1917–1923.

[39] Gyöngyösi M, Blanco J, Marian T, Tron L, Petnehazy Ö, Petrasi Z, Hemetsberger R, Rodriguez J, Font G, Pavo I jr, Kertesz I, Balkay L, Pavo N, Posa A, Emri M, Galuska L, Kraitchman DL, Wojta J, Huber K, Glogar D. Serial non-invasive in vivo positron emmission tomographyc (PET) tracking of percutaneously intramyocardially injected autologous porcine mesenchymal stem cells modified for transgene reporter gene expression Circulation: *Cardiovascular Imaging* 2008:1:94-103.

[40] Krishnan M, Park JM, Cao F, Wang D, Paulmurugan R, Tseng JR, et al. Effects of epigenetic modulation on reporter gene expression: implications for stem cell imaging. *Faseb J.* 2006;20(1):106-8.

[41] Cao F, Lin S, Xie X, Ray P, Patel M, Zhang X, Dylla SJ, Connolly AJ, Chen X, Weissman IL, Gambhir SS, Wu JC. In Vivo Visualization of Embryonic Stem Cell Survival, Proliferation, and Migration After Cardiac Delivery. *Circulation.* 2006; 113;1005-1014.

[42] Wu JC, Chen IY, Sundaresan G, Min JJ, De A, Qiao JH, Fishbein MC, Gambhir SS. Molecular imaging of cardiac cell transplantation in living animals using optical bioluminescence and positron emission tomography. *Circulation.* 2003; 108:1302-1305.

[43] Massoud TF, Gambhir SS. Molecular imaging in living subjects: seeing fundamental biological processes in a new light. *Genes§Dev.* 2003;17:545-580.

[44] Serganova I, Ponomarev V, Blasberg R. Human reporter genes: potential use in clinical studies. *Nucl. Med. Biol.* 2007;34(7):791-807.

[45] Barton KN, Tyson D, Stricker H, Lew YS, Heisey G, Koul S, et al. GENIS: gene expression of sodium iodide symporter for noninvasive imaging of gene therapy vectors and quantification of gene expression in vivo. *Mol. Ther.* 2003;8(3):508-18.

[46] Groot-Wassink T, Aboagye EO, Wang Y, Lemoine NR, Reader AJ, Vassaux G. Quantitative imaging of Na/I symporter transgene expression using positron emission tomography in the living animal. *Mol. Ther.* 2004;9(3):436-42.

[47] Niu G, Gaut AW, Ponto LL, Hichwa RD, Madsen MT, Graham MM, et al. Multimodality noninvasive imaging of gene transfer using the human sodium iodide symporter. *J. Nucl. Med.* 2004;45(3):445-9.

[48] Chance B. Near-infrared images using continuous, phase-modulated, and pulsed light with quantitation of blood and blood oxygenation. *Ann. N. Y. Acad. Sci.* 1998;838:29-45.

[49] Rudin M, Rausch M, Stoeckli M. Molecular imaging in drug discovery and development: potential and limitations of nonnuclear methods. *Mol. Imaging Biol.* 2005; 7(1):5-13.

In: Handbook of Cardiovascular Research
Editors: Jorgen Brataas and Viggo Nanstveit

ISBN 978-1-60741-792-7
© 2009 Nova Science Publishers, Inc.

Chapter XI

Cardiac Effects of Growth Hormone Treatment in Pediatric Populations

Janine Sanchez[1], Adriana Carrillo[1], Shannon Preble[2], Rebecca E. Scully[2] and Steven E. Lipshultz[1,3,4]*

1. Department of Pediatrics, Leonard M. Miller School of Medicine,
University of Miami, Miami, FL, USA
2. Department of Pediatrics, Division of Clinical Research,
Leonard M. Miller School of Medicine, University of Miami, Miami, FL, USA
3. Holtz Children's Hospital of the University of Miami/
Jackson Memorial Medical Center, Miami, FL, USA
4. The University of Miami Sylvester
Comprehensive Cancer Center, Miami, FL, USA

Introduction

While the full extent of the role that growth hormone (GH) and its effector Insulin-like growth factor 1 (IGF-1) play in the development and maintenance of cardiovascular morphology and function is debated, several conditions associated with altered GH activity have characteristic cardiovascular impairments.[1-3] The effects of GH therapy on cardiac function have been studied in the pediatric population, primarily in the setting of GH deficiency. For individuals whose circulating levels of GH are low, GH replacement therapy appears to improve cardiovascular health. GH therapy has also been shown to improve lean body mass and decrease percent body fat, which may further improve overall cardiovascular

* Corresponding author: Steven E. Lipshultz, P.O. Box 016820 (D820), Miami, FL 33101, USA. E-mail: slipshultz@med.miami.edu, Telephone: 305-243-3993, Facsimile: 305-243-3990. Express mail address: Department of Pediatrics, Miller School of Medicine, University of Miami, Medical Campus-MCCD-D820, 1601 NW 12th Avenue, 9th Floor, Miami, FL 33136.

health. However, GH excess may lead to cardiac hypertrophy, as seen in acromegaly. GH therapy may also lead to reduced insulin sensitivity, a pre-diabetic state, in some individuals, particularly women with Turner syndrome. Thus, the systemic effects of GH therapy, specifically its effect on the cardiovascular system, vary by underlying condition.

Background

Growth hormone is a peptide hormone secreted by the anterior pituitary. Growth hormone secretion is pulsatile and controlled directly by the hypothalamus via growth hormone releasing hormone (GHRH), a stimulating factor, and somatostatin, an inhibitory factor. Many metabolic, hormonal, and neuronal factors, reflecting both physiological and pathophysiological processes, effect the interaction between GHRH and somatostatin and impact GH secretion. Growth hormone's tissue-specific effects are mediated by dimerized GH receptors. Growth hormone binding activates the tyrosine kinase

Janus 2 (JAK2), generating a cascade of signaling proteins and pathways activating transcription, the mitogen activated protein kinase (MAPK) pathway, and phosphatidylinositol 3'-kinase pathway. Growth hormone has a variety of metabolic effects and its activity is mediated by insulin growth factor 1 (IGF-1) in some tissues. While GH appears to increase insulin secretion acutely, over the long-term, insulin sensitivity decreases. Growth hormone also increases protein synthesis and lipolysis. IGF-I decreases insulin secretion, but mirrors GH activity in increasing protein synthesis and fat metabolism.

Growth hormone therapy is primarily used to increase vertical growth and improve projected adult height in children with short stature. GH therapy may also help to improve psychological health and quality of life. However, chronic GH elevation may impair central nervous and immune system activity as well as cardiac development and function. Extreme, persistent elevations, as seen in acromegly, are well known to cause significant cardiac dysfunction.[4]

Growth Hormone Therapy in the Cardiac Setting

Dilated cardiomyopathy (DCM) is a disease of the heart muscle characterized by a weakened, enlarged heart with reduced pumping ability. It is one of the most common causes of heart failure among children and is often progressive despite available therapy. Etiology varies widely though mounting evidence implicates both heritable mutations and exposure to toxins or infections. Growth hormone has been proposed as a possible means of reversing some types of left ventricular (LV) dysfunction; [5-9] GH has been shown to increase LV contractility [10, 11] and induce LV hypertrophy [12-14], thereby improving LV performance by decreasing systolic wall stress.[15] Studies conducted with a variety of experimental models of heart failure show that GH treatment is beneficial to the failing heart. [8, 16, 17-22] Further, adults with GH insufficiency have impaired LV structure and function, which improve with GH replacement therapy.[17,23,24] However, the results of clinical studies of GH administration to patients with CHF remain inconsistent. [5, 14, 25-28]

A preliminary study by Fazio et al.[5] found that GH administered over three months increased myocardial mass and improved cardiac function in 7 patients with idiopathic DCM and moderate-to-severe heart failure. The changes in cardiac size and shape, systolic function, and exercise tolerance were, however, partially reversed three months after GH therapy was discontinued. Subsequent studies have yielded mixed results. Treatment over fourteen weeks with synthetic GH increased serum IGF-1 levels but did not affect degree of apoptosis or improve cardiac structure and function in 38 children with dilated cardiomyopathy.[29] Twelve-week treatment with subcutaneous GH in 50 adults with DCM led to a significant increase in left-ventricular mass but did not translate to improved clinical status.[27]

A recent metaregression of available clinical trials attributed these differing results to individual variation in response to GH therapy and induced increases in circulating IGF-I levels.[30] As GH is not known to cause deteriorations in cardiac function or significant arrhythmia, the cardiac effects of GH therapy warrant further investigation in the setting of CHF, particularly in light of apparent improvements in physical exercise capacity following GH therapy.[31]

The safety and efficacy of GH therapy as a means of increasing adult final height following pediatric cardiac transplantation has also been a focus of current research. In a preliminary study, growth velocity increased and rejection frequency did not change with therapy. Increased LV volume was the only measure where elevations persisted following discontinuation of GH therapy and was also increased in control patients who did not receive GH. These results suggest that GH therapy may be a safe and effective way to increase adult height following pediatric heart transplantation.[32]

Isolated GH Deficiency

Abnormal LV diastolic function and impaired systolic function have been reported in growth hormone deficient individuals. Young adults with GHD show significant increases in arterial intima-media thickness, early atherosclerotic changes in the carotid and femoral arteries, and dyslipidemia indicating elevated cardiovascular risk. Children with GHD also show reduced cardiac mass and dimension when compared to controls. [33, 34]

A two year case-control study of 30 children (aged 9.3 +/- 0.5 yrs) with GHD and 30 healthy matched controls found that LV mass index (LVMi) was significantly lower in GHD children (50.2 +/- 1.7 g/m^2) than in controls (60.3 +/- 2.5 g/m^2; P<0.002).[33] A study of 12 prepubertal children with GHD found LV wall thickness (LVPWT) and LV end-diastolic dimension (LVEDD), as well as LVMi, to be significantly lower in GHD children than controls.[35] These deficits were reversed by GH therapy. Twelve months of 30 mcg/kg/day GH therapy in 12 prepubertal GHD children achieved a normal LVMi.

Left ventricular systolic function has been found to be similar in GHD children and controls at baseline and does not change during GH therapy. Adults with childhood onset GHD, however, do have reduced systolic function, though it does appear to be responsive to treatment. Twelve months of GH therapy saw systolic volume fall (P<0.05) and ejection fraction increased(p<0.01) in 16 adults with childhood onset GH deficiency. [36]

Growth hormone deficiency may also affect lipid levels in children. In a study of 12 adolescents with GHD, low density lipoprotein- (LDL) cholesterol levels were increased in untreated GHD patients when compared to healthy controls (P<0.01), although total cholesterol (TC), high density lipoprotein (HDL)-cholesterol, and triglyceride concentrations were similar in both groups.[37] While additional studies have shown mean concentrations of TC and LDL-cholesterol, lipoprotein(a), and apolipoprotein(B) to be significantly higher in patients with GHD than in controls [36,38], results are not uniform and several have found no difference in lipid levels between GHD and healthy children.[33, 35]

Several additional atherosclerotic risk factors are also increased in GHD children and adolescents. While heart rate and blood pressure tend to be similar in GHD patients and controls at baseline, the flow-mediated endothelium-dependent vasodilation of untreated GHD adolescents is depressed, indicating vascular abnormalities.[34, 35] GH therapy was associated with improved endothelial function and reduced arterial stiffness in both studies.

GHD children and adolescents may experience reduced LVMi, significantly elevated IMT levels, dyslipidemia, and increased atherosclerotic risk factors, all of which can increase their cardiovascular morbidity. GH therapy seems to modify these risk factors by normalizing cardiac mass and the atherogenic index and by reducing arterial stiffness and improving endothelial function.

Turner Syndrome

Turner syndrome is the most common chromosomal disorder in women with an incidence of 1 in 2000 live females. Common features include short stature, obesity, congenital cardiac abnormalities, and ovarian failure. Life expectancy is reduced by up to 13 years and cardiovascular disease is the most common cause of death.[39] While the prevalence of congenital cardiac abnormalities in Turner syndrome is well established, recent investigation suggests that the cardiac phenotype may be more complex than initially believed.[38, 40,41] Pseudocoarctation, a kinking at the juncture of the ascending and descending aortas, is common, affecting half of all women with Turner syndrome. Valvular abnormalities and generalized dilation of the major vessels are also prevalent. In total, it appears that nearly 75% of all women diagnosed with Turner syndrome have significant cardiac abnormalities.[42] Aortic size index (diameter standardized to body surface area) is significantly elevated in women with Turner syndrome; in one study one-third of women had aortic size indices above the 95th percentile of 2.0 cm/m^2.[38] Risk of aortic dissection was correlated with aortic size index leading Matura et al. to recommend that women with a descending aortic size index >2.0 cm/m^2 receive close cardiovascular surveillance.

Impaired glucose metabolism has also been reported in 10 to 34% of patients with Turner syndrome. Type 2 diabetes mellitus is 2 to 4 times more common than in the general population, further increasing risk of cardiovascular disease and mortality. High blood pressure is also commonly seen and is a major risk factor for aortic dilation.[36, 41]

Although children with Turner syndrome are not GH deficient, GH has been approved by US Food and Drug Administration to promote somatic growth. Supraphysiological doses of GH are used and cause a sustained increase in growth velocity and improvements in body composition measures. [43-47] However, GH treatment is also associated with increased insulin levels, which may translate to increased incidence of diabetes particularly in a population with elevated rates of obesity.

The effects of long term GH treatment on cardiac function have been evaluated through several studies. Sas et al.[48] monitored 68 girls with Turner syndrome though 7 years of GH treatment. Systolic IVS, end systolic LVID, end-diastolic wall thickness, and end-systolic LVPW did not show significant change. Blood pressure values were normal though slightly elevated when compared to controls and did not change with GH treatment. Matura et al.[49] found that while somatic growth increased with treatment, when adjusted to body size no significant differences in cardiac structural or functional parameters were seen after GH therapy. In a related article, Bondy et al.[50] reported GH treatment increased aortic diameter in 53 girls with Turner syndrome in proportion to somatic growth. These results suggest that even at pharmacologic levels, GH does not produce abnormal cardiac growth or hypertrophy in girls with Turner syndrome and it may be a safe and effective means of increasing adult height.[51]

It appears that GH therapy may also be associated with a reduction in severity of cardiac malformations, suggesting a reduction in risk of aneurysm. While women with Turner syndrome have larger aortic dimension and decreased distendability [52], contributing to the high rate of aortic dissection in this population [53], previous GH replacement therapy was associated with improved aortic function and dimension.

Noonan Syndrome

Noonan syndrome is an autosomal dominant disorder associated with growth retardation and cardiac defects. Mean adult height is 5.3 feet in men and 5.0 feet in women. Variable hypogonadism, cryptorchidism, delayed puberty, deafness, visual problems, and clotting disorders are also seen. Children with Noonan syndrome are not typically GHD, but multiple studies have shown a short to medium-term increase in height velocity in children treated with GH.[51,54-59] However, not all have demonstrated an improvement in final adult height. Approximately 40% of clinical cases with Noonan syndrome have mutations in the PTPN11 gene, which has a role in GH receptor signaling. It is in these children that GH treatment may have a significant effect. In children who are mutation-negative, growth response appears to be much more significant.

Gain in height standard deviation score (SDS) due to growth hormone treatment can range from 0.8 SDS units over 3 yrs to 1.85 SDS units after 2.5 years of therapy.[55,59] In a study of children with Noonan syndrome (aged 5.4 to 17.5 years), patients receiving GH (n=8) had a significantly greater gain in height SDS than in the control group (n=15) over the first year of therapy.[51] However, when patients were taken off GH after two years, they experienced a fall in height SDS of 0.2 SDS units.

Height velocity is also improved in NS patients receiving GH therapy. In a multicenter study of 30 prepubertal children, treatment with GH resulted in an increase in height velocity from 4.9 +/- 0.2 to 8.9 +/- 0.3 cm/yr at 6 months of treatment and 8.1 +/- 0.4 cm/yr (P<0.0001) and an increase in SDS from -0.7 +/- 0.15 to 2.42 +/- 0.32 over one year

(P<0.0001).[56]. A study including 23 patients treated with GH reported an increase in height velocity from 4.4 cm/yr at baseline to 8.4 in the first year, but growth velocity dropped to 6.2cm/yr) in the second year, and 5.8 cm/yr in the third year.[55]

Noonan syndrome children who have an SHP-2 mutation may be mildly GH resistant.[60] After 1 year of GH treatment (0.043 mg/kg.d), the mean difference in height SDS was +0.66 +/- 0.21 in the mutation positive group, but +1.26 +/- 0.36 in the mutation negative group (P = 0.007). Also, specific heart defects, pulmonic stenosis (P = 0.0007) and septal defects (P = 0.02) were more prevalent in the mutation positive group. The cardiac effects of GH therapy in Noonan syndrome children with the SHP-2 mutation should be further investigated in order to determine the safety and efficacy of GH treatment.

Growth hormone therapy has been a concern for Noonan syndrome patients due to its effects on cardiac muscle mass. While no studies have reported worsening cardiac function, many have excluded children with hypertrophic cardiomyopathy from treatment. In a retrospective, multicenter study of 274 patients with Noonan syndrome, 85% of patients had some type of heart defect.[61] Pulmonary valve stenosis (60%), atrial septal defect, ostium secundum type (25%), and stenosis of the peripheral pulmonary arteries (at least 15%) were among the most common congenital heart defects in this population. Baseline echocardiographic measurements were taken in 27 children with Noonan syndrome.[62] LVPW was thicker than average and internal LV diameters were smaller. After one year, there was no significant difference in LV dimensions between children with Noonan syndrome who had received GH and those who did not. After four years, LV dimensions in the GH therapy group were not significantly different from baseline. Other studies have not found an increase in LVPWT or hypertrophic cardiomyopathy during GH treatment.[54,56]

Prader-Willi Syndrome

Prader-Willi syndrome is a genetic syndrome characterized by hyperphagia, morbid obesity, behavioral disturbance and intellectual disability. Prader-Willi syndrome is associated with a high incidence of sudden death of suspected cardiopulmonary. Prader-Willi syndrome is also associated with altered GH secretion [63] potentially leading to reduced cardiac mass and systolic function. A number of cardiovascular risk factors have been reported in PWS patients including elevated highly-sensitive C reactive protein (hsCRP) (> 3.0 mg/l, p < 0.001),, decreased exercise capacity(< 4 metabolic equivalents (METs) on exercise stress testing), abnormal ECG, cardiac tamponade, and coronary artery disease.[64-66]

Growth hormone therapy has been shown to successfully improve adult height, body composition, and agility in Prader-Willi syndrome,[67,68] which may help to decrease cardiac risk, particularly related to long-term obesity. Functional cardiac effects specific to GH treatment in the setting of Prader-Willi syndrome are not well documented, though risk of atherosclerosis appears to improve with therapy. GH therapy was associated with significant improvements in lean mass, fat mass, visceral fat, and hsCRP levels in 13 obese adults with Prader-Willi.[69] Long-term (3 years) GH treatment improved cardiovascular risk factors in 23 children, aged 0.3 to 14.6 years, with Prader-Willi syndrome. Treatment was associated with decreased fat mass and normalized waist to hip ratio. The ratio of LDL-cholesterol to HDL-cholesterol also improved.[70] Growth hormone therapy was, however, associated with increased LV mass and decreased left ventricle ejection fraction (LVEF) in some children, indicating that while GH treatment may significantly improve physical functioning in Prader-Willi syndrome, these patients should be monitored closely during therapy.[69]

Small for Gestational Age (SGA)

Children who are small for gestational age are at elevated risk for increased systolic blood pressure and reduced insulin sensitivity [71], diabetes mellitus type 2, and hyperlipidemia early in adulthood.[72,73] While GH treatment may help to increase somatic growth, it may also increase the risk of cardiovascular disease.

Growth hormone is often used to treat short children born small for gestational age and has been shown to be effective in normalizing the height of these children.[74,75] However, there is some concern regarding the affect on insulin sensitivity.[71] This is an important concern in small for gestational age children, who are more likely to have insulin insensitivity and develop insulin resistance than the normal population. In 78 children born small for gestational age, GH treatment induced higher fasting insulin levels and glucose-stimulated insulin levels, representing relative insulin resistance.[76] However, insulin sensitivity may return to pretreatment values after GH therapy discontinued.[77]

Decreased adiponectin levels and increased resistin, interleukin-6 (IL-6), and CRP levels are associated with increased prevalence of obesity, cardiovascular disease, and diabetes mellitus type 2 in adults.[71] Ninety prepubertal children born small for gestational age were randomized to either 1 or 2 mg/m^2/day of GH. Adiponectin levels decreased in both dosage groups at near adult height, and continued to decrease in the higher-dosage group after discontinuation of GH therapy. Despite this decrease, adiponectin levels remained in the normal range compared with age-matched controls throughout treatment. At near adult height, the 1 mg GH/m^2/d dosage group had higher levels of resistin than at baseline (P<0.01). After discontinuation of GH treatment, both groups had higher levels of resistin than at baseline (P<0.01 for 1 mg GH/m^2/d; P<0.05 for 2 mg GH/m^2/d). Both IL-6 and CRP were not significantly different before, during, or after treatment.[71] While adiponectin and resistin levels were both affected by GH treatment, they remained normal compared to age-matched controls, and therefore may not increase risk of cardiovascular disease and DMT2. Another study of 50 GH treated children found that neither adiponectin nor resistin levels changed significantly during 2 years of GH therapy.[78] GH may increase systemic inflammation. Twenty-nine short children born small for gestational age assigned to receive GH treatment experienced a rise in neutrophil counts, a marker of inflammation. Neutrophil counts rose significantly by 1.1 x 1000.mm^3 (P=0.004) compared to short children born small for gestational age who remained untreated. Therefore, GH treatment may increase inflammation and lead to a poor adipocytokine profile, both of which increase the risk for developing cardiovascular disease and DMT2.[79]

Other cardiovascular risks factors have also been examined in short children born small for gestational age. Seventy-nine children born SGA were divided into two dosage groups (3 vs. 6 $IU/m^2/d$) and data was collected on BMI, skinfolds, blood pressure, and lipid levels. BMI SDS increased significantly in both GH-treated groups to values not significantly different from zero. Skinfold values were not significantly different from pretreatment values, but were significantly lower than zero (P<0.001). Mean pretreatment systolic blood pressure SDS was significantly higher than zero, but over the course of 4 years GH treatment lowered to values not significantly different from zero. In contrast, mean pretreatment diastolic blood pressure SDS was significantly lower than zero, and over the course of GH treatment was lowered further. Total serum cholesterol, LDL-cholesterol, and the atherogenic index also decreased significantly. In this study, GH had a positive effect on height, lipid levels, and systolic blood pressure.[74]

Another study found that total serum cholesterol, LDL-cholesterol, and HDL-cholesterol levels significantly decreased after 6 yr of GH treatment (P<0.01). After discontinuation of GH, total cholesterol levels showed no change in both boys and girls, and LDL-cholesterol and HDL-cholesterol increased for girls only (P=0.01). Systolic and diastolic blood pressure also decreased significantly after 6 years of GH treatment (P<0.05, P<0.001, respectively).[77]

In conclusion, growth hormone therapy is an effective agent in increasing height for short children born small for gestational age. However, long-term follow-up studies are necessary to truly understand the effects of GH on the heart in this population.

Induced GH Deficiency

Radiation is an important tool in the treatment of several childhood cancers including Hodgkin's disease and leukemia. It is, however, associated with increased cardiovascular risk, particularly that of atherosclerosis, and induced hypothalamic-pituitary hormone insufficiency. While cardiotoxicity varies depending on concurrent chemotherapy and field of exposure, restrictive cardiomyopathy, systolic dysfunction, and atherosclerosis are common. Compared with controls, long-term survivors of childhood ALL who receive cranial radiation therapy show significantly higher fat mass and lower lean body mass and elevated circulating levels of insulin, glucose, LDL-cholesterol, apolipoprotein (Apo) B, triglycerides, fibrinogen, and leptin. [80] The peak GH response to stimulus of 44 GH deficient survivors of childhood ALL was negatively correlated to total body fat mass (r = -0.48, P = 0.001) and waist to hip ratio (r = -0.32, P = 0.03) years after treatment. [80] These data suggest that cranial radiotherapy has a lasting impact on the hypothalamic-pituitary axis which translates to increased cardiac risk over the long-term.

Fortunately, GH replacement therapy appears to be successful in treating the cardiac and metabolic sequelae of cranial radiotherapy. Of 18 long-term survivors of childhood ALL that received cranial radiotherapy and subsequently developed GHD, all showed significant improvements in cardiac function following 2 years of GH treatment including increases in left ventricular mass index ($P = 0.06$), fractional shortening ($P = 0.03$), and ejection fraction ($P = 0.03$). Metabolic syndrome was reversed in 6 of 6 patients suggesting that while short-term treatment may yield changes in only anthropometric variables [81], longer treatment times may be needed to improve metabolic function.

Anthracycline chemotherapy is associated with progressive abnormalities of LV structure and function unrelated to induced GH deficiency.[82-85] As many as 65% of children treated for ALL with an anthracycline develop increased LV afterload attributable to reduced LV wall thickness, decreased contractility, or both at a mean of 6.4 years after the completion of chemotherapy.[85] Growth hormone therapy among 34 anthracycline-treated childhood cancer survivors produced transient improvements in cardiac function.[82] Left ventricular wall thickness and contractility were lower than the age adjusted mean (-1.38 SD and -1.08 SD, respectively) prior to GH therapy. While wall thickness increased during GH therapy (from -1.38 SD to -1.09 SD after 3 years of GH therapy) , the effect was lost shortly after GH therapy ended and continued to diminished over time (-1.50 SD at 1 year after therapy and -1.96 SD at 4 years). Further, increased thickness did not translate into functional gains; LV contractility remained depressed throughout treatment and follow-up (-1.08 SD before therapy and -1.88 SD 4 years post therapy).

Conclusion

Growth hormone is an effective treatment to restore growth velocity and to improve final height in diverse pediatric populations. Growth hormone therapy may also help to improve cardiovascular parameters in patients with Turner syndrome and isolated GH deficiency among others. GH effects such as improving lean body mass and decreasing percent body fat may also further improve overall cardiovascular risk profile. In pediatric patients with CMP and heart failure related to cancer treatment GH may delay progression, but will not alter the course of cardiac dysfunction. In all incidences, pediatric patients receiving GH therapy should be monitored carefully and treatment decision and monitoring should include a multidisciplinary medical team.

References

[1]   Bates, A.S., et al., The effect of hypopituitarism on life expectancy. *J. Clin. Endocrinol. Metab,* 1996. 81(3): p. 1169-72.

[2]   Rosen, T. and B.A. Bengtsson, Premature mortality due to cardiovascular disease in hypopituitarism. *Lancet,* 1990. 336(8710): p. 285-8.

[3]   Tomlinson, J.W., et al., Association between premature mortality and hypopituitarism. *The Lancet,* 2001. 357(9254): p. 425-431.

[4]   Bengtsson, B.A., et al., Epidemiology and long-term survival in acromegaly. A study of 166 cases diagnosed between 1955 and 1984. *Acta Med. Scand,* 1988. 223(4): p. 327-35.

[5]   Fazio, S., et al., A preliminary study of growth hormone in the treatment of dilated cardiomyopathy. *N. Engl. J. Med,* 1996. 334(13): p. 809-14.

[6]   Cuneo, R.C., et al., Cardiac failure responding to growth hormone. *Lancet,* 1989. 1(8642): p. 838-9.

[7]   Volterrani, M., et al., Haemodynamic effects of intravenous growth hormone in congestive heart failure. *Lancet,* 1997. 349(9058): p. 1067-8.

[8]   Yang, R., et al., Growth hormone improves cardiac performance in experimental heart failure. *Circulation,* 1995. 92(2): p. 262-7.

[9]   Moran, A.M., et al., Exogenous growth hormone: a new therapy for dilated cardiomyopathy. *Prog. Pediatr. Cardiol,* 2000. 12(1): p. 125-132.

[10] Mayoux, E., et al., Mechanical properties of rat cardiac skinned fibers are altered by chronic growth hormone hypersecretion. *Circ. Res,* 1993. 72(1): p. 57-64.

[11] Thuesen, L., et al., Increased myocardial contractility following growth hormone administration in normal man. An echocardiographic study. *Dan. Med. Bull,* 1988. 35(2): p. 193-6.

[12] Sacca, L., A. Cittadini, and S. Fazio, Growth hormone and the heart. *Endocr. Rev,* 1994. 15(5): p. 555-73.

[13] Ito, H., et al., Insulin-like growth factor-I induces hypertrophy with enhanced expression of muscle specific genes in cultured rat cardiomyocytes. *Circulation,* 1993. 87(5): p. 1715-21.

[14] Perrot, A., et al., Growth hormone treatment in dilated cardiomyopathy. *J. Card. Surg,* 2001. 16(2): p. 127-31.

[15] Fazio, S., et al., Growth hormone and heart performance. A novel mechanism of cardiac wall stress regulation in humans. *Eur. Heart J,* 1997. 18(2): p. 340-7.

[16] Cittadini, A., et al., Impaired cardiac performance in GH-deficient adults and its improvement after GH replacement. *Am. J. Physiol,* 1994. 267(2 Pt 1): p. E219-25.

[17] Duerr, R.L., et al., Cardiovascular effects of insulin-like growth factor-1 and growth hormone in chronic left ventricular failure in the rat. *Circulation,* 1996. 93(12): p. 2188-96.

[18] Duerr, R.L., et al., Insulin-like growth factor-1 enhances ventricular hypertrophy and function during the onset of experimental cardiac failure. *J. Clin. Invest,* 1995. 95(2): p. 619-27.

[19] Cittadini, A., et al., Growth hormone attenuates early left ventricular remodeling and improves cardiac function in rats with large myocardial infarction. *J. Am. Coll. Cardiol,* 1997. 29(5): p. 1109-16.

[20] Tajima, M., et al., Treatment with growth hormone enhances contractile reserve and intracellular calcium transients in myocytes from rats with postinfarction heart failure. *Circulation,* 1999. 99(1): p. 127-34.

[21] Houck, W.V., et al., Effects of growth hormone supplementation on left ventricular morphology and myocyte function with the development of congestive heart failure. *Circulation,* 1999. 100(19): p. 2003-9.

[22] Omerovic, E., et al., Growth hormone improves bioenergetics and decreases catecholamines in postinfarct rat hearts. *Endocrinology,* 2000. 141(12): p. 4592-9.

[23] Amato, G., et al., Body composition, bone metabolism, and heart structure and function in growth hormone (GH)-deficient adults before and after GH replacement therapy at low doses. *J. Clin. Endocrinol. Metab,* 1993. 77(6): p. 1671-6.

[24] Merola, B., et al., Cardiac structural and functional abnormalities in adult patients with growth hormone deficiency. *J. Clin. Endocrinol. Metab,* 1993. 77(6): p. 1658-61.

[25] Isgaard, J., et al., A placebo-controlled study of growth hormone in patients with congestive heart failure. *Eur. Heart J,* 1998. 19(11): p. 1704-11.

[26] Spallarossa, P., et al., Evaluation of growth hormone administration in patients with chronic heart failure secondary to coronary artery disease. *Am. J. Cardiol,* 1999. 84(4): p. 430-3.

[27] Osterziel, K.J., et al., Randomised, double-blind, placebo-controlled trial of human recombinant growth hormone in patients with chronic heart failure due to dilated cardiomyopathy. *Lancet,* 1998. 351(9111): p. 1233-7.

[28] Smit, J.W., et al., Six months of recombinant human GH therapy in patients with ischemic cardiac failure does not influence left ventricular function and mass. *J. Clin. Endocrinol. Metab,* 2001. 86(10): p. 4638-43.

[29] Ibe, W., et al., Cardiomyocyte apoptosis is related to left ventricular dysfunction and remodelling in dilated cardiomyopathy, but is not affected by growth hormone treatment. *Eur. J. Heart Fail,* 2007. 9(2): p. 160-7.

[30] Le Corvoisier, P., et al., Cardiac effects of growth hormone treatment in chronic heart failure: A meta-analysis. *J. Clin. Endocrinol. Metab,* 2007. 92(1): p. 180-5.

[31] Fazio, S., et al., Effects of growth hormone on exercise capacity and cardiopulmonary performance in patients with chronic heart failure. *J. Clin. Endocrinol. Metab,* 2007. 92(11): p. 4218-23.

[32] Mital, S., et al., Effects of growth hormone therapy in children after cardiac transplantation. *J. Heart Lung Transplant,* 2006. 25(7): p. 772-7.

[33] Salerno, M., et al., Improvement of cardiac performance and cardiovascular risk factors in children with GH deficiency after two years of GH replacement therapy: an observational, open, prospective, case-control study. *J. Clin. Endocrinol. Metab,* 2006. 91(4): p. 1288-95.

[34] Lanes, R., et al., Endothelial function, carotid artery intima-media thickness, epicardial adipose tissue, and left ventricular mass and function in growth hormone-deficient adolescents: apparent effects of growth hormone treatment on these parameters. *J. Clin. Endocrinol. Metab,* 2005. 90(7): p. 3978-82.

[35] Salerno, M., et al., Left ventricular mass and function in children with GH deficiency before and during 12 months GH replacement therapy. *Clin. Endocrinol. (Oxf),* 2004. 60(5): p. 630-6.

[36] Minczykowski, A., et al., The influence of growth hormone (GH) therapy on cardiac performance in patients with childhood onset GH deficiency. Growth Horm IGF Res, 2005. 15(2): p. 156-64.

[37] Lanes, R., et al., Cardiac mass and function, carotid artery intima-media thickness, and lipoprotein levels in growth hormone-deficient adolescents. *J. Clin. Endocrinol. Metab,* 2001. 86(3): p. 1061-5.

[38] Matura, L.A., et al., Aortic dilatation and dissection in Turner syndrome. *Circulation,* 2007. 116(15): p. 1663-70.

[39] Price, W.H., et al., Mortality ratios, life expectancy, and causes of death in patients with Turner's syndrome. *J. Epidemiol. Community Health,* 1986. 40(2): p. 97-102.

[40] Saenger, P., Turner's syndrome. *N. Engl. J. Med*, 1996. 335(23): p. 1749-54.

[41] Elsheikh, M., et al., Hypertension is a major risk factor for aortic root dilatation in women with Turner's syndrome. *Clin. Endocrinol.* (Oxf), 2001. 54(1): p. 69-73.

[42] Ostberg, J.E., et al., A comparison of echocardiography and magnetic resonance imaging in cardiovascular screening of adults with Turner syndrome. *J. Clin. Endocrinol. Metab*, 2004. 89(12): p. 5966-71.

[43] Rosenfeld, R.G., et al., Six-year results of a randomized, prospective trial of human growth hormone and oxandrolone in Turner syndrome. *J. Pediatr*, 1992. 121(1): p. 49-55.

[44] Stephure, D.K., Impact of growth hormone supplementation on adult height in turner syndrome: results of the Canadian randomized controlled trial. *J. Clin. Endocrinol. Metab*, 2005. 90(6): p. 3360-6.

[45] Gravholt, C.H., et al., Short-term growth hormone treatment in girls with Turner syndrome decreases fat mass and insulin sensitivity: a randomized, double-blind, placebo-controlled, crossover study. *Pediatrics*, 2002. 110(5): p. 889-96.

[46] Ari, M., et al., The effects of growth hormone treatment on bone mineral density and body composition in girls with turner syndrome. *J. Clin. Endocrinol. Metab*, 2006. 91(11): p. 4302-5.

[47] Davenport, M.L., et al., Growth hormone treatment of early growth failure in toddlers with Turner syndrome: a randomized, controlled, multicenter trial. *J. Clin. Endocrinol. Metab*, 2007. 92(9): p. 3406-16.

[48] Sas, T.C., et al., The effects of long-term growth hormone treatment on cardiac left ventricular dimensions and blood pressure in girls with Turner's syndrome. Dutch Working Group on Growth Hormone. *J. Pediatr*, 1999. 135(4): p. 470-6.

[49] Matura, L.A., et al., Growth hormone treatment and left ventricular dimensions in Turner syndrome. *J. Pediatr*, 2007. 150(6): p. 587-91.

[50] Bondy, C.A., et al., Growth hormone treatment and aortic dimensions in Turner syndrome. *J. Clin. Endocrinol. Metab*, 2006. 91(5): p. 1785-8.

[51] Noordam, C., et al., Growth hormone treatment in children with Noonan's syndrome: four year results of a partly controlled trial. *Acta Paediatr*, 2001. 90(8): p. 889-94.

[52] van den Berg, J., et al., Aortic distensibility and dimensions and the effects of growth hormone treatment in the turner syndrome. *Am. J. Cardiol*, 2006. 97(11): p. 1644-9.

[53] Sybert, V.P., Cardiovascular malformations and complications in Turner syndrome. *Pediatrics*, 1998. 101(1): p. E11.

[54] Kelnar, C.J., Growth hormone therapy in noonan syndrome. *Horm. Res*, 2000. 53 Suppl 1: p. 77-81.

[55] MacFarlane, C.E., et al., Growth hormone therapy and growth in children with Noonan's syndrome: results of 3 years' follow-up. *J. Clin. Endocrinol. Metab*, 2001. 86(5): p. 1953-6.

[56] Cotterill, A.M., et al., The short-term effects of growth hormone therapy on height velocity and cardiac ventricular wall thickness in children with Noonan's syndrome. *J. Clin. Endocrinol. Metab*, 1996. 81(6): p. 2291-7.

[57] Brown, D.C., et al., Growth hormone therapy in Noonan's syndrome: non-cardiomyopathic congenital heart disease does not adversely affect growth improvement. *J. Pediatr. Endocrinol. Metab*, 2002. 15(6): p. 851-2.

[58] Osio, D., et al., Improved final height with long-term growth hormone treatment in Noonan syndrome. *Acta Paediatr*, 2005. 94(9): p. 1232-7.

[59] Walton-Betancourth, S., et al., Excellent growth response to growth hormone therapy in a child with PTPN11-negative Noonan syndrome and features of growth hormone resistance. *J. Endocrinol. Invest*, 2007. 30(5): p. 439-41.

[60] Kirk, J.M., et al., Short stature in Noonan syndrome: response to growth hormone therapy. *Arch Dis. Child*, 2001. 84(5): p. 440-3.

[61] Sznajer, Y., et al., The spectrum of cardiac anomalies in Noonan syndrome as a result of mutations in the PTPN11 gene. *Pediatrics,* 2007. 119(6): p. e1325-31.

[62] Noordam, C., et al., Effects of growth hormone treatment on left ventricular dimensions in children with Noonan's syndrome. *Horm. Res*, 2001. 56(3-4): p. 110-3.

[63] Angulo, M., et al., Growth hormone secretion and effects of growth hormone therapy on growth velocity and weight gain in children with Prader-Willi syndrome. *J. Pediatr. Endocrinol. Metab*, 1996. 9(3): p. 393-400.

[64] Patel, S., et al., Characteristics of cardiac and vascular structure and function in Prader-Willi syndrome. *Clin. Endocrinol.* (Oxf), 2007. 66(6): p. 771-7.

[65] Kuramochi, Y., et al., Cardiac tamponade due to systemic lupus erythematosus in patient with Prader-Willi syndrome after growth hormone therapy. *Lupus,* 2007. 16(6): p. 447-9.

[66] Lamb, A.S. and W.M. Johnson, Premature coronary artery atherosclerosis in a patient with Prader-Willi syndrome. *Am. J. Med. Genet*, 1987. 28(4): p. 873-80.

[67] Hoybye, C., et al., Growth hormone treatment improves body composition in adults with Prader-Willi syndrome. *Clin. Endocrinol.* (Oxf), 2003. 58(5): p. 653-61.

[68] Myers, S.E., et al., Sustained benefit after 2 years of growth hormone on body composition, fat utilization, physical strength and agility, and growth in Prader-Willi syndrome. *J. Pediatr,* 2000. 137(1): p. 42-9.

[69] Marzullo, P., et al., Conditional cardiovascular response to growth hormone therapy in adult patients with Prader-Willi syndrome. *J. Clin. Endocrinol. Metab*, 2007. 92(4): p. 1364-71.

[70] l'Allemand, D., et al., Cardiovascular risk factors improve during 3 years of growth hormone therapy in Prader-Willi syndrome. *Eur. J. Pediatr,* 2000. 159(11): p. 835-42.

[71] Willemsen, R.H., et al., Long-term GH treatment is not associated with disadvantageous changes of inflammatory markers and adipocytokines in children born small for gestational age. *Clin. Endocrinol.* (Oxf), 2007.

[72] Barker, D.J., et al., Type 2 (non-insulin-dependent) diabetes mellitus, hypertension and hyperlipidaemia (syndrome X): relation to reduced fetal growth. *Diabetologia*, 1993. 36(1): p. 62-7.

[73] Cutfield, W.S., et al., Reduced insulin sensitivity during growth hormone therapy for short children born small for gestational age. *J. Pediatr*, 2003. 142(2): p. 113-6.

[74] Sas, T., P. Mulder, and A. Hokken-Koelega, Body composition, blood pressure, and lipid metabolism before and during long-term growth hormone (GH) treatment in

children with short stature born small for gestational age either with or without GH deficiency. *J. Clin. Endocrinol. Metab*, 2000. 85(10): p. 3786-92.

[75] Van Pareren, Y., et al., Adult height after long-term, continuous growth hormone (GH) treatment in short children born small for gestational age: results of a randomized, double-blind, dose-response GH trial. *J. Clin. Endocrinol. Metab*, 2003. 88(8): p. 3584-90.

[76] Sas, T., et al., Carbohydrate metabolism during long-term growth hormone treatment in children with short stature born small for gestational age. *Clin. Endocrinol.* (Oxf), 2001. 54(2): p. 243-51.

[77] van Pareren, Y., et al., Effect of discontinuation of growth hormone treatment on risk factors for cardiovascular disease in adolescents born small for gestational age. *J. Clin. Endocrinol. Metab*, 2003. 88(1): p. 347-53.

[78] Willemsen, R.H., et al., Effect of growth hormone therapy on serum adiponectin and resistin levels in short, small-for-gestational-age children and associations with cardiovascular risk parameters. *J. Clin. Endocrinol. Metab*, 2007. 92(1): p. 117-23.

[79] Ibanez, L., et al., Neutrophil count in small-for-gestational age children: contrasting effects of metformin and growth hormone therapy. *J. Clin. Endocrinol. Metab*, 2005. 90(6): p. 3435-9.

[80] Link, K., et al., Growth hormone deficiency predicts cardiovascular risk in young adults treated for acute lymphoblastic leukemia in childhood. *J. Clin. Endocrinol. Metab*, 2004. 89(10): p. 5003-12.

[81] Follin, C., et al., Improvement in cardiac systolic function and reduced prevalence of metabolic syndrome after two years of growth hormone (GH) treatment in GH-deficient adult survivors of childhood-onset acute lymphoblastic leukemia. *J. Clin. Endocrinol. Metab*, 2006. 91(5): p. 1872-5.

[82] Lipshultz, S.E., et al., Cardiac changes associated with growth hormone therapy among children treated with anthracyclines. *Pediatrics*, 2005. 115(6): p. 1613-22.

[83] Lipshultz, S.E., et al., Late cardiac effects of doxorubicin therapy for acute lymphoblastic leukemia in childhood. *N. Engl. J. Med*, 1991. 324(12): p. 808-15.

[84] Lipshultz, S.E., et al., Female sex and drug dose as risk factors for late cardiotoxic effects of doxorubicin therapy for childhood cancer. *N. Engl. J. Med*, 1995. 332(26): p. 1738-43.

[85] Lipshultz, S.E., et al., Chronic progressive cardiac dysfunction years after doxorubicin therapy for childhood acute lymphoblastic leukemia. *J. Clin. Oncol*, 2005. 23(12): p. 2629-36.

In: Handbook of Cardiovascular Research   ISBN 978-1-60741-792-7
Editors: Jorgen Brataas and Viggo Nanstveit   © 2009 Nova Science Publishers, Inc.

Chapter XII

Oxytocin and Cardiovascular System[*]

Hossein Pournajafi-Nazarloo[†], Maryam Esmaeilzadeh,
Habibollah Saadat and C. Sue Carter
Brain-Body Center, College of Medicine, University of Illinois at Chicago,
Chicago, IL 60612, USA

Introduction

The neurohypophysial hormone oxytocin (OT) was the first peptide hormone to be chemically synthesized in biologically active form [1]. OT is synthesized primarily in magnocellular neurons in the paraventricular and supraoptic nuclei of the hypothalamus. It is also produced in peripheral tissues [2], including the heart [3]. In addition to OT effects on reproductive functions and induction of maternal behavior, it is involved in endocrine and neuroendocrine regulation of the heart, vasculature, and kidneys [4-6]. It has been reported that OT acts via neuroendocrine-endocrine-paracrine pathways to regulate blood volume via its natriuretic properties and to modulate blood pressure by stimulating the release of atrial natriuretic peptide (ANP) [4, 6]. In addition, it was demonstrated that in isolated, perfused hearts, an OT antagonist (OTA) blocks basal ANP release [4]. ANP induces vasorelaxation of coronary arteries, inhibition of L-type Ca^{2+} channels in the myocardium, and suppression of the renin-angiotensin system [7]. These effects are recognized as being protective to the cardiovascular system and are also induced by estrogen [8]. Empirical studies suggest that OT may affect or regulate the function of the heart through several different mechanisms.

OT stimulates release of nitric oxide (NO) from human umbilical vein endothelial cells in culture [5]. These findings have led to the suggestion that OT may be an important mediator of vascular function [9]. NO is synthesized from L-arginine in an enzymatic reaction

---

[*]   A version of this chapter was also published in *Leading-Edge Messenger RNA Research Communications,* edited by Martin H. Ostrovskiy published by Nova Science Publishers, Inc. It was submitted for appropriate modifications in an effort to encourage wider dissemination of research

[†] Address Correspondence to: Hossein Pournajafi-Nazarloo, M.D., Ph.D. Brain-Body Center, College of Medicine, University of Illinois at Chicago, 1601 W. Taylor St., Chicago, Illinois 60612, USA. Phone No.; (312) 996-3348. Fax No.; (312) 413-4544. Email; nazarloo@uic.edu.

catalyzed by nitric oxide synthase (NOS) [10]. Three different isoforms of NOS catalyze the oxidation of L-arginine to citrulline and NO: endothelial (eNOS), neuronal (nNOS), and inducible (iNOS) NOS. Myocardial eNOS appears to be important under physiologic conditions in pregnancy, where it is involved in cardiac hypertrophy [11].

Estrogen (E) stimulates NOS in various organs, including cardiac tissue, in association with an increase of cyclic guanosine monophosphate (cGMP) [12], the second messenger of NO. Recent observations suggest that E's effects in vascular cells, and possibly in the myocardium, depend on the relative expression of alpha and beta estrogen receptors (ERα and ERβ) [13]. Interactions between OT and E have been reported in several systems. In MCF7 breast cancer cell lines treatment with OT inhibited the ability of E to stimulate mitosis [14]. OT treatment had a number of effects on ERα in the MCF7 cell line, including changes in the production of ERα mRNA, binding affinity, and ERα transcriptional activity [15].

In rats, neonatal treatment with OT produced marked changes in weight and responses to pain [16] and placental and fetal growth during pregnancy as adults [17]. In prairie voles, a single treatment on the day of birth with OT or OTA affected partner preference formation, aggression and reproductive competency in adults [18-20]. In addition, a single injection of OT or OTA on the day of birth produced a significant increase in OT immunoreactivity in the brain by postnatal day 21 [21].

Based on previous studies from our laboratory and others showing that neonatal exposure to exogenous OT can have long-term effects on the subsequent expression of adult behavior and physiology [16-19, 21, 22], we used female and male rats, in an attempt to define the possible role of OTR, ANP, NOS and ERs during the early postnatal effects of OT on the heart, animals were treated with OT or OTA on the day of birth and the mRNAs expression for OTR, ANP, iNOS, eNOS, ERα and ERβ in postnatal day 1 (D1) and day 21 (D21) rats were measured utilizing real time reverse transcription-polymerase chain reaction (RT-PCR) [23]. We have also used female and male prairie voles to define the possible role of OTR and ERs during the early postnatal effects of OT on the heart. The animals were treated with OT or OTA on the day of birth and the mRNAs expression for OTR, ERα and ERβ in postnatal day 1 (D1), postnatal day 8 (D8) and day 21 (D21) were measured [24].

Modulation of Oxytocin Receptor, Atrial Natriuretic Peptide, Nitric Oxide Synthase and Estrogen Receptor Mrnas Expression in Rat

Effect of OT Injection on Cardiac OTR mRNA

We examined the possible involvement of cardiac OTR mRNA expression in the OT actions on the heart in postnatal D1 and D21 female and male rats. The results indicated that OTR mRNA expression can be modulated by OT exposure in early postnatal life. In addition to the potential effects of OT on cardiac development we also found that there were significant changes in the expression of mRNA for OTR from the day of birth until weaning on D21.

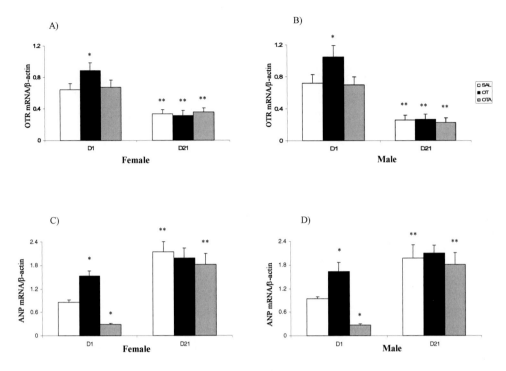

Figure 1. Effect of neonatal treatment with SAL, OT or OTA on heart OTR (A, B) and ANP (C, D) mRNAs expression on postnatal day 1 or 21 in female and male rats. Data represent the mean ± SEM (n=5). * represents significant alteration at p<0.05, when compared to SAL groups within the same age and sex, ** represents significant alteration at p<0.01, when compared to D1 groups within the same treatment and sex. Reproduced [23] with permission from Elsevier.

In this study we observed an age-dependent decline in cardiac OTR mRNA expression in female and male rats, suggesting that cardiac OTR may be functional in the fetal life. The importance of the OT system during rodents development was validated by a study showing that OT and OTR are expressed in the fetal rat heart and decrease to relatively low levels in adulthood [25]. These findings suggest that cardiac OT may be functional in fetal life, in contrast to low OT synthesis [26] and the low concentration of biologically active OT in the hypothalamus [25]. It might be speculated that OT production in the heart during fetal life and early maturation may supplement low OT production in hypothalamic nuclei. This hypothesis is supported by high plasma OT levels in newborn rats that exceed those of adult rats [27]. We found that early neonatal OT administration caused a significant increase in cardiac OTR mRNA expression of postnatal D1 female and male rats, and OTA treatment elicited no changes in cardiac OT receptors mRNA expression, suggesting that OTR may be one factor that mediates the effects of OT on the cardiovascular system in early life (Figure 1A, B). This is in agreement with a previous study in which P19 embryonic carcinoma cells, a model of mouse embryonic stem cells, express OT receptors, and OT stimulates the differentiation of these cells [28]. It was reported that isolated rat heart perfusion with OT induced significant bradycardia [4]. Perfusion of isolated rat hearts with OT results in a dose-dependent negative chronotropic effect while exerting a positive inotropic effect [29].

Further, it was reported that perfusion with OTA alone did not have any effect on heart rate and force of contraction. However, co-administration with OTA completely inhibited the effects of OT on beating rate and force, which suggested that these effects are mediated by OT receptors [30].

Oxytocin receptors in the heart may be localized on intrinsic cholinergic neurons, and upon activation, they release acetylcholine (ACh) to decrease heart rate and force of contraction [30]. Oxytocin may act in an autocrine/paracrine manner to modulate the release of ACh from intrinsic cardiac cholinergic neurons [30], to clarify the OTR localization. It has been shown that stimulation of oxytocin receptors leads to elevation of intracellular Ca^{2+}. Increased Ca^{2+} stimulate cellular exocytosis [31] and also stimulate ANP secretion by the heart [32].

Effect of OT Injection on Cardiac ANP mRNA Expression

Because ANP transcription changes during maturation, we have investigated ANP mRNA expression in early postnatal life (D1) and at weaning (D21) in female and male rats. We found that OT administration to female and male rats on the first day of life caused a significant increase in cardiac ANP mRNA expression on postnatal D1 in both sexes, suggesting that ANP may play a role on the effects of OT in rat heart (Figure 1C, D). Haanwinckel and collaborators have shown that OT administration in rats promotes an increase in ANP plasma levels [6]. In our study neonatal treatment with OTA decreased basal ANP mRNA expression. Several studies have demonstrated that perfusion of isolated rat hearts with OT stimulates ANP release, and an OT receptor antagonist after prolonged perfusion decreases the OT-induced ANP release below that of control hearts [3, 4, 9].

Taken together, our results, and others in which OTA attenuates ANP release, suggest the presence of an intracardiac oxytocinergic system controlling basal ANP release. OT may contribute to the natriuretic action via stimulation of ANP release. Presumably, blood volume expansion via baroreceptor input to the brain causes the release of OT that circulates to the heart. OT-induced ANP release in the heart may be achieved after activation of OT receptors and subsequent elevation of intracellular $[Ca^{2+}]$, which in turn could stimulate exocytosis and ANP secretion [3]. ANP then exerts a negative chrono- and inotropic effect via activation of guanylyl cyclase and release of cGMP [3].

Effect of OT Injection on Cardiac NOS mRNA Expression

We have also measured rat heart iNOS and eNOS mRNAs expression in different ages and sexes. We found no changes in cardiac iNOS mRNA expression, but a significant increase in cardiac eNOS mRNA expression following OT treatment and a significant decrease after OTA treatment in female and male postnatal day 1 rats, suggesting that OTR may play a role in OT-induced eNOS mRNA expression in heart (Figure 2).

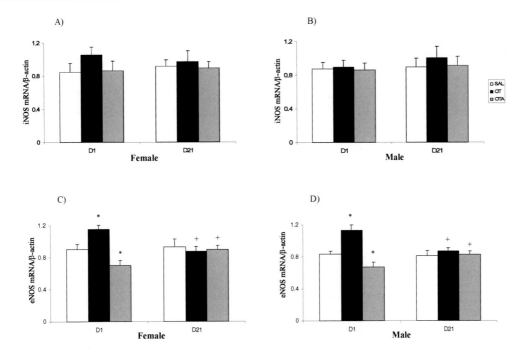

Figure 2. Effect of neonatal treatment with SAL, OT or OTA on heart iNOS (A, B) and eNOS (C, D) mRNAs expression on postnatal day 1 or 21 in female and male rats. Data represent the mean ± SEM (n=5). * represents significant alteration at p<0.05, when compared to SAL groups within the same age and sex, + represents significant alteration at p<0.05, when compared to D1 groups within the same treatment and sex. Reproduced [23] with permission from Elsevier.

In a study using isolated right atria, it was shown that oxytocin effects on beating rate and force of contraction are totally blocked by the muscarinic blocking drug atropine [27]. Because atropine suppresses transmission from the postganglionic fiber to the cardiac effecter cells, these results imply that oxytocin may primarily act on oxytocin receptors present on parasympathetic postganglionic fibers to stimulate the release of acetylcholine, which consequently acts on muscarinic receptors and results in lower rate and force of contraction. Activation of cardiac muscarinic receptors may influence cardiac functions through regulation of the activity of several ion channels. Muscarinic receptor activation inhibits cardiac L-type calcium channel through interaction with G Proteins [33]. This inhibition is mediated in part via activation of NO synthase and generation of NO, which stimulates soluble guanylyl cyclase to produce cGMP [34], subsequent activation of cGMP-dependent protein kinase G, and dephosphorylation of potassium and calcium channel proteins. We have shown that neonatal OT treatment caused a significant increase in cardiac OTR and eNOS mRNAs expression on postnatal D1. OT-induced activation of OTR would generate NO that would activate guanylyl cyclase, leading to production of cGMP that would dilate the vascular smooth muscle [35], suggesting that the physiological action of OT is vasodilatory and its action is mediated by OT receptors.

It seems that different mechanisms and/or factors may be involved differentially in the effects of OT on the heart.

Effect of OT Injection on Cardiac Estrogen Receptors mRNA Expression

Because of the abundance of estrogen receptors on the heart in rats [36] and the presence of estrogen receptors in myocytes secreting ANP [37], it was hypothesized that estrogen induces ANP synthesis and release from the heart through an ER-dependent mechanism. Since interactions between OT and estrogen have been reported in several systems, we also investigated ERα and ERβ mRNAs expression in early postnatal life and in juvenile female and male rats. Utilizing Real Time PCR analysis, we found that ERs are developmentally regulated in the rat heart. We observed that ERα expression rises from low levels on postnatal D1, whereas ERβ mRNA decreases by postnatal D21 in the rat heart, suggesting a specific role for both receptors in heart maturation (Figure 3).

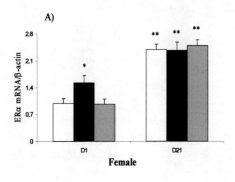
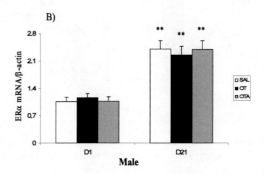

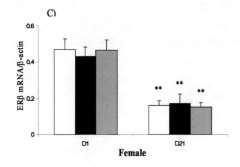
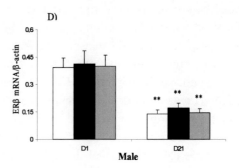

Figure 3. Effect of neonatal treatment with SAL, OT or OTA on heart ERα (A, B) and ERβ (C, D) mRNAs expression on postnatal day 1 or 21 in female and male rats. Data represent the mean ± SEM (n=5). * represents significant alteration at $p<0.05$, when compared to SAL groups within the same age and sex, ** represents significant alteration at $p<0.01$, when compared to D1 groups within the same treatment and sex. Reproduced [23] with permission from Elsevier.

These results are in agreement with previous study in which high ERβ expression was observed in the newborn heart and at 4 days of postnatal life [38], when extensive hyperplasia of the rat heart occurs and the heart grows more rapidly than the body [29]. In adult rats, ERβ expression is low, in contrast to relatively high ERα mRNA levels. Age-dependent increases in ERα suggest that this receptor plays a role in heart maturation. We found no changes in cardiac ERβ mRNA expression, but a significant increase in cardiac ERα mRNA expression following OT treatment only in females on postnatal day 1, suggesting that ERα mRNAs expression can be modulated by OT exposure in early postnatal life, and this modulation is sexually dimorphic. Additional studies will be required to determine the mechanisms of differential modulation of ERs mRNA across age and sex in response to neonatal OT manipulation. Moreover, since maternal OT sharply rises during labor, this OT elevation might modulate expression of OTR, ERs or NOS mRNAs in the neonatal rat heart. Perhaps due to the short time effect of OT on gene expression in the neonatal heart, we could not detect the possible modulation of these mRNAs expression in our studies. However, additional studies will be required also to evaluate the possible effect of maternal OT on the neonatal cardiovascular system.

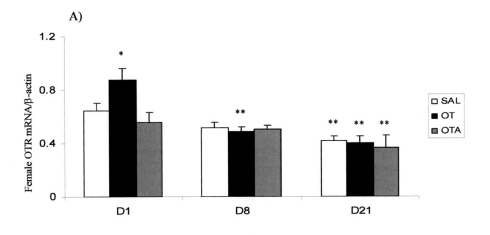

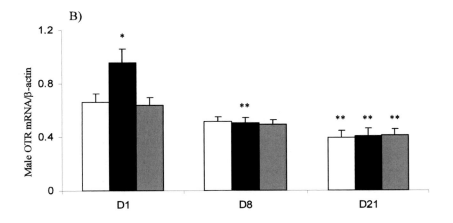

Figure 4. Effect of neonatal treatment with OT or OTA on heart OTR mRNA expression on postnatal day 1, 8 or 21 in female (A) and male (B) prairie voles. Data represent means ± SEM (n=5). * represents significant alteration at $p<0.05$, when compared to SAL groups within the same age and sex; ** represents significant alteration at $p<0.01$, when compared to D1 animals within the same treatment and sex. Reproduced [24] with permission from Springer.

Modulation of Cardiac Oxytocin Receptor and Estrogen Receptor Alpha mRNAs Expression Following Neonatal Oxytocin Treatment in Prairie Vole

We have also used as a model the prairie vole *(Microtus ochrogaster)*. This socially monogamous species exhibits behavioral characteristics that are similar to humans, including an active engagement in and reliance on the social environment, the formation of male-female pair bonds, display of biparental care, and a tendency to live in extended families [22, 39, 40]. In addition, recent evidence indicates remarkable parallels in mechanisms responsible for cardiovascular function in prairie voles and humans. For example, the neural control of the heart in prairie voles, as in humans, is strongly influenced by parasympathetic activity [41] and is highly sensitive to chronic isolation, as well as acute social stressors [42].

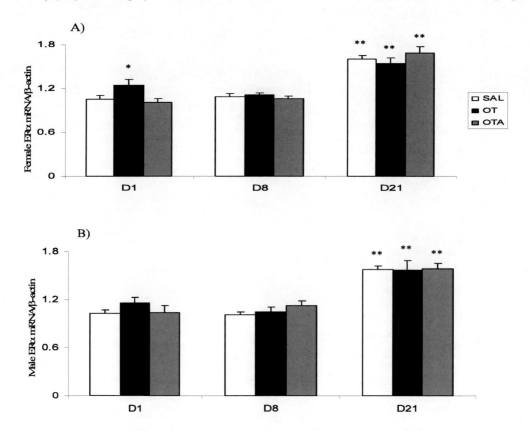

Figure 5. Effect neonatal treatment with OT or OTA on cardiac ERα mRNA expression on postnatal day 1, 8 or 21 in female (A) and male (B) prairie voles. Data represent means ± SEM (n=5). * represents significant alteration at p<0.05, when compared to SAL group within the same age and sex; ** represents significant alteration at p<0.01, when compared to D1 and D8 animals within the same treatment and sex. Reproduced [24] with permission from Springer.

In this study we examined the possible involvement of cardiac OTR, ERα and ERβ mRNAs expression in the neonatal OT actions on the heart of postnatal D1, D8 and D21 female and male prairie voles. The results indicated that OTR mRNA expression (Figure 4) and ERα mRNA expression (Figure 5) can be modulated by OT exposure in early postnatal life and this modulation is sexually dimorphic for ERα mRNA expression, with OT effects seen only in females. In addition to the potential effects of OT on cardiac development, we also found that there were significant changes in the expression of mRNAs for OTR, ERα and ERβ between D1 and D21. We observed that the basal level of heart OTR mRNA expression was significantly decreased by postnatal day 21, suggesting that cardiac OTR may be particularly functional in the fetal life, playing a lesser role as the animals develop (Figure 4). We found that OT administration caused a significant increase in heart OTR mRNA on D1, but not on D8 and D21, and OTA treatment elicited no changes in heart OTR mRNA expression, suggesting that OTR may mediates the effects of OT on the cardiovascular system in early life. Utilizing RT-PCR analysis, we found that ERs are developmentally regulated in the prairie vole heart. We observed that ERα expression rises from low levels on postnatal D1, whereas ERβ mRNA decreases by postnatal D21, suggesting a specific role for both receptors in heart maturation (Figure 6). We also found that OT administration on the first day of life caused a significant increase in heart ERα, but not in ERβ mRNA expression, and OTA treatment elicited no changes in heart ERs mRNAs expression, suggesting that ERα may be involved in the effects of OT on the cardiovascular system.

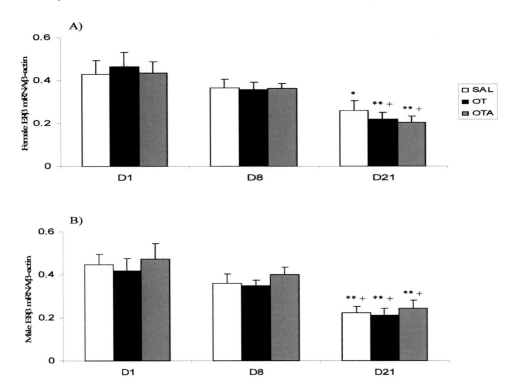

Figure 6. Effect neonatal treatment with OT or OTA on heart ER□ mRNA expression on postnatal day 1, 8 or 21 in female (A) and male (B) prairie voles. Data represent means ± SEM (n=5). * and ** represent significant alteration at p<0.05 and p<0.01, respectively, when compared to D1 animals within the same treatment and sex; + represents significant alteration at p<0.05, when compared to D8 animals within the same treatment and sex. Reproduced [24] with permission from Springer.

Summary and Conclusions

In summary, we have investigated the effect of early postnatal OT manipulation on cardiac OTR, ANP, iNOS, eNOS and ERs mRNAs expression in neonatal or juvenile female and male rats. We have also investigated the effect of early postnatal OT manipulation on cardiac OTR and ERs mRNAs expression in neonatal or juvenile female and male prairie voles. We observed that cardiac OTR, ANP, eNOS and ERα mRNAs expression can be modulated by OT exposure in early postnatal life and this modulation is sexually dimorphic for ERα mRNA expression. Additional studies will be required to determine the mechanisms of differential modulation of ERs mRNA across age and sex in response to neonatal OT manipulation. Moreover, since maternal OT sharply rises during labor, this OT elevation might modulate expression of OTR, ERs or NOS mRNAs in the neonatal rat/prairie vole heart.

References

[1]   Du Vigneaud V, Ressler C, Trippett S. The sequence of amino acids in oxytocin, with a proposal for the structure of oxytocin. *J. Biol. Chem.* 1953;205:949–957.

[2]   Lefebvre DL, Giaid A, Bennett H, Lariviere R, Zingg HH. Oxytocin gene expression in rat uterus. *Science* 1992;256:1553–1555.

[3]   Jankowski M, Hajjar F, Al-Kawas S, Mukaddam-Daher S, Hoffman G, McCann S, Gutkowska J. Rat heart: a novel site of oxytocin production and action. *Proc. Nat. Acad. Sci. USA* 1998;95:14558 –14563.

[4]   Gutkowska J, Jankowski M, Lambert C, Mukaddam-Daher S, Zingg HH, McCann SM. Oxytocin releases atrial natriuretic peptide: evidence for oxytocin receptors in the heart. *Proc. Nat. Acad. Sci. USA* 1997;94:11704–11709.

[5]   Thibonnier M, Conarty DM, Preston JA, Plesnicher CL, Dweik RA, Erzurum SC. Human vascular endothelial cells express oxytocin receptors. *Endocrinology* 1999;140:1301–1309.

[6]   Haanwinckel MA, Elias Lk, Favaretto ALV, Gutkowska J, McCann SM, Antunes-Rodrigues J. Oxytocin mediates atrial natriuretic peptide release and natriuresis after volume expansion in the rat. *Proc. Nat. Acad. Sci. USA* 1995;92:7902–7906.

[7]   Tohse N, Nakaya H, Takeda Y, Kanno M. Cyclic GMP-mediated inhibition of L-type Ca2+ channel activity by human natriuretic peptide in rabbit heart cells. *Br. J. Pharmacol.* 1995;114:1076–1082.

[8]   Mendelsohn ME, Karas RH. The protective effects of estrogen on the cardiovascular system. *N. Engl. J. Med.* 1999;340:1801–1811.

[9]   Gutkowska J, Jankowski M, Mukaddam-Daher S, McCann SM. Oxytocin is a cardiovascular hormone. *Braz. J. Med. Biol. Res.* 2000;33:625– 33.

[10]   Palmer RM, Ashton DS, Moncada S. Vascular endothelial cells synthesize nitric oxide from L-arginine. *Nature* 1988;333:664–6.

[11] Trochu JN, Bouhour JB, Kaley G, Hintze TH. Role of endothelium-derived nitric oxide in the regulation of cardiac oxygen metabolism: implications in health and disease. *Circ. Res.* 2000;87:1108–1117.

[12] Weiner CP, Knowles RG, Moncada S. Induction of nitric oxide synthases early in pregnancy. *Am. J. Obstet. Gynecol.* 1994;171:838–843.

[13] Hodges YK, Tung L, Yan XD, Graham JD, Horwitz KB, Horwitz LD. Estrogen receptors alpha and beta: prevalence of estrogen receptor beta mRNA in human vascular smooth muscle and transcriptional effects. *Circulation* 2000;101:1792–1798.

[14] Cassoni P, Sapino A, Fortunati N, Munaron L, Chini B, Bussolati G. Oxytocin inhibits the proliferation of MDA-MB231 human breast-cancer cells via cyclic adenosine monophosphate and protein kinase A. *Int. J. Oncol.* 1997;72:340–344.

[15] Cassoni P, Catalano MG, Sapino A, Marrocco T, Fazzari A, Bussolati G, Fortunati N. Oxytocin modulates estrogen receptor alpha expression and function in MCF7 human breast cancer cells. *Int. J. Oncol.* 2002;21:375–378.

[16] Uvnas-Moberg K, Alster P, Petersson M, Sohlstrom A, Bjorkstrand E. Postnatal oxytocin injections cause sustained weight gain and increased nociceptive thresholds in male and female rats. *Ped. Res.* 1998;43:344–9.

[17] Sohlstrom A, Olausson H, Brismar K, Uvnas-Moberg K. Oxytocin treatment during early life influences reproductive performance in ad libitum fed and food-restricted female rats. *Biol. Neonate* 2002; 81:132– 8.

[18] Bales KL, Carter CS. Oxytocin facilitates parental care in female prairie voles (but not in males). *Horm. Behav.* 2002;41:456.

[19] Pfeifer L, Bales KL, Carter CS. Neonatal manipulation of oxytocin affects alloparental behavior in male prairie voles. *Horm. Behav.* 2001;39:344.

[20] Bales KL, Abdelnabi M, Carter CS. Neonatal injections affect reproductive parameters in male prairie voles. *Horm. Behav.* 2001;39:324.

[21] Yamamoto Y, Cushing BS, Kramer KM, Epperson P, Hoffman GE, Carter CS. Neonatal manipulations of oxytocin alter expression of oxytocin and vasopressin immunoreactive cells in the paraventricular nucleus of the hypothalamus in a gender specific manner. *Neuroscience* 2004;125:947–955.

[22] Carter CS. Developmental consequences of oxytocin. *Physiol. Behav.* 2003;79:383–397.

[23] Pournajafi Nazarloo H, Perry A, Partoo L, Papademetriou E, Azizi F, Carter, CS, Cushing B. Neonatal oxytocin treatment modulates oxytocin receptor, atrial natriuretic peptide, nitric oxide synthase and estrogen receptor mRNAs expression in rat heart. *Peptides* 2007;28:1170-7.

[24] Pournajafi Nazarloo H, Papademetriou E, Partoo L, Saadat H, Cushing B. Modulation of cardiac oxytocin receptor and estrogen receptor alpha mRNAs expression following neonatal oxytocin treatment. *Endocrine* 2007;31:154-60.

[25] Jankowski M, Danalache B, Wang D, Bhat P, Hajjar F, Marcinkiewicz M, Paquin J, McCann SM, Gutkowska J. Oxytocin in cardiac ontogeny. *Proc. Nat. Acad. Sci. USA* 2004;101:13074–13079.

[26] Almazan G, Lefebvre DL, Zingg HH. Ontogeny of hypothalamic vasopressin, oxytocin and somatostatin gene expression. *Dev. Brain Res.* 1989;45:69–75.

[27] Hartman RD, Rosella-Dampman LM, Emmert SE, Summy-Long JY. Ontogeny of opioid inhibition of vasopressin and oxytocin release in response to osmotic stimulation. *Endocrinology* 1986;119:1–11.

[28] Paquin J, Danalache BA, Jankowski M, McCann AM, Gutkowska J. Oxytocin induces differentiation of P19 embryonic stem cells to cardiomyocytes. *Proc. Nat. Acad. Sci. USA* 2002;99:9550-9555.

[29] Coulson CC, Thorp Jr JM, Mayer DC, Cefalo RC. Central hemodynamic effects of oxytocin and interaction with magnesium and pregnancy in the isolated perfused rat heart. *Am. J. Obstet. Gynecol.* 1997;177:91–93.

[30] Mukaddam-Daher S, Yin YL, Roy J, Gutkowska J, Cardinal R. Negative inotropic and chronotropic effects of oxytocin. *Hypertension* 2001;38:292–296.

[31] Knight DE, von Grafenstein H, Athayde CM. Calcium-dependent and calcium-independent exocytosis. *Trends Neurosci.* 1989;12:451–458.

[32] Ruskoaho H, Toth M, Lang RE. Atrial natriuretic peptide secretion: synergistic effect of phorbol ester and A23187. *Biochem. Biophys. Res. Commun.* 1985;133:581–8.

[33] Robishaw JD, Hansen CA. Structure and function of G proteins mediating signal transduction pathways in the heart. *Alcohol. Clin. Exp. Res.* 1994;18:115–120.

[34] Han X, Shimoni Y, Giles WR. A cellular mechanism for nitric oxidemediated cholinergic control of mammalian heart rate. *J. Gen. Physiol.* 1995;106:45– 65.

[35] Soares TJ, Coimbra TM, Martins AR, Pereira AG, Carnio EC, Branco LG, Albuquerque-Araujo WI, de Nucci G, Favaretto AL, Gutkowska J, McCann SM, Antunes-Rodrigues J. Atrial natriuretic peptide and oxytocin induce natriuresis by release of cGMP. *Proc. Natl. Acad. Sci. USA.* 1999;96:278-83.

[36] Stumpf WE, Sar M, Aumuller G. The heart: a target organ for estradiol. Science 1977;196:319–321.

[37] Back H, Forssmann WG, Stumpf WE. Atrial myoendocrine cells (cardiodilatin/atrial natriuretic polypeptide-containing myocardiocytes) are target cells for estradiol. *Cell Tissue Res.* 1989;255:673–674.

[38] Jankowski M, Rachelska G, Wang D, McCann SM, Gutkowska J. Estrogen receptors activate atrial natriuretic peptide in the rat heart. *Proc. Nat. Acad. Sci. USA* 2001;98:11765–11770.

[39] Carter CS, DeVries AC, Getz LL. Physiological substrates of mammalian monogamy: the prairie vole model. *Neurosci. Biobehav. Rev.* 1995;19:303-314.

[40] Keverne EB, Curley JP. Vasopressin, oxytocin and social behaviour. *Curr. Opin. Neurobiol.* 2004;14:777-83.

[41] Grippo AJ, Lamb DG, Carter CS, Porges SW. Cardiac regulation in the socially monogamous prairie vole. *Physiol. Behav.* 2007;90:386-93.

[42] Grippo AJ, Cushing BS, Carter CS. Depression-like behavior and stressor-induced neuroendocrine activation in female prairie voles exposed to chronic social isolation. *Psychosom. Med.* 2007; 69:149-57.

In: Handbook of Cardiovascular Research   ISBN 978-1-60741-792-7
Editors: Jorgen Brataas and Viggo Nanstveit   © 2009 Nova Science Publishers, Inc.

Chapter XIII

Diagnosis of Cardiomyopathies and Rare Diseases: From "Phenocopy" to "Genocopy" Era

Giuseppe Limongelli*, Giuseppe Pacileo, Paolo Calabro',
Alessandra Rea, Valeria Maddaloni,
Raffaella D'Alessandro and Raffaele Calabro'
Monaldi Hospital, Second University of Naples, Naples, Italy

Abstract

Cardiomyopathies represent an heterogeneous group of inherited diseases, characterized by different signs and symptoms, natural history, and clinical outcome. The genetic knowledge regarding this class of diseases is rapidly growing in the last two decades. The genetics of cardiomyopathies has born in 1989 with a single gene theory (identification of beta myosin mutations in hypertrophic cardiomyopathy: one gene=one disese), but the complexity and wide heterogeneity of the disease has moved toward a different direction (sarcomeric genes in hypertrophic cardiomyopathy: many genes=one diseases; beta myosin as disease causing for hypertrophic, dilated, restrictive and noncompaction cardiomyopathy: one gene=many diseases or genocopies). Elucidation of the molecular basis of cardiomyopathies has led to a categorization of the phenotypes according to their genetic etiology. The American Hearth Association and the European Society of Cardiology have recently proposed a different scheme of classification based on a distinction between primary (genetic, mixed, non genetic types) and secondary cardiomyopathies, or between the familial and non familial types, respectively. The possibility of a different approach of intervention (i.e. enzyme replacement therapy in metabolic cardiomyopathies) underlies the need to make an early and precise etiologic diagnosis.

---

* Address for Correspondence: Giuseppe Limongelli, Department of Cardiothoracic Sciences, Second University of Naples, Monaldi Hospital, Via L Bianchi, 80131, Naples, Italy. Email: limongelligiuseppe@libero.it, Work-phone:+390817062852, Mobile: +393381041147, FAX:+390817062683.

Family history, physical examination, electrocardiogram and non-invasive imaging techniques are the essential methods for a "first step" toward an etiologic diagnosis, followed by biochemical and, eventually, genetic investigations which can help the final discriminations between similar pathologic conditions (phenocopies).

Keywords: cardiomyopathies, phenocopy, genocopy, diagnosis, management

Introduction

Cardiomyopathies are diseases of heart muscle. They represent an important and heterogeneous group of diseases. The awareness of cardiomyopathies in both the public and medical communities historically has been impaired by persistent confusion surrounding definitions and nomenclature. However, many classifications offered in the literature and in textbooks are to some degree contradictory in presentation. For more than 30 years, the term "cardiomyopathies" has been used to describe disorders of the heart with particular morphological and physiological characteristics.

Old Classifications

In 1980, the World Health Organization (WHO) in defined cardiomyopathies as "heart muscle diseases of unknown cause," to distinguish cardiomyopathy (including: Hypertrophic cardiomyopathy, Dilated cardiomyopathy, and Restrictive cardiomyopathy) from cardiac dysfunction due to known diseases such as hypertension, ischemic heart disease, or valvular disease. Heart muscle disorders of known aetiology (eg, ischemic or hypertensive cardiomyopathy) were classified as secondary diseases [1].

In1995, the WHO/International Society and Federation of Cardiology (ISFC) Task Force on the Definition and Classification of the Cardiomyopathies expanded the classification to include all diseases affecting heart muscle and to take into consideration etiology as well as the dominant pathophysiology. Cardiomyopathies were defined as "diseases of the myocardium associated with cardiac dysfunction", and they were classified according to anatomy and physiology into the following four types: Hypertrophic cardiomyopathy, HCM; Dilated cardiomyopathy, DCM; Restrictive cardiomyopathy, RCM; Arrhythmogenic right ventricular cardiomyopathy, ARVC, and Unclassified cardiomyopathies. Cardiomyopathies that are associated with specific cardiac or systemic disorders generally fall into one of these categories. These include ischemic, valvular, hypertensive, inflammatory, toxic, mitochondrial, neuromuscular, metabolic, and inherited disorders (Figure 1) [2].

These disorders have been also indicated as "phenocopies". The term "specific cardiomyopathy" or "phenocopies" was probably the first important step toward a new classification, reflecting the fact that the genetic basis of the cardiomyopathies was being elucidated. Indeed, over the last two decades, clinical and molecular insights helped to better understand aetiology and management of cardiomyopathies. Many disorders considered before as "idiopathic" or "primary" disorders have been associated to specific genetic or non genetic defects, clinical features and outcome.

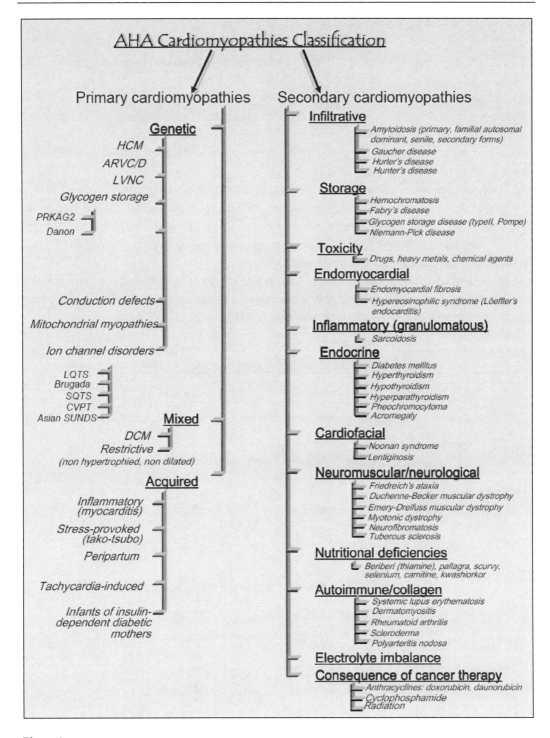

Figure 1.

The American Heart Association Classification

In 2006, an expert committee of the American Heart Association proposed the following definition of cardiomyopathies: "Cardiomyopathies are a heterogeneous group of diseases of the myocardium associated with mechanical and/or electrical dysfunction that usually (but not invariably) exhibit inappropriate ventricular hypertrophy or dilatation and are due to a variety of causes that frequently are genetic. Cardiomyopathies either are confined to the heart or are a part of generalized systemic disorders, often leading to cardiovascular death or progressive heart failure-related disability."

They also proposed a new scheme of classification, in which the term "primary" is used to describe diseases in which the heart is the sole or predominantly involved organ and "secondary" to describe diseases in which myocardial dysfunction is part of a systemic disorder. Primary cardiomyopathies have been sub-classified in genetic forms, mixed forms (genetic and non genetic), or acquired forms.

The main departure of the proposed AHA Scientific Statement definition from previous classifications is the inclusion of the ion channelopathies as primary cardiomyopathies, despite the absence of gross structural abnormalities (Figure 2) [3].

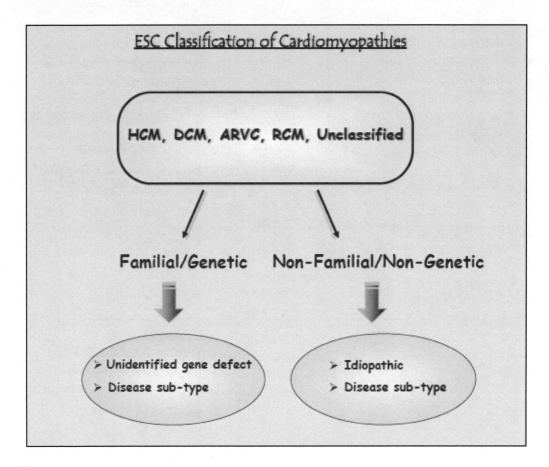

Figure 2.

The European Classification

In 2007, the Working Group on Myocardial and Pericardial Diseases of the European Society of Cardiology proposed an update of the WHO/ISFC classification, defining cardiomyopathy as: "A myocardial disorder in which the heart muscle is structurally and functionally abnormal in the absence of coronary artery disease, hypertension, valvular disease and congenital heart disease sufficient to explain the observed myocardial abnormality." Cardiomyopathies are grouped into specific morphological and functional phenotypes: each phenotype is then subclassified into familial/genetic and non-familial/non genetics forms. Like the 2006 AHA proposal, it focuses on the established morphological distinctions (hypertrophic cardiomyopathy, dilated cardiomyopathy, arrhythmogenic right ventricular cardiomyopathy, restrictive cardiomyopathy). Unlike the AHA classification, heart disease secondary to coronary heart diseases, valvular and congenital disorders are not included. Channelopathies are excluded as well (Figure 3) [4].

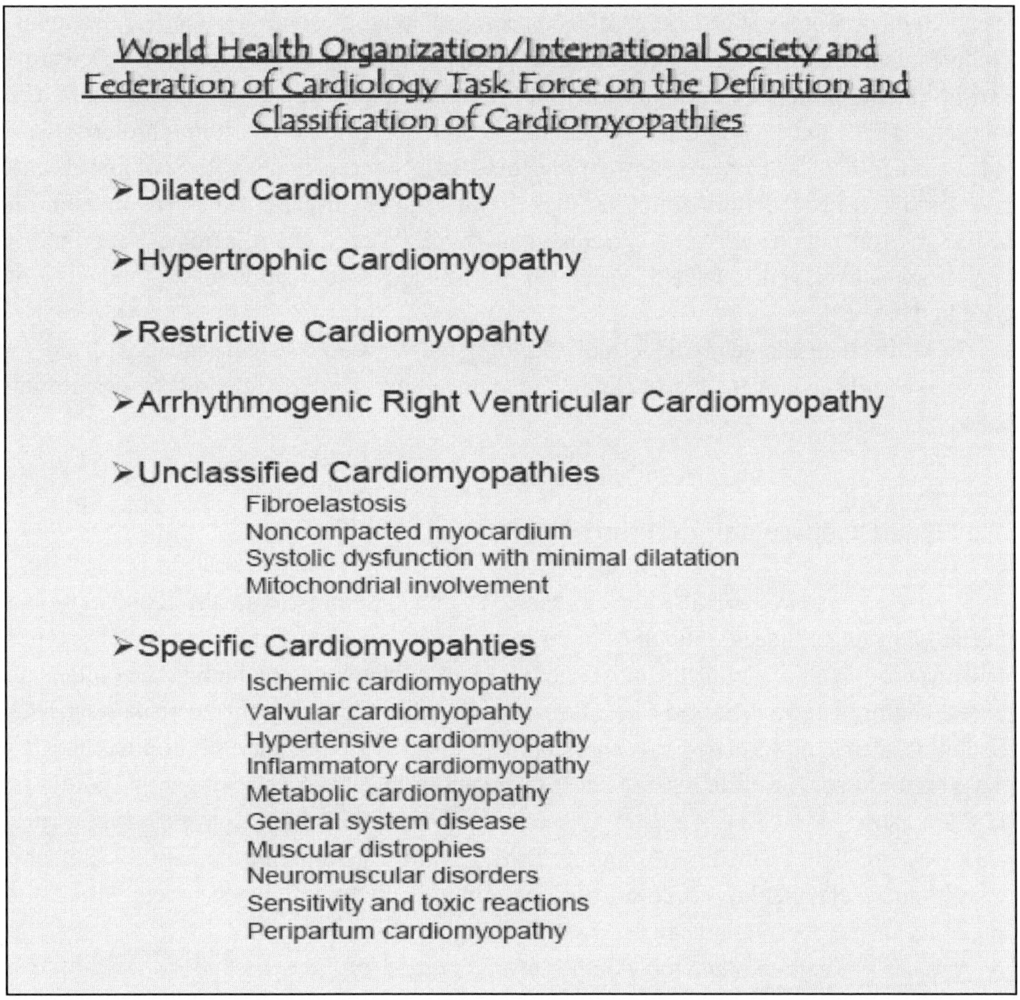

World Health Organization/International Society and Federation of Cardiology Task Force on the Definition and Classification of Cardiomyopathies

> Dilated Cardiomyopahty

> Hypertrophic Cardiomyopathy

> Restrictive Cardiomyopahty

> Arrhythmogenic Right Ventricular Cardiomyopathy

> Unclassified Cardiomyopathies
  Fibroelastosis
  Noncompacted myocardium
  Systolic dysfunction with minimal dilatation
  Mitochondrial involvement

> Specific Cardiomyopahties
  Ischemic cardiomyopathy
  Valvular cardiomyopahty
  Hypertensive cardiomyopathy
  Inflammatory cardiomyopathy
  Metabolic cardiomyopathy
  General system disease
  Muscular distrophies
  Neuromuscular disorders
  Sensitivity and toxic reactions
  Peripartum cardiomyopathy

Figure 3.

Genetics of Cardiomyopathy: A Long Way to Go

From "One Gene-One Disease"...

In 1989, Christine and Jon Seidman and co-workers reported the first association between an inherited gene defect and a primary cardiomyopathy [5]. In a subsequent study, they reported the first beta myosin missense mutation in a French Canadian family with hypertrophic cardiomyopathy, leading to the equation "one gene=one disease" [6].

...To "One Disease-Many Genes"...

Since then, substantial progress has been made in elucidating further (sarcomeric and non sarcomeric) gene defects in cardiomyopathies. To date, over 450 mutations in sarcomere protein genes (thick and thin filaments) have been identified in patients with HCM: β-myosin heavy chain (chromosome 14); cardiac troponin T (chromosome 1); cardiac troponin I (chromosome 19); troponin C (chromosome 3); α-tropomyosin (chromosome 15); cardiac myosin-binding protein C (chromosome 11); the essential and regulatory myosin light chains (chromosomes 3 and 12, respectively); cardiac actin (chromosome 15), titin (chromosome 2), and α-cardiac myosin heavy chain (chromosome 14). Some patients with sporadic disease, have similar genetic abnormalities as those with familial disease. De novo mutations in cardiac myosin binding protein-C, cardiac beta-myosin heavy chain, cardiac troponin T or alpha-tropomyosin genes have been found in isolated case reports of individuals with sporadic HCM [7].

HCM was then characterized as a disease of the sarcomere. As a consequence, DCM was indicated as a disease of the cytoskeleton and extracellular matrix, ARVC of the desmosome, and so on.

...To "One Disease-Many (Different) Genes"...

However, this "systematic" view became, again, in contrast with the rapidly growing genetic knowledge. Indeed, mutations in sarcomeric genes account for approximately 50-60% of all cases of HCM, which is the most know form of cardiomyopathy both in the clinical and genetic setting, so far. The absence of sarcomeric gene mutations in the remaining HCM population seems to be related to a shortcomings in current mutation detection methods and strategies, or to be a result of disease-causing mutations in yet unidentified genes[7].

Rare causes of HCM have been associated with mutations in sarcomere-related protein genes (myosin light chain kinase, muscle LIM protein, LIM binding domain 3, telethonin, vinculin and metavinculin, caveolin, titin, α-actinin 2, myozenin 2, and junctophilin 2), or functional genes (phospholamban, RAF-1) [7].

Another possible explanation for the low proportion of cases thought to be caused by sarcomere gene mutations is that the population of hypertrophic cardiomyopathy without sarcomeric gene mutations may carry one of the several diseases that mimic the phenotypic expression of sarcomeric hypertrophic cardiomyopathy (the so called "phenocopies" of the disease), including metabolic-mitochondrial-neuromuscular diseases, inherited syndromes, and chromosomal abnormalities [7].

Mutations in the genes encoding the gamma-2 regulatory subunit of adenosine monophosphate (AMP)-activated protein kinase (PRKAG2) and lysosome-associated membrane protein 2 (LAMP2) have been associated with hypertrophic cardiomyopathy in association with Wolff-Parkinson-White (WPW) syndrome [7,8]. Similar to PRKAG2 and LAMP2, Fabry's disease, an X-linked lisosomial disorder, can express predominant cardiac features of left ventricular hypertrophy. Over the years, mutations in GLA-encoded alpha-galactosidase A have been found in patients with this multisystem disorder[7,9]. Friedreich ataxia, an autosomal-recessive disease involving sclerosis of the spinal cord, is often associated with cardiomyopathies, and its cardiovascular manifestations may precede the neurological symptoms by up to a decade in some cases [7,10]. Chromosome Abnormalities, including Down syndrome and trisomy 18, Autosomal Dominant Cardiofacial Disorders (Noonan syndrome, LEOPARD syndrome, Cardiofaciocutaneous syndrome Costello syndrome) or Phakomatoses (Neurofibromatosis, Tuberous sclerosis) have been associated with a variety of cardiac defects, including hypertrophic cardiomyopathy[7,11-14].

...To "One Gene-Many Diseases"

The major cardiomyopathies are genetically heterogeneous diseases for which the causative genes are partially overlapping. The evidence that a complex of genes (i.e. sarcomeric protein genes) may be responsible of a "spectrum" of different phenotypes, including HCM, DCM, RCM and recently LVNC, represent a further step in the knowledge and understanding of cardiomyopathies[15]. The identification of sarcomeric mutations in familial LVNC, and an alpha-actin mutation in HCM with LVNC and atrial septal defect together with the observation of late onset LVNC in a Duchenne patient, suggests that the aetiology of LVNC extends beyond an arrest in embryonic cardiac development (i.e. the possibility of late onset LVNC[16,17]. The current findings expand the genetic heterogeneity of LVNC, and the identification of sarcomeric defects in familial LVNC suggests that LVNC may be part of a cardiomyopathy spectrum including HCM, RCM, and DCM[16,17]. Whether this means that these are different diseases or rather different manifestations (phenotypes) of the same pathological mechanism is presently not clear.

... Or to "One Gene-Many (Different) Diseases"...

It is now evident that a large number of mutations in different genes, albeit largely within the same class, could cause the same phenotype. Moreover, mutations in one gene could cause multiple phenotypes, as best illustrated in the case of lamin A/C, whereby mutations can cause 13 different diseases, including DCM, conduction defects, Emery Dreifuss muscular dystrophy, familial partial lipodystrophy, premature aging, axonal neuropathy, and insulin resistance [18]. In addition, SCN5A (sodium channel) gene mutations may cause phenotypes that combine features of LQT3 (Long QT Syndrome 3), Brugada syndrome, conduction disease and dilated cardiomyopathy ("one gene-different diseases") [19].

One Disease or Many Diseases? From " Phenocopy" To " Genocopy"

Genomic medicine has entered clinical practice, and the recognition of the diagnostic utility of genetic testing for cardiomyopathies (particularly, hypertrophic cardiomyopathy) is growing. With expanding knowledge of the genetic background of these diseases, primary cardiomyopathies have recently been subclassified into genetic, mixed, and acquired cardiomyopathies (AHA 2006) or familial and non familial disease (ESC 2007), shifting the general view of cardiomyopathies from a "phenocopy" to a "genocopy" model.

However, although a number of cardiomyopathies susceptibility genes involving different pathways have been identified, the search for novel mutations in new genes continues. As a result of the increasing genetic heterogeneity of HCM, a classification based on functional genetics might seem very helpful, but in the light of the low yield of mutations in a large number of these genes as well as the commercial availability of just a small number of these genes, a phenotypic classification might be a more useful tool in looking at this disease from a clinical-practice vantage point. With the growing number of cardiomyopathy-associated genes discovered, strategic choices have to be made in clinical practice.

Diagnosis of Cardiomyopathy

The utility of an accurate diagnosis and distinction from a phenocopy state is well illustrated in certain circumstances, such as Fabry disease, which could be clinically indistinguishable from HCM caused by mutations in sarcomeric proteins [9]. Enzyme replacement therapy with alpha-galactosidase, the enzyme responsible for Fabry disease, has been shown to impart considerable clinical benefit in management of patients with Fabry disease, while the conventional treatment offered for true HCM would render no significant benefit in such patients [20].

The age of onset (infancy, childhood, adolescency, or adulthood), the pattern of inheritance (autosomic, X linked or matrilinear), symptoms/signs at onset, physical abnormalities (dysmorphic features, myopathy, mental retardation), ECG abnormalities (i.e. short PR in metabolic or mitochondrial disorders), the echocardiographic pattern (i.e. left ventricular non-compaction cardiomyopathy associated with specific neuromuscular disorders), and other biochemical or functional tests (i.e. premature lactic acidosis and flat oxigen pulse during metabolic stress test in mitochondrial disorders) may be relevant to discriminate between different causes of cardiomyopathies. Detailed clinical evaluation and mutation analysis are, therefore, important to provide an accurate diagnosis in order to enable genetic counselling, prognostic evaluation and appropriate clinical management [21].

Physical Examination

Physical abnormalities can be characteristics of specific disorders and lead to the final clinical diagnosis. Macroglossia, carpal tunnel syndrome, reticular lung infiltrates and Bence-Jones proteinuria may be hallmarks of plasma-cell-dyscrasia-related systemic amyloidosis. Metabolic disorders and syndromes are associated with characteristic physical abnormalities (dysmorphic features, myopathy, mental retardation) and symptoms at onset. Patients with inborn errors of metabolism involving impaired energy production or the accumulation of toxic metabolites often have signs and symptoms of multiple organ dysfunction. Dysmorphic features may characterize malformation syndromes as well as storage diseases, and therefore other minor and major malformations should also be sought. In patients with primary neuromuscular disorder, skeletal muscle weakness usually precedes the cardiomyopathy and dominates the clinical picture. Occasionally, however, skeletal myopathy is subtle, and the first symptom of disease may be cardiac failure. Encephalopathy is characteristically seen in the mitochondrial syndromes MELAS (Mitochondrial Encephalopathy, Lactic Acidosis, and Strokelike episodes), MERRF (Myoclonic Epilepsy, Ragged Red Fibers), Kearns-Sayre syndrome, and Leigh disease. Acute worsening can occur in these syndromes in association with intercurrent illness or metabolic stressors. In general, the neurological features of these syndromes (epilepsy, strokelike episodes, dementia, and ophthalmoplegia) predominate, and the cardiomyopathy typically occurs later in the clinical course[21,22].

Electrocardiogramm

Almost all (95%) patients with hypertrophic cardiomyopathy have an abnormal ECG. The most frequent ECG changes are left atrial enlargement, repolarization abnormalities, and pathologic Q waves, most commonly in the inferolateral leads. Voltage criteria for left ventricular hypertrophy alone are non-specific and are often seen in normal young adults. Giant negative T waves in the mid-precordial leads are characteristic of hypertrophy confined to the left ventricular apex. Some patients have a short PR interval, including metabolic/storage (Danon, PRKAG2, Fabry disease) or mitochondrial disorders. Patients with amyloidosis often show low voltages in the precordial leads[7-10, 21-23].

Non Invasive Imaging Technology

Standard echocardiography, new echocardiographic technologies, and Cardiac magnetic resonance (CMR) provide information on myocardial structure and have been suggested as a potential tool to discriminate between different phenocopy states.

Standard Echo

Left ventricular hypertrophy associated to congenital heart defects is frequently seen in malformation syndromes (such as pulmonary valve abnormalities in Noonan and LEOPARD syndrome). An abnormal texture of the interventricular septum ("granular sparkling" aspect), especially if associated with biatrial dilation, pericardial effusion and restrictive phenotype, may be diagnostic of amyloid. However, other infiltrative diseases (i.e. metabolic myopathies, Gaucher, Hunter's, and Hurler's diseases) or storage cardiomyopathies (haemochromatosis, Fabry's disease, glycogen storage, and Niemann-Pick disease) should be considered. In advanced haemochromatosis all cardiac chambers may be dilated. Mucopolysaccharidosis and Gaucher's disease may lead to aortic and mitral stenosis. In hypothyroidism, other than amyloidosis, a pericardial effusion can be present. Pieroni et al. showed in 83% of Fabry's cardiomyopathy patients (95% of FC patients with LVH) a binary appearance of endocardial border absent in all HCM, hypertensive, and healthy subjects (sensitivity 94%; specificity 100%), reflecting an endomyocardial glycosphingolipids compartmentalization, consisting of thickened glycolipid-rich endocardium, free glycosphingolipid subendocardial storage, and an inner severely affected myocardial layer with a clear subendocardial-midwall layer gradient of disease severity. On the other hand, Kounas et al. showed the binary sign in 8/28 patients with HCM (3 patients) and with Fabry's cardiomyopathy (5 patients). The sensitivity and specificity of the binary sign as a discriminator of AFD from HCM were 35% and 79%, respectively. The authors suggest that the binary endocardial appearance lacks sufficient sensitivity and specificity to be used as an echocardiographic screening tool. In neuromuscular disorders like glycogenosis, mitochondriopathy and myotonic dystrophy, myocardial thickening, hypertrabeculation/ noncomnpaction and systolic dysfunction are found. The coexistence of left ventricular non-compaction and localised inferobasal left ventricular akinesia are almost pathognomonic of dystrophinopathies. Finally, a diagnosis of neuromuscular/metabolic/ mitochondrial cardiomyopathy is favored in presence of concentric/asymmetric/apical, non-obstructive hypertrophic cardiomyopathy, with or without hypertrabeculation of the apex, especially when associated with an early onset impairment of LV systolic function. However, metabolic and mitochondrial cardiomyopathy might also be presented with dilated type, and hypertrophy may become dilated in the later stage [7,9,10-12, 24-26].

Recently, genotype–phenotype studies from the Majo Clinic Cardiomyopathy Group have discovered an important relationship between the morphology of the left ventricle, its underlying genetic substrate and the long-term outcome of this disease. They observed that the septal contour was the strongest predictor of the presence of a myofilament mutation, regardless of age. Intriguing conclusions can be drawn from these observations. Whereas in initial morphological studies, sigmoidal HCM seemed to be associated with older age, the underlying genotype rather than age appears to be the predominant determinant of septal morphology. Furthermore, Z-disc HCM seems to have a predilection for sigmoidal contour status These observations may facilitate echo-guided genetic testing by enabling informed genetic counseling about the a-priori probability of a positive genetic test based upon the patient's expressed anatomical phenotype[27].

New Imaging Techonologies

Weidemann et al. have investigated in a prospective study whether regional non-ischaemic fibrosis in hypertrophic myocardium can also be detected by ultrasonic strain-rate imaging based on specific visual features of the myocardial deformation traces. This diagnostic study aimed to define left ventricular fibrotic segments in 30 patients with hypertrophic cardiomyopathy (n = 10), severe aortic valve stenosis (n = 10), Fabry disease cardiomyopathy (n = 10), and 10 healthy controls. In total, 42 segments showed late enhancement by magnetic resonance imaging. Using strain-rate imaging, all late enhancement positive segments displayed a characteristic pattern consisting of a first peak in early systole followed by a rapid fall in strain rate close to zero and a second peak during isovolumetric relaxation. This 'double peak sign' was never seen in segments of healthy controls. However, it was detected in 10 segments without late enhancement. These 'false-positive' segments belonged to Fabry patients who often develop a fast progressing fibrosis. In a follow-up magnetic resonance imaging study after 2 years, all these segments had developed late enhancement. Therefore, the 'double peak sign' in strain-rate imaging tracings seems to be a reliable tool to diagnose regional fibrosis[26].

CMR

Moon JC et al. have shown that late gadolinium enhancement cardiovascular magnetic resonance can visualize myocardial interstitial abnormalities. Late enhancement was demonstrated in nine patients with different specific cardiomyopathies, with a mean signal intensity of 390 +/- 220% compared with normal regions. The distribution pattern of late enhancement was unlike the subendocardial late enhancement related to coronary territories found in myocardial infarction. The affected areas included papillary muscles (sarcoid), the mid-myocardium (Anderson-Fabry disease, glycogen storage disease, myocarditis, Becker muscular dystrophy) and the global sub-endocardium (systemic sclerosis, Loeffler's endocarditis, amyloid, Churg-Strauss). Focal myocardial late gadolinium enhancement have been found in these specific cardiomyopathies, and the pattern is distinct from that seen in infarction. CMR hyperenhancement pattern is very characteristic for cardiac involvement of amyloidosis and can therefore be used to discriminate this disease from other forms of restrictive or hypertrophic cardiomyopathies. Although most profound in the subendocardial layer of myocardium, amyloid deposition occurs throughout the entire myocardium, causing the entire myocardium to have a higher signal on delayed contrast enhancement images than normal myocardium [28].

Biochemical/Metabolic Tests

Biochemical analysis represents an step for the diagnosis of mitochondrial, metabolic and neuromuscular cardiomyopathies. The presence of hypoglycemia, primary metabolic acidosis with an increased anion gap, or hyperammonemia should alert the physician to the possibility of a metabolic disorder. The insulin-excess states of Beckwith-Wiedemann syndrome and the infant of a diabetic mother can produce hypoketotic hypoglycemia but are distinguished by low free fatty acid levels by characteristic clinical features. Disorders in fatty acid metabolism can be identified as defects of fatty acid ß-oxidation or of carnitine-dependent transport depending on quantitative carnitine levels in blood, urine, and tissue; acylcarnitine profile in blood; and urine organic acids (fatty acids, dicarboxylic, and hydroxydicarboxylic acids). In Fabry disease, electrolyte imbalances and proteinuria reflecting renal failure may be seen. Level of globotriaosylceramide (Gb3 or GL-3) a glycosphingolipid may be elevated. Enzymatic analysis performed by using plasma or leukocytes may show a deficiency of alpha-galactosidase A. However, levels of Gb3 and alpha-galactosidase A may be normal in female heterozygote Fabry patients. Therefore, genetic and/or molecular diagnosis is necessary to confirm Fabry disease if suspected based on clinical features of proteinuria and acroparesthesias that were invariably present in both men and women with Fabry mutation and cryptogenic stroke. Elevated serum creatine kinase levels can be associated with diagnosis of a neuromuscular disease. Although clinical signs and laboratory tests are useful for identifying and classifying diseases of the lower motor unit, in isolation, they rarely lead to a specific diagnosis. However, a markedly elevated serum creatine kinase level (10 to 100 times higher than normal) is invariably found early in the clinical course of Duchenne muscular dystrophy and almost always in its milder allelic form, Becker-type muscular dystrophy, whereas the serum creatine kinase level is usually lower in other muscular dystrophies and myopathies (1 to 10 times higher than normal). Because creatine kinase levels can vary markedly among different patients with the same disease and may fluctuate in a given patient over time, clinical judgment is necessary to interpret these values. A premature lactic acidosis, a very low VO_2 and a flat oxygen pulse may represent markers of metabolic/mitochondrial diseases. The diagnosis can be confirmed on measurement of blood and cerebrospinal fluid lactate and pyruvate levels, histological analysis of skeletal muscle, assay of respiratory chain enzymes, and/or mitochondrial DNA analysis[21, 29].

Genetic Testing

The clinical application of mutation analysis is technically possible, but has been hindered by logistics and high cost. Given the cost of mutation analysis, however, a strategic approach based on probabilities should be employed where possible. Careful phenotyping should identify the most common phenocopies of cardiomyopathies.

The major goals of genetic testing in patients with cardiomyopathies are:

- to contribute to diagnosis;
- to provide prognostic and therapeutic benefits;
- most important, to detect relatives affected or at risk to develop the disease (carriers).

Once a mutation has been detected in a proband, the possibility of genetic testing should be suggested to first-degree relatives (who have a 50% probability of being gene-positive in autosomal disorders: 'cascade' screening). This type of screening enables close clinical management of mutation carriers, and identifies genetically normal family members, obviating the need for them to undergo clinical screening and repeat follow-up examinations. Appropriate genetic counselling, performed by a well trained physician (clinicians, geneticist) or genetic counsellor, should precede and follow genetic testing to help the patient and his/her family to comprehend the reasons to perform the test and the clinical significance and impact of a positive/negative diagnosis. A specially trained and experienced nurse may serve as coordinator of the investigations and as contact person for the family [3,4,7,15,22].

Organ-specific and Skeletal Muscle Biopsy

Biopsy with Congo red staining and immunostaining is the procedure of choice for the diagnosis of amyloidosis. Stain the tissue with an alkaline solution of Congo red, and examine it under polarized light, where positive (green) birefringence is detectable in the presence of amyloidosis of any type. The nature of the fibril precursor can be established by immunohistochemical staining with antibodies specific for the major amyloid precursors (Amyloid A, immunoglobulin L chains of k or l type, antitransthyretin). In Amyloid A amyloidosis, only the Amyloid A is positive. The amyloid nature of the deposit can by confirmed by staining with an antiserum specific for serum amyloid P-component. In amyloidosis, the tissue with the highest yield, particularly in the presence of proteinuria or renal failure, is the kidney (technically adequate samples have a diagnostic yield close to 100%). If renal biopsy is deemed too risky for a specific patient or if amyloidosis without renal disease is suspected, 2 sites have been shown to be useful in obtaining tissue for histologic and immunochemical analysis. Subcutaneous fat aspiration is positive in approximately 60% of individuals with Amyloid A amyloidosis, except in the case of familial Mediterranean fever, when it rarely, if ever, is positive. Rectal biopsy is more useful than subcutaneous fat aspiration in Amyloid A amyloidosis. It has been found to produce positive results (assuming that submucosa is included in the biopsy specimen) in 80-85% of patients ultimately found to have tissue amyloid at a clinically relevant site. Samples from either the subcutaneous fat aspirate or the rectal biopsy can be stained as conventional tissue biopsies to determine the presence and nature of the amyloid precursor. Occasionally, patients have positive results on subcutaneous fat aspirates in the presence of a negative result on rectal biopsy, while others may have deposits in the rectal tissue and not in the aspirate. Use of both procedures may increase the yield to 90%. Abdominal subcutaneous fat biopsy results are not very sensitive in Amyloid A caused by familial Mediterranean fever and in dialysis-related amyloidosis. The results are usually negative, probably because beta2-microglobulin does not accumulate in this tissue.

A skeletal muscle biopsy is often necessary, especially in infants, when the clinical and laboratory findings are nonspecific. If a muscular dystrophy is suspected, particularly in a boy, molecular analysis of the dystrophin gene and/or protein is indicated. Dystrophin, a cytoskeletal protein normally found in all muscle cell types, is thought to stabilize the plasma membrane of the muscle cell and may be important in the regulation of intracellular calcium. Approximately 65% of patients with Duchenne muscular dystrophy or Becker-type muscular dystrophy have deletions of the dystrophin gene that can be detected by PCR in blood lymphocytes. In the other 35% of patients, including manifesting female carriers for whom PCR results are difficult to interpret, a muscle biopsy is required to detect a reduced amount of the dystrophin protein or abnormalities of its size. The presence of dystrophic changes in a skeletal muscle biopsy specimen is also an indication for molecular analysis of dystrophin [22,30,31].

Endomyocardial Biopsy

Although the role of endomyocardial biopsy (EMB) in the diagnosis and treatment of adult and pediatric cardiovascular disease remains controversial, a recent joint AHA/ACC/ESC statement recommends endomyocardial biopsy (class I, evidence B) in patients with suspected myocarditis, including

1) new onset heart failure of less than two weeks duration associated with a normal sized or dilated left ventricle and haemodynamic compromise;
2) new onset heart failure of 2 weeks to 3 months duration associated with a dilated left ventricle and new ventricular arrhythmias, second- or third-degree heart block, or failure to respond to usual care within 1 to 2 weeks. In addition, endomyocardial biopsy is reasonable (IIA; evidence C):
   - in the clinical setting of unexplained heart failure of >3 months' duration associated with a dilated left ventricle and new ventricular arrhythmias, Mobitz type II second- or third-degree AV heart block, or failure to respond to usual care within 1 to 2 weeks;
   - in the setting of unexplained heart failure associated with suspected anthracycline cardiomyopathy;
   - in the setting of heart failure associated with unexplained restrictive cardiomyopathy;
   - in the setting of unexplained heart failure associated with a DCM of any duration that is associated with suspected allergic reaction in addition to eosinophilia.
   - in the setting of suspected cardiac tumors, with the exception of typical myxomas whereas adenovirus is most commonly associated with histological [32].

Conclusions

In 1968, the World Health Organization defined cardiomyopathies as "diseases of different and often unknown etiology in which the dominant feature is cardiomegaly and heart failure". This statement was updated in 1980 and defined cardiomyopathies as "heart muscle diseases of unknown cause", thereby differentiating them from specific identified heart muscle diseases of known cause such as myocarditis. In 1995, a World Health Organization/International Society and Federation of Cardiology Task Force on cardiomyopathies classified the different cardiomyopathies by the dominant pathophysiology or by etiological/pathogenetic factors *(Phenocopy era)*. Over the last two decades, the importance of gene defects in the etiology of cardiomyopathies has been recognized, and several new disease entities have been identified with the introduction of molecular biology into clinical medicine *(Genocopy era)*, rendering previous classifications and formal cardiomyopathies concepts obsolete, and leading to different reclassification of cardiomyopathies by the AHA and the Working Group of the ESC.

However, given the extreme heterogeneity of cardiomyopathies, there probably is no single classification or "model" that can be regarded as generally acceptable to all the interested parties from diverse disciplines (researchers, clinicians, epidemiologists, geneticists). Nevertheless, cardiologists and cardiomyopathy specialists need to become familiar with the basic principles of molecular biology and clinical genetics, in order to generally understand the basis of the disease, to provide a correct characterization of the clinical phenotype and to eventually guide the genotype, to understand and manage the implications of a positive genetic diagnosis for the proband and his/her family.

References

[1] Report of the WHO/ISFC task force on the definition and classification of cardiomyopathies. *Br. Heart J.* 1980; 44:672–673.

[2] Richardson P, McKenna W, Bristow M, et al. Report of the 1995 World Health Organization/International Society and Federation of Cardiology Task Force on the definition and classification of cardiomyopathies. *Circulation* 1996; 93:841–842.

[3] Maron BJ, Towbin JA, Thiene G, et al. Contemporary definitions and classification of the cardiomyopathies: an American Heart Association Scientific Statement from the Council on Clinical Cardiology, Heart Failure and Transplantation Committee; Quality of Care and Outcomes Research and Functional Genomics and Translational Biology Interdisciplinary Working Groups; and Council on Epidemiology and Prevention. *Circulation* 2006; 113:1807–1816

[4] Elliott P, Andersson B, Arbustini E, et al. Classification of the cardiomyopathies: a position statement from the European society of cardiology working group on myocardial and pericardial diseases. *Eur. Heart J.* 2007; 29(2):270-6.

[5] Jarcho JA, McKenna W, Pare JA, et al. Mapping a gene for familial hypertrophic cardiomyopathy to chromosome 14q1. *N. Engl. J. Med.* 1989; 321: 1372–1378.

[6] Geisterfer-Lowrance AA, Kass S, Tanigawa G, et al. A molecular basis for familial hypertrophic cardiomyopathy: a beta cardiac myosin heavy chain gene missense mutation. *Cell* 1990; 62:999–1006.

[7] Keren A, Syrris P, McKenna WJ. Hypertrophic cardiomyopathy: the genetic determinants of clinical disease expression. Nat Clin Pract Card Med 2008;5:158-168.

[8] Arad M, Maron BJ, Gorham JM, et al. Glycogen storage diseases presenting as hypertrophic cardiomyopathy. *N. Engl. J. Med.* 2005; 352:362–372.

[9] Sachdev B, Takenaka T, Teraguchi H, et al. Prevalence of Anderson–Fabry disease in male patients with late onset hypertrophic cardiomyopathy. *Circulation* 2002; 105: 1407–1411.

[10] Van Driest SL, Gakh O, Ommen SR, et al. Molecular and functional characterization of a human frataxin mutation found in hypertrophic cardiomyopathy. *Mol. Genet Metab.* 2005; 85:280–285.

[11] Limongelli G, Hawkes L, Calabro R, et al. Mutation screening of the PTPN11 gene in hypertrophic cardiomyopathy. *Eur. J. Med. Genet.* 2006;49(5):426-30.

[12] Limongelli G, Pacileo G, Marino B, et al. Prevalence and clinical significance of cardiovascular abnormalities in patients with the LEOPARD syndrome. *Am. J. Cardiol.* 2007; 100:736-41.

[13] Limongelli G, Pacileo G, Digilio MC, et al. Severe, obstructive biventricular hypertrophy in a patient with Costello syndrome: Clinical impact and management. *Int. J. Cardiol.* 2008; 130: e108-e110.

[14] Limongelli G, Pacileo G, Melis D, et al. Trisomy 18 and hypertrophy cardiomyopathy in an 18-year-old woman. *Am. J. Med. Genet A.* 2008;146(3):327-9.

[15] Marian AJ. Phenotypic plasticity of sarcomeric protein mutations. *J. Am. Coll Cardiol.* 2007 Jun 26;49:2427-9.

[16] Klaassen S, Probst S, Oechslin E, et al. Mutations in Sarcomere Protein Genes in Left Ventricular Noncompaction. *Circulation* 2008;117;2893-2901.

[17] Hoedemaekers YM, Caliskan K, Majoor-Krakauer D et al. Cardiac b-myosin heavy chain defects in two families with non-compaction cardiomyopathy: linking non-compaction to hypertrophic, restrictive, and dilated cardiomyopathies. *Eur. Heart J.* 2007 Nov;28(22):2732-7.

[18] Capell BC, Collins FS. Human laminopathies: nuclei gone genetically awry. *Nat. Rev. Genet* 2006;7:940 –52.

[19] Remme CA, Wilde AA, Bezzina CR. Cardiac sodium channel overlap syndromes: different faces of SCN5A mutations. *Trends Cardiovasc. Med.* 2008 Apr;18(3):78-87.

[20] Wilcox WR, Banikazemi M, Guffon N, et al. Long-term safety and efficacy of enzyme replacement therapy for Fabry disease. *Am. J. Hum. Genet.* 2004;75:65–74.

[21] Schwartz ML, Cox GF, Lin AE. Clinical Approach to Genetic Cardiomyopathy in Children. *Circulation* 1996;94:2021-2038.

[22] Anan R, Nakagawa M, Miyata M, et al. Cardiac involvement in mitochondrial diseases: a study on 17 patients with documented mitochondrial DNA defects. *Circulation* 1995; 91:955-961.

[23] Stern S. Electrocardiogram: Still the Cardiologist's Best Friend. *Circulation* 2006;113: 753-756.

[24] Cueto-Garcia L, Reeder GS, Kyle RA, et al. Echocardiographic findings in systemic amyloidosis: spectrum of cardiac involvement and relation to survival. *J. Am. Coll. Cardiol.* 1985; 6:737–743.

[25] C Rapezzi, O Leone, E Biagini et al. Echocardiographic clues to diagnosis of dystrophin related dilated cardiomyopathy. *Heart* 2007;93:10.

[26] Weidemann F, Strotmann JM. Use of tissue Doppler imaging to identify and manage systemic diseases. *Clin. Res. Cardiol.* 2007; 96:1–9 .

[27] Bosa JM, Ommen SR, Ackerman MJ. Genetics of hypertrophic cardiomyopathy: one, two, or more diseases? *Curr. Opin. Cardiol.* 22:193–199.

[28] Silva C, Moon JC, Elkington AG, et. al. Myocardial late gadolinium enhancement in specific cardiomyopathies by cardiovascular magnetic resonance: a preliminary experience. *J. Cardiovasc. Med.* (Hagerstown). 2007;8:1076-9.

[29] Di Lenarda A, Arbustini E. Diagnosis of dilated cardiomyopathy: how to improve clinical and etiological definition. *Ital. Heart J. Suppl.* 2002; 3:375-7.

[30] Obici L, Perfetti V, Palladini G, et al. Clinical aspects of systemic amyloid diseases. *Biochim. Biophys. Acta* Nov 10 2005;1753(1):11-22.

[31] Finsterer J, Stöllbergerb C. The Heart in Human Dystrophinopathies. *Cardiology* 2003; 99:1-19.

[32] Cooper LT, Baughman KL, Feldman AM, et al. The role of endomyocardial biopsy in the management of cardiovascular disease: a scientific statement from the American Heart Association, the American College of Cardiology, and the European Society of Cardiology. *Circulation* 2007;116:2216-33.

In: Handbook of Cardiovascular Research   ISBN 978-1-60741-792-7
Editors: Jorgen Brataas and Viggo Nanstveit   © 2009 Nova Science Publishers, Inc.

Chapter XIV

Transient Left Ventricular Apical Ballooning Syndrome or Takotsubo Cardiomyopathy: A Systematic Review

E. Vizzardi*, P. Faggiano, G. Zanini, E. Antonioli, I. Bonadei,
C. Fiorina, R. Raddino and L. Dei Cas
Section of Cardiovascular Disease,
Department of Applied Experimental Medicine
Department of Cardiology, Brescia
University Study of Brescia, Brescia, Italy

Introduction

Tako-tsubo cardiomyopathy (TC) is a recently described acute cardiac syndrome that mimics acute myocardial infarction and is characterized by ischemic chest symptoms, an elevated ST segment on electrocardiogram, increase levels of cardiac disease markers and transient left apical and middle ventricular walls disfunction (apical "ballooning"). In contrast to the acute coronary arterial syndromes (ACS), patients with TC have no angiographically detectable or nonobstructive coronary arterial disease [1].

This syndrome can be triggered by profound psychological stress and is also known as "stress cardiomyopathy" or "broken-heart syndrome" [2].

The onset of the transient LV apical ballooning syndrome is often preceded by emotional or physical stress. An emotional stressor, such as unexpected death of a relative or friend, domestic abuse, a catastrophic medical diagnosis, devastating business, or gambling losses, was identified and a physical stressor, such as exhausting work, asthma attack, gastric

* Corrisponding author: Vizzardi Enrico, Department of Cardiology, University of Brescia Italy, Pzz.le Spedali
Civili 1 25124 Brescia, Tel 049303995659, Email: enrico.vizzardi@tin.it.

endoscopy, exacerbated systemic disorders in about 70% (Table 1); drugs poisoning such as nortriptyline are potential stressors and cocaine binge was described in a case report [3].

However in 30% there was no preceding emotional or physical stressful event identified.

The occurrence of a reversible cardiomyopathy in familial member is a sporadic event signalled and it induce to speculate on the possibility of a familial predisposition to this entity or its variants but the association cannot be ascertained until specific genetic tests have evolved and statistical correlation be established with more such observations. What has not been delved into much is the possibility of a familial predisposition towards stress-induced cardiomyopathy. A review of literature notes the recent observation by Japanese investigators of CD 36 deficiency in a patient with stress-; induced cardiomiopathy [4] suggesting an association between this entity and certain genetic profiles.

Further studies of tako-tsubo-shaped cardiomyopathy and CD36 deficiency may reveal an association between this cardiomyopathy and specific genetic profiles.

Epidemiology and Clinical Presentations

The TC was initially recognized in the Japanese population (first described in 1991) but has recently been reported in the USA and Europe [5]. The term "tako-tsubo" was proposed by Dote et al and means "fishing pot for trapping octopus," and the left ventricle disfunction, in this syndrome, resembles that shape [6] (Figure 1). The true prevalence of the apical ballooning syndrome remains uncertain. In the last few years, the number of published reports of patients presenting with this syndrome is constantly increasing. Only six series assessed the prevalence of this syndrome among consecutive patients presenting with suspected ACS. Klinceva M et al. evaluated the prevalence of stress-induced myocardial stunning during a four-year period (2002-2005), and it was estimated as 0.07% and the annual population incidence of this disorder was as 0.00006% [7]; also Pillière et al. assess same results [8]. In a study from the USA, Bybee et al. [9] reported that the apical ballooning syndrome accounted for 2.2% of the ST-segment elevation ACS presenting to the investigators' institution. Three series evaluated the prevalence of this syndrome in Japan. Among patients presenting with suspected ACS, Ito et al. [10] reported that the apical ballooning syndrome accounted for 1.7% of cases and Matsuoka et al. [11] for 2.2%. Akashi et al. [12] diagnosed apical ballooning syndrome in 2.0% of patients with sudden onset of heart failure and abnormal Q waves or ST-T changes suggestive of acute myocardial infarction (AMI) on admission.

This cardiomyopathy has been documented prevalently in postmenopausal women of an advanced age and the explanation for this gender and age incidence is still unresolved [13].

In a recent review, Gianni et al. [1] reported a history of hypertension in 43% of patients, diabetes in 11.0%, dyslipidaemia in 25.45% and current or past smoking in 23%. The most common presenting clinical symptoms were chest pain and dyspnoea. Chest pain was reported to be a cardinal presenting symptom in 67.8%, and dyspnoea in 17.8%. However, more serious clinical presentations such as cardiogenic shock and ventricular fibrillation are frequent, 4.2% and 1.5% respectively. In one case there was a fatal left ventricular rupture [14]. Isolated cases of syncope as the presenting symptom have been reported [8].

Table 1.

Physical stress (60%)
External injury
Heavy labor
Travel
Electrophysiologic study
Emotional stress (35%)
Human relations
Death of spouse
Public performance
Medical examination (5%)

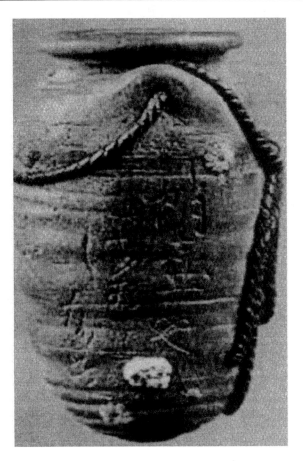

Figure 1. an antique TakoTsubo.

Electrocardiographic Features and Cardiac Biomarkers

Electrocardiographic changes in the acute phase comprise ST-elevations. These changes may be present only for several hours. Then, normalization of the ST- segment occurs, followed by negative T-waves in V1-V6, I and aVL, which persist for weeks to months. The QT interval is initially often prolonged and may shorten over weeks [15, 16]. ST-elevation was detected in 81.6%,, usually involving the precordial leads (83.9%); T wave abnormalities were seen in 64.3% patients and Q waves were present in 31.8% patients. Only rarely ST − depression and the development of Q waves have been observed [17]. (Figure 2). However, a recent study shows ECG findings in TC patients are significantly different from those in patients with acute myocardial infarction (AMI). At initial presentation, the extent of ST-segment elevation and the number of abnormal Q waves are greater in AMI. During follow-up, no Q wave, a longer QTc interval and a greater extent of T-wave inversion are typical findings in TC patients [18].

Six studies measured serum levels of troponin I and three CK-MB fraction levels. Troponin I was positive in 86.2% and CK-MB levels were elevated in 73.9%.

However, in this particular syndrome, cardiac biomarker levels were usually only slightly elevated compared to the extension of segment involved with a rapid decrease to normal enzymatic plasmatic level suggesting a reversible myocardial dysfunction, compared to the ordinary kinetic of a "normal" acute myocardial infarction. Frequently, an increase of plasma brain natriuretic peptide can be observed in the acute phase [11] but is not associated with a poor prognosis in this condition [19].

Cardiac Catheterization and Echocardiography

The coronary angiographic pattern usually shows the absence of coronary disease or only mild coronary atherosclerosis (<50%); coronary spasm may be visible or may be provoked by acetylcholine or ergonovine administration in up to 80% of patients [20]. Left ventriculography documents akinesis in the apical, diaphragmatic and/or anterolateral segments, and hyperkinesis in the basal segments (Figure 3). According to the proposed diagnostic criteria, demonstration of ruptured atherosclerotic plaques in the major coronary arteries by angiography or intracoronary ultrasound examination (IVUS) formally excludes tako-tsubo.

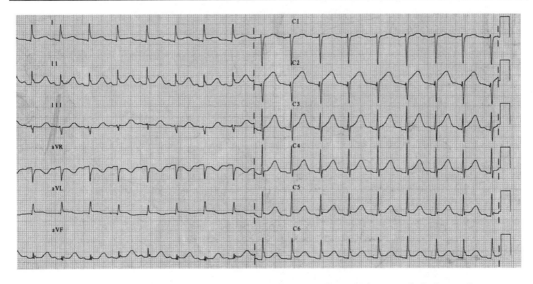

Figure 2. example of tako-tsubo syndrome electrocardiogram of one patient at admission and demission.

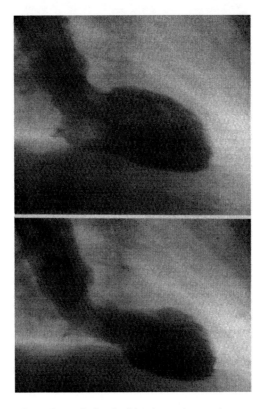

Figure 3. Ventriculography of a patient admitted with tako-tsubo syndrome.

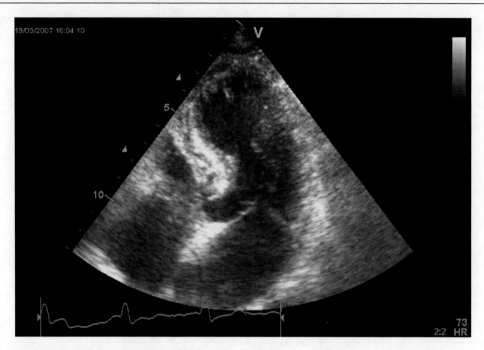

Figure 4. Echocardiographic aspect of tako-tsubo with hypercontractility of the basal segments and akinesia and apical expansion.

Table 2. Proposed Mayo Clinic Criteria for the Clinical Diagnosis of tako-tsubo syndrome

1. Transient hypokinesis, akinesis, or dyskinesis of the left ventricular mid segments with or without apical involvement. The regional wall-motion abnormalities extend beyond a single epicardial vascular distribution.*
2. Absence of obstructive coronary disease or angiographic evidence of acute plaque rupture.†
3. New ECG abnormalities (either ST-segment elevation and/or T-wave inversion) or elevated cardiac troponin.
4. Absence of: recent significant head trauma intracranial bleeding, pheochromocytoma, myocarditis, hypertrophic cardiomyopathy.

*There are rare exceptions to these criteria, such as those patients in whom the regional wall-motion abnormality is limited to a single coronary territory.
†It is possible that a patient with obstructive coronary atherosclerosis may also develop tako-tsubo syndrome. However, this is very rare in our experience and in the published literature, perhaps because such cases are misdiagnosed as an acute coronary syndrome.
In both of the above circumstances, the diagnosis of tako-tsubo syndrome should be made with caution, and a clear stressful precipitating trigger must be sought.

During the acute phase, all patients had an abnormal left ventricular ejection fraction (mean, 0.39 to 0.49) that improve rapidly over a period of days to weeks (mean follow- up left ventricular ejection fraction, 0.60 to 0.76) [21].

Echocardiogram shows also the apical ballooning of the left ventricle akinesis or diskinesis with the basal function preserved or hyperkinetic (Figure 4). The akinesia is more extensive than the area supplied by any one coronary vessel [22]. Occasionally, a left intraventricular gradient with high velocity in the basal segment may be detected [23]. Mild-ventricle and apical wall-motion abnormalities completely resolved in all surviving patients.

Some studies evidenced that reversible right ventricular (RV) dysfunction is common in this syndrome and involves about one-quarter of patients. Its presence seems to be associated with a more severe impairment in LV function. Pleural effusion, especially when significant or bilateral, is a reliable clinical indicator of RV involvement [24].

Clinical experience with cardiovascular magnetic resonance (CMR) in this entity is still limited. CMR may be a valuable tool in the diagnosis work up of patients with classical as well as variant tako-tsubo cardiomyopathy and seems to be superior to echocardiography in this regard; it may be useful in differentiating this entity from those with similar clinical presentation such as myocardial infarction and myocarditis and, which commonly exhibit typical patterns of delayed hyperenhancement and it provides information on extent and reversibility of left ventricular wall motion abnormality. Furthermore, absence of delayed hyperenhancement indicates good functional recovery [25]. There was some criteria for the clinical diagnosis of tako-tsubo syndrome (see Table 2).

Pathophysiological Mechanisms

The cause of the transient left ventricular apical ballooning syndrome is unknown. However, speculatively, it may represent a catecholamine-mediated myocardial stunning that results from a combination of myocardial ischemia related to diffuse microvascular dysfunction and, in some cases, multivessel epicardial spasm and metabolic injury; however the presence of a myocardial bridge is possibly associated with focal abnormalities in the myocardial architecture [26].

The explanation for a female predominance of TC is also unclear. However, the reason may be related to postmenopausal alterations of endothelial function in response to reduced estrogen levels [27] and microcirculatory vasomotor reactivity in response to catecholamine-mediated stimuli [28].

Many studies have evaluated the presence of either spontaneous or provocable multivessel epicardial spasm during angiography. Only few patients experienced spontaneous multivessel epicardial spasm during coronarography (1.4%). Coronary flow reserve, which assesses coronary microvascular function, has been reported in a few patients, and results were conflicting [20, 29]. Frame counts from the Thrombolysis in Myocardial Infarction (TIMI) study, a quantization method of the time required for injected intracoronary contrast to reach predefined distal landmarks, were reported in 2 series. In these reports they saw an abnormal TIMI frame counts, a validated index of coronary blood flow, in all 3 major epicardial coronary arteries during the acute phase of the syndrome; this finding suggests widespread coronary microvascular dysfunction [30, 19].

Abe et al. evaluated the coronary microcirculation using Doppler guidewire or contrast echocardiography. Although based only on few patients, their findings suggest that abnormalities in the coronary microcirculation do not contribute significantly to the syndrome [24]. In contrast, Kurisu et al. found that the TIMI frame count was significantly higher in patients with transient LV apical ballooning syndrome when compared with controls both during acute phase and follow-up [26]. Bybee et al. confirmed these findings, evaluating coronary angiograms on admission. They also evaluated the TIMI frame counts in 16 patients with this syndrome, who were compared with 16 age and gender matched controls, without coronary atherosclerosis but who underwent coronary angiography before valve surgery. They found that all patients with transient LV apical ballooning syndrome had significantly abnormal TIMI frame counts in one or more epicardial coronary vessels [27]. These investigators interpreted their findings as indicative of diffuse coronary microvascular dysfunction and suggested that this abnormality may play a significant role in the pathogenesis of this syndrome. However, it remains unclear whether microvascular dysfunction is the primary cause of the syndrome or a secondary phenomenon.

Some investigators used provocative tests, such as infusion of ergonovine or acetylcholine, to evaluate inducible coronary spasm, with conflicting results. Overall 28.6% experienced multivessel spasm after infusion of a provocative agent. Considering only the reports from Japan, where vasospastic ischaemia may be more common, the presence of spontaneous coronary spasm was ranging from 1.8 to 27.7%.

Catecholamines probably play a role in the syndrome. Some researchers have suggested that the syndrome could be a result of catecholamine-associated stunning of the myocardium, which is provoked by emotional or physiologic stress [31]. Patients presenting with the syndrome appear to have abnormalities of cardiac sympathetic innervation with evidence of sympathetic hyperactivity at the cardiac apex; a recent study shows a functional alteration in presynaptic sympathetic neurotransmission in these patients [32].

Local release of catecholamines from cardiac sympathetic efferent neurons seems to be an unlikely explanation because of the higher norepinephrine content and greater density of sympathetic nerves at the base of the heart when compared with the apex [10, 33]. The distribution of apical wall-motion abnormalities in the syndrome is similar to the distribution reported with catecholamine-induced cardiomyopathy [34]. Of note, the wall-motion abnormalities in the syndrome are not typical of those found with subarachnoid or intracranial hemorrhage in which the apex is generally spared and the basal left ventricular segments are affected [35, 36]. However, isolated reports describe transient apical sistolic dysfunction associated with subarachnoid hemorrhage [30, 37, 38, 39]. Measurements of circulating catecholamine levels in patients presenting with the syndrome have shown inconsistent results [15, 28]. In some studies plasma levels of catecholamines and their metabolites were measured and it has been found that catecholamines levels were two to three times higher in patients with transient LV apical ballooning syndrome [40].

However, several case reports of patients with pheochromocytoma-related cardiomyopathy described a similar distribution of LV wall-motion abnormalities [41], catecholamine excess can result in cAMP-mediated calcium overload via activation of β-adrenergic receptors, which leads to cardiocyte damage through a decrease in RNA, protein synthesis and cell viability [42].

Furthermore, there is some evidence suggesting that the apical myocardium may be more responsive to sympathetic stimulation and may be more vulnerable to sudden catecholamine surges. A longitudinal, base-to-apex decline in LV myocardial perfusion, as described in patients with coronary risk factors, was also proposed as a possible alternative explanation. A longitudinal, base-to-apex decline in LV myocardial perfusion, as described in patients with coronary risk factors, was also proposed as a possible alternative explanation.

An acute coronary syndrome with early reperfusion and extensive left ventricular stunning is a further pathogenic theory, substantiated by IVUS atherosclerotic plaques findings in a small series of Tako-Tsubo patients [43]. This hypothesis need to be tested by further studies comprising a large number of patients [44].

Four studies evaluated myocardial perfusion using single photon emission computed tomography (SPECT) [9, 14, 16, 20]. Results of these studies showed moderate or severe myocardial ischaemia. Thus, Abe et al. reported that 11 of 13 patients (85%), in whom resting technetium-99m tetrofosmin tomographic myocardial imaging was performed during the acute phase, had decreased radioisotope uptake at the LV apex [20]. Ito et al. reported that myocardial perfusion assessed by the SPECT imaging was impaired immediately after hospital admission, but improved considerably at 3–5 days. They interpreted the nuclear imaging findings of decreased myocardial perfusion in the absence of obstructive coronary lesions as direct evidence for impaired coronary microcirculation as a causative mechanism of this syndrome [8].

Results of these studies showed moderate or severe myocardial ischaemia decreased myocardial perfusion in the absence of obstructive coronary lesions as direct evidence for impaired coronary microcirculation as a causative mechanism of this syndrome.

Recent studies have provided initial evidence that patients with TC may show subtle metabolic abnormalities. Reduced myocardial glucose metabolism has been reported to occur in the left ventricular apex in patients with transient apical ballooning [45]. Moreover, myocardial fatty acid metabolism is suggested as being impaired in this clinical entity [8]. The resultant lipid overstorage (ie, cardiac steatosis) may produce lipotoxic intermediates that stimulate formation of reactive oxygen species and cause cardiomyocyte apoptosis [46]. Notably, TC has been reported to co-occur with mitochondrial pathology [47], thereby suggesting that apical ballooning may be exacerbated by dysfunctional cardiac bioenergetics. Moreover, myocardial stunning, a paramount feature of takotsubo cardiomyopathy [48], has been associated with important metabolic abnormalities on a cellular level, such as increased free radical production, intracellular calcium overload, and altered myofilament calcium sensitivity due to troponin-I degradation. Reactive oxygen species in particular have been implicated in myocardial stunning, and antioxidants have been shown to potently improve contractile force in *ex vivo* animal models [49].

Penas-Lado et al. suggest a possible role of a transient dynamic left ventricular outflow tract (LVOT) obstruction in the pathogenesis of this syndrome [50]. In fact, a transient dynamic LVOT gradient was detected at initial evaluation in a substantial proportion of the patients described by Tsuchihashi et al., and in other cases described elsewhere. In these patients, the clinical and hemodynamic situation improved after gradient disappearing. Moreover, in some of the patients presenting with cardiogenic shock, this situation persisted until the dynamic obstruction was diagnosed and specifically treated [51]. Thus, at least in some patients, a possible mechanism for tako-tsubo syndrome could be a dynamic LVOT obstruction preceding the ischemic event. Once present, the dynamic obstruction elevates left ventricular filling pressures, increasing myocardial oxygen demand at the mid-to-apical cavity. If this situation persists, apical hypoperfusion and ischemia may worsen, with eventual apical infarction. In fact, it is well known that, even in normal hearts, exposure to an exogenous catecholamine, such as dobutamine infusion, can precipitate dynamic LVOT obstruction [52]. Some patients, primarily women, may have geometric predisposition (sigmoid interventricular septum, small LVOT, reduced left ventricular volume) to dynamic LVOT obstruction, which may manifest only in the setting of intense adrenergic stimulation or hypovolemia. In these susceptible patients, increate adrenergic tone might produce primary LVOT obstruction leading to secondary ischemia and focal wall-motion abnormalities. Thus, the intense physical or emotional stress that precedes apical ischemia in most patients with apical ballooning syndrome could be the trigger for the acute development of LVOT obstruction capable of producing severe apical ischemia.

Myocarditis could have characteristics similar to those seen with the transient left ventricular apical ballooning syndrome but results of endomyocardial biopsies and paired serum tests for viral serology have been always resulted negative in the patients studied [15, 20].

Patients with the transient left ventricular apical ballooning syndrome seem to often present in the setting of an acute mental stress, a time of enhanced sympathetic outflow. This association could be linked to mental stress– induced transient coronary endothelial dysfunction [53, 54]. It is unclear why the apex of the heart is affected and the basal segments are spared. However, this may be partly explained by increased adrenergic receptor density in cardiac apical segments or increased apical myocardial responsiveness to adrenergic stimulation [55]. Transient apical and mid-ventricular wall-motion abnormalities have been induced in rats through physical immobilization, a model of emotional stress [56]. In this model, the wall-motion abnormalities could not be reproduced after pretreatment with the α- and β- adrenoreceptor antagonist. Notably estradiol supplementation has been reported to attenuate emotional stress–induced changes in left ventricular function in ovariectomized female rats [25].

In literature there are a lot of cases describing TC activated by a number of different situations. Adrain Ionescu [57] and Merli et al [58] reported that all their patients had mid-septal thickening contribution to the development of subaortic obstruction. Low-dose dobutamine stress echo showed regional stunning. Intraventricular gradients are not universally present thought suggesting a complex, non homogenous pathophysiology. Widespread subendocardial ischaemia (from excess catecholamines and high intracavitary pressures, potentially exacerbated by relative or absolute hypovolemia) may lead to loss of apical ventricular function, perhaps with a contribution from microvascular dysfunction.

Lentschener et al [59] diagnosed transient left ventricular apical wall motion abnormalities after non cardiac surgery; Satoro Sakuragi et al [60] described TC associated with epileptic seizure while Wadi Mawad et al [61] observed this syndrome following transcatheter radiofrequency ablation of the atrioventricular node.

Complications and Prognosis

Left ventricular apical ballooning may have the same complications of myocardial infarction, adding the early ventricular fibrillation to the previous findings of left ventricular wall rupture, ventricular arrhythmias during hospitalization and complete atrio-ventricular block. Moreover, left ventricular apical ballooning may have different and unusual clinical onsets, including sudden cardiac death due to ventricular tachyarrhythmias in the absence of associated symptoms [62].

Most patients, however, experience improvements in left ventricular function within 2–4 weeks of symptom onset. Prognosis seems to be good and the in-hospital death rate ranged from 0% to 8% in the various studies. The largest group, 88 patients, had a 1% death rate [52]. The presence of acute pulmonary oedema or acute heart failure was represented by a variable patient incidence of 3-46% and some of them were treated with aortic counterpulsation. Systolic dysfunction usually regresses in an average time of a few days or weeks, with complete recovery of normal ventricular contractility and geometry.

Only 3.5% of cases experienced a recurrence. However, evaluation of the true recurrence rate is limited, as follow-up is not reported in all patients, and in patients assessed during follow-up, timing of the follow-up assessment varied widely.

There is no evidence in the literature of therapy and short/long-term follow-up yet.

Recently a new syndrome has been described called "inverted Tako-Tsubo syndrome" ("squid syndrome") [63]. This is less frequent than *tako-tsubo* syndrome even more mind boggling syndrome. This syndrome can also be transient and reversible.

How about the inverted tako-tsubo syndrome that has been recently described in patients with severe intra cranial process or with pheochromocytoma crisis. In those rare cases, instead of the tip of the left ventricle becoming stunned and "paralyzed", the tip of the left ventricle is hyperdynamic ("hypercontracting") while it is the base of the heart that is stunned and "paralyzed".

Cherien et al. recently reported a case of an older patient who had two episodes with features that satisfy proposed current diagnostic criteria for TC [64]. Her daughter had reversible inferior wall akinesia that did not span the distribution of more than one epicardial coronary artery. Hence this would not be classified today as TC although variant forms have been described in literature very recently [65]. These variant forms or 'acute reversible heart injury syndromes', which have spared the apex, have been multi vessels in distribution. However, since coronary microvascular spasm and/ or cardiac autonomic dysfunction have been shown to be probable mechanisms involved in tako-tsubo cardiomyopathy, they would like to cautiously speculate on the possibility that the younger patient described may have experienced a variant form of tako-tsubo cardiomyopathy involving a smaller portion of myocardium. As in the variant forms, anatomic variations in sympathetic innervation in their younger patient would explain the difference in the portion of the myocardium that was 'stunned'. So in that patient if one were to consider the scenario of a takotsubo-like cardiomyopathy in terms of etiopathogenesis, the question arise [66].

Therapy

In the absence of studies specifically evaluating different therapies, the treatment of this syndrome remains entirely empirical and should be individualized according to the patient characteristics at the time of presentation. No consensus exists regarding appropriate therapy for Takotsubo cardiomyopathy because the number of reported cases is low and the disorder is possibly underdiagnosed. Patients with tako-tsubo syndrome should be monitored like patients with myocardial infarction. Ventilators support may be necessary in up to 77% of the patients due to respiratory failure [67].

Most data regarding treatment have been derived by observing patients initially treated for STEMI, and diagnosed later as having TC. Since differentiation between this cardiomyopathy and an acute coronary syndrome is often difficult at initial presentation, we tend to treat patients conservatively to avoid complications that might arise by failing to treat an anterior wall myocardial infarction. Patients receive aspirin, β-blockers, angiotensin-converting-enzyme inhibitors, cardiac catheterization and intravenous diuretics if needed; it has been suggested that β-blockers and ACE inhibitors may need to be continued indefinitely due to the chance of a late recurrence [68].

Whether anticoagulation should be administered in cases with large apical akinesia is controversial [69, 70] but short-term anticoagulation may be considered to prevent left ventricular mural thrombus formation in patients with markedly depressed left ventricular function [71]. Patients with TC must be monitored for symptoms of cardiogenic shock, heart failure and arrhythmias. Heart failure may require aggressive pharmacological treatment with inotropics drugs and mechanical circulatory support such as intra-aortic balloon pumps and left ventricular assist devices. Those with hypotension should be evaluated by echocardiography or cardiac catheterization to exclude intra-cavitary gradient, which in this case was exacerbated by dobutamine and resulted in a dynamic left ventricular mid-cavity obstruction. If a dynamic outflow pressure gradient is identified, nitroglycerine, inotropic drugs, and ACE inhibitors should be immediately discontinued to avoid gradient increasing and intravenous beta-blockers, should be administered to suppress contractility in basal segments and increase left ventricular diastolic filling time and end-diastolic volume.

However, an intravenous β-blocking agent must be used under careful monitoring because numerous contraindications to its use may exist, including bronchial asthma, respiratory failure, diabetic coma, uncontrolled pheochromocytoma, vasospasm, and bradyarrhythmias, which may be masked by the presence of transient LV apical ballooning. In fact, in a study, a beta blocker was only indicated in 38% of patients [72]; an alternative intravenous ultra-short-acting β-blocker might be considered because intravenous β-blocker produces short-term remission.

The optimal long-term management of the syndrome has not been defined [3, 7, 15, 21, 73]. Thickening of the mid ventricular septum is reported to be a predisposing factor for developing an intracavitary gradient.

Although no randomized studies are available, it seems reasonable to give beta-blockers to patients in the acute and chronic phases, and possibly indefinitely, to prevent recurrences [51, 74].

References

[1] Gianni M, Dentali F, Grandi AM et al. Apical ballooning syndrome or takotsubo cardiomyopathy: a systematic review. *European Heart Journal* (2006) 27, 1523–1529

[2] Pavin D, LeBreton H, Daubert C. Human stress cardiomyopathy mimicking acute myocardial syndrome. *Heart.* 1997;78:509 –511

[3] Daka MA, Khan RS, Deppert EJ. Transient left ventricular apical ballooning after a cocaine binge. *J. Invasive Cardiol.* 2007 Dec;19(12):E378-80.

[4] Kushiro T, Saito F, Kusama J et al. Takotsubo-shaped cardiomyopathy with type I CD36 deficiency. *Heart Vessels* May 2005;20(3):123–5.

[5] Desmet WJ, Adriaenssens BF, Dens JA. Apical ballooning of the left ventricle: first series in white patients. *Heart* 2003;89:1027–1031.

[6] Dote K, Sato H, Tateishi H, Uhida T, Ishihara M. Myocardial stunning due to simulataneous multivessel coronary spasm: a review of 5 cases. *J. cardiol.* 1991;21: 203–214.

[7] Klinceva M, Widimský P, Pesl L, Stásek J, Tousek F, Vambera M, Bílková D. Prevalence of stress-induced myocardial stunning (Tako-Tsubo cardiomyopathy) among patients undergoing emergency coronary angiography for suspected acute myocardial infarction. *Int. J. Cardiol.* 2007 Sep 3;120(3):411-3.

[8] Pillière R, Mansencal N, Digne F, Lacombe P, Joseph T, Dubourg O. Prevalence of tako-tsubo syndrome in a large urban agglomeration. *Am. J. Cardiol.* 2006 Sep 1;98(5): 662-5.

[9] Bybee KA, Prasad A, Barsness GW, Lerman A, Jaffe AS, Murphy JG, Wright RS, Rihal CS. Clinical characteristics and thrombolysis in myocardial infarction frame counts in women with transient left ventricular apical ballooning syndrome. *Am. J. Cardiol.* 2004;94:343–3

[10] Ito K, Sugihara H, Katoh S, Azuma A, Nakagawa M. Assessment of Takotsubo (ampulla) cardiomyopathy using 99mTc-tetrofosmin myocardial SPECT-comparison with acute coronary syndrome. *Ann. Nucl. Med.* 2003;17:115–122.

[11] Matsuoka K, Okubo S, Fujii E, Uchida F, Kasai A, Aoki T, Makino K, Omichi C, Fujimoto N, Ohta S, Sawai T, Nakano T. Evaluation of the arrhythmogenicity of stress-induced 'takotsubo cardiomyopathy' from the time course of the 12-lead surface electrocardiogram. *Am. J. Cardiol.* 2003;92:230–233.

[12] Akashi YJ, Nakazawa K, Sakakibara M, Miyake F, Musha H, Sasaka K. 123I-MIBG myocardial scintigraphy in patients with 'takotsubo' cardiomyopathy. *J. Nucl. Med.* 2004;45:1121–1127.

[13] Lindberg, Terrence F. Longe and Barry J. Maron Scott W. Sharkey, John R. Lesser, Andrey G. Zenovich, Martin S. Maron, Jana Acute and Reversible Cardiomyopathy Provoked by Stress in Women From the United States *Circulation* 2005;111;472-479

[14] Akashi Y, Tejma T et al. Left Ventricular Rupture Associated With Takotsubo Cardiomyopathy Mayo Clin Proc. 2004;79:821-824

[15] Ogura R, Hiasa Y, Takahashi T et al. Specific findings on the standard 12-lead ECG in patients with Takotsubo cardiomyopathy. Comparison with the findings of acute anterior myocardial infarction. *Circ. J.* 2003; 67: 687-90

[16] Kurisu S, Inoue I, Kawagoe T et al. Time course of electrocardiographic changes in patients with tako-tsubo syndrome. Comparison with acute myocardial infarction with minimal enzymatic release. *Circ. J.* 2004; 68: 77-81

[17] Akashi YJ, Nakazawa K, Sakakibara M et al. The clinical features of takotsubo cardiomyopathy. *QJ. Med.* 2003; 96:563-73

[18] Peters K, Stein J, Schneider B.Electrocardiographic changes in patients presenting with an acute coronary syndrome: "apical ballooning" versus anterior myocardial infarction. *Dtsch Med. Wochenschr.* 2008 Apr;133(16):823-8.

[19] Akashi YJ, Musha H, Nakazawa K, Miyake F. Plasma brain natriuretic peptide in takotsubo cardiomyopathy. *QJM* 2004 Sep;97(9):599-607

[20] Yamasa T, Ikeda S, Ninomiya A et al. Characteristic clinical findings of reversibile left ventricular dysfunction. *Intern. Med.* 2002;41: 789-92

[21] Bybee K, Kara T, Prasad A et al. Systematic Review: Transient Left Ventricular Apical Ballooning: A Syndrome That Mimics ST-Segment Elevation Myocardial Infarction. *Ann. Intern. Med.* 2004;141:858-865.

[22] Abe Y, Kondo M, Matsuoka R et al . Assessment of clinical features in transient left ventricular apical ballooning. *J. Am. Coll. Cardiol.* 2003; 41: 737-42

[23] Villareal RP, Achari A, Wilansky S et al. Anteroapical stunning and left ventricular out flow tract obstruction. *Mayo Clinic Proc.* 2001; 76: 79-83

[24] Haghi D, Athanasiadis A, Papavassiliu T et al. Right ventricular involvement in Takotsubo Cardiomyopathy. *Eur. Heart J.* 2006 Oct;27(20):2433-9.

[25] Haghi D , Fluechter S, Suselbeck T et al. Cardiovascular magnetic resonance findings in typical versus atipical forms of the acute apical ballooning syndrome (Takotsubo cardiomyopathy). *International Journal of Cardiology* 120 (2007) 205–211

[26] Salerno D, Lisi M, Gori T. The Tako-Tsubo syndrome: No evidence of peripheral endothelial or microvascular dysfunction. *Int. J. Cardiol.* 2008 Mar 19

[27] Celermajer DS, Sorensen KE, Spiegelhalter DJ, Georgakopoulos D, Robinson J, Deanfield JE. Aging is associated with endothelial dysfunction in healthy men years before the age-related decline in women. *J. Am. Coll. Cardiol.* 1994;24: 471-6.

[28] Ueyama T, Hano T, Kasamatsu K, Yamamoto K, Tsuruo Y, Nishio I. Estrogen attenuates the emotional stress-induced cardiac responses in the animal model of Tako-tsubo (Ampulla) cardiomyopathy. *J. Cardiovasc. Pharmacol.* 2003;42 Suppl 1:S117-9

[29] Ako J, Takenaka K, Uno K, Nakamura F, Shoji T, Iijima K, et al. Reversible left ventricular systolic dysfunction—reversibility of coronary microvascular abnormality. *Jpn. Heart J.* 2001;42:355-63

[30] Kurisu S, Sato H, Kawagoe T, Ishihara M, Shimatani Y, Nishioka K, et al. Tako-tsubo-like left ventricular dysfunction with ST-segment elevation: a novel cardiac syndrome mimicking acute myocardial infarction. *Am. Heart J.* 2002;143: 448-55.

[31] Kono T, Morita H, Kuroiwa T, Onaka H, Takatsuka H, Fujiwara A. Left ventricular wall motion abnormalities in patients with subarachnoid hemorrhage: neurogenic stunned myocardium. *J. Am. Coll. Cardiol.* 1994;24:636-40

[32] Burgdorf C, von Hof K, Schunkert H, et al. Regional alterations in myocardial sympathetic innervation in patients with transient left-ventricular apical ballooning (Tako-Tsubo cardiomyopathy). *J. Nucl. Cardiol.* 2008 Jan-Feb;15(1):65-72.

[33] Owa M, Aizawa K, Urasawa N, Ichinose H, Yamamoto K, Karasawa K, et al. Emotional stress-induced "ampulla cardiomyopathy": discrepancy between the metabolic and sympathetic innervation imaging performed during the recovery course. *Jpn. Circ. J.* 2001;65:349-52.

[34] Scott IU, Gutterman DD. Pheochromocytoma with reversible focal cardiac dysfunction. *Am. Heart J.* 1995;130:909-1

[35] Dujardin KS, McCully RB, Wijdicks EF, Tazelaar HD, Seward JB, McGregor CG, et al. Myocardial dysfunction associated with brain death: clinical, echocardiographic, and pathologic features. *J. Heart Lung Transplant* 2001; 20:350-7.

[36] Zaroff JG, Rordorf GA, Ogilvy CS, Picard MH. Regional patterns of left ventricular systolic dysfunction after subarachnoid hemorrhage: evidence for neurally mediated cardiac injury. *J. Am. Soc. Echocardiogr.* 2000;13:774-9.

[37] Yoshikawa D, Hara T, Takahashi K, Morita T, Goto F. An association between QTc prolongation and left ventricular hypokinesis during sequential episodes of subarachnoid hemorrhage. *Anesth. Analg.* 1999;89:962-4

[38] Chang PC, Lee SH, Hung HF, Kaun P, Cheng JJ. Transient ST elevation and left ventricular asynergy associated with normal coronary artery and Tc-99m PYP Myocardial Infarct Scan in subarachnoid hemorrhage [Letter]. *Int. J. Cardiol.* 1998;63: 189-92.

[39] Pollick C, Cujec B, Parker S, Tator C. Left ventricular wall motion abnormalities in subarachnoid hemorrhage: an echocardiographic study. *J. Am. Coll. Cardiol.* 1988;12: 600-5.

[40] Wittstein I, Thiemann D, Lima J et al. Neurohumoral Features of Myocardial Stunning Due to Sudden Emotional Stress *N. Engl. J. Med.* 2005;352:539-48.

[41] Sarsedai SH, Mourant AJ, Sivathan Y et al. Pheocromocytoma and catecholamine induced cardiomyopathy presentino as heart failure. *Br. Heart J.* 1990; 63: 234-7

[42] Mann DL , Kent RL, Parsons B, et al. Adrenergic effects on the biology of the adult mammalian cardiocyte. *Circulation* 1991;85: 790 - 804

[43] Ibanez B, Navarro F, Cordoba M et al. Tako-tsubo transient left ventricular apical ballooning: is intravascular ultrasound the key to resolve the enigma? *Heart* 2005; 91:102-4

[44] Briguori C, Tobis J, Nishida T et al. Discrepancy between angiography and intravascular ultrasound when analysing small coronary arteries. *Eur. Heart J.* 2002; 23: 247-54

[45] Bybee KA, Murphy J, Prasad A et al: Acute impairment of regional myocardial glucose uptake in the apical balloonong (takotsubo) syndrome. *J. Nucl. Cardiol,* 2006; 13:244-50

[46] McGavock JM, Lingvay I, Zib I et al: Cardiac steatosis in diabetes mellitus: a 1H-magnetic resonance spectroscopy study. *Circulation,* 2007; 116: 1170-75

[47] Finsterer J, Stöllberger C, Sehnal E, et al. : Apical ballooning (Takotsubo syndrome) in mitochondrial disorder during mechanical ventilation. *J. Cardiovasc. Med.* (Hagerstown). 2007 Oct;8(10):859-63.

[48] Cheng TO. Takotsubo cardiomyopathy represents a stress-induced myocardial stunning. *J. Cardiol.* 2007 Feb;49(2):106-7.

[49] Kaplan P, Matejovicova M, Herijgers P, et al .Effect of free radical scavengers on myocardial function and Na+, K+-ATPase activity in stunned rabbit myocardium. *Scand. Cardiovasc. J.* 2005 Sep;39(4):213-9.

[50] Penas-Lado M, Barriales-Villa R, Goicolea J. Transient Left Ventricular Apical Ballooning and Outflow Tract Obstruction *JACC* Vol. 42, No. 6, 2003 September 17, 2003:1140–6

[51] Haley JH, Sinak LJ, Tajik AJ, Ommen SR, Oh JK. Dynamic left ventricular outflow tract obstruction in acute coronary syndromes: an important cause of new systolic murmur and cardiogenic shock. *Mayo Clin. Proc.* 1999;74:901–6.

[52] Luria D, Klutstein MW, Rosenmann D, Shaheen J, Sergey S, Tzivoni D. Prevalence and significance of left ventricular outflow gradient during dobutamine echocardiography. *Eur. Heart J.* 1999;20:386–92

[53] Spieker LE, Hurlimann D, Ruschitzka F, Corti R, Enseleit F, Shaw S, et al. Mental stress induces prolonged endothelial dysfunction via endothelin-A receptors. *Circulation* 2002;105:2817-20

[54] Ghiadoni L, Donald AE, Cropley M, Mullen MJ, Oakley G, Taylor M, et al. Mental stress induces transient endothelial dysfunction in humans. *Circulation* 2000;102:2473-8.

[55] Mori H, Ishikawa S, Kojima S, Hayashi J, Watanabe Y, Hoffman JI, et al. Increased responsiveness of left ventricular apical myocardium to adrenergic stimuli. *Cardiovasc. Res.* 1993;27:192-8.

[56] Ueyama T, Kasamatsu K, Hano T, Yamamoto K, Tsuruo Y, Nishio I. Emotional stress induces transient left ventricular hypocontraction in the rat via activation of cardiac adrenoceptors: a possible animal model of 'tako-tsubo' cardiomyopathy. *Circ. J.* 2002; 66:712-3

[57] Ionescu A. Subaortic dynamic obstruction: A contributing factor to hemodynamic instability in tako-tsubo syndrome? *Eur. J. Echocardiogr.* 2007 Jan 3

[58] Merli E, Sutcliffe S, Gori M, Sutherland GG. Tako-Tsubo cardiomyopathy: new insights into the possible underlying pathophysiology. *Eur. J. Echocardiogr.* 2006 Jan; 7(1): 53-61.

[59] Lentschener C, Vignaux O, Spaulding C, Bonnichon P, Legmann P, Ozier Y. Early postoperative tako-tsubo-like left ventricular dysfunction: transient left ventricular apical ballooning syndrome. *Anesth. Analg.* 2006 Sep;103(3):580-2.

[60] Sakuragi S, Tokunaga N, Okawa K et al. A case of takotsubo cardiomyopathy associated with epileptic seizure: reversible left ventricular wall motion abnormality and ST-segment elevation. *Heart Vessels* 2007 Jan;22(1):59-63.

[61] Mawad W, Guerra PG, Dubuc M, Khairy P. Tako-tsubo cardiomyopathy following transcatheter radiofrequency ablation of the atrioventricular node. *Europace* 2007 Nov; 9(11): 1075-6.

[62] Raddino R, Pedrinazzi C, Zanini G et al. Out-of-hospital cardiac arrest caused by transient left ventricular apical ballooning syndrome. *Int. J. Cardiol.* 2007 Aug 9.

[63] Bulut A, Rav-Acha M, Aydin O, et al. "Inverted Tako-Tsubo": Transient apical-sparing cardiomyopathy. *Int. J. Cardiol.* 2008 Apr 3.

[64] Kevin B, Kara Tomas, Abhiram P, et al. Systematic review: transient left ventricular apical ballooning: a syndrome that mimics ST-segment elevation myocardial infarction. *Ann. Intern. Med.* 2004;141:858–65

[65] Haghi D, Papavassiliu T, Flüchter S, et al. Variant form of the acute apical ballooning syndrome (takotsubo cardiomyopathy): observations on a novel entity. *Heart* 2006;92: 392–4.

[66] Cherian J, Angelis D, Filiberti A, Saperia G. Can takotsubo cardiomyopathy be familial? *Int. J. Cardiol.* 2007 Sep 14;121(1):74-5.

[67] Seth PS, Aurigemma GP, Krasnow JM et al. A syndrome of transient left ventricular apical wall motion abnormality in the absence of coronary disease: a perspective from the United States. *Cardiology* 2003; 100:61.6

[68] Dec GW. Recognition of the apical ballooning syndrome in the United States. *Circulation* 2005; 111:388-90

[69] Sasaki N, Kinugawa T, Yamawaki M, et al. Transient left ventricular apical ballooning in a patient with bicuspid aortic valve created a left ventricular thrombus leading to acute renal infarction. *Circ. J.* 2004; 68:1081-3

[70] Akashi Yj, Tejima T, Sakurada H, et al. Takotsubo cardiomyopathy with a significant pressure gradient in the left ventricle. *Heart Vessels* 2000; 15:203

[71] Andò G, Saporito F, Trio O, Cerrito M et al.. Systemic embolism in takotsubo syndrome. *Int. J. Cardiol.* 2008 Mar 24

[72] Yoshioka T, Hashimoto A, Tsuchihashi K, et al. Clinical implications of midventricular obstruction and intravenous propranolol use in transient left ventricular apical ballooning (Takotsubo cardiomyopathy). *Am. Heart J.* 2008 Mar;155(3):526.e1-7

[73] Tsuchihashi K, Ueshima K, Uchida T, et al. Angina Pectoris- Miocardial Infarction Investigations in Japan. Transient left ventricular apical ballooning without coronary artery stenosis: aA novel heart syndrome mimicking acute myocardial infarction. *J. Am. Coll. Cardiol.* 2001; 38: 11-8

[74] Kyuma M, Tsuchihashi K, Shinshi Y, et al. Effect of intravenous propanolol on left ventricular apical ballooning without coronary artery stenosis (ampulla cardiomyopathy): Three cases. *Circ. J.* 2002;66:1181-4

In: Handbook of Cardiovascular Research ISBN 978-1-60741-792-7
Editors: Jorgen Brataas and Viggo Nanstveit © 2009 Nova Science Publishers, Inc.

Chapter XV

Chest Pain: Causes, Diagnosis, and Treatment

Giovanni Fazio
Department of Cardiology, University of Palermo

Chest pain is one of the most frightening symptoms a person can have. It is sometimes difficult even for a doctor or other medical professional to tell what is causing chest pain and whether it is life-threatening.

Chest pain can be defined as discomfort or pain that you feel anywhere along the front of your body between your neck and upper abdomen.

Any part of the chest can be the cause of the pain including the heart, lungs, esophagus, muscle, bone, and skin (table 1).

Table 1. Differential Diagnoses of Patients Admitted to Hospital with Acute Chest Pain Ruled Not Myocardial Infarction

Diagnosis	Percent
Gastroesophageal diseases	42%
Gastroesophageal reflux	
Esophageal motility disorders	
Peptic ulcer	
Gallstones	
Ischemic heart disease	31%
Chest wall syndromes	28%
Pericarditis	4%
Pleuritis/pneumonia	2%
Pulmonary embolism	2%
Lung cancer	1.5%
Aortic aneurysm	1%
Aortic stenosis	1%
Herpes zoster	1%

The causes of chest pain fall into two major categories: Cardiac and Non-cardiac causes.

The main cardiac causes of chest pain are: Heart attack, Angina, Aortic dissection, Acute pericarditis, Mitral valve prolapse.

Potentially life-threatening cardiac causes of chest pain are as follows:

Heart attack (acute myocardial infarction) A heart attack [1] occurs when blood flow to the arteries that supply the heart (coronary arteries) becomes blocked. The muscle of the heart does not receive enough oxygen. This can cause damage, deterioration, and death of the heart muscle. A heart attack is caused by coronary heart disease, or coronary artery disease. Heart disease may be caused by cholesterol build up in the coronary arteries (atherosclerosis), blood clots, or spasm of the vessels that supply blood to the heart. Typical heart attack pain occurs in the mid to left side of the chest and may also extend to the left shoulder, the left arm, the jaw, the stomach, or the back. Other associated symptoms are shortness of breath, increased sweating, nausea, vomiting, heartburn, sweatiness, lightheadedness, dizziness, or unexplained fatigue [2]. *Diagnosis:* in the hospital emergency department, the healthcare providers use three basic procedures to decide if a patient is having a heart attack. The first is the symptoms reported by the patient. The second is an electrocardiogram (ECG or EKG), an electrical tracing of the heart's activity. On the ECG, it may be possible to tell which vessels in the heart are blocked or narrowed. The third is measurement of enzymes produced by the heart muscle cells when they do not receive enough oxygen. These enzymes are detectable with blood tests and are called cardiac enzymes. *Treatment* for a heart attack is aimed at increasing blood flow by opening arteries blocked or narrowed by a blood clot. Medicines used to achieve this include aspirin, heparin, and clot-busting (thrombolytic) drugs [3]. Other medications can be used to slow the heart rate, which decreases the workload of the heart and reduces pain. Angioplasty [4] is a way of unblocking an artery. Angiography is done first to locate narrowing or blockages. A very thin plastic tube called a catheter is inserted into the artery. A tiny balloon on the end of the catheter is inflated. This expands the artery, providing a wider passage for blood. The balloon is then deflated and removed. Sometimes a small metal scaffold called a stent is placed in the artery to keep it expanded. Surgery may be required if medical treatment is unsuccessful. This could include angioplasty or cardiac bypass.

Angina: Angina is chest pain related to an imbalance between the oxygen demand of the heart and the amount of oxygen delivered via the blood [5]. It is caused by blockage or narrowing of the blood vessels that supply blood to the heart. Angina is different from a heart attack [6] in that the arteries are not completely blocked, and it causes little or no permanent damage to the heart. "Stable" angina occurs repetitively and predictably while exercising and goes away with rest. "Unstable" angina results in unusual and unpredictable pain not relieved totally by rest, or pain that actually occurs at rest. Angina is similar to heart attack pain but occurs with physical exertion or exercise and is relieved by rest or nitroglycerin. Angina becomes life-threatening when pain occurs at rest, has increased in frequency or intensity, or is not relieved with at least three nitroglycerin tablets taken five minutes apart.This is considered to be unstable angina, which may be a warning sign of an impending heart attack. *Diagnosis:* Angina is diagnosed [7] by the same methods doctors use to diagnose heart attacks. In angina, the test results reveal no permanent damage to the heart. The diagnosis is made only after the possibility of a heart attack has been ruled out, usually by negative results on three sets of cardiac enzyme tests [8]. Although the ECG may show abnormalities, these changes are often reversible. Another way to diagnose angina is the stress test: these tests monitor your ECG during exercise or other stress to identify blockages in blood vessels to the heart. Cardiac catheterization is used to identify blockages. This is a special type of x-ray (angiography or arteriography) that uses a harmless dye to highlight blockages or other abnormalities in blood vessels. *Treatment* of angina is directed at relieving chest pain that occurs as the result of reduced blood flow to the heart. The medication nitroglycerin is the most widely used treatment. Nitroglycerin dilates (widens) the coronary arteries. It is often taken under the tongue (sublingually). People with known angina may be treated with nitroglycerin for three doses, five minutes apart. If the pain remains, nitroglycerin is given by IV, and the patient is admitted to the hospital and monitored to rule out a heart attack. Long-term treatment after the first episode of angina focuses on reducing risk factors for atherosclerosis and heart disease.

Aortic dissection: The aorta is the main artery that supplies blood to the vital organs of the body, such as the brain, heart, kidneys, lungs, and intestines Aortic dissection may be caused by conditions that damage the innermost lining of the aorta. These include uncontrolled high blood pressure, connective-tissue diseases, cocaine use, advanced age, pregnancy, congenital heart disease, and cardiac catheterization. . Men are at higher risk than women. The chest pain associated with aortic dissection occurs suddenly and is described as "ripping" or "tearing." The pain may radiate to the back or between the shoulder blades. Symptoms may also include: angina-type pain, shortness of breath, fainting, abdominal pain, or symptoms of stroke. A similar condition is aortic aneurysm. This is an enlargement of the aorta that can rupture, causing pain and bleeding. Aneurysms can occur in the aorta in the chest or the abdomen. *Diagnosis:* the diagnosis of aortic dissection [9] is based on the symptoms the patient describes, chest x-ray, and other special imaging tests. On a chest x-ray, the aorta will have an abnormal contour or appear widened. Transesophageal echocardiography is a specialized ultrasound of the heart in which a probe is inserted into the esophagus. The technique is performed under sedation or general anesthesia. The dissection may be identified very accurately by a CT scan of the chest or angiography. *Treatment:* Suspected aortic dissection often is treated with medications that reduce blood pressure. Medications that slow the heart rate and dilate the arteries are the most widely used. Close monitoring is required to avoid lowering the blood pressure too much, which can be dangerous. Surgical repair is required for any dissection that involves the ascending (upward) portion of the aorta.

Cardiac causes of chest pain that are not immediately life-threatening include the following:

Acute pericarditis: This is an inflammation of the pericardium, which is the sac that covers the heart. Pericarditis can be caused by viral infection, bacterial infection, cancer, connective-tissue diseases, certain medications, radiation treatment, and chronic renal failure. One life-threatening complication of pericarditis is cardiac tamponade. Cardiac tamponade is an accumulation of fluid around the heart. This prevents the heart from effectively pumping blood to the body. Symptoms of cardiac tamponade include sudden onset of shortness of breath, fainting, and chest pain. The pain of pericarditis is typically described as a sharp or stabbing pain in the mid-chest, worsened by deep breaths. This pain may mimic the pain of a heart attack, because it may radiate to the left side of the back or shoulder. One distinguishing factor is that the pain is worsened by lying flat and improved by leaning forward. When lying flat, the inflamed pericardium is in direct contact with the heart and causes pain. When leaning forward, there is a space between the pericardium and the heart.Many people report a recent cold, fever, shortness of breath, or pain when swallowing just before developing pericarditis. *Diagnosis:* acute pericarditis is usually diagnosed by the patient's symptoms, serial ECGs, and echocardiography. Certain lab tests may be helpful in determining the cause. *Treatment:* Viral pericarditis usually improves with 7-21 days of therapy with nonsteroidal anti-inflammatory agents such as aspirin and ibuprofen (for example, Motrin).

Mitral valve prolapse: Mitral valve prolapse is an abnormality of one of the heart valves in which the "leaves" of the valve bulge into the upper heart chamber during contraction. When this occurs, a small amount of blood flows backward in the heart. Mitral valve prolapse usually has no symptoms, but some people experience palpitations (sensation of rapid or strong heartbeat) and chest pain. Chest pain associated with mitral valve prolapse differs from that of typical angina in that it is sharp, does not radiate, and is not related to physical exertion. Other symptoms include fatigue, lightheadedness [10], and shortness of breath. Complications include infection of the heart valves, mitral valve regurgitation (an abnormal blood flow within the chambers of the heart), and abnormal heart rhythms, witch rarely cause sudden death.

The main Non-cardiac causes of chest pain are: pulmonary embolism, pneumonia, spontaneous pneumothorax, perforated viscus, pleuris, disorders of the esophagus, costochondritis, herpes zoster, shingles, gallbladder or pancreas problems, cancer and panic attack.

Potentially life-threatening cardiac causes of chest pain are as follows:

Pulmonary embolism: A pulmonary embolus is a blood clot in one of the major blood vessels that supplies the lungs. It is a potentially life-threatening cause of chest pain but is not associated with the heart. Pulmonary embolism risk factors include: sedentary lifestyle, obesity, prolonged immobility, fracture of a long bone of the legs, pregnancy, cancer, history or family history of blood clots, irregular heartbeat (arrhythmias), heart attack, or congestive heart failure. Symptoms of a pulmonary embolus include: the sudden onset of shortness of breath, rapid breathing, and sharp pain in the mid chest, which increases with deep breaths. *Diagnosis:* The diagnosis of pulmonary embolism is made from a variety of sources. Description of the patient's symptoms and results of ECG and chest x-ray all may contribute to the diagnosis, but are not definitive. The healthcare provider may draw blood drawn from the patient's artery to check the levels of oxygen and other gases. Abnormalities in blood gases indicate a problem in the lungs that is preventing the patient from getting enough oxygen. A ventilation-perfusion scan (V/Q scan) compares blood flow to oxygen intake in different segments of the lung. An irregularity in just one segment can indicate an embolism. A CT scan of the lungs is another way to determine if a patient has a pulmonary embolus. It may be done instead of the V/Q scan. Anyone with a presumed or documented pulmonary embolism requires admission to the hospital. *Treatment* usually includes supplemental oxygen and medication to prevent further clotting of blood, typically heparin. If the embolism is very large, clot-busting medications are given in some situations to dissolve the clot. Some people undergo surgery to place an umbrella-like filter in a blood vessel to prevent blood clots from the lower extremities from moving to the lungs.

Spontaneous pneumothorax: (collapsed lung) occurs when the pressure balance between the sac that contains the lung and the outside atmosphere is disrupted. Injury to the chest that pierces through to the lung sac is the most common cause of this condition. This can be caused by trauma, as in a car wreck, bad fall, gunshot wound or stabbing, or in surgery. Other risk factors for pneumothorax include AIDS-related pneumonia, emphysema, severe asthma, cystic fibrosis, cancer, and marijuana and crack cocaine use. Symptoms of pneumothorax include: the sudden onset of shortness of breath,sharp chest pain, rapid heart rate, dizziness, lightheadedness, or faintness. Normally, negative pressure in the chest cavity allows the lungs to expand. When a spontaneous pneumothorax occurs, air enters the chest cavity. When the pressure balance is lost, the lung is unable to re-expand. This cuts off the normal oxygen supply in the body. *Diagnosis:* spontaneous pneumothorax is diagnosed by physical exam and chest x-ray. A CT scan may be helpful in locating a small pneumothorax. *Treatment:* A pneumothorax without symptoms involves six hours of hospital observation and repeat chest x-rays. If the size of the pneumothorax remains unchanged, the patient is usually discharged with a follow-up appointment in 24 hours. If the patient develop symptoms or the pneumothorax enlarges, they will be admitted to the hospital. The patient will undergo catheter aspiration or have a chest tube inserted to restore negative pressure in the lung sac.

Perforated viscus: A perforated viscus is a hole or tear in the wall of any area of the gastrointestinal tract. This allows air to enter the abdominal cavity, which irritates the diaphragm, and can cause chest pain. Risk factors not related to trauma are: untreated ulcers, prolonged or forceful vomiting, swallowing a foreign body, cancer, appendicitis, long-term steroid use, infection of the gallbladder, gallstones, and AIDS. Perforated viscus comes on suddenly with severe abdominal, chest, and/or back pain. Abdominal pain may increase with movement or when breathing in and may be accompanied by a rigid, boardlike abdominal wall. *Diagnosis:* Perforated viscus usually can be identified by a chest x-ray with the patient standing upright or an abdominal x-ray lying on the left side. X-rays in these positions allow air to rise to the diaphragm, where it can be detected. The symptoms and the results of the physical exam and other lab tests also assist in diagnosis. *Treatment:* Any disruption or perforation of the intestinal tract (viscus) is a potentially life-threatening emergency. Immediate surgery may be required.

Causes of chest pain that are not immediately life-threatening include the following:

Pneumonia: It is an infection of the lung tissue. Chest pain occurs because of inflammation to the lining of the lungs [11] The pain is usually one-sided an is worsened by coughing. Other associated symptoms include fever, coughing up mucus (sputum), and shortness of breath. *Diagnosis:* Pneumonia is diagnosed by the patient's symptoms and medical history, physical examination, and chest x-ray. *Treatment:* Pneumonia is treated with antibiotics, and pain medication is given for chest wall tenderness.

Pleurisy. This sharp, localized chest pain that's made worse when you inhale or cough occurs when the membrane that lines your chest cavity and covers your lungs becomes inflamed. Pleurisy may result from a wide variety of underlying conditions, including pneumonia and, rarely, autoimmune conditions, such as lupus. An autoimmune disease is one in which your body's immune system mistakenly attacks healthy tissue. *Diagnosis:* It is diagnosed by the patient's symptoms and medical history, physical examination, and chest x-ray. *Treatment:* Pleurisy is treated with antibiotics, and pain medication is given for chest wall tenderness.

Disorders of the esophagus: Chest pain from esophageal disorders can be an alarming symptom because it often mimics chest pain from a heart attack.

- *Acid reflux disease* (gastroesophageal reflux disease, GERD, heartburn) occurs when acidic digestive juices flow backward from the stomach into the esophagus. Acid reflux (GERD) may be caused by any factors that decrease the pressure on the lower part of the esophagus, decreased movement of the esophagus, or prolonged emptying of the stomach. This condition may be brought on by: consumption of high-fat foods, nicotine use, alcohol use, caffeine, pregnancy, certain medications, diabetes, or scleroderma. The resulting heartburn is sometimes experienced as chest pain. Symptoms include: heartburn, painful swallowing, excessive salivation, dull chest discomfort, chest pressure, or severe squeezing pain across the mid chest. Pain from GERD is often relieved with antacids
- *Esophagitis* is an inflammation of the esophagus. Esophagitis may be caused by yeast, fungi, viruses, bacteria, or irritation from medications. The symptoms include difficulty swallowing, painful swallowing, or symptoms of GERD. The chest pain comes on suddenly and is not relieved by antacids.
- *Esophageal spasm* is defined as excessive, intensified, or uncoordinated contractions of the smooth muscle of the esophagus. It is caused by excessive, intensified, or uncoordinated contractions of the smooth muscle of the esophagus. Spasm may be triggered by emotional upset or swallowing very hot or cold liquids The pain of esophageal spasm is usually intermittent and dull. It is located in the mid-chest and may radiate to the back, neck, or shoulders. Disorders of the esophagus causing chest pain are diagnosed by a process of elimination. The diagnosis is made on the basis of the patient's symptoms and medical history, after ruling out cardiac causes and observing whether the patient experiences pain relief from antacids.

Treatment: The three major esophageal disorders that cause chest pain are treated with antacid therapy; antibiotic, antiviral, or antifungal medication; medication to relax the muscles of the esophagus; or some combination of these.

Costochondritis: This is an inflammation of the cartilage between the ribs. Pain is typically located in the mid-chest, with intermittently dull and sharp pain that may be increased with deep breaths, movement, and deep touch. Treatment: Costochondritis is usually treated with nonsteroidal anti-inflammatory medication such as ibuprofen.

Herpes zoster: Also known as shingles, this is a reactivation of the viral infection that causes chickenpox. With shingles, a rash occurs, usually only on one small part of the body. The pain, often very severe, is usually confined to the area of the rash. The pain may precede the rash by 4-7 days. Risk factors include any condition in which the immune system is compromised, such as advanced age, HIV, or cancer. Herpes zoster is highly contagious to people who have not had chickenpox or have not been vaccinated against chickenpox for the five days before and the five days after the appearance of the rash.

Shingles: This infection of the nerves caused by the chickenpox virus can produce pain and a band of blisters from your back around to your chest wall.

Gallbladder or pancreas problems: Gallstones or inflammation of your gallbladder (cholecystitis) or pancreas can cause acute abdominal pain that radiates to your chest.

Cancer. Rarely, cancer involving the chest or cancer that has spread from another part of the body can cause chest.

Panic attack. If you experience periods of intense fear accompanied by chest pain, rapid heartbeat, rapid breathing (hyperventilation), profuse sweating and shortness of breath, you may be experiencing a panic attack - a form of anxiety [12].

The evaluation of the patient with chest discomfort must accommodate two goals—determining the diagnosis and assessing the safety of the immediate management plan.

Considerations in the Assessment of the Patient with Chest Pain

1. Could the chest discomfort be due to an acute, potentially lifethreatening condition that warrants immediate hospitalization and aggressive evaluation?
   - Acute ischemic heart disease Pulmonary embolism
   - Aortic dissection Spontaneous pneumothorax
2. If not, could the discomfort be due to a chronic condition likely to lead to serious complications?
   - Stable angina
   - Aortic stenosis
   - Pulmonary hypertension
3. If not, could the discomfort be due to an acute condition that warrants specific treatment?
   - Pericarditis
   - Pneumonia/pleuritis
   - Herpes zoster
4. If not, could the discomfort be due to another treatable chronic condition?
   - Esophageal reflux Cervical disk disease
   - Esophageal spasm Arthritis of the shoulder or spine
   - Peptic ulcer disease Costochondritis
   - Gallbladder disease Other musculoskeletal disorders
   - Other gastrointestinal conditions
   - Anxiety state

Follow-up

No matter what the cause of chest pain, regular follow-up visits with your healthcare provider are important. This will help you remain as healthy as possible and prevent worsening of your condition.

Prevention

Heart Attack Prevention: Prevention of heart attack and angina [13] involves living what the American Heart Association calls a "heart healthy" lifestyle. Reducing your risk factors has a significant effect on reducing your risk. Don't smoke, maintain a healthy weigh, eat nutritious, low-fat foods in moderate quantities, if you drink alcohol, use alcohol moderately, engage in physical activity or exercise for at least 30 minutes every day, control high blood pressure and high cholesterol.

Aortic Dissection Prevention: Aortic dissection may be prevented by controlling high blood pressure and getting proper screening if the patient has a familial disposition to this disorder [14].

Pulmonary Embolism Prevention: Prevention of pulmonary embolism includes living a heart healthy lifestyle.No one should smoke, but women older than 35 years who use birth control pills are at especially high risk from smoking, when traveling on extended trips that require sitting for long periods of time (plane, car, train, etc.) or other times of leg immobilization, get up and allow time for stretching and movement of the legs. Isometric contractions of the calves are helpful if getting out of the seat is not possible.You should always receive preventive anticoagulant medication after surgery, especially after orthopedic surgery.

Spontaneous Pneumothorax Prevention: Smoking cessation decreases the risk of spontaneous pneumothorax.

Perforated Viscus Prevention: treating peptic ulcers appropriately and avoiding swallowing foreign bodies reduces the risk of perforated viscus.

Pericarditis Prevention: because many cases of acute pericarditis are caused by viruses, effective handwashing may reduce transmission of infectious viral agents.

Pneumonia Prevention: effective handwashing and good hygiene will help reduce the transmission of infectious viruses and bacteria that can cause pneumonia.

Esophagus Disease Prevention: Acid reflux (GERD) can be prevented to a certain extent in most people. Avoid foods and other substances that bring on or worsen symptoms, especially fatty foods. Stop smoking, use alcohol in moderation, avoid eating large meals, avoid eating for three hours before bedtime, avoid lying down right after eating.

Whatever may be the cause of chest pain, cardiac cause and extracardiac cause, or potentially life threatening, chest pain remains a symptom of very difficult approach, petitioner the maximum attention in the nosografic organization and the early treatment, to the aim to avoid diagnostic errors and to resolve the pain.

References

[1]   Cannon CP et al: National Heart Attack Alert Program (NHAAP) Coordinating Committee Critical Pathways Writing Group. Critical pathways for management of patients with acute coronary syndromes: An assessment by the National Heart Attack Alert Program. *Am. Heart J.* 143:777, 2002

[2]   Pope JH, et al: Missed diagnoses of acute cardiac ischemia in the emergency department. *N. Engl. J. Med.* 342:1163, 2000

[3]   Pollack CV Jr. 2004 American College of Cardiology/American Heart Association guidelines for the management of patients with ST-elevation myocardial infarction: implications for emergency department practice. *Ann. Emerg. Med.* 2005; 45(4): 363-76.

[4]   Boden WE, O'rourke RA, Teo KK, et al. Optimal Medical Therapy with or without PCI for Stable Coronary Disease. *N. Engl. J. Med.* 2007 Mar 26; [Epub ahead of print].

[5]   Gibson PB, et al: Low event rate for stress-only perfusion imaging in patients evaluated for chest pain. *J. Am. Coll. Cardiol.* 39:999, 2002

[6]   Braunwald E et al: ACC/AHA guideline update for the management of patients with unstable angina and non-ST-segment elevation myocardial infarction, 2002: Summary article. *J. Am. Coll. Cardiol.* 40:1366, 2002

[7]   Stein RA, et al: Safety and utility of exercise testing in emergency room chest pain centers: An advisory from the Committee on Exercise, Rehabilitation, and Prevention Council on Clinical Cardiology, American Heart Association. *Circulation* 102:1463, 2000

[8]   Hamm CW: Cardiac biomarkers for rapid evaluation of chest pain. *Circulation* 104: 1454, 2001

[9]   NG SM, et al: Ninety-minute accelerated critical pathway for chest pain evaluation. *Am. J. Cardiol.* 88:611:2001

[10] Weber BE, Kapoor WN: Evaluation and outcomes of patients with palpitations. *Am. J. Med.* 100:138, 1996

[11] Van Peski-Oosterbaan AS et al: Cognitive-behavioral therapy for non cardiac chest pain: A randomized trial. *Am. J. Med.* 106:424, 1999

[12] Barsky AJ et al: Somatized psychiatric disorder presenting as palpitations. *Arch Intern. Med.* 156:1102, 1996

[13] Mosca L, Banka CL, Benjamin EJ, et al. Evidence-Based Guidelines for Cardiovascular Disease Prevention in Women: 2007 Update. *Circulation.* 2007; Published online before print February 19, 2007.

[14] The Seventh Report of the Joint National Committee on Prevention, Detection, Evaluation, and Treatment of High Blood Pressure. *Clinical Guidelines/Evidence Reports.* 2003 May; 3(5233); 1.

In: Handbook of Cardiovascular Research
Editors: Jorgen Brataas and Viggo Nanstveit

ISBN 978-1-60741-792-7
© 2009 Nova Science Publishers, Inc.

Chapter XVI

Stem Cells and Repair of the Heart: Current Limitations and Future Perspectives of Cell-Releasing Epicardial Scaffolds

Enrico Vizzardi [1], Roberto Lorusso [2], Giuseppe De Cicco [2],
Gregoriana Zanini [1], Pompilio Faggiano [1]
and Livio Dei Cas [1]

1. Department of Cardiology,
University of Brescia, Brescia, Italy
2. Experimental Cardiac Surgery Laboratory,
Cardiac Surgery Unit, Civic Hospital, Brescia, Italy

Chronic heart failure(CHF) has emerged as a major worldwide epidemic. Recently, a fundamental shift in the underlying etiology of CHF is becoming evident, in which the most common cause is no longer hypertension or valvular disease, but rather long-term survival after acute myocardial infarction (AMI) [1,2].

The costs of this syndrome, both in economic and personal terms, are considerable [3]. American Heart Association statistics indicate that CHF affects 4.7 million patients in the United States and is responsible for approximately one million hospitalizations and 300,000 deaths annually.

The total annual costs associated with this disorder have been estimated to exceed $22 billion. The societal impact of CHF is also remarkable. Patients with CHF often suffer a greatly compromised quality of life. About 30% of diagnosed individuals (i.e.,1.5 million in U.S.) experience difficulty breathing with little or no physical exertion, and are very restricted in their daily functions. This forced sedentary lifestyle inevitably leads to further physical and mental distress.

The CHF problem is growing worse. While CHF already represents one of our greatest health care problems, it is expected to become even more severe in the future. By 2010, the number of patients suffering from HF will have grown to nearly 7 million, a more than 40% increase.

Coronary artery disease (CAD) is the cause of CHF in the majority of patients, and CHF is the only mode of CAD presentation associated with increasing incidence and mortality.

However, it is evident, running through the different therapeutical strategies of CHF, that the appropriate treatment of patients with ischemic heart failure is still unknown [4,5].

After myocardial infarction, injured cardiomyocytes are replaced by fibrotic tissue promoting the development of heart failure. Cell transplantation has emerged as a potential therapy and stem cells may be an important and powerful cellular source.

Cell transplantation represents the last frontier within the treatment of cardiac diseases. Cell transplantation is currently generating a great deal of interest since the replacement of akinetic scar tissue by viable myocardium should improve cardiac function, impede progressive LV remodelling, and revascularize ischemic area. The goals of cell therapy are multiple and non exclusive, leading to the formation of a new tissue.

One should expect to replace a scar tissue by living cells and/or to block or reverse the remodelling process or change its nature and/or to restore the contractility of the cardiac tissue and/or to induce neoangiogenesis that would favour the recruitment of hibernating cardiomyocytes or to enhance transplanted cell engraftment, survival, function, and, ultimately, synergistic interaction with resident cells.

From the first paper published in 1992 that has documented the potentials of the transplantation of autologous skeletal muscle to treat the damage induced by acute myocardial infarction [5], innumerable techniques, types of cells, myocardial pathologies, and techniques of implantation have been reported, greatly expanding this innovative and appealing field of search in cardiovascular medicine.

Different stem cell populations have been intensively studied in the last decade as a potential source of new cardiomyocytes to ameliorate the injured myocardium, compensate for the loss of ventricular mass and contractility and eventually restore cardiac function. An array of cell types has been explored in this respect, including skeletal muscle, bone marrow derived stem cells, embryonic stem cells (ESC) and more recently cardiac progenitor cells. The best-studied cell types are mouse and human ESC cells, which have undisputedly been demonstrated to differentiate into cardiomyocyte and vascular lineages and have been of great help to understand the differentiation process of pluripotent cells. However, due to their immunogenicity, risk of tumor development and the ethical challenge arising from their embryonic origin, they do not provide a suitable cell source for a regenerative therapy approach.

Embryonic stem cells can differentiate into true cardiomyocytes, making them in principle an unlimited source of transplantable cells for cardiac repair, although immunological and ethical constraints exist. Somatic stem cells are an attractive option to explore for transplantation as they are autologous, but their differentiation potential is more restricted than embryonic stem cells. Currently, the major sources of somatic cells used for basic research and in clinical trials originate from the bone marrow. The differentiation capacity of different populations of bone marrow-derived stem cells into cardiomyocytes has been studied intensively. Only mesenchymal stem cells seem to form cardiomyocytes, and only a small percentage of this population will do so in vitro or in vivo. A newly identified cell population isolated from cardiac tissue, called cardiac progenitor cells, holds great potential for cardiac regeneration.

New approaches for cardiac repair have been enabled by the discovery that the heart contains its own reservoir of stem cells. These cells are positive for various stem/progenitor cell markers, are self-renewing, and exhibit multilineage differentiation potential. Recently has been developed a method for ex vivo expansion of cardiac-derived stem cells from human myocardial biopsies with a view to subsequent autologous transplantation for myocardial regeneration.

Despite original promises and expectations, current evidences of stem cell transplantation are still weak and controversial. The use of trypsin to detach the cells from the culture dish disrupts their microintercellular communication and extracellular matrix, restricts cell survival and growth, and thus appears deleterious to cell transplantation theraphy. Intercellular communication factors play a key role in cell adhesion, migration, proliferation, differentiation, and death and must be maintained for optimal cellular benefits. Therefore, alternative line of research are being explored, particularly in the field of techniques of cell implantation and engraftment.

Besides direct implantation or myocardial colonization by bone marrow stimulation, epicardial application of cell-delivering systems (scaffold and patches) have gained popularity due to the possibility to apply selectively a cell-containing device which may gradually release the chosen cell type, alone or in combination with trophic substances.

The scaffolds have proven to be successful in this respect and may represent a valid alternative to coronary, intra-myocardial, or venous injection of stem cells, or to stem cell stimulating factors.

Several materials have been assessed for generate scaffold. Li and associates produced 3-D contractile cardiac grafts using gelatin sponges and synthetic biodegradable polymers [6]. Leor and colleagues reported the formation of bioengineered cardiac grafts with 3-D alginate scaffolds [7] Eschenhagen and coworkers engineered 3-D heart tissue by gelling a mixture of cardiomyocytes and collagen [8]. Robinson et al experimented urinary bladder matrix (UBM) and demonstrated UBM superiority to synthetic material for cardiac patching and trends toward myocardial replacement at 3 months [9].

Biological patches may, moreover, show enormous advantages, particularly in congenital diseases, where the existence of a growing tissue might reduce or limit the postoperative complications linked to not-growing material, ultimately leading to stenosis or patient/material mismatch with the need of replacement with all the risks related to redo surgery.

The engineered heart tissue survived and matured after implantation on uninjured hearts. Shimizu and colleagues have developed a novel approach of culturing cell sheets without scaffolds using a temperature-responsive polymer [10]. Several cell sheets were layered on top of each other to create thicker grafts. Ishii et al as an alternative approach, developed an in vitro system for creating sheets of cardiomyocytes on a mesh consisting of ultrafine fibers. This device consists of a thin, highly porous, nonwoven fibrous mesh stretched across a wire ring. This novel scaffold can be fabricated in specific shapes and is easy to handle. However, thicker grafts are required to obtain sufficient function. It is hypothesized that a clinically relevant cardiac graft will require a vasculature to provide sufficient perfusion of oxygenated blood. As an intermediate step toward a thick, vascularized cardiac graft, it is important to assess the ability to increasing the thickness without a vasculature and determine the maximum thickness before core ischemia is observed in the graft. So is essential the development of a multilayer system as an intermediate step toward functional cardiac grafts.

Kochupura et al matured a novel finding that a tissue-engineered myocardial patch (TEMP) derived from extra cellular matrix (ECM) contributes to regional function 8 weeks after implantation in the canine heart [11]. In addition, they confirmed cardiomyocyte population of ECM. The etiology of these cells has been under investigation, with possible explanations including the deposition of circulating bone marrow-derived progenitor cells and the fusion of cardiac progenitor cells with host cells.

The regional mechanical benefit with ECM patch report an active contraction of the ECM and not passive elastic recoil. This contraction is also in synchrony with native myocardium. Microscopic evaluation of Dacron patches did not demonstrate the presence of cardiomyocytes nor do the mechanical data indicate that Dacron implantation contributes to regional function. Increasing the number of ECM layers could be an alternative, but it is unclear if the physiological benefit, ie, cardiomyocyte population, would still be evident. Grossly, Dacron elicited far greater fibrosis than ECM, correlating with more mediastinal adhesions and epicardial connective tissue deposition. On placement, the Dacron patch was clearly under tension. In sharp contrast, ECM triggered far less fibrosis. The patch was neither wrinkled nor aneurismal and appeared to share the same surface tension as adjacent native myocardium. Finally, after removal of adhesions, it was difficult to grossly distinguish ECM from native myocardium The quantitative and qualitative differences between ECM and Dacron could be explained by an inherent ability of ECM to house cellular elements that facilitate remodeling.

The modulus of elasticity of Dacron is at least 4 orders of magnitude greater than healthy myocardium, ie, Dacron is stiffer than myocardium. Thus, the use of Dacron as a myocardial patch may have a "tethering effect" that would reduce the mechanical function of surrounding myocardium. Furthermore, the cellular response to Dacron was primarily diffuse fibroblast proliferation, an observation also seen with remodeling after myocardial infarction. In contrast, ECM stimulated less fibrosis and was populated by different cell types, including cardiomyocytes.

Atkins et al have shown that the reduction of infarct stiffness via cell transplantation leads to increased diastolic function [12]. Similarly, Quarterman et al created a detailed finite element model to show that cell transplantation alone will result in changes in compliance that result in mechanical benefit [13]. The potential clinical applications of ECM as a scaffold are many and would have a powerful impact on the management of cardiac disease. These would include instances in which Dacron is presently used as a myocardial patch: repair of ventricular aneurysms, repair of congenital heart defects, and most recently, surgical restoration of a dyskinetic or akinetic ventricle. By its contribution to regional systolic function, ECM provides true restoration of the ventricle rather than nonfunctional substitution of defective tissue, as is the case with Dacron.

Limits and Perspectives

The use of scaffold for tissue engineering is supportive for myocardial regeneration but subject to biocompatibility, biodegradability, and cytotoxicity, including inflammatory response and surface adhesion molecule loss issues, and this limits its efficacy. Eliminating such disadvantages, is necessary to establish cell sheet engineering technology without using scaffolds. The engineered cell sheets from this technique showed preserved cellular communication junctions, endogenous extracellular matrix, and integrative adhesive agents. Nonligature implantation of these engineered neonatal cardiomyocyte sheets to infarcted myocardium showed their integration with impaired myocardium and improved cardiac performance. For clinical application, use of skeletal myoblasts averts ethical and cell source issues. Recent findings suggested that locally or transgenically delivered stromal-derived factor 1 (SDF-1) expression plays a role in mobilizing and recruiting stem cells with neovascularization [14]. Because SDF-1 is secreted in skeletal muscle tissue, grafted myoblasts might beneficially attract hematopoietic stem cells (HSCs) to home in the infarct heart area for heart regeneration and angiogenesis [15].

The use of engineered patches, therefore, represents an appealing frontier which, in several formats, may provide material and solutions for some complex and inoperable disease. These devices, appropriately designed, may also allow the release of any kind of compounds and material, from cells to drugs, from factor to solution, ad programmed speed, ranging from transient and quick release (high biodegradability) to slow release (low degradability, several months). Last, but not least, the material chosen for realising such a device may also represent a containing structure, variably ranging from pure passive to slightly active action, which may play a role in the mechanical effect on cardiac dilatation in the case of heart containment procedure.

Finally, some treatments, particularly drug-related, showed promising results, but the potential disadvantages of systemic administration hampered a clinical or wider application. The possibility to deliver a specifc agent only locally, with obvious reduction in systemic effects, might be appealing and allow higher and focused concentration only to the target organ, that is the heart, or area of the heart.

References

[1]   Ansari M, Massie BM. Heart failure : how big is the problem ? Who are the patients ? What does the future hold ? *Am. Heart J.* 2003;146:1-4

[2]   Berry C, Murdoch DR, McMurray JJ. Economics of chronic heart failure. *Eur. J. Heart Fail* 2001;3:283-91

[3]   Doenst T, Velazquez EJ, Beyerdorf F, Michler R, Menicanti L, Di Donato , Gradinac S, Sun B, Rao V (STITCH Investigators). To STITCH or not to STITCH : we know the answer, but do we understand the question ? *J. Thorac. Cardiovasc. Surg.* 2005;129: 246-9

[4]   Buckberg GD. Early and late results of left ventricular reconstruction in thin-walled chambers : is this our patient population ? *J. Thorac. Cardiovasc. Surg.* 2004;128:21-6

[5]   Marelli D, Desrosiers C, el-Alfy M, Kao RL, Chiu RC. Cell transplantation for myocardial repair: an experimental approach. *Cell Transplant* 1992;1:383-90.

[6]   Li RK, Jia ZQ, Weisel RD, Mickle DA, Choi A, Yau TM. Survival and function of bioengineered cardiac grafts. *Circulation* 1999;100(suppl II):II63-9.

[7]   Leor J, Aboulafia-Etzion S, Dar A, Shapiro L, Barbash IM, Battler A, et al. Bioengineered cardiac grafts: a new approach to repair the infarcted myocardium? *Circulation* 2000; 102 (suppl 3):III56-61.

[8]   Eschenhagen T, Fink C, Remmers U, Scholz H, Wattchow J, Weil J, et al. Three-dimensional reconstitution of embryonic cardiomyocytes in a collagen matrix: a new heart muscle model system. *FASEB J.* 1997;11:683-94.

[9]   Robinson K, Li J, Mathison M, Redkar A, Cui J, Chronos F, Matheny RG, Badylak S. Extracellular Matrix Scaffold for Cardiac Repair. *Circulation* 2005;112[suppl I]:I-135–I-143.)

[10] Shimizu T, Yamato M, Isoi Y, Akutsu T, Setomaru T, Abe K, et al. Fabrication of pulsatile cardiac tissue grafts using a novel 3-dimensional cell sheet manipulation technique and temperature responsive cell culture surfaces. *Circ. Res.* 2002;90:e40.

[11] Kochupura; Azeloglu E; Kelly D, Doronin S; Badylak S, Krukenkamp I et al. Tissue-Engineered Myocardial Patch Derived FromExtracellular Matrix Provides Regional Mechanical Function. *Circulation* 2005;112[suppl I]:I-144–I-149

[12] Atkins BZ, Hueman MT, Meuchel J, Hutcheson KA, Glower DD, Taylor DA. Cellular cardiomyoplasty improves diastolic properties of injured heart. *J. Surg. Res.* 1999;85: 234–242.

[13] Quarterman RL, Moonly S, Wallace AW, Guccione J, Ratcliffe MB. A finite element model of left ventricular cellular transplantation in dilated cardiomyopathy. *ASAIO J.* 2002; 48:508–513.

[14] Askari AT, Unzek S, Penn MS, et al. Effect of stromal-cell-derived factor 1 on stem-cell homing and tissue regeneration in ischemic cardiomyopathy. *Lancet* 2003;362:697-703.

[15] Ratajczak MZ, Peiper S, Janowska WA, et al. Expression of functional CXCR4 by muscle satellite cells and secretion of SDF-1 by musclederived fibroblasts is associated with the presence of both muscle progenitors in bone marrow and hematopoietic stem/progenitor cells in muscles. *Stem Cells* 2003;21:363-71.

In: Handbook of Cardiovascular Research
Editors: Jorgen Brataas and Viggo Nanstveit

ISBN 978-1-60741-792-7
© 2009 Nova Science Publishers, Inc.

Chapter XVII

Among More than 100 Sources of Chest Pain: Angina Pectoris

William H. Wehrmacher
Loyola University of Chicago,
Stritch School of Medicine, Maywood, IL

Among the more that a hundred known types of pain in the chest, angina ranks at the top of the list for seriousness as well as for reckless diagnosis -- too frequently diagnosed when absent and too dangerously when overlooked.. Failure to recognize it in an emergency facility leading to risky discharge becomes a source for both litigation and patient injury; faulty targeting the diagnosis for one of the many other sources becomes both expensive and provocative of unnecessary anxiety. The diagnosis is certain to be overlooked if all the sources fail to be considered.

Such oversight has been responsible for most of the treatment failures that have been encountered in my consultation practice. Identification of the specific cause for pain or distress in the chest in clinical practice is ordinarily more difficult than specific treatment. Proper recognition becomes the first step in clinical management; more than 100 different disorders have been identified to produce pain or discomfort in the chest.

Pain considered to arise within the chest may actually originate in the wall of the chest as well as in its viscera. It can also arise from disorders from within the head, neck, or abdomen. Diagnosis may ordinarily be fairly simply established when the significant details from the clinical history taking, from physical examination, and from laboratory investigation are adequately evaluated. Special investigations, ordinarily available in university and diagnostic centers, sometimes become essential; although details of the more readily available diagnostic facilities become more important safeguards for correct diagnosis than are the reports from referral centers.

Detailed analysis of the pain itself provides the essential guide through the perplexing labyrinth of a lot of possible causes. Unfortunately the patient readily abandons his essential leadership role through that labyrinth when forced into a rigid inquiry prematurely. With skill and experience, however, the patient can be enticed to go all the way through that labyrinth when the physician and patient work adequately together. Both must appreciate the diagnostic significance of the entire trip. The patient can ordinarily take the physician almost directly to the correct diagnosis. Even when the patient is personally mistaken at the outset, often fearfully mistaken, about the real significance of the symptoms, the diagnostic target cam still be struck by combined physician-and-patient skill.

I have found seven characteristics of the pain -- *location, radiation, quality, duration, intensity, fluctuation and periodicity, and the circumstances of its occurrence and subsidence* essential not only for proper diagnosis but also for the patient's own appreciation of the problem and the assurance that I also actually understand it too..

These seven characteristics often emerge during the patient-physician encounter in variable order and detail. To keep the record straight and free from interruption until the patient has done his best, I have found a grid on my note pad listing these characteristics useful during the inquiry. After the patient has done his best, I can complete the record with a minimum of direct questions. Ordinarily the information fills in rather well and promptly when one is equipped to deal with it as it spills forth from the distraught patient.

As one listens to a patient with Angina pectoris describe symptoms, one ordinarily hears words describing deep *sub-sternal* pain, perhaps inclined slightly to the left, perhaps *radiating* into the anterior cords of the neck or down the medial surface of the left or both arms. The patient may say that the pain is of pressing or crushing *quality,* but ordinarily experiences difficulty finding appropriate words to describe it. The pain almost always *lasts* less than 30 minutes and ordinarily only 1-3 minutes after the end of the provocative exertion. To the patient, and particularly when fearful, the distress may seem to last much longer. The pain of myocardial infarction ordinarily does last longer. Timing is best done with a watch and the patient will use it when recognizing the importance of measuring its duration. The *severity* of the pain is variable and of relatively little value either diagnostically or as a measure of the seriousness of the illness but perhaps of considerable importance in determining the amount of disability. If one were to insist upon finding pain commensurate with the seriousness of the illness, he would miss more cases of angina than he would find. As the patient records the *fluctuation and periodicity* of the distress, one can identify the *circumstances* under which these fluctuations occur. Angina is ordinarily *precipitated* by exercise, not by movement as of the chest or arms. It is *aggravated* by anything that increases the work of the heart, including emotional disturbances and fear. It is ordinarily *relieved* by rest or nitroglycerin.

As one carefully scrutinizes the fluctuation and periodicity of the distress, it is important to steer-clear of inconsistent and clang-like associations. One must clearly identify the actual causal relationships within the circumstances of occurrence and subsidence. It becomes too seductive to ask whether it is stress related and relaxation corrected, prompting an easy response from the patient when, in fact, that relationship does not actually exist. Diurnal variations in angina frequently are related to eating, walking, working and other habits of daily living. Eating predisposes to anginal attacks: (1) by reflex coronary constriction. (2) by increasing the work demand upon the heart called forth by the digestive process, and (3) by alterations in blood viscosity resulting from agglutination of the red cells following ingestion of the fats in the meal. Ingestion of food decreases the time required to produce anginal attacks by 20 to 40% under stressful con-ditions. On the other hand. some protection sometimes results from eating for those patients who benefit from resulting greater concentrations of sugar in the blood. Angina decubitus occurs during recumbency, usually at night when nocturnal increase of the blood volume results from hydrostatic pressure changes.

When the fluctuation and periodicity are independently analyzed, one can usually identify the circumstances of occurrence and subsidence and correlate them with amount of provocative stress occurring within the cardiovascular system.

As one listens to a patient with one of the innocent pains of the chest wall, such as Tietze's syndrome, slipping rib, or tussive fracture of a rib, one expects complaints of pain directly over the offending lesion and of radiation into the same sclerotome rather than into the classical distribution of angina pectoris. Usually the pain is sharp, but depending upon the nature of the lesion, it may resemble a muscular pain or rheumatic pain. It is not so difficult for the intelligent patient to describe as the pain of angina is. Innocent chest wall pain may come and go in a flash or be a catch-in-the-side like pleurisy. It may be prolonged and resemble rheumatic pain but rarely exactly duplicates the pattern of the pain of coronary artery disease. Referred pain to the chest wall that sometimes complicates coronary artery disease, on the other hand, and may exactly simulate other chest wall pain because it is a chest-wall pain and related to pectoral and intercostal muscular spasm. Severity varies and is often commensurate with the disturbance responsible. Chest wall pains are likely to be brought on by movement of the chest, particularly by deep breathing, coughing, sneezing, or stretching and are relieved by immobilizing the involved area. Many pains of chest wall origin and particularly that pain resulting from tussive fracture of the rib may be called pleurisy erroneously because they may feel so much like a stitch-in-the-side. Pericarditis does. All these pains have much in common with one another and each must be considered along with diseases of the underlying pleura and pericardium in making a differential diagnosis whenever the characteristic pain appears because it is a chest-wall pain and related to pectoral and intercostal muscular spasm.

Severity varies and is often commensurate with the disturbance responsible. Chest wall pains are likely to be brought on by movement of the chest, particularly by deep breathing, coughing, sneezing, or stretching and are relieved by immobilizing the involved area. Many pains of chest wall origin and particularly that pain resulting from tussive fracture of the rib may be called pleurisy erroneously because they may feel so much like a stitch-in-the-side. Pericarditis does. All these pains have much in common with one another and each must be considered along with diseases of the underlying pleura and pericardium in making a dif-ferential diagnosis whenever the characteristic pain appears because it is a chest-wall pain and related to pectoral and intercostal muscular spasm.

Chest wall pains are likely to be brought on by movement of the chest, particularly by deep breathing, coughing, sneezing, or stretching and are relieved by immobilizing the involved area. Many pains of chest wall origin and particularly that pain resulting from tussive fracture of the rib may be called pleurisy erroneously because they may feel so much like a stitch-in-the-side. Pericarditis does. All these pains have much in common with one another and each must be considered along with diseases of the underlying pleura and pericardium in making a differential diagnosis whenever the characteristic pain appears.

As one listens to a patient with pulmonary pain one may hear complaints suggesting the deep, difficult-to-describe pain of myocardial ischemia. As a pulmonary embolism lodges in the artery, the quality of the pain is likely to be deceptive until pulmonary infarction results and produces an overlying pleuritis or until the diagnostically helpful haemoptysis appears.

As the patient whose pain originates outside the chest as in the head, neck or abdomen relates his symptoms, the patient will ordinarily refer to some distress over the offending lesion even when most of the pain is felt within the chest. If suffering from Cervical Nerve Root Compression by spurs from the uncovertebral joint of Luschka or by other masses the patient should be expected to complain about his neck even when most of the pain is felt in his chest. The pain often exhibits a shooting character and extends into the anatomical distribution of the involved nerve roots. It may be shock-like and simulate the distress after hitting the ulnar nerve (the "crazy-bone") at the elbow.

Summary

Seven characteristics of any pain -- *location, radiation, quality, duration, intensity, fluctuation and periodicity, and the circumstances of its occurrence and subsidence* --become essential not only for accurate diagnosis but also for the patient's own appreciation of the problem and for the assurance that the examiner actually understands it too.

References for Further Study

Wehrmacher, W.H. Pain in the Chest. (book)Springfield:Charles C. Thomas Co., 403p, 1964;

Wehrmacher, W.H. Unstable Angina Treatment. *2006 Update. Comp. Ther.* 2006 32(3): 144-146.

Wehrmacher, W.H. Acute Myocardial Infarction 2000 Recognition. *Comprehensive Therapy* Vol. 27, 2001, p. 140-143

Wehrmacher, W.H. Myocardial Infarction Patterns in Clinical Electrocardiography. Postgraduate Institute for Medicine, Parker Colorado. 1981

Wehrmacher, W.H. and K.A. Wetklo. Schmerzen im Thoraxbereich. *Diagnostik* 9:38-40, 1977

Wehrmacher, W.H. Pain in the chest. In: *Current Diagnosis*, Chapter 4. Eds., H.F. Conn and R.B. Conn. Philadelphia: W. B. Saunders Company, 1974

Wehrmacher, W.H. Clinical clues in the diagnosis of cardiac disease. in:*Therapeutic Advances in the Practice of Cardiology*, Chap.1. Eds., C.P. Bailey, A.G. Shapiro and S. Gollub, NY: Grune and Stratton, 1970.

Wehrmacher, W.H. and C.A. Vera. Causa de dolor de pecho:: pericarditis. *La Prensa Medica,* Argentina 55:1977, 1968.

Wehrmacher, W.H. Anterior chest pain. *JAMA* 194:217, 1965.

Blonsky, E.,. Kezdi, P and WEHRMACHER, W.H. Pain in the chest associated with hypertension of the lesser circulation.I.Mitral valvular disease. *Quarterly Bulletin, NW U Med School,* 35 241-247, 1961.

Wehrmacher, W.H., K. Kuroda and P. Kezdi. Pain in the chest associated with hypertension of the lesser circulation. II. Congenital heart disease. *Minn. Med.* 44:347-379, 1961.

.Wehrmacher, W.H. Chest pain-significant or insignificant? Proceedings of the 49th Annual Meeting of the American Life Convention, Hot Springs, Virginia, 1961.

Wehrmacher, W.H. Musculo-skeletal pain masquerading as angina pectoris. Sixth International Congress of Internal Medicine, Basel, 1960.

Wehrmacher, W.H. The painful anterior chest wall syndromes. *Med. Clin. N. A.* 1958; 42:111-118.

Wehrmacher, W.H. Significance of Tietze's syndrome in differential diagnosis of chest pain. *JAMA* 1955; 157: 505-507.

In: Handbook of Cardiovascular Research
Editors: Jorgen Brataas and Viggo Nanstveit

ISBN 978-1-60741-792-7
© 2009 Nova Science Publishers, Inc.

Chapter XVIII

Evaluation of a Smoking Relapse Prevention Program for Cardiovascular Patients

Warren R. Stanton[1,2,*], John B. Lowe[1,3], Kevin P. Balanda[1,4]
and Christopher B. Del Mar[5]

1. Cancer Prevention Research Centre, School of Population Health,
University of Queensland, Australia
2. Division of Physiotherapy, School of Health and Rehabilitation Sciences,
University of Queensland, Australia
3. Department of Community and Behavioral Health,
College of Public Health, University of Iowa
4. Institute of Public Health, Redmond's Hill,
Dublin, Republic of Ireland
5. Centre for General Practice, Department of Social and Preventive Medicine,
University of Queensland, Australia

Abstract

Smoking cessation reduces both the mortality and re-infarction rate amongst smokers who have experienced a myocardial infarction (MI). Smoking cessation programs have tended to be conducted with post-operative or seriously ill patients. In this study, we examined the efficacy of a relapse prevention program for hospital cardiovascular patients who did not require operative procedures or extensive hospitalization. A pre-post, two groups, control trial involving 208 patients (103 in the intervention group) recruited from three coronary care units in large metropolitan hospitals was used to assess the effect of the intervention. Smoking status of self-reported quitters were verified using CO concentrations in expired air. Complete follow-

---

[*]Address for correspondence and reprints: Dr Warren Stanton, School of Health and Rehabilitation Science, University of Queensland, St. Lucia, Queensland 4006, Australia.

up was obtained from 129 (62.0%) of initial participants. At three months after discharge, the self-report quite rate in the intervention group was 19.4%, significantly higher than in the control group (7.6%) (p = 0.046). This difference persisted at nine months after discharge, when the self reported quit rate was 27.3% in the intervention group and 12.9% in the control group (p = 0.043). A behavior-based smoking cessation program was effective for less serious cardiovascular patients and the effect persisted for nine months after discharge.

Keywords: smoking; relapse-prevention; cardiovascular

Smoking is a risk factor in half the major causes of death for older adults, in particular heart disease (Orleans, Jepson, Resch and Rimer, 1994; Guilmette, Motta, Shadel, Mukand and Niaura, 2001). An increased risk of myocardial infarction (MI) is associated with an increase in amount smoked, and is considerably elevated for heavy smokers (Rosenburg and Shapiro, 1990). By comparison to post MI non-smokers, post MI smokers have more non-fatal MI's, increased arteriosclerosis peripheral vascular disease and more severe and extensive atherosclerosis of the aorta and coronary arteries (Chowdhury, Lasker and Dyer, 1999; Milei and Grana, 1998). Cessation of smoking reduces both mortality and re-infarction rate by 50% (Burling, Singleton, Bigelow, Baile and Gottlieb 1984; Jajich, Ostfeld and Freeman, 1984; Squires, Gau, Miller, Allison and Lavie, 1990). After 5 - 10 years of cessation (less than 5 years according to Rosenberg et al, 1990 and Gottlieb, 1992), ex-smokers exhibit coronary heart disease mortality ratios similar to that of non-smokers (Burling et al, 1984). Opportunities to quit and the availability of suitable resources are therefore essential for all patients who have had a myocardial infarction.

The immediate post-hospitalisation period is a critical stage of rehabilitation (Moller, Pedersen, Villebro, et al., 2003). Patients are receptive to changes in lifestyle and are motivated by a clear recollection of the acute event (Squires et al, 1990). A longer period of smoking cessation has been found to be associated with higher severity of the MI, previous heart problems, higher degree of perceived threat, smoking history, belief that smoking contributed to their cardiac problem, extent of the disease, age and occupation, being married and male (Baile, Bigelow, Gottlieb, Stitzer and Sacktor, 1982; Ockene et al, 1985a, 1985b; Scott and Lamparski, 1985; Havik and Maeland, 1988; Frid et al, 1991; Rice et al, 1994). In these first few weeks, relapse is strongly associated with anxiety and depression; later it is primarily associated with poorer general cardiac knowledge and understanding of smoking as a risk factor (Havik and Maeland, 1988). Long-term quitting is related to steady gain in basic cardiac knowledge.

There are a variety of behavioural reasons for relapse by smokers. Smokers may start smoking again because of the presence and frequency of smoking in their environment (learning theory), because smoking is used as a behaviour to cope with stress (stress-coping theories), or because of the relationship between attitudes and behaviour itself (cognitive - attitudinal theories eg. health belief model) (Oldenburg and Pope, 1990). In the immediate post-quitting phase, which for many smokers occurs when they are admitted to hospital with MI, behavioural programs should include social support, reinforcement and coping skills. In the later phase of long-term maintenance, emphasis can be given to ongoing monitoring and vigilance, lifestyle change, cue exposure, stress management and weight control (Oldenburg and Pope, 1990) Multi-component, self-management packages have been found to consistently aid smoking control (Kamarck and Lichtenstein, 1985).

A number of studies have examined the behaviour of smokers after myocardial infarction. Factors such as personality traits and perceived self control (Maiani, Callegari and Sanavio, 1990) smoking history, health beliefs and demographic characteristics (Baile et al, 1982) are unrelated to cessation or relapse in this population group. In the absence of an intervention program, between 16% and 32% of MI patients stop smoking initially for part of the first 12 months after hospitalisation (Scott and Lamparski, 1985; Rigotti, Singer, Mulley and Thibault, 1991; Emmons and Goldstein, 1992). Positive health beliefs are associated with post-MI cessation maintenance, though experience of the MI was seen as the main motivational factor (Marshall, 1990). (Scott and Lamparski, 1985) concluded that the best time to intervene was immediately after a patient's first cardiac event.

Smoking interventions for MI patients have yielded different levels of success. The short-term cessation rate (5-6 weeks) for hospitalised post-operative patients given three structured cessation sessions and follow-up phone calls over 5 weeks, was 12% higher than the 'usual care' group in a study by Wewers, Bowen, Stanislaw and Desimone (1994). A nurse-managed program which consisted of a manual focussing on identification and coping with high risk situations and follow-up phone calls, resulted in a 12-month cessation rate which was 29% higher in the intervention group compared to the 'usual care' group (Taylor, Houston-Miller, Killen and Debusk, 1990). A more recent and rigorous randomised control trial conducted by the same group (Miller et al, 1997) incorporated a nurse-mediated, behaviourally-oriented, relapse prevention counselling with follow-up telephone calls, and produced a more modest effect size of 7%. A study by Rice et al, (1994) found that nurse-patient interactions were more effective than self-help materials, but they also found a higher 12-month cessation rate among the non-intervention group (possibly due to other group differences). A behavioural multi-component intervention delivered to seriously ill MI patients Ockene et al, (1985a), achieved an 11% increase in cessation compared to a group who received advice only. The cessation rates for validated smoking status were 45% and 34% respectively.

Studies to date have generally been conducted with post-operative or seriously ill patients and have produced varied levels of success. The aim of this study is to examine the efficacy of a relapse prevention program for cardiovascular patients with less serious illness, who were hospitalised with heart problems that did not require operative procedures or an extensive period of hospitalisation. This group may be less motivated to quit smoking and provide a more conservative test of the efficacy of a behavioural program for cardiovascular patients.

Methods

Sample

The eligible sample consisted of patients admitted to the coronary care unit of three Brisbane hospitals, who had been regular smokers and had smoked in the month prior to hospitalisation. The criteria for inclusion of smokers in the eligible sample included those with myocardial infarction, ischemic heart problems or unstable angina. Patients who required oxygen or narcotic pain control (or other drugs potentially inhibiting cognitive function) were excluded from the sample. Over the recruitment period of four years, which was required to achieve a sufficiently large sample size to detect an estimated 20% effect size with 80% power at the 5% level of significance allowing for loss to follow-up, 208 patients were enrolled in the project (105 in the control group and 103 in the intervention group).

The socio-demographic characteristics of the enrolled sample was as follows: 75% male, 25% female; 63% married or de facto, 21% separated or divorced, 7% widowed, 9% single; 56% skilled or professional, 36% semi-skilled, 8% unskilled; age range 20-76 years (mean = 53.6, standard deviation = 11.0).

Procedure

After ethical approval was obtained from the hospitals, two focus group interviews were conducted with 12-15 coronary care patients, in order to gauge the range of issues relevant to patients who were smokers and to obtain information that would inform the development of the intervention. The intervention was developed from a cognitive behavioural approach fostering individuals' responsibility for their behavioural choices. The theoretical basis of the intervention was drawn from Roger's Protection Motivation Theory (Rogers, 1983), which holds that for behaviour change to occur the individual must be sufficiently motivated, but also hold a high belief in their ability to achieve the desired change, that is high self-efficacy to quit smoking (Maddux and Rogers, 1983). Components of the intervention were developed in accord with other cited smoking prevention programs delivered to cardiovascular patients.

Each morning of the recruitment period, coronary care units of the participating hospitals were contacted or made contact with the research team, and patients who were admitted in the past 24 hours and had been regular smokers were identified. If a past or current smoker had been admitted, a registered nurse visited the hospital, screened the patient for eligibility in the study, and if eligible, sought written informed consent and administered a baseline self-completed questionnaire (assisted by the nurse blind to group allocation, if the patient was having difficulty). Information was obtained about a range of topics including socio-demographic characteristics, their admission and prognosis, past and current health status, smoking history and environment, history and opinions about quitting cigarette smoking and knowledge of the health risks of smoking. The cardiologist of each patient enrolled in the study was informed of their patient's participation in order to ensure that the program was suitable for their medical condition.

The study was conducted as a two group, pre-post, control design. Allocation to the intervention group was based on alternate week blocks of eligible admissions, which in combination with low weekly recruitment rates effectively minimised the possibility of contamination. Patients allocated to the control group received the usual care of the hospitals and were provided with an efficacious self-help, smoking cessation booklet (Balanda, Lowe and O'Connor-Fleming, 1999). Patients allocated to the intervention group received the program described below.

Delivery of the intervention was based on two sessions with the patient in hospital where they were not permitted to smoke, and weekly follow-up phone calls for a month post-discharge. The content of each session, based on commonly used behavioural strategies, was as follows:

Session 1 was designed to develop the patient's motivation and self-efficacy to stop smoking. The material included two audio-tapes of motivational and educational material produced by the research team. The content for the tapes was drawn from the results of the focus groups and findings reported in the relevant literature. The first tape dealt with ambivalence towards quitting as well as the known positive and negative factors related to quitting, discussed by a group of blue-collar workers during a work break. The second tape encouraged positive attitudes and exemplified appropriate strategies, in a scene of a doctor discussing with an intern doctor the approach to be taken with patients wishing to quit smoking. After listening to the tapes, patients completed a self-administered quiz (Situational Competency Test) which allowed patients to identify high-risk situations, viewed a booklet containing cognitive strategies targeting each of these situations, and signed a "Stop Smoking" contract designed to develop the patient's commitment to not smoking while in hospital.

Session 2 continues to build the patient's motivation and self-efficacy and teach the patient skills for dealing with high risk situations for smoking relapse. The material consisted of an audio-taped discussion of cardiac patients views on quitting and the difficulties they encountered, a self-scored quiz (Behavioural Competency Test) dealing with behavioural issues related to high risk situations, a booklet providing behavioural activities which complemented the cognitive strategies developed in Session 1, a 'daily plan' to deal with these situations during the week following discharge which incorporated (a) gradually revealing hidden messages as a reward for each day of success and (b) a self nominated reward for staying quit for the week, and a letter requesting support sent to a nominated friend or partner. A letter was also sent to their General Practitioner informing them of the patients involvement in the project.

After discharge from hospital, a series of 4 follow-up phone calls were conducted weekly in order to provide the patient with continued support following discharge. The nurse enquired as to their progress in staying quit, provided support for positive activities and encouragement to quit if they had lapsed, and asked about use of the components of the intervention (cognitive and behavioural strategies booklets, daily plan completed in hospital, and support by friend and partner).

Among the 208 patients enrolled in the study 138 (66.3%) were followed up at 3 months after discharge from hospital (T2); among the remainder 52 did not return the questionnaire after 3 contacts from research staff, 12 could not be contacted and 6 had died. At 9 month follow-up (T3) 129 (62.0%) were surveyed; 43 did not reply, 30 could not be contacted and 6 had died. Similar proportions of participants in the two intervention groups were followed up. A number of patients (n=16) who did not participate.at T2 did so at T3. Self-reported quit rates were calculated on the basis of triangulating answers to three questions; "Have you changed your level of smoking since you were admitted to hospital with your heart problem" (answered 'stopped altogether') and "Have you had even one puff of a cigarette since you left hospital" (answered 'no') and "How long is it since you have smoked (even a puff)" (where the number of reported days was greater than the days to follow-up assessment). In addition, internal consistency for the group identified as quitters at T2 was obtained by a requirement that the number of days between the recorded discharge date and the follow-up date was less than the number of days since they reported they last smoked. Those who were self reported smokers at T2 but became non-smokers were coded as 'quitters' at T3. A subset of the participants who indicated they had quit smoking (50 at T2 and 44 at T3) were tested for verification of self report by a measure of carbon monoxide in expired air. Those contacted who refused to provide a measure of CO or had readings above 9ppm were classed as smokers.

Results

Data from the baseline questionnaire showed that the intervention and control groups were statistically similar across the broad range of variables examined in the study, including socio-demographics (gender, age, education and occupation), rating of current health, family history of heart disease, advice to stop smoking from GP, smoking history, partners who smoke, intentions to stay quit, amount smoked in the week before admission, number of previous admissions and length of hospital stay (p>0.05).

A 'process' survey conducted with the 70 intervention cases followed up at 3 months indicated that the program was well received. Questions about each component of the program showed that two-thirds of the intervention group thought the tape recordings, cognitive and behavioural quiz with resource booklets, contract and daily plan were helpful to them in their efforts to quit. A larger proportion (more than 80%) thought the conversations with the nurse while in hospital and follow-up phone calls after discharge were helpful.

At 3 month follow-up, complete data was obtained from 133 participants (67 from the intervention group). Chi-square analysis of self-report of quitting (based on the 4 criteria described above), indicated that 7.6% of the comparison group had quit smoking completely, compared to 19.4% of the intervention group (x^2=3.97, df=1, p=.046). Apart from those who had quit, a notable trend was evident in which 23.2% of the intervention group indicated they had puffed on a cigarette since they left hospital but had stopped again, compared with only 3.0% of the comparison group. Examination of CO readings for the subset of 50 quitters (and 3 refusals) whose smoking status was verified or assumed to be a smoker, confirmed that approximately 92% of both groups were non-smokers, the adjusted quit rates based on 'intention to treat' were 4.8% and 12.6% respectively.

At 9 month follow-up, complete data was obtained from 128 participants (66 from the intervention group). The rate of self-reported quitting was 12.9% in the comparison group and 27.3% in the intervention group (X^2=4.3, df=1, p=.043). The effect across groups of a different level of quitting after a lapse was not evident at 9 month follow-up. Verification of smoking status for 44 quitters (and 5 refusals) confirmed that 90% were not smoking, and was similar for both groups the adjusted quit rates based on 'intention to quit' were 7.6% and 17.5% respectively.

A loglinear analysis (multiway contingency) with a saturated model was used to test for change in smoking status between 3 month and 9 month followup for 108 participants who provided complete data at both follow-up assessments. Results of the analysis indicated that a significant proportion of respondents changed their smoking status (X^2=5.6, df=1, p=.018). Among those who were smokers at 3 months follow-up (T2), proportionally more of the intervention group (26.1%) than the comparison group (10.4%) quit smoking between the 3 month and 9 month follow-up assessments.

Variables in the baseline survey which were significantly (p<.05) correlated with 'number of weeks since they had smoked or puffed on a cigarette' at 3 month follow-up were; GP had advised them to stop smoking (r=.19), greater confidence staying quit after leaving hospital (r=.21) and perception of self as a non-smoker (r=.24). Variables from the baseline questionnaire which predicted 'more weeks without smoking' at 9 month follow-up were; the amount of pain experienced before admission (r=.24), GP had offered help to stop smoking (r=.22) and perceived ease of staying quit (r=.21). The rates of quitting were not sufficiently high to examine a dichotomous measure of quitting. The factor of 'group' was partialled out of these reported correlations.

Correlations of the measure of quitting with variables from the follow-up surveys are shown in Table 1. A range of variables were correlated with quitting, but knowledge of the health risks of smoking and ratings of helpfulness of each of the components of the program (intervention group only) were not related to quitting, and are not listed in the table. Notably, perceived 'state of health', 'seriousness of condition' (T3) and rating of heart problem and hospital stay as a 'frightening experience', were not related to the variable of 'number of weeks without smoking' (p>.05).

Discussion

Results of previous studies of smoking cessation among cardiovascular patients have produced inconsistent results, in part because the seriousness of the illness may have an impact on the outcome of smoking relapse prevention programs. This study indicated that a behavioural-based program is effective for patients not requiring operative procedures for heart problems. A multi-component program containing motivational material, cognitive restructuring, cognitive and behavioural skills development, social support and use of behavioural strategies including reinforcement, was effective in producing a quit rate significantly higher than achieved with 'usual care' which included a self-help quit book. The impact of the program was evident at 3 months (T2) and 9 months (T3) post discharge and also resulted in an increased quit rate after the 3 month period. Confirmation of non-smoking status by measurement of CO in expired air indicated that self-report of quitting was reliable.

The predictors of quitting identified in the study provide a profile of the type of patient who may benefit from this type of program. Variables such as 'education level', 'perceived difficulty staying quit' and 'age of onset of smoking' are supported by the results of previous research, but the significance of a number of variables such as 'self perception as a non-smoker' and 'GP offered assistance with quitting' provide avenues for new initiatives which would support this type of behavioural program. Notably, variables related to perceived severity of the health problem predicted patients efforts to quit. Commonly reported reasons for wanting to continue smoking were also related to failed quit efforts (Table 1).

Table 1. Correlates of patient's reports of number of weeks since smoking or puffing a cigarette, at three month follow-up (T2) and nine month follow-up (T3), adjusted for the factor of 'group'

Variable	Correlates of more weeks without smoking at T2	Correlates of more weeks without smoking at T3
1. How important are each of the following for you continuing to smoke. (4 point Likert scale, 1 = very, 4 = not at all)		
a) Enjoyment	.20*	.31*
b) Social reasons; family and friends do	.20*	.18
c) Relieve stress	.27*	.41*
d) Addicted to cigarettes	.28*	.43*
e) fills in time when bored	.16	.36*
2. How would you describe your state of health at the moment? (7 point scale; 1 = extremely poor, 7 = extremely good)	.03	.07
3. How serious do you think your current condition is? (4 point scale: 1 = very serious, 4 = not at all serious)	-.20*	.01
4. How frightening was your heart problem at stay in hospital? (4 point scale; 1 = not at all frightening, 4 = the most frightening experience ever)	.13	.13
5. How hard or easy do you think it will be to stay off cigarettes now that you have left hospital? (4 point scale; 1 = very easy, 4 = very hard)	-.24*	-.64*
6. How sure are you that you can stay off cigarettes? (4 point scale; 1 = very unsure, 4 = very sure)	.32*	.52*
7. Have you asked your family or friends to help you stop smoking (1 = No, 2 = Yes)	-.03	.25*
8. How much encouragement have you been getting from family to stop smoking (4 point scale; 1 = none at all, 4 = very much)	.04	.19*

*=p<.05

The program as presented by the study nurse appears to be of assistance in helping patients remain abstinent from smoking. Further research needs to be conducted to determine whether the program as currently designed can continue to be effective when delivered by nursing staff in the wards. Recent debate about nicotine replacement therapy (NRT) for patients with cardiovascular disease favours its use (McRobbie and Hajek, 2001; Joseph and Fu, 2003) and should be included in future behavioural-based programs. In addition, as this was principally an efficacy trial, cost data was not collated. Further research needs to incorporate a comprehensive cost study to determine whether the addition of this program to the cost of the health care system can be measured against the possible cost saving of maintaining this group of high risk patients smoke free.

Acknowledgments

The authors wish to acknowledge the contribution of Michelle Willis, Romana Madl and Sandra Chippindall to this project. The authors also thank the hospital staff and patients for their participation. This project was funded by the National Heart Foundation of Australia.

References

Baile, W.F., Bigelow, G.E., Gottlieb, S.H., Stitzer, M.L., Sacktor, J.D. (1982): Rapid resumption of cigarette smoking following myocardial infarction: Inverse relation to MI severity. *Addictive Behaviours* 7, 373-380.

Balanda, K.P., Lowe, J.B., O'Connor-Fleming, M.L. (1999): Which booklet to use: A comparison of two self-help smoking cessation booklets. *Tobacco Control* 8, 57-61.

Burling, T.A., Singleton, E.G., Bigelow, G.E., Baile, W.F., Gottlieb, S.H.(1984): Smoking following myocardial infarction: A critical review of the literature. *Health Psychology* 3, 83-96.

Chowdhury, T.A., Lasker, S.S., Dyer, P.H.(1999): Comparison of secondary prevention measures after myocardial infarction in subjects with and without diabetes mellitus. *Journal of Internal Medicine* 254, 565-570.

Emmons, K.M., Goldstein, M.G.(1992): Smokers who are hospitalized: A window of opportunity for cessation interventions. *Preventive Medicine* 21, 262-269.

Frid, D., et al. (1991): Severity of angiographically proven artery disease predicts smoking cessation. *American Journal of Preventive Medicine* 7, 131-135.

Gottlieb, S.O. (1992): Cardiovascular benefits of smoking cessation. *Heart Disease and Stroke* 1, 173-175.

Guilmette, T.J., Motta, S.I., Shadel, W.G., Mukand, J., Niaura, R. (2001): Promoting smoking cessation in the rehabilitation setting. *American Journal of Physical Medicine and Rehabilitation* 80, 560-562.

Havik, O.E., Maeland, J.G.(1988): Changes in smoking behavior after myocardial infarction. *Health Psychology* 7, 3-20.

Jajich, C.L., Ostfeld, A.M., Freeman, D.H.(1984): Smoking and coronary heart disease mortality in the elderly. *Journal of the American Medical Association* 252, 2831-2834.

Joseph, A.M., Fu, S.S. (2003): Safety issues in pharmacotherapy for smoking in patients with cardiovascular disease. *Progress in Cardiovascular Diseases* 45, 429-441.

Kamarck, T.W., Lichtenstein, E.(1985): Current trends in clinic-based smoking control. *Annals of Behavioural Medicine* 7, 19-23.

Maddux, J.E., Rogers, (1983): R.W., Protection motivation and self-efficacy: A revised theory of fear appeals and attitude change. *Journal of Expermental Social Psychology* 19, 469-479.

Maiani, G., Callegari, S., Sanavio, E. (1990): Smoking after myocardial infarction. *New Trends in Experimental Clinical Psychiatry* 6, 207-215.

Marshall, P.(1990): "Just one more...!" A study into the smoking attitudes and behavior of patients following first myocardial infarction. *International Journal of Nursing Studies* 27, 375-387.

McRobbie, H., Hajek, P. (2001): Nicotine replacement therapy in patients with cardiovascular disease: Guidelines for health professionals. *Addiction* 2001, 1547-1551.

Milei, J., Grana, D.R.(1998): Mortality and morbidity from smoking-induced cardiovascular diseases: the necessity of the cardiologist's involvement and commitment. *International Journal of Cardiology* 67, 95-109.

Miller, N.H., et al. (1997): Smoking cessation in hospitalized patients. Results of a randomized trial. *Archives of Internal Medicine* 157, 409-415.

Moller, A.M., Pedersen, T., Villebro, N., Schnaberich, A., Haas, M., Tonnesen, R. (2003): A study of the impact of long-term tobacco smoking on postoperative intensive care admission. *Anaesthesia* 58, 55-59.

Ockene, J.K., et al.(1985a): Factors affecting cigarette smoking status in patients with ischemic heart disease. *Journal of Chronic Disease* 38, 985-994.

Ockene, J., et al. (1985b): Smoking cessation and severity of disease: the Coronary Artery Smoking Intervention Study. *Health Psychology* 11, 119-126.

Oldenburg, B., Pope, J. (1990): A critical review of determinan0ts of smoking cessation. *Behavior Change* 7, 101-109.

Orleans, C.T., Jepson, C., Resch, N., Rimer, B.K. (1994): Quitting motives and barriers among older smokers. The 1986 Adult Use of Tobacco Survey revisited. *Cancer* 74(7 suppl), 2055-2061.

Rice, V.H., et al. (1994): A comparison of nursing interventions for smoking cessation in adults with cardiovascular health problems. *Heart and Lung* 23, 473-486.

Rosenberg, L.P., Shapiro, J.R. (1990): Decline in the risk of myocardial infarction among women who stop smoking. *New England Journal of Medicine* 322, 213-217.

Rigotti, N.A., Singer, D.E., Mulley, A.G., Thibault, G.E. (1991): Smoking cessation following admission to a coronary care unit. *Journal of General Internal Medicine* 6, 305-311.

Rogers, R.W. (1983): Cognitive and physiological processes in fear appeals and attitude change: A revised theory of protection motivation. *In: Cacioppo and Petty, eds. Social Psychophysiology.* New York;

Scott, R.R., Lamparski, D.(1985): Variables related to long-term smoking status following cardiac events. *Addictive Behaviours* 10, 257-264.

Squires, R.W., Gau, G.T., Miller, T.D., Allison, T.G., Lavie, L.J. (1990): Cardiovascular rehabilitation status. *Mayo Clinic Proceedings* 65, 731-755.

Taylor, C.B., Houston-Miller, N., Killen, J.D., Debusk, R.F. (1990): Smoking cessation after acute myocardial infarction: Effects of a nurse-managed intervention. *Annals of Internal Medicine* 113, 118-123.

Wewers, M.E., Bowen, J.M., Stanislaw, A.E., Desimone, V.B. (1994): A nurse-delivered smoking cessation intervention among hospitalized postoperative patients--influence of a smoking-related diagnosis: A pilot study. *Heart and Lung* 23, 151-156.

In: Handbook of Cardiovascular Research
Editors: Jorgen Brataas and Viggo Nanstveit

ISBN 978-1-60741-792-7
© 2009 Nova Science Publishers, Inc.

Chapter XIX

The Role of Caspases in Cardiovascular Diseases

*Yuchi Han** and Peter M. Kang*

Cardiovascular Division, Beth Israel Deaconess Medical Center
and Harvard Medical School, Boston, MA, USA

Abstract

Apoptosis is implicated in wide variety of physiological and pathological processes, and the role of apoptosis in cardiovascular diseases is also becoming more evident. In this paper, we review the current literature on the known caspases and their role in the heart. The importance of the categories of initiator and effector caspases are well recognized in the heart and role of the inflammatory caspases is emerging. Furthermore, we present specific studies that are being done in our laboratory as well as others in elucidating the mechanism of inhibiting apoptosis in cardiac myocytes. The inhibition of apoptosis as a potential therapeutic tool is emerging for various forms of cardiovascular disease, and the inhibition of caspases is an important target for anti-apoptotic therapy in the heart.

A. Introduction

Apoptosis is a highly regulated process of cell death that plays a fundamental role in physiological processes in multi-cellular organisms, from nematodes to humans [1]. This process is also implicated in a wide variety of pathological processes. In the last decade, the basic mechanisms of apoptosis have been discovered in greater depth and the role of apoptosis in pathogenesis has been increasingly elucidated. In the heart, apoptosis has been

---

* Correspondence concerning this article should be addressed to Peter M. Kang, Cardiovascular Division, Beth Israel Deaconess Medical Center, 330 Brookline Ave., SL-423C, Boston, MA 02215. TEL: (617) 667-4865; FAX: (617) 975-5201; E-mail: pkang@bidmc.harvard.edu.

shown to play an important role in numerous pathologic processes, such as myocardial infarction (MI), reperfusion injury, development of both acute and chronic heart failure, plaque rupture, and various forms of cardiomyopathies [2-4]. In fact, the inhibition of apoptosis as a potential therapeutic strategy is emerging in cardiovascular disease. Residing in the central stage of apoptosis is a family of cysteine proteases called caspases. In this review, we will examine the molecular mechanisms of cardiac apoptosis, especially focusing on the caspases, and the potential therapeutic strategies to inhibit caspases to treat various cardiovascular diseases.

B. Molecular Mechanisms
of Caspase-Dependent Apoptosis

Molecularly, apoptosis results from complex interactions between various pro- and anti-apoptotic molecules that modulate cell death pathways. Generally, apoptosis is mediated through two central pathways, mitochondria or death receptor mediated pathways. (Figure 1) In the mitochondria-mediated pathway, which is also known as the intrinsic apoptotic pathway, an apoptotic insult induces the mitochondria to release cytochrome c into the cytosol [5]. An activation complex, the apoptosome, is formed with apoptotic protein activating factor-1 (Apaf-1), cytochrome c, dATP, and caspase-9 [6,7]. Apoptosome formation results in the autoprocessing of caspase-9, as well as the activation of downstream caspases, such as caspase-3, to execute the final morphological and biochemical alterations [6,8]. Activation of mitochondrial pathway components has been demonstrated in various models of cardiac apoptosis, and may be the primary apoptotic pathway associated with oxidative stress in the heart [9-12].

The death receptor-mediated, or extrinsic, apoptotic pathway involves binding a death ligand, for example, FasL, to a death receptor, such as Fas [13]. This binding recruits the death domain, e.g., the Fas-associated death domain (FADD), which activates caspase-8 that in turn is responsible for the subsequent activation of downstream caspases. Both pathways, in fact, ultimately converge on a common downstream pathway when effector caspases are activated, where the final morphological and biochemical alterations characteristic of apoptosis take place [14].

Further studies indicate that one of the pro-apoptotic members of the Bcl-2 protein family, BH3 interacting domain death agonist (Bid), may regulate the interaction between death receptor and mitochondria pathways. Bid is usually located in the cytosol, but translocates to the mitochondria when it is cleaved into truncated Bid (tBid) by activated caspase-8 [15]. In mitochondria, translocated tBid triggers cytochrome c release most likely by interacting with two other pro-apoptotic family member of Bcl-2 family - Bak and Bax, and subsequently activate mitochondria mediated pathway [16].

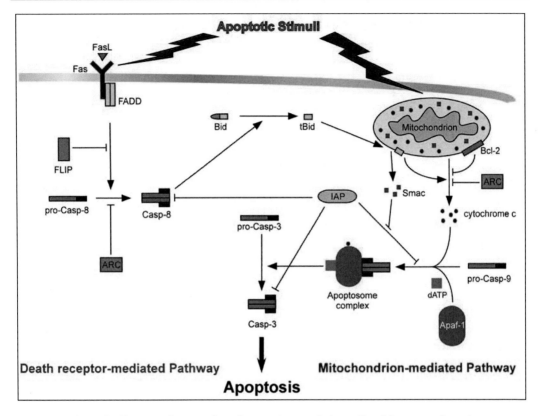

Figure 1. Schematic diagram of apoptosis pathways. Apoptosis is mediated by two main pathways, mitochondrion- and death receptor-mediated pathways, which than converge on a common downstream pathway to cause apoptosis. These pathways may also interact upstream via Bid. Death receptor pathway is initiated by activation of death receptor (e.g. Fas) and Fas associated death receptor (FADD), which activate caspase-8, which in turn activates caspase-3. Mitochondrial pathway is initiated by release of cytochrome c, which interacts with apaf-1 and caspase-9 in presence of dATP to form apoptosome complex that activates caspase 3. These pathways are subject to modulation by numerous inhibitors, such as Bcl-2, IAP, ARC and FLIP. Pro-apoptotic molecule Smac could inhibit IAP, resulting in lifting of inhibition by IAP.

C. Caspases

1. Classification of Caspases

The caspases are a family of cysteine proteases that cleave target proteins at specific aspartate residues [14]. Caspases are produced as zymogens, or pro-caspases, which are activated via cleavage of their prodomains. Caspases can be grouped into three categories by their function: the initiator, the effector, and the inflammatory caspases. Initiator caspases, caspase-2, -8, -9, and -10, possess a long prodomain with a functionally important interacting domain. (Figure 2) They act upstream to initiate and regulate apoptosis, and also activate the downstream effector caspases. By contrast, effector caspases, caspase-3, -6, and -7, are characterized by a short prodomain. They generally depend on the initiator caspases for activation, and they act downstream to carry out the final biochemical changes seen in apoptosis. Inflammatory caspases include caspase-1, -4, -5, and -11 to -14, which are thought to be more involved in the pro-inflammatory cellular response which includes key steps of interleukin processing. However, there are more recent data elucidating their key roles in apoptosis, and this will be discussed in detail later.

2. Caspase Deficient Mice

The roles of the various caspases, which have been studied by generating lines of caspase-deficient mice using homologous recombination, have revealed important functions of caspases in apoptosis, cytokine maturation, and cell growth and differentiation. A summary of various caspase knockout mice, as outlined in Table 1, shows a range of phenotypic variability from no phenotype to embryonic lethality [15,17-28]. Interestingly, the majority of caspase knockouts exhibit tissue- and cell type-specific or stimulus-dependent effects, rather than a global suppression of cell death. For example, caspase-1$^{-/-}$, caspase-2$^{-/-}$ and caspase-11$^{-/-}$ mice have no significant overall abnormalities, except for minor functional defects related to lack of apoptosis processing in specific tissues [15,17-19,21,24,26]. These preferential apoptosis defects suggest that different sets of caspases may be involved in specific apoptotic pathways and act in tissue-specific manners.

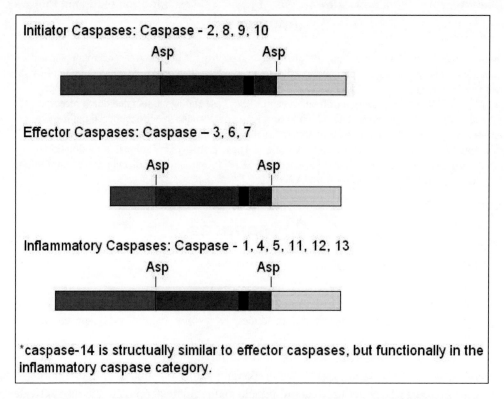

Figure 2. Structure of two different family of caspases. Initiator caspases and inflammatory caspases contain long pro-domains, but effector caspases contain short pro-domains. These caspases contain protease domains that contain large subunits and small subunits that are cleaved at Asp sites. Dark area is an active catalytic site of caspase that determines the specificity and the activity.

Table 1. Phenotypes of various homozygous caspase knockout mice

Caspases	Viable	Phenotype
Caspase-1	Yes	No IL-1β and IL-18 processing
Caspase-2	Yes	Oocytes resistant to drug-induced apoptosis
Caspase-3	Yes, if bred in C57BL/6	Resistant to apoptosis in neuronal cells
Caspase-7	Yes	Fibroblasts slightly resistant
Caspase-3/7	No. Perinatally lethal	Dilated cardiomyopathy with noncompaction
Caspase-8	No. Embryonic lethal	Fibroblasts resistant to death receptor mediated apoptosis
Caspase-9	No. Perinatally lethal	Severe brain abnormality; Defective mitochondria-mediated apoptosis
Caspase-11	Yes	Defective IL-1α and IL-1β processing
Caspase-12	Yes	Defective ER mediated apoptosis

In contrast, caspase-3, -8 and -9, deficiencies led to profound apoptotic defects associated with perinatal mortality [20,22,23,25,29]. Caspase-3 knockout mice generated on a 129/Sv background die perinatally; bred on a C57BL/6 background, however, they survive to adulthood [22,30-32]. In this case, they exhibit a more restrained apoptotic defect, which manifests as nerve cell resistance to oxidative stress-induced apoptosis *in vivo* and *in vitro* [32]. There is evidence that increased caspase-7 expression was able to compensate for caspase-3 function developmentally in these C57BL/6 mice [33]. However, in the caspase-3/7 double knockout, the brain still developed normally on the C57BL/6 genetic background, but the mice die of non-compaction of the ventricle perinatally [28].

Caspase-9$^{-/-}$ mice, are characterized by severe brain abnormalities and die perinatally; they exhibit defective apoptosis through the mitochondria-mediated pathway [20,23], which is consistent with the finding that caspase-9 is activated by the Apaf-1/cytochome c complex. Caspase-8$^{-/-}$ mice are characterized by severe developmental defects including cardiac non-compaction and a dramatic reduction in the number of hematopoietic precursors, and they die as embryos [25]. Thus caspase-8 and caspase-9, both "initiation caspases," are critical components of apoptosis pathways. Until we are able to achieve postnatal, tissue-specific deletions of caspase-8 and -9 in the adults, their functional significance in specific adult tissues remains unclear.

3. Initiator Caspases (2, 8, 9, 10)

a. Caspase 2

Caspase 2 has two forms, caspase-2L and caspase-2S, derived from two distinct caspase-2 mRNA variants result from alternative splicing. Caspase-2L seems to be pro-apoptotic, whereas caspase-2S can be anti-apoptotic with overexpression [34]. Caspase-2L is the dominant isoform that is expressed in most tissues [34]. Caspase-2$^{-/-}$ develop normally; however, their sympathetic and motor neurons are more sensitive to death than neurons of wild type mice when deprived of nerve growth factor. In contrast, B lymphoblasts, germ cells, and oocytes are found to be resistant to cell death [15].

Physiological levels of purified caspase-2 can cleave cytosolic Bid protein, which in turn can trigger the release of cytochrome c from isolated mitochondria. Caspase-2 can also induce directly the release of cytochrome c, AIF (apoptosis-inducing factor), and Smac (second mitochondria-derived activator of caspases protein) from isolated mitochondria independent of Bid [35]. Caspase-2 could provoke the activation of caspase-7 and it is not subject to inhibition by members of the IAP family of apoptosis inhibitors [36]. In rat neonatal endothelial cells, caspase-2 is the earliest activated caspase in norepinepherine (NE) induced apoptosis, followed by caspase-3 and caspase-9 activation [37]. Caspase-2 and -3 inhibitors had the most significant effect on the inhibition of NE-induced apoptosis as well as over-expression of Bcl-2 [37]. B-adrenergic blockers only partially inhibited apoptosis in these cells. It remains unclear the different pathways that are involved in the activation of caspase-2 and its relationship to Bcl-2 activation. In cardiac myocytes, Communal et al reported NE-induced cardiac apoptosis via β-adrenergic pathways [38] and Zaugg et al [39] reported that is selectively mediated by the β1 adrenergic pathway. Whether caspase-2 is involved in NE-induced cardiac myocyte apoptosis remains unknown. In a pacing dog model for dilated cardiomyopathy, caspase-2 and caspase-3 were found to be elevated in both atrial and ventricular cardiac myocytes undergoing apoptosis while Bcl-2 level was significantly decreased [40]. For staurosporine induced chick cardiac myocyte apoptosis, caspase-2 inhibitor produced a significant despite small reduction in apoptosis, which was additive to and greater than the inhibition of caspase-3 [41]. From these studies, we can conclude that caspase-2 plays a potentially important role in cardiac myocyte apoptosis, but its relative importance and its interaction with other caspase pathways remain to be clarified.

b. Caspase-8 and -10

Caspase-8 is an initiator caspase involved in death receptor-mediated apoptosis. Caspase-8 and caspase-10 contain two tandem repeats of death effector domains. Death receptors are some members of the TNFR family with conserved death domain in the intracellular domains [42]. Binding of the death ligand to the death receptors leads to the formation of the death-inducing signaling complex (DISC) containing the death receptors, adaptor proteins (FADD /TRADD (TNFR-associated death domain)), which recruits procaspase-8 and/or procaspase-10 [42]. Procaspase-8 dimerizes and becomes activated caspase-8, which then cleaves and activates the downstream caspase-3 and Bid [16,43,44].

Death receptor mediated pathway is an important apoptosis pathway in many cell types, however, cardiac myocytes are generally resistant to Fas-mediated apoptosis under normal conditions [45-47]. When subjected to hypoxia [46], hydrogen peroxide [47], and in the presence of nonlethal dose of doxorubicin [45], neonatal cardiac myocytes became susceptible to FasL induced apoptosis. In a rat model of adriamycin-induced cardiomyopathy, a neutralizing FasL antibody reduced cardiac apopotosis [48]. Furthermore, isolated hearts from mice lacking functional Fas displayed marked reduction in infarct size following ischemia/reperfusion [49]. In humans, soluble FasL was elevated in advanced congestive heart failure [50,51] and myocarditis [52]. Soluble Fas antagonists was suppressed in failing human myocardium [53]. The importance of low grade apoptosis leading to a lethal dilated cardiomyopathy was elegantly demonstrated by an inducible cardiac restricted caspase-8 allele in transgenic mice [54]. Mice carrying an inactive mutant were resistant and a pancaspase inhibitor was able to delay the effect of caspase-8 activation in the heart [54].

There are three major factors that regulate caspase-8 activity. The first and the best studied caspase inhibitors in mammalian systems are the inhibitor of apoptosis proteins (IAPs). They comprise a family of evolutionarily-conserved, homologous proteins first discovered in baculovirus [55,56]. IAPs directly bind caspase-3, -8 and -9 to inhibit their activity. The knockout of one of the IAP molecules, XIAP, resulted in no identifiable abnormalities, suggesting the presence of redundant IAP family members that can compensate for the lack of XIAP [57]. In addition, another level of control is provided by Smac/Diablo, a mitochondrial protein that promotes caspase activation by eliminating IAP inhibition [58]. Upon apoptotic stimulation, Smac/Diablo escapes into the cytosol, where it promotes caspase-8, -9, and -3 activations by binding to IAP. Caspase-8 is also inhibited by Apoptosis Repressor with CARD domain (ARC). ARC is expressed at high levels in skeletal and cardiac muscle, and specifically blocks caspase-8 and caspase-2 [59]. In addition, ARC also blocks cytochrome c release from the mitochondria and suppresses hypoxia-induced apoptosis in a caspase-independent manner [60]. In addition, under physiological conditions, another inhibitor of the Fas signaling pathway is FLICE-inhibitory Protein (FLIP), which is an anti-apoptotic protein highly expressed in the muscle and lymphoid tissues [61,62]. FLIP is a cytoplasmic protein, and has a short form (FLIP$_S$) and a long form (FLIP$_L$), both of which interact with the adaptor protein FADD and the protease FLICE, and potently inhibit apoptosis induced by all known human death receptors [61]. FLIP down-regulation in the cardiac myocytes has been reported in the ischemia/reperfusion [62] as well as after doxorubicin treatment [63].

Caspase-10 is the only other caspase that has death effector domain homology with caspase-8 [64]. Two isoforms of caspase-10 were identified. The caspase-10$_L$ isoform is identical to capase-10$_S$ except an additional 43 amino acids between the prodomain and protease domain [42]. Caspase-10 is highly expressed in lymphocytes and dendritic cells [64]. Activation of caspase-10, -3, and -7 as well as Bid cleavage and cytochrome c release in caspase-8-deficient Jurkat cells treated with FasL was reported [64,65]. Apoptosis was inhibited by a broad spectrum caspase inhibitor as well as a caspase-10 specific inhibitor [65]. In addition, caspase-10 was able to cleave Bid to generate active tBid in vitro [65]. These experiments strongly support the notion that caspase-10 is an initiator caspase in its own right in Fas signaling leading to Bid processing, caspase cascade activation, and apoptosis.

c. Caspase 9

Caspase-9 plays a critical role in the mitochondria-mediated apoptotic pathway. Pro-caspase-9 has a long prodomain (~13kDa) containing a caspase-recruitment domain (CARD) that interacts with other CARD-containing adaptor molecules (Apaf-1), in the presence of dATP and cytochrome c to undergo adaptor-mediated aggregation and self-activation, thus the formation of apoptosome [6,66]. Mutation of the interface residue in either pro-caspase-9 or Apaf-1 prevents pro-caspase-9 activation in a cell free system [67].

The regulation of caspase-9 involves several mechanisms. The first level of regulation involves mitochondria. The most extensively studied mechanism is the regulation of pro-caspase-9 activation by controlling the release of cytochrome c from mitochondria by the anti-apoptotic (e.g. Bcl-2 and Bcl-x_L) and pro-apoptotic (e.g. Bad and Bax) Bcl-2 family of proteins [43,68-72]. In heart, our laboratory as well as other investigators have shown that Bcl-2 over-expression protects against apoptosis during oxidative stress [58,73-75]. Similar to caspase-8, IAPs provide another level of control of caspase-9 activity by direct binding. Similar to the IAP inhibitor Smac/Diablo, a serine protease Omi/HtrA2 is released from mitochondria upon apoptotic stimulation and induces apoptosis by inhibiting IAP, thus activating caspase by releasing it from IAP inhibition [76-81]. A recent study suggests that inhibition of Omi/HtrA2 by ucf-101, a specific Omi/HtrA2 inhibitor, significantly blocks ischemia/reperfusion-induced cardiac myocyte cell death and decreases myocardial loss [82]. The mechanism appears to be mediated via the mitochondrial apoptosis pathway, since there was attenuation of XIAP degradation and inhibition of caspase-9 and caspase-3 activities. Additional mechanisms of caspase inhibition include Aven, which prevents the activation of the apoptosome by interfering with Apaf-1 self association [83], and the inactivation of caspase-9 by Akt phosphorylation of procaspase-9 [84].

Another important inhibitor of caspase-9 may be HAX-1 (hematopoietic lineage specific protein-1 (HS-1) associated protein), a 35kDa intracellular protein ubiquitously expressed in all tissues, but with significantly greater expression in skeletal muscle, heart, pancreas, and the liver [85,86]. In our lab, we observed that adult cardiac myocytes are relatively resistant to caspase-9 induced apoptosis, and significantly lack pro-caspase-9 processing when caspase-9 is over-expressed. This suggested that adult cardiac myocytes possess factor(s) that inhibit caspase-9 processing. We identified HAX-1 as a protein that binds with caspase-9 using a yeast-2-hybrid system. We further demonstrated that the recombinant HAX-1 protein specifically inhibits the processing of pro-caspase-9 as well as pro-caspase-3 in a concentration-dependent manner in a cell-free system [87]. The over-expression of HAX-1 in cardiac myocytes resulted in significant attenuation of caspase-9 processing and hypoxia/reoxygenation-induced cell death [87]. In fact, knockdown of HAX-1 expression using siRNA resulted in significantly decreased cell survival compared to the control. Thus, these findings suggest that HAX-1 is another newly identified caspase-9 inhibitor, particularly in adult cardiac myocytes.

4. Effector Caspases (3, 6, 7)

Proteolytic activation of caspase-3, -6, -7 results in the cleavage of a variety of substrates and characteristic apoptosis findings such as PARP cleavage, and DNA laddering [88]. Among these effector caspases, caspase-3 is the most extensively studied. Caspase-3 has a short prodomain and composed of subunits of 17 kDa and 12 kDa [88]. It is widely distributed with high expressions in lymphoid cells [89]. Caspase-6 gene encodes a 34 kDa protein, and is highly homologous to caspase-3 [90]. Activated caspase-6 and caspase-3 can cleave each other and result in each other's activation, thus result in a protease amplification cycle [91]. Caspase-7 gene encodes a 35 kDa protein, with the highest degree of homology to caspase-3 as compared to other caspases, is localized in the cytoplasm and is expressed in a variety of tissues and cell lines [92]. It has two splice variant, alpha and beta [92]. Of interest, recombinant caspase-3 17 kDa subunit can form an active heteromeric enzyme complex with recombinant caspase-7 alpha 12 kDa subunit and vice versa, as determined by the ability of the heteromeric complexes to induce apoptosis in cell lines [92].

Caspase -3 are generally activated by DISC complex containing caspase-8 or apoptosome containing caspase-9. In cells containing high levels of DISC complexes, activated caspase-8 can directly activate downstream caspase-3 [93]. In cells with low levels of DISC complexes, low level of caspase-8 cleaves Bid into tBid, which releases cytochrome c from the mitochondria and activates apoptosome [93]. Activated caspase-9 then cleaves downstream caspase-3 [93]. Caspase-3 can be inhibited by XIAP via its BIR2 domain [94]. Procaspase 7 has been shown to be cleaved and activated by an apoptosome complex [95]. Procaspase-9 recruitment to the apoptosome and processing are accelerated in lysates supplemented with caspase-3 [95]. In lysates containing very low levels of Smac and Omi/HtrA2, XIAP binds tightly to caspase-9 in the apoptosome complex and inhibits procaspase-7 processing [95]. With higher level of Smac and Omi/HtrA2, active caspase-7 is released from the apoptosome and its function is inhibited by a stable XIAP-caspase-7 complex [95].

Caspase-3 and caspase-7 double knockout (DKO) was published recently revealing a number of interesting insights into the overlapping but yet unique roles of caspase -3 and caspase-7 in apoptosis [28]. Caspase-3$^{-/-}$ MEFs showed complete lack of DNA fragmentation and poly(ADP-ribose) polymerase (PARP) cleavage [28]. Caspase-7$^{-/-}$ MEFs showed increased viability although the DKO conferred the most resistance to apoptotic stimuli, including staurosporine, FasL, and TNF-α; they were nearly completely resistant to UV irradiation induced apoptosis [28]. DKO MEFs also exhibited delayed Bax translocation, cytochrome c release, and complete lack of AIF release from the mitochondria [28]. This provides evidence for "caspase-independent mechanism" may be caspase-8 or -9 independent, but are not truly independent of all caspases. The combined action of caspase-3 and caspase-7 is critical in cardiac muscle organization and compaction, however, the pathways involved still need further elucidation [28].

5. Inflammatory Caspases (1, 4, 5, 11, 12, 13, 14)

Human caspase-1, -4, -5, mouse caspase-11 (homologue of human caspase-4 and -5 [96]) and -12, are considered caspase-1 subfamily, with prime function of regulation of inflammatory process. Caspase-1, initially discovered as interleukin converting enzyme (ICE), is expressed as a proform and activated through proteolytic cleavage of an amino-terminal 11kDa prodomain to release p20 and p10, which forms an active tetramer $(p20/p10)_2$ protease [97] (Figure 3). Caspase-1 forms its activation complex, known as inflammasome by oligomerization with scaffold adaptor proteins such NALP1 and a second adaptor protein ASC via the CARD domain [61,98]. Composed of three domains: a leucine-rich repeat, a NACHT domain, and a pyrin domain [61,98], NALP family proteins have structure similarities to Apaf-1 [61]. ASC contains both a pyrin and a CARD domain. Murine caspase-

11 or human caspase-5 are necessary constituents for the activation of inflammasome upon lipopolysaccharide binding to its receptor TLR-4 [26]. However, the formation of the inflammasome in response to hypoxia or oxidative stress is not well understood.

Caspase-1 is critical in interleukin-1β (IL-1β) and -18 (IL-18) processing as demonstrated by lack of active forms of these two cytokines in the knock out mice [24]. IL-1β is one of the principal pro-inflammatory cytokines. IL-18 is essential for full expression of INFγ, TNF, and a number of chemokines, which are involved in the maladaptive ventricular remodeling process after myocardial injury [99]. IL-18 has also been implicated in the acceleration and vulnerability of atherosclerotic plaques [100]. Higher serum level of IL-18 was found to be a strong independent predictor of cardiovascular death in stable and unstable angina [101]. Frantz et al compared caspase-1 knock-out mice with wild type mice in the left coronary artery ligation myocardial infarction model, and showed decreased level of metalloproteinase 3, IL-18, rate of apoptosis by TUNEL staining, and decreased left ventricular end-diastolic area on 2D echocardiography [102]. In an ischemia/reperfusion (I/R) model of suprafused human atrial myocardium, inhibition of capase-1 has been shown to improve myocardial contractile function after I/R via inhibition of IL-18 and IL-1β [99].

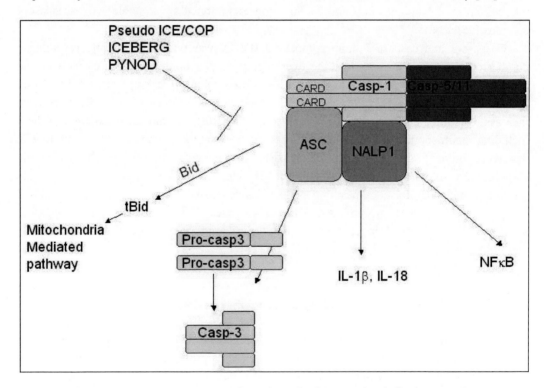

Figure 3. Inflammatory caspases. Caspase-1 forms its activation complex, inflammasome, by oligomerization with NALP1 and ASC. Caspase-11 and/or caspase-5 are necessary constituents for the activation of inflammasome. The inflammasome is involved in interleukin-1β (IL-1β) and -18 (IL-18) processing as well as apoptosis via caspase-3. Several inhibitors, such as pseudo-ICE/COP, ICEBERG and PYNOD, may modulate its action.

In addition to mediating the pro-inflammatory effect through interleukin processing, caspase-1 has also been reported to be directly involved in apoptosis of cardiac myocytes.

Caspase-1 has been found to be up-regulated in myocardial hypertrophy and heart failure [103-105]. Over-expression (30 fold) of pro-caspase-1 had no noticeable pathology in unstressed mouse hearts, however, under endotoxic or hypoxic stress, excess pro-caspase-1 was activated in the heart to induce increased apoptosis via direct or indirect activation of effector caspase-3, resulting in exaggerated myocardial injury [106]. Cardiac depression is a well-known phenomenon in sepsis. In a study of human fetal myocytes exposed to human septic serum, caspase-1 processing was induced in these human fetal myocytes, and apoptosis could be reduced by caspase-1,-4,-5 inhibitor Ac-YVAD-FMK, as well as inhibitors of other caspases [107]. Myocarditis has been associated with multiple infectious agents with no current therapeutic interventions. Most patients recover their regional wall motions, but a number of patients present with acute heart failure, reduced ejection fraction, and do not recover. An interesting study by Londono *et al* studied cardiac apoptosis in severe relapsing fever Borreliosis in antibody deficient mice, and found evidence of apoptosis of macrophages as well as cardiac myocytes with significant up-regulation of caspases, most notably caspase-1 [108]. Caspase-1 has also been shown to process Bid to tBid, and activates caspase-9 via the mitochondria pathway [42].

Inhibitors of caspase-1, ICEBERG and COP (pseudo-ICE) are found near caspase-1 on the chromosome 11q22. They both consist of a single CARD domain and negatively regulate caspase-1 and inhibit cytokine production, but not apoptosis [35]. Other inhibitors include DASC (decoy ASC) and proteinase inhibitor 9, which are inducible by proinflammatory agents, likely constitute a negative feedback loop [109,110]. PYNOD, a member of Apaf-1-like molecules (close relationship to NALP family proteins), expressed in high levels in heart, skeletal muscle, and brain, was found to bind ASC and inhibit apoptosis and IL-1β maturation [37]. In human atherosclerotic lesion, restenosis may reflect a resistance of apoptosis [111]. Caspase-1 and caspase-8 were found to have lower expression levels in these resistant cells in addition to higher level of Bcl-Xs expression and cyclin D1 expression [112].

Many questions still remain in the role of caspase-1 in cardiac apoptosis. Caspase-1 is at the center of many inflammatory and apoptotic pathways. The details of its activating stimulus, its interactions with other caspases, and its contribution to cardiac apoptosis in different disease states still need clarification. Nonetheless, with inflammation increasingly being recognized as an important component in coronary artery disease and heart failure in addition to the traditionally recognized sepsis and myocarditis states, caspase-1 maybe an important drug target to prevent and treat myocardial injury.

Caspase-5 may have a regulatory role in tumorgenesis in addition to participating in the inflammasome formation [113]. Very little is known about caspase-4, other than it is induced by interferon and it can be activated when cells are treated with ER stress [114,115]. Accumulation of misfolded proteins and alteration in calcium homeostasis in the ER leads to ER stress [27]. Murine caspase-12 is involved in ER-stress induced apoptosis [27]. Polymorphism in caspase-12 in humans results either a truncated CARD only protein, or an enzymatically inactive molecule, which are more related to ICEBERG and COP in its function [55]. However, the exact role of these two forms of human caspase-12 requires further investigation. Murine caspase-11 has also been shown to be part of the inflammasome formation and is also activated in the setting of caspase-1 activation [26,116].

Caspase-13 is constitutively expressed mainly in peripheral blood lymphocytes, spleen, and placenta [117]. Caspase-13 can be activated by caspase-8, is able to induce apoptosis when over-expressed, and can be blocked by caspase inhibitors baculovirus protein p35 and pox virus cytokine response modifier protein CrmA [117]. There has been no report of caspase-13 activity in cardiovascular cells.

Caspase-14 was identified as a developmentally active caspase as it is highly expressed in embryonic tissues but present only in adult epidermal keratinocytes [118]. Caspase-14 has an unusually short prodomain, preferentially associates with large prodomain caspases, including caspase-1, -2, -4, -8, and -10 [118]. Caspase-14 processes caspase activity and was able to induce apoptosis in human breast cancer cells, which was attenuated by pan-caspase inhibitors [118]. Human caspase-14 seems to have a substrate preference similar to a cytokine activator, which groups it functionally in the inflammatory caspases, while mouse caspase-14 seems to have a substrate preference similar to caspase-8 and -9 [119]. Its developmental role remains unclear and it does not seem to have a role in adult cardiac myocyte apoptosis.

D. Caspase-Dependent and Caspase-Independent Apoptosis Mechanisms

The activation of caspase is central to the regulation and execution of the apoptotic program and is most likely the predominant mechanism involved in apoptosis. However, there is accumulating evidence to suggest that apoptosis can be mediated by caspase-independent mechanisms [120-123]. (Figure 4) The best demonstrated example of caspase-independent apoptosis involves apoptosis inducing factor (AIF). AIF is an NADH-oxidase produced as a 67-kDa protein containing an N-terminal mitochondrial localization signal sequence [124-126]. In mitochondria, AIF is processed into a 57-kDa mature form. AIF is then released into the cytosol upon apoptotic stimulation and may translocate into the nucleus and induce DNA fragmentation without caspase activation [124,126]. This notion is supported by the fact that microinjection of AIF into cells induced apoptotic changes, such as chromatin condensation, that could not be blocked by zVAD.fmk or the over-expression of Bcl-2 [124,127,128]. Furthermore, AIF can still trigger DNA fragmentation in Apaf-1 and caspase-9 deficient cells [122], which is possibly mediated through direct activation of caspase-3 [28].

The mechanisms that regulate AIF release from mitochondria are complex and controversial. For example, AIF release may be regulated by Bcl-2 proteins-dependent as well as Bcl-2 proteins-independent mechanisms. Several studies have shown that Bcl-2 over-expression prevents both the release of AIF and cell death [126,129]. Furthermore, Bax over-expression triggers AIF release [130,131] and AIF release is blocked in Bax-deficient neurons upon apoptotic induction [129]. In contrast, the Bcl-2-independent mechanism of AIF release involves a PARP-1, which has been shown to facilitate the release of AIF from mitochondria and AIF nuclear translocation independent of the Bcl-2 protein family and caspase activation [132-134]. In addition, there is considerable debate over the relationship of AIF to caspase activation. Initial studies showed that AIF functions upstream and independent of caspase activation [126,135,136]. However, several studies in C. elegans, as well as in mammalian cells, suggest that caspase activation is needed for AIF release in certain model of apoptosis stimuli, including staurosporine or actinomycin D, or hydrogen peroxide [128,130,131]. In the caspase-3 and -7 double knockout mice, no AIF release is observed under UV irradiation, which provides further evidence for the dependence of the combined caspase action for AIF release [28]. The contribution of caspase-independent apoptosis in the heart is unknown, and how these complicated and somewhat conflicting mechanisms might be coordinated has not yet been satisfactorily addressed.

Other evidence of caspase-independent apoptosis comes from studies of endonuclease G (EndoG). Similar to AIF, EndoG translocates from the mitochondria to the nucleus during apoptosis and induces DNA fragmentation independent of the caspases [64,137]. During development, caspase-9 is down regulated in cardiac myocytes [87,138], EndoG and truncated AIF become the essential mediators of apoptosis in a caspase-independent manner in ischemia induced cardiac myocyte apoptosis [138]. Furthermore, Omi/HtrA2, a mitochondrial serine protease with pro-apoptotic properties, may also contributes to caspase-independent apoptosis [76], however, this mechanism of action is less well defined. In addition, since caspases are proteases, it has been suggested that caspase-independent cell death may utilize other proteases, such as cathepsin, the calpains, or granzyme B [94,139-141]. Lastly, BH3-domain only proteins, such as tBid, Bim and Bad, which have been shown to promote caspase activation, have also been shown to kill cells independent of Apaf-1 and caspase activation [142].

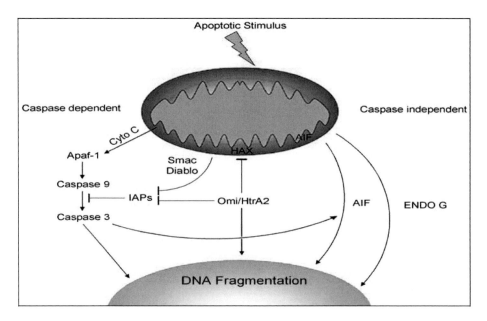

Figure 4. Caspase-dependent and caspase-independent mitochondrial pathways. In response to an apoptotic stimulus, mitochondria release various pro-apoptotic factors to initiate apoptosis that may be caspase-dependent (e.g. cytochrome c), caspase-independent (e.g. AIF and Endo G) or both (e.g. Omi/HtrA2).

E. Therapeutic Implications

Since apoptosis is implicated in the pathogenesis of many different cardiovascular diseases, the inhibition of apoptosis promises to be an extraordinarily important target for therapeutic intervention [4,143,144]. The critical role of the caspases in the apoptotic program puts them at the focus of anti-apoptotic therapies. Caspase inhibition has already been shown to reduce myocardial loss and improve cardiac function in various animal models [145,146]. However, caspase inhibition strategy is complicated by the activation of caspase-independent apoptosis pathways accompanied by the release of cytochrome c, AIF, EndoG, and Omi/HtrA2 in the absence of caspase activation. Furthermore, the molecular mechanism of cardiac apoptosis, especially the role of critical caspases in heart, is not completely understood. With the emerging possibility of chronic systemic use of apoptosis inhibitors, we also need to be particularly aware of potential safety concerns that may arise from their prolonged application, which include the induction of cancer and autoimmune diseases [11]. Thus, a better understanding of the regulation of the caspases, their relationship with caspase-independent pathways, as well as achieving a more targeted approach to caspase modulation, will be critical to developing caspase modulation as an effective therapeutic option.

Table 2. Tissue and apoptotic stimuli specificities of the caspases

Caspases	Tissue/cell type specificity	Apoptotic Stimuli in Heart
Caspase-1 (h+m)	Whole heart [116], mononuclear cells [97]	Hypertrophy, heart failure [103-106], sepsis [107], ischemia/infarction [99], myocarditis [108]
Caspase-2 (h+m)	Endothelial cells [37] cardiac myocytes [40,41], most tissues [34]	Staurosporine [41], Pacing [40]
Caspase-3 (h+m)	Whole heart [116], neurons and glia [119], most tissues	Multiple stimuli
Caspase-4 (human)	monocytes [88]	
Caspase-5 (human)	monocytes [88]	
Caspase-6 (h+m)	Neurons and glia [119]	
Caspase-7 (h+m)	T-lymphocytes [92], most tissues	
Caspase-8 (h+m)	Neurons and glia [119], cardiac myocytes [45-47], most tissues	hypoxia [46], hydrogen peroxide [47], doxorubicin [45], ischemia/reperfusion [49]
Caspase-9 (h+m)	Neurons [147], cardiac myocytes [82], most tissues.	Ischemia/reperfusion [82], multiple stimuli
Caspase-10	Neurons and glia [119], lymphocytes [42]	
Caspase-11 (murine)	Whole heart [116]	
Caspase-12, (h+m) ER/SR	Cardiac myocytes [148]	Doxorubicin, ER stress [27]
Caspase-13	Peripheral lymphocytes, spleen, placenta [117]	
Caspase-14 (h+m)	Epidermis, neurons, and glia [119]	

h+m = human and murine.

Acknowledgments

This study was supported by the grants from National Heart, Lung and Blood Institutes HL65742 (PMK), HL67091 (PMK) and American Heart Association Northeast Affiliate Post-doctoral fellowship 0225612T (YH).

References

[1]   Kerr JF, Wyllie AH, Currie AR. Apoptosis: a basic biological phenomenon with wide-ranging implications in tissue kinetics. *Br. J. Cancer* 1972;26(4):239-257.

[2]   Gottlieb RA, Burleson KO, Kloner RA, et al. Reperfusion injury induces apoptosis in rabbit cardiomyocytes. *J. Clin. Invest.* 1994;94(4):1621-1628.

[3]   Kang PM, Izumo S. Apoptosis in heart: basic mechanisms and implications in cardiovascular diseases. *Trends Mol. Med.* Apr 2003;9(4):177-182.

[4]   Kang PM, Izumo S. Apoptosis and heart failure: A critical review of the literature. *Circ. Res.* Jun 9 2000;86(11):1107-1113.

[5]   Liu X, Kim CN, Yang J, et al. Induction of apoptotic program in cell-free extracts: requirement for dATP and cytochrome c. *Cell* 1996;86(1):147-157.

[6]   Li P, Nijhawan D, Budihardjo I, et al. Cytochrome c and dATP-dependent formation of Apaf-1/caspase-9 complex initiates an apoptotic protease cascade. *Cell* Nov 14 1997;91(4):479-489.

[7]   Zou H, Henzel WJ, Liu X, et al. Apaf-1, a human protein homologous to C. elegans CED-4, participates in cytochrome c-dependent activation of caspase-3 [see comments]. *Cell* 1997;90(3):405-413.

[8]   Slee EA, Harte MT, Kluck RM, et al. Ordering the cytochrome c-initiated caspase cascade: hierarchical activation of caspases-2, -3, -6, -7, -8, and -10 in a caspase-9-dependent manner [In Process Citation]. *J. Cell Biol.* 1999;144(2):281-292.

[9]   Adams JW, Armstrong RC, Kirshenbaum LA, et al. Bcl-2 expression inhibits Gaq-induced mitochondrial cytochrome c release and prevents caspase-dependent apoptosis. *Circulation (supp).* 1999;100:I-282.

[10]   Bialik S, Cryns VL, Drincic A, et al. The mitochondrial apoptotic pathway is activated by serum and glucose deprivation in cardiac myocytes. *Circ. Res.* 1999;85(5):403-414.

[11]   Kang PM, Haunstetter A, Aoki H, et al. Morphological and molecular characterization of adult cardiomyocyte apoptosis during hypoxia and reoxygenation. *Circ. Res.* Jul 21 2000; 87(2):118-125.

[12]   Narula J, Pandey P, Arbustini E, et al. Apoptosis in heart failure: release of cytochrome c from mitochondria and activation of caspase-3 in human cardiomyopathy [see comments]. *Proc. Natl. Acad. Sci. USA* 1999;96(14):8144-8149.

[13]   Nagata S. Apoptosis by death factor. *Cell.* 1997;88(3):355-365.

[14]   Nicholson DW, Thornberry NA. Caspases: killer proteases. *Trends Biochem. Sci.* 1997; 22(8): 299-306.

[15]   Bergeron L, Perez GI, Macdonald G, et al. Defects in regulation of apoptosis in caspase-2-deficient mice. *Genes Dev.* 1998; 12(9):1304-1314.

[16] Gross A, Yin XM, Wang K, et al. Caspase cleaved BID targets mitochondria and is required for cytochrome c release, while BCL-XL prevents this release but not tumor necrosis factor-R1/Fas death. *J. Biol. Chem.* Jan 8 1999;274(2):1156-1163.

[17] Fantuzzi G, Puren AJ, Harding MW, et al. Interleukin-18 regulation of interferon gamma production and cell proliferation as shown in interleukin-1beta-converting enzyme (caspase-1)-deficient mice. *Blood* 1998;91(6):2118-2125.

[18] Ghayur T, Banerjee S, Hugunin M, et al. Caspase-1 processes IFN-gamma-inducing factor and regulates LPS-induced IFN-gamma production. *Nature* 1997;386(6625):619-623.

[19] Gu Y, Kuida K, Tsutsui H, et al. Activation of interferon-gamma inducing factor mediated by interleukin-1beta converting enzyme. *Science* Jan 10 1997;275(5297):206-209.

[20] Hakem R, Hakem A, Duncan GS, et al. Differential requirement for caspase 9 in apoptotic pathways in vivo. *Cell* Aug 7 1998;94(3):339-352.

[21] Kuida K, Lippke JA, Ku G, et al. Altered cytokine export and apoptosis in mice deficient in interleukin-1 beta converting enzyme. *Science* 1995;267(5206):2000-2003.

[22] Kuida K, Zheng TS, Na S, et al. Decreased apoptosis in the brain and premature lethality in CPP32-deficient mice. *Nature* 1996;384(6607):368-372.

[23] Kuida K, Haydar TF, Kuan CY, et al. Reduced apoptosis and cytochrome c-mediated caspase activation in mice lacking caspase 9. *Cell* Aug 7 1998;94(3):325-337.

[24] Li P, Allen H, Banerjee S, et al. Mice deficient in IL-1 beta-converting enzyme are defective in production of mature IL-1 beta and resistant to endotoxic shock. *Cell* 1995; 80(3):401-411.

[25] Varfolomeev EE, Schuchmann M, Luria V, et al. Targeted disruption of the mouse Caspase 8 gene ablates cell death induction by the TNF receptors, Fas/Apo1, and DR3 and is lethal prenatally. *Immunity* 1998;9(2):267-276.

[26] Wang S, Miura M, Jung YK, et al. Murine caspase-11, an ICE-interacting protease, is essential for the activation of ICE. *Cell* 1998;92(4):501-509.

[27] Nakagawa T, Zhu H, Morishima N, et al. Caspase-12 mediates endoplasmic-reticulum-specific apoptosis and cytotoxicity by amyloid-beta. *Nature* 2000;403(6765):98-103.

[28] Lakhani SA, Masud A, Kuida K, et al. Caspases 3 and 7: key mediators of mitochondrial events of apoptosis. *Science* Feb 10 2006;311(5762):847-851.

[29] Zheng TS, Hunot S, Kuida K, et al. Caspase knockouts: matters of life and death. *Cell Death Differ.* Nov 1999;6(11):1043-1053.

[30] Zheng TS, Hunot S, Kuida K, et al. Deficiency in caspase-9 or caspase-3 induces compensatory caspase activation. *Nat. Med.* Nov 2000;6(11):1241-1247.

[31] Leonard JR, Klocke BJ, D'Sa C, et al. Strain-dependent neurodevelopmental abnormalities in caspase-3-deficient mice. *J. Neuropathol. Exp. Neurol.* Aug 2002; 61(8): 673-677.

[32] Le DA, Wu Y, Huang Z, et al. Caspase activation and neuroprotection in caspase-3-deficient mice after in vivo cerebral ischemia and in vitro oxygen glucose deprivation. *Proc. Natl. Acad. Sci. USA* Nov 12 2002;99(23):15188-15193.

[33] Houde C, Banks KG, Coulombe N, et al. Caspase-7 expanded function and intrinsic expression level underlies strain-specific brain phenotype of caspase-3-null mice. *J. Neurosci.* Nov 3 2004;24(44):9977-9984.

[34] Wang L, Miura M, Bergeron L, et al. Ich-1, an Ice/ced-3-related gene, encodes both positive and negative regulators of programmed cell death. *Cell* Sep 9 1994;78(5):739-750.

[35] Guo Y, Srinivasula SM, Druilhe A, et al. Caspase-2 induces apoptosis by releasing proapoptotic proteins from mitochondria. *J. Biol. Chem.* Apr 19 2002;277(16):13430-13437.

[36] Ho PK, Jabbour AM, Ekert PG, et al. Caspase-2 is resistant to inhibition by inhibitor of apoptosis proteins (IAPs) and can activate caspase-7. *Febs J.* Mar 2005;272(6):1401-1414.

[37] Fu YC, Chi CS, Yin SC, et al. Norepinephrine induces apoptosis in neonatal rat endothelial cells via down-regulation of Bcl-2 and activation of beta-adrenergic and caspase-2 pathways. *Cardiovasc. Res.* Jan 1 2004;61(1):143-151.

[38] Communal C, Singh K, Pimentel DR, et al. Norepinephrine stimulates apoptosis in adult rat ventricular myocytes by activation of the beta-adrenergic pathway. *Circulation* Sep 29 1998;98(13):1329-1334.

[39] Zaugg M, Xu W, Lucchinetti E, et al. Beta-adrenergic receptor subtypes differentially affect apoptosis in adult rat ventricular myocytes. *Circulation* Jul 18 2000;102(3):344-350.

[40] Heinke MY, Yao M, Chang D, et al. Apoptosis of ventricular and atrial myocytes from pacing-induced canine heart failure. *Cardiovasc. Res.* Jan 2001;49(1):127-134.

[41] Rabkin SW. Prevention of staurosporine-induced cell death in embryonic chick cardiomyocyte is more dependent on caspase-2 than caspase-3 inhibition and is independent of sphingomyelinase activation and ceramide generation. *Arch Biochem. Biophys.* Jun 1 2001;390(1):119-127.

[42] Guegan C, Vila M, Teismann P, et al. Instrumental activation of bid by caspase-1 in a transgenic mouse model of ALS. *Mol. Cell Neurosci.* Aug 2002;20(4):553-562.

[43] Luo X, Budihardjo I, Zou H, et al. Bid, a Bcl2 interacting protein, mediates cytochrome c release from mitochondria in response to activation of cell surface death receptors. *Cell* Aug 21 1998;94(4):481-490.

[44] Li H, Zhu H, Xu CJ, et al. Cleavage of BID by caspase 8 mediates the mitochondrial damage in the Fas pathway of apoptosis. *Cell* 1998;94(4):491-501.

[45] Yamaoka M, Yamaguchi S, Suzuki T, et al. Apoptosis in rat cardiac myocytes induced by Fas ligand: priming for Fas-mediated apoptosis with doxorubicin. *J. Mol. Cell Cardiol.* Jun 2000;32(6):881-889.

[46] Yaniv G, Shilkrut M, Lotan R, et al. Hypoxia predisposes neonatal rat ventricular myocytes to apoptosis induced by activation of the Fas (CD95/Apo-1) receptor: Fas activation and apoptosis in hypoxic myocytes. *Cardiovasc. Res.* Jun 2002;54(3):611-623.

[47] Yaniv G, Shilkrut M, Larisch S, et al. Hydrogen peroxide predisposes neonatal rat ventricular myocytes to Fas-mediated apoptosis. *Biochem. Biophys. Res. Commun.* Oct 28 2005;336(3):740-746.

[48] Holly TA, Drincic A, Byun Y, et al. Caspase inhibition reduces myocyte cell death induced by myocardial ischemia and reperfusion in vivo. *J. Mol. Cell Cardiol.* 1999; 31(9): 1709-1715.

[49] Lee P, Sata M, Lefer DJ, et al. Fas pathway is a critical mediator of cardiac myocyte death and MI during ischemia-reperfusion in vivo. *Am. J. Physiol. Heart Circ. Physiol.* Feb 2003;284(2):H456-463.

[50] Nishigaki K, Minatoguchi S, Seishima M, et al. Plasma Fas ligand, an inducer of apoptosis, and plasma soluble Fas, an inhibitor of apoptosis, in patients with chronic congestive heart failure. *J. Am. Coll. Cardiol.* 1997;29(6):1214-1220.

[51] Yamaguchi S, Yamaoka M, Okuyama M, et al. Elevated circulating levels and cardiac secretion of soluble Fas ligand in patients with congestive heart failure. *Am. J. Cardiol.* May 15 1999;83(10):1500-1503, A1508.

[52] Toyozaki T, Hiroe M, Tanaka M, et al. Levels of soluble Fas ligand in myocarditis. *Am. J. Cardiol.* Jul 15 1998;82(2):246-248.

[53] Schumann H, Morawietz H, Hakim K, et al. Alternative splicing of the primary Fas transcript generating soluble Fas antagonists is suppressed in the failing human ventricular myocardium. *Biochem. Biophys. Res. Commun.* Oct 29 1997; 239(3):794-798.

[54] Fujio Y, Nguyen T, Wencker D, et al. Akt promotes survival of cardiomyocytes in vitro and protects against ischemia-reperfusion injury in mouse heart. *Circulation* 2000; 101(6): 660-667.

[55] Srinivasula SM, Hegde R, Saleh A, et al. A conserved XIAP-interaction motif in caspase-9 and Smac/DIABLO regulates caspase activity and apoptosis. *Nature* Mar 1 2001;410(6824):112-116.

[56] Takahashi R, Deveraux Q, Tamm I, et al. A single BIR domain of XIAP sufficient for inhibiting caspases. *J. Biol. Chem.* Apr 3 1998;273(14):7787-7790.

[57] Harlin H, Reffey SB, Duckett CS, et al. Characterization of XIAP-deficient mice. *Mol. Cell Biol.* May 2001;21(10):3604-3608.

[58] Brocheriou V, Hagege AA, Oubenaissa A, et al. Cardiac functional improvement by a human Bcl-2 transgene in a mouse model of ischemia/reperfusion injury. *J. Gene Med.* Sep-Oct 2000;2(5):326-333.

[59] Koseki T, Inohara N, Chen S, et al. ARC, an inhibitor of apoptosis expressed in skeletal muscle and heart that interacts selectively with caspases. *Proc. Natl. Acad. Sci. USA* 1998; 95(9):5156-5160.

[60] Ekhterae D, Lin Z, Lundberg MS, et al. ARC inhibits cytochrome c release from mitochondria and protects against hypoxia-induced apoptosis in heart-derived H9c2 cells. *Circ. Res.* Dec 9 1999;85(12):e70-77.

[61] Van de Craen M, Van den Brande I, Declercq W, et al. Cleavage of caspase family members by granzyme B: a comparative study in vitro. *Eur. J. Immunol.* May 1997; 27(5): 1296-1299.

[62] Rasper DM, Vaillancourt JP, Hadano S, et al. Cell death attenuation by 'Usurpin', a mammalian DED-caspase homologue that precludes caspase-8 recruitment and activation by the CD-95 (Fas, APO-1) receptor complex. *Cell Death Differ.* Apr 1998; 5(4): 271-288.

[63] Nitobe J, Yamaguchi S, Okuyama M, et al. Reactive oxygen species regulate FLICE inhibitory protein (FLIP) and susceptibility to Fas-mediated apoptosis in cardiac myocytes. *Cardiovasc. Res.* Jan 2003;57(1):119-128.

[64] Li LY, Luo X, Wang X. Endonuclease G is an apoptotic DNase when released from mitochondria. *Nature* Jul 5 2001;412(6842):95-99.

[65] Milhas D, Cuvillier O, Therville N, et al. Caspase-10 triggers Bid cleavage and caspase cascade activation in FasL-induced apoptosis. *J. Biol. Chem.* May 20 2005;280(20): 19836-19842.

[66] Salvesen GS, Dixit VM. Caspase activation: the induced-proximity model. *Proc. Natl. Acad. Sci. USA* 1999;96(20):10964-10967.

[67] Qin H, Srinivasula SM, Wu G, et al. Structural basis of procaspase-9 recruitment by the apoptotic protease-activating factor 1. *Nature* 1999; 399(6736):549-557.

[68] Adams JM, Cory S. The Bcl-2 protein family: arbiters of cell survival. *Science* 1998; 281(5381): 1322-1326.

[69] Chen G, Cizeau J, Vande Velde C, et al. Nix and Nip3 form a subfamily of pro-apoptotic mitochondrial proteins. *J. Biol. Chem.* Jan 1 1999;274(1):7-10.

[70] Chao DT, Korsmeyer SJ. BCL-2 family: regulators of cell death. *Annu. Rev. Immunol.* 1998; 16:395-419.

[71] Ray R, Chen G, Vande Velde C, et al. BNIP3 heterodimerizes with Bcl-2/Bcl-X(L) and induces cell death independent of a Bcl-2 homology 3 (BH3) domain at both mitochondrial and nonmitochondrial sites. *J. Biol. Chem.* Jan 14 2000; 275(2):1439-1448.

[72] Scorrano L, Oakes SA, Opferman JT, et al. BAX and BAK regulation of endoplasmic reticulum Ca2+: a control point for apoptosis. *Science* Apr 4 2003;300(5616):135-139.

[73] von Harsdorf R, Li PF, Dietz R. Signaling pathways in reactive oxygen species-induced cardiomyocyte apoptosis. *Circulation* Jun 8 1999;99(22):2934-2941.

[74] Chen Z, Chua CC, Ho YS, et al. Overexpression of Bcl-2 attenuates apoptosis and protects against myocardial I/R injury in transgenic mice. *Am. J. Physiol. Heart Circ. Physiol.* May 2001;280(5):H2313-2320.

[75] Cook SA, Sugden PH, Clerk A. Regulation of bcl-2 family proteins during development and in response to oxidative stress in cardiac myocytes: association with changes in mitochondrial membrane potential. *Circ. Res.* Nov 12 1999;85(10):940-949.

[76] Suzuki Y, Imai Y, Nakayama H, et al. A serine protease, HtrA2, is released from the mitochondria and interacts with XIAP, inducing cell death. *Mol. Cell.* Sep 2001; 8(3): 613-621.

[77] Hegde R, Srinivasula SM, Zhang Z, et al. Identification of Omi/HtrA2 as a mitochondrial apoptotic serine protease that disrupts inhibitor of apoptosis protein-caspase interaction. *J. Biol. Chem.* Jan 4 2002;277(1):432-438.

[78] Martins LM, Iaccarino I, Tenev T, et al. The serine protease Omi/HtrA2 regulates apoptosis by binding XIAP through a reaper-like motif. *J. Biol. Chem.* Jan 4 2002; 277(1):439-444.

[79] Verhagen AM, Silke J, Ekert PG, et al. HtrA2 promotes cell death through its serine protease activity and its ability to antagonize inhibitor of apoptosis proteins. *J. Biol. Chem.* Jan 4 2002;277(1):445-454.

[80] Yang QH, Church-Hajduk R, Ren J, et al. Omi/HtrA2 catalytic cleavage of inhibitor of apoptosis (IAP) irreversibly inactivates IAPs and facilitates caspase activity in apoptosis. *Genes Dev.* Jun 15 2003;17(12):1487-1496.

[81] Srinivasula SM, Gupta S, Datta P, et al. Inhibitor of apoptosis proteins are substrates for the mitochondrial serine protease Omi/HtrA2. *J. Biol. Chem.* Aug 22 2003;278(34): 31469-31472.

[82] Liu HR, Gao E, Hu A, et al. Role of Omi/HtrA2 in apoptotic cell death after myocardial ischemia and reperfusion. *Circulation* Jan 4 2005;111(1):90-96.

[83] Chau BN, Cheng EH, Kerr DA, et al. Aven, a novel inhibitor of caspase activation, binds Bcl-xL and Apaf-1. *Mol. Cell.* Jul 2000;6(1):31-40.

[84] Cardone MH, Roy N, Stennicke HR, et al. Regulation of cell death protease caspase-9 by phosphorylation [see comments]. *Science* 1998;282(5392):1318-1321.

[85] Mirmohammadsadegh A, Tartler U, Michel G, et al. HAX-1, identified by differential display reverse transcription polymerase chain reaction, is overexpressed in lesional psoriasis. *J. Invest Dermatol.* Jun 2003;120(6):1045-1051.

[86] Suzuki Y, Demoliere C, Kitamura D, et al. HAX-1, a novel intracellular protein, localized on mitochondria, directly associates with HS1, a substrate of Src family tyrosine kinases. *J. Immunol.* Mar 15 1997;158(6):2736-2744.

[87] Han Y, Chen YS, Liu Z, et al. Overexpression of HAX-1 Protects Cardiac Myocytes From Apoptosis Through Caspase-9 Inhibition. *Circ. Res.* Jul 20 2006.

[88] Munday NA, Vaillancourt JP, Ali A, et al. Molecular cloning and pro-apoptotic activity of ICErelII and ICErelIII, members of the ICE/CED-3 family of cysteine proteases. *J. Biol. Chem.* Jun 30 1995;270(26):15870-15876.

[89] Fernandes-Alnemri T, Litwack G, Alnemri ES. CPP32, a novel human apoptotic protein with homology to Caenorhabditis elegans cell death protein Ced-3 and mammalian interleukin-1 beta-converting enzyme. *J. Biol. Chem.* Dec 9 1994;269(49): 30761-30764.

[90] Fernandes-Alnemri T, Litwack G, Alnemri ES. Mch2, a new member of the apoptotic Ced-3/Ice cysteine protease gene family. *Cancer Res.* Jul 1 1995;55(13):2737-2742.

[91] Srinivasula SM, Ahmad M, Fernandes-Alnemri T, et al. Molecular ordering of the Fas-apoptotic pathway: the Fas/APO-1 protease Mch5 is a CrmA-inhibitable protease that activates multiple Ced-3/ICE-like cysteine proteases. *Proc. Natl. Acad. Sci. USA* Dec 10 1996;93(25):14486-14491.

[92] Fernandes-Alnemri T, Takahashi A, Armstrong R, et al. Mch3, a novel human apoptotic cysteine protease highly related to CPP32. *Cancer Res.* Dec 15 1995;55(24): 6045-6052.

[93] Scaffidi C, Fulda S, Srinivasan A, et al. Two CD95 (APO-1/Fas) signaling pathways. *Embo J.* Mar 16 1998;17(6):1675-1687.

[94] Pennacchio LA, Bouley DM, Higgins KM, et al. Progressive ataxia, myoclonic epilepsy and cerebellar apoptosis in cystatin B-deficient mice. *Nat. Genet.* Nov 1998; 20(3):251-258.

[95] Twiddy D, Cohen GM, Macfarlane M, et al. Caspase-7 is directly activated by the approximately 700-kDa apoptosome complex and is released as a stable XIAP-caspase-7 approximately 200-kDa complex. *J. Biol. Chem.* Feb 17 2006;281(7):3876-3888.

[96] Lin XY, Choi MS, Porter AG. Expression analysis of the human caspase-1 subfamily reveals specific regulation of the CASP5 gene by lipopolysaccharide and interferon-gamma. *J. Biol. Chem.* Dec 22 2000;275(51):39920-39926.

[97] Thornberry NA, Bull HG, Calaycay JR, et al. A novel heterodimeric cysteine protease is required for interleukin-1 beta processing in monocytes. *Nature* Apr 30 1992; 356(6372):768-774.

[98] Martinon F, Tschopp J. Inflammatory caspases: linking an intracellular innate immune system to autoinflammatory diseases. *Cell* May 28 2004;117(5):561-574.

[99] Pomerantz BJ, Reznikov LL, Harken AH, et al. Inhibition of caspase 1 reduces human myocardial ischemic dysfunction via inhibition of IL-18 and IL-1beta. *Proc. Natl. Acad. Sci. USA* Feb 27 2001;98(5):2871-2876.

[100] Mallat Z, Corbaz A, Scoazec A, et al. Expression of interleukin-18 in human atherosclerotic plaques and relation to plaque instability. *Circulation* Oct 2 2001; 104(14): 1598-1603.

[101] Blankenberg S, Tiret L, Bickel C, et al. Interleukin-18 is a strong predictor of cardiovascular death in stable and unstable angina. *Circulation* Jul 2 2002;106(1):24-30.

[102] Frantz S, Ducharme A, Sawyer D, et al. Targeted deletion of caspase-1 reduces early mortality and left ventricular dilatation following myocardial infarction. *J. Mol. Cell Cardiol.* Jun 2003;35(6):685-694.

[103] Aronow BJ, Toyokawa T, Canning A, et al. Divergent transcriptional responses to independent genetic causes of cardiac hypertrophy. *Physiol. Genomics* Jun 6 2001; 6(1):19-28.

[104] Yussman MG, Toyokawa T, Odley A, et al. Mitochondrial death protein Nix is induced in cardiac hypertrophy and triggers apoptotic cardiomyopathy. *Nat. Med..* Jul 2002; 8(7):725-730.

[105] Kubota T, Miyagishima M, Frye CS, et al. Overexpression of tumor necrosis factor-alpha activates both anti- and pro-apoptotic pathways in the myocardium. *J. Mol. Cell Cardiol.* Jul 2001;33(7):1331-1344.

[106] Syed FM, Hahn HS, Odley A, et al. Proapoptotic effects of caspase-1/interleukin-converting enzyme dominate in myocardial ischemia. *Circ. Res.* May 27 2005;96(10): 1103-1109.

[107] Kumar A, Kumar A, Michael P, et al. Human serum from patients with septic shock activates transcription factors STAT1, IRF1, and NF-kappaB and induces apoptosis in human cardiac myocytes. *J. Biol. Chem.* Dec 30 2005;280(52):42619-42626.

[108] Londono D, Bai Y, Zuckert WR, et al. Cardiac apoptosis in severe relapsing fever borreliosis. *Infect Immun.* Nov 2005;73(11):7669-7676.

[109] Stehlik C, Krajewska M, Welsh K, et al. The PAAD/PYRIN-only protein POP1/ASC2 is a modulator of ASC-mediated nuclear-factor-kappa B and pro-caspase-1 regulation. *Biochem. J.* Jul 1 2003;373(Pt 1):101-113.

[110] Annand RR, Dahlen JR, Sprecher CA, et al. Caspase-1 (interleukin-1beta-converting enzyme) is inhibited by the human serpin analogue proteinase inhibitor 9. *Biochem. J.* Sep 15 1999;342 Pt 3:655-665.

[111] Rembold C. Could atherosclerosis originate from defective smooth muscle cell death (apoptosis)? *Perspect. Biol. Med.* Spring 1996;39(3):405-408.

[112] Gagarin D, Yang Z, Butler J, et al. Genomic profiling of acquired resistance to apoptosis in cells derived from human atherosclerotic lesions: potential role of STATs, cyclinD1, BAD, and Bcl-XL. *J. Mol. Cell Cardiol.* Sep 2005;39(3):453-465.

[113] Krippner-Heidenreich A, Talanian RV, Sekul R, et al. Targeting of the transcription factor Max during apoptosis: phosphorylation-regulated cleavage by caspase-5 at an unusual glutamic acid residue in position P1. *Biochem. J.* Sep 15 2001;358(Pt 3):705-715.

[114] Belke DD, Betuing S, Tuttle MJ, et al. Insulin signaling coordinately regulates cardiac size, metabolism, and contractile protein isoform expression. *J. Clin. Invest.* Mar 2002; 109(5):629-639.

[115] Hitomi J, Katayama T, Eguchi Y, et al. Involvement of caspase-4 in endoplasmic reticulum stress-induced apoptosis and Abeta-induced cell death. *J. Cell Biol.* May 10 2004;165(3):347-356.

[116] Wang M, Tsai BM, Turrentine MW, et al. p38 mitogen activated protein kinase mediates both death signaling and functional depression in the heart. *Ann. Thorac. Surg.* Dec 2005;80(6):2235-2241.

[117] Humke EW, Ni J, Dixit VM. ERICE, a novel FLICE-activatable caspase. *J. Biol. Chem.* Jun 19 1998;273(25):15702-15707.

[118] Hu S, Snipas SJ, Vincenz C, et al. Caspase-14 is a novel developmentally regulated protease. *J. Biol. Chem.* Nov 6 1998;273(45):29648-29653.

[119] Krajewska M, Rosenthal RE, Mikolajczyk J, et al. Early processing of Bid and caspase-6, -8, -10, -14 in the canine brain during cardiac arrest and resuscitation. *Exp. Neurol.* Oct 2004;189(2):261-279.

[120] Abraham MC, Shaham S. Death without caspases, caspases without death. *Trends Cell Biol.* Apr 2004;14(4):184-193.

[121] Cregan SP, Dawson VL, Slack RS. Role of AIF in caspase-dependent and caspase-independent cell death. *Oncogene* Apr 12 2004;23(16):2785-2796.

[122] Cande C, Cecconi F, Dessen P, et al. Apoptosis-inducing factor (AIF): key to the conserved caspase-independent pathways of cell death? *J. Cell Sci.* Dec 15 2002;115(Pt 24):4727-4734.

[123] Lockshin RA, Zakeri Z. Caspase-independent cell death? *Oncogene* Apr 12 2004; 23(16):2766-2773.

[124] Lorenzo HK, Susin SA, Penninger J, et al. Apoptosis inducing factor (AIF): a phylogenetically old, caspase-independent effector of cell death. *Cell Death Differ.* Jun 1999; 6(6):516-524.

[125] Penninger JM, Kroemer G. Mitochondria, AIF and caspases--rivaling for cell death execution. *Nat. Cell Biol.* Feb 2003;5(2):97-99.

[126] Susin SA, Lorenzo HK, Zamzami N, et al. Molecular characterization of mitochondrial apoptosis-inducing factor. *Nature* Feb 4 1999;397(6718):441-446.

[127] Susin SA, Lorenzo HK, Zamzami N, et al. Mitochondrial release of caspase-2 and -9 during the apoptotic process. *J. Exp. Med.* Jan 18 1999;189(2):381-394.

[128] Wang X, Yang C, Chai J, et al. Mechanisms of AIF-mediated apoptotic DNA degradation in Caenorhabditis elegans. *Science* Nov 22 2002;298(5598):1587-1592.

[129] Cregan SP, Fortin A, MacLaurin JG, et al. Apoptosis-inducing factor is involved in the regulation of caspase-independent neuronal cell death. *J. Cell Biol.* Aug 5 2002;158(3): 507-517.

[130] Arnoult D, Parone P, Martinou JC, et al. Mitochondrial release of apoptosis-inducing factor occurs downstream of cytochrome c release in response to several proapoptotic stimuli. *J. Cell Biol.* Dec 23 2002;159(6):923-929.

[131] Arnoult D, Gaume B, Karbowski M, et al. Mitochondrial release of AIF and EndoG requires caspase activation downstream of Bax/Bak-mediated permeabilization. *Embo J.* Sep 1 2003;22(17):4385-4399.

[132] Joseph B, Marchetti P, Formstecher P, et al. Mitochondrial dysfunction is an essential step for killing of non-small cell lung carcinomas resistant to conventional treatment. *Oncogene* Jan 3 2002;21(1):65-77.

[133] Alonso M, Tamasdan C, Miller DC, et al. Flavopiridol induces apoptosis in glioma cell lines independent of retinoblastoma and p53 tumor suppressor pathway alterations by a caspase-independent pathway. *Mol. Cancer Ther.* Feb 2003;2(2):139-150.

[134] Pieper AA, Brat DJ, Krug DK, et al. Poly(ADP-ribose) polymerase-deficient mice are protected from streptozotocin-induced diabetes. *Proc. Natl. Acad. Sci. USA.* Mar 16 1999; 96(6): 3059-3064.

[135] Yu SW, Wang H, Poitras MF, et al. Mediation of poly(ADP-ribose) polymerase-1-dependent cell death by apoptosis-inducing factor. *Science* Jul 12 2002;297(5579):259-263.

[136] Daugas E, Susin SA, Zamzami N, et al. Mitochondrio-nuclear translocation of AIF in apoptosis and necrosis. *Faseb J.* Apr 2000;14(5):729-739.

[137] van Loo G, Schotte P, van Gurp M, et al. Endonuclease G: a mitochondrial protein released in apoptosis and involved in caspase-independent DNA degradation. *Cell Death Differ.* Dec 2001;8(12):1136-1142.

[138] Bahi N, Zhang J, Llovera M, et al. Switch from caspase-dependent to -independent death during heart development: Essential role of EndoG in ischemia-induced DNA processing of differentiated cardiomyocytes. *J. Biol. Chem.* Jun 5 2006.

[139] Mathiasen IS, Sergeev IN, Bastholm L, et al. Calcium and calpain as key mediators of apoptosis-like death induced by vitamin D compounds in breast cancer cells. *J. Biol. Chem.* Aug 23 2002;277(34):30738-30745.

[140] Syntichaki P, Xu K, Driscoll M, et al. Specific aspartyl and calpain proteases are required for neurodegeneration in C. elegans. *Nature* Oct 31 2002;419(6910):939-944.

[141] Heibein JA, Barry M, Motyka B, et al. Granzyme B-induced loss of mitochondrial inner membrane potential (Delta Psi m) and cytochrome c release are caspase independent. *J. Immunol.* Nov 1 1999;163(9):4683-4693.

[142] Cheng EH, Wei MC, Weiler S, et al. BCL-2, BCL-X(L) sequester BH3 domain-only molecules preventing BAX- and BAK-mediated mitochondrial apoptosis. *Mol. Cell.* Sep 2001;8(3):705-711.

[143] Garg S, Narula J, Chandrashekhar Y. Apoptosis and heart failure: clinical relevance and therapeutic target. *J. Mol. Cell Cardiol.* Jan 2005;38(1):73-79.

[144] Logue SE, Gustafsson AB, Samali A, et al. Ischemia/reperfusion injury at the intersection with cell death. *J. Mol. Cell Cardiol.* Jan 2005;38(1):21-33.

[145] Yaoita H, Ogawa K, Maehara K, et al. Attenuation of ischemia/reperfusion injury in rats by a caspase inhibitor [In Process Citation]. *Circulation* 1998;97(3):276-281.

[146] Laugwitz KL, Moretti A, Weig HJ, et al. Blocking caspase-activated apoptosis improves contractility in failing myocardium. *Hum. Gene Ther.* Nov 20 2001;12(17): 2051-2063.

[147] Krajewski S, Krajewska M, Ellerby LM, et al. Release of caspase-9 from mitochondria during neuronal apoptosis and cerebral ischemia. *Proc. Natl. Acad. Sci. USA.* May 11 1999; 96(10):5752-5757.

[148] Jang YM, Kendaiah S, Drew B, et al. Doxorubicin treatment in vivo activates caspase-12 mediated cardiac apoptosis in both male and female rats. *FEBS Lett.* Nov 19 2004; 577(3):483-490.

In: Handbook of Cardiovascular Research
Editors: Jorgen Brataas and Viggo Nanstveit

ISBN 978-1-60741-792-7
© 2009 Nova Science Publishers, Inc.

Chapter XX

Vitamins E and C for Prevention of Cardiovascular Disease

F. Violi*, R. Cangemi and L. Loffredo
IV Division of Clinical Medicine, University of Rome
"La Sapienza", Italy

Abstract

Oxidative stress seems to play a key-role in the pathogenesis of atherosclerosis. Agents that prevent LDL from oxidation have been shown to reduce initiation of atherosclerosis. Among these, the antioxidant micronutrients, including the carotenoids and vitamins C and E, have gained wide interest because of the potential for prevention of atherosclerotic vascular disease in humans. Lipid-soluble antioxidants present in LDL, including α-tocopherol (vitamin E), and water-soluble antioxidants present in the extracellular fluid, including ascorbic acid (vitamin C), inhibit LDL oxidation through an LDL-specific antioxidant action. Moreover antioxidants present in the cells of the vascular wall decrease cellular production and release of reactive oxygen species (ROS), inhibit endothelial activation (expression of adhesion molecules and monocyte chemoattractants), and improve the biologic activity of endothelium-derived nitric oxide (EDNO) through a cell- or tissue-specific antioxidant action. [1] In the last decade many trials with antioxidants have been planned in patients with cardiovascular disease but the results are equivocal. The reason for the disappointing findings is unclear but one possible explanation is the lack of identification criteria of patients who are potentially candidates for antioxidant treatment. Several studies have been done in patients at risk of cardiovascular disease indicating that enhanced oxidative stress is associated with the presence of the classical risk factors for atherosclerosis, like diabetes, hypercholesterolemia, hypertension, smoking and obesity.

---

* Correspondence concerning this article should be addressed to: Francesco Violi, IV Divisione di Clinica Medica, Viale del Policlinico 155, Roma, 00161, Italy. Voice: +39-064461933; fax +39-064461933; email: francesco.violi@uniroma1.it.

In this chapter the data so far reported will be analyzed to see if there is a clear support the hypothesis that patients at risk of cardiovascular may be candidates for antioxidant treatment.

Keywords: oxidative stress; atherosclerosis; α-tocopherol; ascorbic acid; antioxidant; cardiovascular disease.

Introduction

Oxidative stress is believed to play a crucial role in initiation and progression of atherosclerosis disease. Steinberg et al. [2] were among the first to postulate that modified low-density lipoprotein (LDL) could account for the accumulation of lipid within macrophages, a critical early step in the formation of the atherosclerotic plaque. In the early phases, native LDL may amass in the subendothelial arterial space and may be minimally oxidized by resident vascular cells through the activity of such enzymes as 12/15-lipoxygenase. In turn, this minimally modified LDL leads to the production of chemotactic factors and granulocyte and macrophage colony-stimulating factors, which enhance recruitment of circulating monocytes and their differentiation to macrophages in the vessel wall. Plaque stability is believed to be influenced by levels of inflammatory mediators locally, which may stimulate expression of a number of proteolytic enzymes that lead to plaque fragility and rupture. These inflammatory actions encourage further oxidization of LDL, leading to both structural and functional changes in the vessel. [3] Macrophages avidly accumulate LDL particles modified by oxidation or acetylation through a number of scavenger receptors, including CD36 and scavenger receptors A-I/II, leading to the accumulation of foam cells and development of the atherosclerotic plaque. [4] At the same time, oxidized LDL species are directly toxic to vascular cells, and lead to endothelial injury and dysfunction, disabling, among other things, the intrinsic antiplatelet effects of this protective barrier, as well as the generation of nitric oxide, with deleterious effects on vascular tone and reactivity. [3] The importance of oxidized LDL in atherogenesis has been further confirmed by the use of specific antibodies to oxidized LDL, which have been shown to localize to atherosclerotic lesions in the vessel wall. [5] Oxidative stress may contribute to atherogenesis by mechanisms that are not necessarily linked to LDL oxidation. For example, free radical oxygen species such as superoxide anion can rapidly react with and inactivate nitric oxide, enhancing proatherogenic mechanisms (e.g. leukocyte adherence to endothelium, impaired vasorelaxation, platelet aggregation).[6]

Although enzymatic and non enzymatic oxidation of LDL seems to be involved its relevance in the evolution of human atherosclerosis is still unclear.

An important matter of discussion is the evident discrepancy between experimental and clinical trials with antioxidants that, in fact, provided divergent results. Most trials with antioxidants in experimental models of atherosclerosis demonstrated that this treatment is able to retard the progression of atherosclerosis while the results of clinical trials are conflicting, [6] inasmuch as positive as well as negative effects have been reported. Investigation of antioxidants for prevention of atherosclerosis stems from observational trials that demonstrated the existence of an inverse relationship between the consumption of antioxidant vitamins and the risk of cardiovascular events.

On the basis of these data almost all the trials have planned on the assumption that supplementation with vitamin E and C would represent a useful approach for preventing cardiovascular disease. However, candidates for antioxidant treatment were not accurately defined: any patient at risk of cardiovascular events has been indiscriminately enrolled in those trials. We argue, on the contrary that, as antioxidant status represents an important marker of oxidative stress, [7] its determination may useful for better identifying candidates for antioxidant treatment. In order to substantiate this hypothesis data inherent to oxidative stress and antioxidant status in patients at risk for cardiovascular disease and in patients included in observational and interventional trials have been reviewed. As antioxidant vitamins, vitamins E and C have been object of the most important researches in this field, our analysis is essentially concentrated on the clinical relevance of this vitamin in patients with cardiovascular disease.

CHD Risk Factors and Oxidative Stress

Endothelial dysfunction and intimal-medial thickness are considered the early steps in atherosclerosis. Russel Ross [8] has modified atherosclerosis pathogenetical theories because numerous pathophysiologic observations in humans and animals led to the formulation of the response-to injury hypothesis of atherosclerosis. Each characteristic lesion of atherosclerosis represents a different stage in a chronic inflammatory process in the artery: in fact the lesions of atherosclerosis represent a series of highly specific cellular and molecular responses that can be described as an inflammatory disease. Possible causes of endothelial dysfunction leading to atherosclerosis include hypercholesterolemia, hypertension, diabetes mellitus, cigarette smoking, elevated plasma homocysteine concentrations, infectious microorganisms, ageing. Framingham's studies have shown how each factor and combination of them are associated with the atherosclerotic diseases. [9] We should like to pay attention to the association of all these factors with oxidative stress. [10-15]

Cigarette smoking, hypertension, diabetes mellitus, genetic alterations, elevated plasma homocysteine concentrations, infectious microorganisms, such as herpes viruses or Chlamydia pneumoniae, have proinflammatory actions, increasing the formation of hydrogen peroxide and free radicals such as superoxide anion and hydroxyl radicals in plasma.

These substances reduce the formation of nitric oxide (NO) by endothelium. Nitric oxide is a free radical with an unpaired electron in the highest orbital. This is why behaves as a potential antioxidant agent by virtue of its ability to reduce other molecules. In vitro experiments support this concept inasmuch as NO is able to inhibit lipid peroxidation. However, NO is rapidly inactivated by the peroxide anion (O_2^-) to form peroxynitrite (NO_3^-) which is a potent oxidant. Therefore, in the presence of O_2^-, NO behaves as a potent pro-oxidant. This is the mechanism that accounts for the low density lipoprotein LDL oxidation that occurs when NO and O_2^- are simultaneously present in the medium. As NO and O_2^- are simultaneously released by cells, such as endothelial cells, the balance between these two radicals is crucial in understanding the net effect of NO on lipid peroxidation. Thus an excess of NO will favor lipid peroxidation inhibition, while an excess of O_2^- or equimolar concentrations of NO and O_2^- will induce lipid peroxidation. [16] Modulation of this balance may have important clinical implications, particularly in the atherosclerotic process in which oxidative stress seems to play a pivotal role in the onset and progression of vascular lesions.

Several studies strongly suggested that enhanced oxidative stress may represent an important trigger for atherogenesis elicited by Angiotensin II. Free radical formation mediates some of the effects of hypertension. Angiotensin II concentrations are often elevated in patients with hypertension and it is a potent vasoconstrictor. It also increases smooth-muscle hypertrophy and lipoxygenase activity that, in turn, can increase inflammation and the oxidation of LDL.

Griendling et al. [17] examined the effect of Ag II on superoxide anion (O_2^-) production by smooth muscle cells and demonstrated that 4 to 6 hour exposure of these cells to Ag II elicited enhanced production of O_2^-. Such effect was mediated by NADH and NADPH oxidase activation likely via intracellular mobilization of fatty acids such as arachidonic acid. Experimental study in animals demonstrated that Ag II infusion enhanced simultaneously blood pressure and vascular production of O_2^-; this last effect was dependent upon NADH/NADPH oxidase, further suggesting the role of this pathway in Ag II mediated O_2^- production. These data have important pathophysiologic implications due to the effect of O_2^- on vascular motility. The oxidative stress may have a role in hypertensive patients, in whom a reduced vasodilating response to acetylcholine has been demonstrated. Thus, in patients with hypertension, the administration of the antioxidant, vitamin C, has been able to restore acetylcholine induced vasorelaxation, suggesting a role for oxygen free radicals in inducing vascular dysfunction in patients with hypertension. [18]

Cigarette smoke contains large amounts of free radicals which may degrade nitric oxide release from the endothelium and also produce highly reactive intermediates resulting in endothelial injury. Antioxidants, such as vitamin E, can also reduce free-radical formation by modified LDL.[19]

Blood analysis of lipid peroxides or measurement of urinary excretion of isoprostanes provided evidence that oxidative stress is enhanced in patients with diabetes. [20] The impact of these data in the context of atherosclerosis progression is still unclear but there is some evidence supporting a role for oxidative stress in contributing to deteriorate vascular disease. For instance, an important finding is the demonstration that endothelium-dependent vasodilation is reduced in patients with diabetes and that vitamin C is able to prevent it, so indicating a role for oxygen free radicals in reducing vasodilatory property of endothelium. [21] Oxidative stress could also contribute to worse metabolic disturbance by interfering with glycemic control. Thus it has been demonstrated that in diabetes oxidative stress impairs insulin activity and antioxidants prevent it. [22] That hyperglycemia is a risk for enhanced oxidative stress has been further corroborated by a study in patients with type II diabetes, in whom an increased urinary excretion of PGF2m-III, that derives from arachidonic and interaction with oxygen free radicals, has been demonstrated. [23] It is of note that a significant reduction of urinary PGF2cx-III was observed when patients underwent a strict glycemic control further reinforcing the relationship between hyperglycemia and oxidative stress.

Hyperglycemia may enhance oxidative stress and in turn induce vascular damage via several pathways, including the formation of the advanced glycated end products that are proatherogenic and prothrombotic substance (Fig. 1 panel C). [24] Furthermore glucose may alter the balance between free radicals such as O_2^- and NO in endothelial cells; thus NO exerts its vasodilatory and antioxidant effect unless it is converted to $ONOO^-$ by interaction with O^o. This deleterious effect occurs in endothelial cells exposed to glucose, that, in fact, favors the formation of O_2^- and in turn promotes oxidation.[25]

An interesting mechanism potentially accounting for enhanced production of ROS by glucose is reported in Fig.1. Hyperglycemia could enhance endothelial O_2^- generation via activation of cyclooxygenase pathway which is known to generate ROS with a mechanism involving NAD(P)H oxidase. [26] The potential role of this enzyme in inducing oxidative stress has been recently demonstrated by Guzik at al. who studied the expression of NAD(P)H oxidase in the vessel wall of diabetic and healthy subjects. [27] They found that, compared to control, vascular expression of NAD(P)H oxidase submits, p22 phox and p47 phox, were overexpressed in diabetic patients. [27]

There are experimental and clinical evidences indicating that hypercholesterolemia is associated with enhanced oxidative stress. Oxygen free radicals, such as O_2^-, and F2-isoprostanes, have been found elevated in the artery of hypercholesterolemic animals or in the urine of patients with high serum cholesterol respectively. [28,29] The relevance of these findings in the contest of pathophysiology of atherosclerosis is unclear even if there are some evidence that in this setting oxidative stress may have a role in reducing the vasodilatory propriety of endothelium. [30] Conversely we have not yet evidence that the increase of these markers actually represents a marker of progression of atherosclerotic disease.

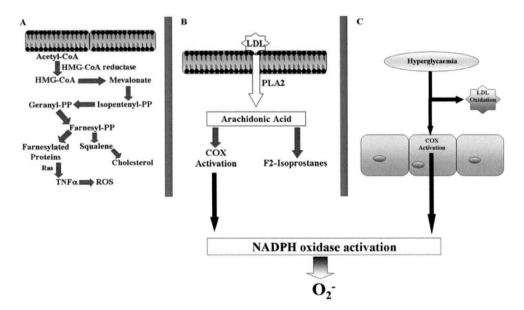

Figure 1.

Two hypotheses can be done for explaining why hypercholesterolemia enhances oxidative stress (Fig. 1, panel A,B). Cholesterol has been recently shown to activate the metabolism of arachidonic acid pathway, [31] that in turn seems to be associated with NAD(P)H oxidase activation. [24] This hypothesis has been recently underscored by our group showing that platelet incubation with cholesterol enhanced O_2^- production and that inhibition of PLA2 or NADPH oxidase enzymes significantly reduced O_2^- formation (Fig. 1 panel B). [31]

The cascade of cholesterol biosynthesis may represent per se another pathway leading to enhanced oxidative stress. Intracellular metabolism of mevalonate leads, in fact, to the formation of protein farnesylation, that has a key role in the production of proinflammatory and pro-oxidant cytokines such as Tumor Necrosis Factor alpha (TNF) /Fig. 1, panel A). [32] Accordingly, treatment of hypercholesterolemic patients with an inhibitor of HMG-CoA-reductase was associated with reduced monocytes formation of TNF, suggesting a relationship between cholesterol and intracellular formation of pro-oxidant cytokines. [33] The association between hypercholesterolemia and oxidative stress has been further corroborated by an interventional study with statin in hypercholesterolemic patients in whom simvastatin reduced the urinary excretion of PGF2cx-III likely by lowering serum cholesterol; [34] however, the existence of mechanism independent of cholesterol lowering was not investigated. The relationship between hypertriglyceridaemia and oxidative stress has been not fully investigated. We found only one report aimed at analyzing if patients with hypertriglyceridaemia had enhanced oxidative stress. Pronai et al measured scavenging property and O_2^- formation by peripheral monocytes of hypertriglyceridaemic patients with and without diabetes. [35] They found a significant positive correlation between O_2^- generation and plasma triglycerides and a significant negative correlation between superoxide scavenging property and plasma triglycerides. [35]

Role of Antioxidants

Human plasma contains a vast array of antioxidant defenses. There are a number of antioxidant proteins, like metal-binding proteins (albumin, transferrin, ceruloplasmin, etc.), enzymes, such as superoxide dismutase, glutathione peroxidase, catalase, and small molecule antioxidants. However, these antioxidant enzymes are mainly intracellular, so in plasma, the transport medium of LDL, an important role seems to have the small molecule antioxidants. They can be separated into water-soluble antioxidants and lipid-soluble or lipoprotein-associated antioxidants. [1] The water-soluble antioxidants include mainly uric acid, ascorbic acid and bilirubin. The most abundant lipid-soluble antioxidant in LDL is α-tocopherol, [36] which is the chemically and biologically most active form of vitamin E. Other lipid-soluble antioxidants, such as ubiquinol-10, lycopene, β-carotene and other carotenoids, are present in much smaller amounts, usually less than $1/20^{th}$ of the α-tocopherol concentration.

Many basic research studies have investigated how effectively and by what mechanisms the endogenous antioxidants in human plasma and LDL inhibit lipid peroxidation and oxidative modification of LDL. These studies have focused mainly on two antioxidants, ascorbic acid, α-tocopherol.

Vitamin C

Vitamin C (ascorbic acid) is a six-carbon lactone that is synthesized from glucose in the liver of most mammalian species, but not by humans. Vitamin C is an electron donor and therefore a reducing agent. As an electron donor, vitamin C acts as a cofactor for 8 enzymes involved in collagen hydroxylation, biosynthesis of carnitine and norepinephrine, tyrosine metabolism and amidation of peptide hormones. [37] Vitamin C is called an antioxidant because, by donating its electrons, it prevents other compounds from being oxidized. When a reactive and possibly harmful free radical can interact with ascorbate. the reactive free radical is reduced, and the ascorbyl radical formed in its place is less reactive. Reduction of a reactive free radical with formation of a less reactive compound is sometimes free radical scavenging. [38].

When given orally, ascorbic acid is well absorbed at lower doses, but absorption decreases as the dose increases. Thus, median bioavailability following an oral dose is 87% for 30 mg, 80% for 100 mg, 72% for 200 mg and 63% for 500 mg. Less than 50% of a 1250-mg dose is absorbed, and most of the absorbed dose is excreted in the urine. Decreased bioavailability and renal excretion keep plasma vitamin C at less than 100 μmol/L, even with an oral dose of 1000 mg.. When ascorbic acid is administered intravenously, the limiting absorptive mechanism is bypassed and very high plasma levels are attained. Following the administration of 1.25 g intravenously, a peak plasma level of 1000 μmol/L is reached, even though 100 μmol/L is not exceeded by oral dosing of 1000 mg. Brain, adrenal cortex, liver, spleen, pancreas and kidney tissues concentrate vitamin C for unknown reasons. [39]

There is convincing evidence from in vitro studies that physiological concentrations of ascorbate strongly inhibit LDL oxidation by vascular cells and neutrophils, [40] as well as in cell-free systems. [41] Ascorbate prevents oxidative modification of LDL primarily by scavenging free radicals and other reactive species in the aqueous milieu. Thus, direct and rapid trapping of these aqueous reactive species by ascorbate prevents them from interacting with and oxidizing LDL. Ascorbyl radicals formed in this process may be reduced back to ascorbate by dismutation, chemical reduction (e.g., by glutathione), or enzymatic reduction (e.g., by thioredoxin reductase).[42]

In vitro studies show that ascorbic acid prevents oxidative modification of LDL by several distinct mechanisms, which may act in concert free radical scavenging; [43] preventing aqueous oxidants from initiating lipid peroxidation in LDL; modification of histidine residues and other copper-binding sites on apo-B; [44] imparting increased resistance to Cu^{2+}-induced LDL oxidation; destruction of preformed lipid hydroperoxides; [45] preventing propagation of lipid peroxidation in LDL. [1]

Moreover vitamin C has been indicated as one of the most important co-antioxidant that could prevent α-tocopherol-mediated peroxidation of LDL. In vitro studies have suggested that under some circumstances vitamin E could act as a pro-oxidant. [46] The regeneration of α –TOH (α-tocopherol) from α -TO• (α-tocopheroxyl radical) by ascorbate, with concomitant generation of the ascorbyl radical, is well established. [47, 48]

Addition of ascorbate to LDL undergoing oxidation induced by aqueous radicals results in immediate cessation of α-TOH consumption and lipid oxidation. Upon removal of ascorbate, consumption of α-TOH and oxidation of LDL resumes, attaining the same rates as those prior to the addition of ascorbate. [49]

In addition to protecting LDL directly against oxidation, ascorbic acid may inhibit cell-mediated LDL oxidation by reducing the cellular production and release of reactive oxygen species.

Many studies have focused on the importance of vitamin C on the endothelium. Some evidence suggests that increased vascular oxidative stress contributes to the pathophysiology of endothelial dysfunction and hypertension. Low plasma vitamin C concentrations have been associated with hypertension and impaired endothelial function. In healthy subjects the administration of high doses of vitamin C restored endothelium-dependent vasodilatation that was impaired by acute hyperglycemia [50] or hyperhomocysteinemia due to ingestion of methionine. [51] Similar beneficial effects of vitamin C with normalization of the vasodilatory response were observed in patients with coronary spastic angina, [52] chronic heart failure, [53] hypercholesterolemia, [30] or hypertension. [54,18] Thus vitamin C may have favorable effects on vascular dilatation, possibly through its antioxidant effects on sparing NO by scavenging superoxide radicals. [55]

Extracellular ascorbic acid also has been reported to inhibit neutrophil-endothelial cell interactions. [56] Physiologic concentrations of ascorbic acid abolish cigarette smoke- or ox-LDL-induced leukocyte adhesion to endothelium in vivo. [57] In addition, smokers have lower plasma levels of vitamin C, and monocytes isolated from smokers exhibit increased adhesiveness to cultured human endothelial cells. [58] Following supplementation of the smokers with vitamin C, their monocytes exhibited normal endothelial adhesiveness. This finding indicates that upregulation of ligands on monocytes is inhibited by ascorbate and it has been supported by studies with animal models in which ascorbate showed an important role in inhibiting leukocyte–endothelial cell interactions induced by cigarette smoke [57] or oxidized LDL, [59] likely by antioxidant mechanisms.

Vitamin E

Vitamin E includes several tocopherols having the biological activity of RRR-α-tocopherol, the most abundant form in foods. Vitamin E circulates in the blood as free tocopherol bound to beta-lipoproteins and is present in cell membrane where it exerts a potent defense against lipid peroxidation. [60] Blood concentration of vitamin E in humans ranges from 25 to 30 M, depending on daily intake and body's ability to absorb fat. [60].

Vitamin E is the main lipid-soluble chain-breaking antioxidant in plasma and tissues and converts the peroxyl-free radical to hydroperoxide, a less reactive radical. It acts as a first-line anti-oxidative defense of LDL particles, protecting unsaturated fatty acids from peroxidation. [61] Polyunsaturated fatty acids are highly susceptible to peroxidation because methylenic hydrogens, which are positioned upon the carbon between two double bonds, have low bond energy and can be abstracted by a free radical. [62] Hydrogen abstraction is followed by molecular rearrangement and formation of a conjugated diene system in the molecule. The following step is reaction with oxygen and formation of the peroxyl radical (LOO°) intermediate. Peculiar of the lipid peroxidation is the chain reaction with recruitment of additional polyunsaturated fatty acids by intermediate radicals like carbon centered lipid radicals (L°), alkoxyl radicals (LO°), and peroxyl radicals (LOO°), which perpetuate the reaction in presence of oxygen supply. The chain reaction can be interrupted if the radical-carrying lipid molecule is intercepted by an hydrogen donor having peculiar chemical-physical characteristics. By virtue of this action, these molecules are currently named chain-breaking antioxidants and the prototypical molecule in biological system is vitamin E. Lipid peroxidation products, isoprostanes and oxidized epitopes of Apo B100, as a result of LDL oxidation, have been found in the atherosclerotic plaque, [63, 64] and antioxidants have been shown to inhibit atherosclerosis in animal models [65, 66].

This problem was specifically investigated in a study, that simultaneously analyzed the relationship among oxidative stress, vitamin E supplementation and atherosclerosis in Apo E-deficient mice [67]. This study showed an early increase in isoprostanes, indices of oxidant stress, in cholesterol-fed animals and its significant decrease after vitamin E supplementation, along with a significant decrease of atherosclerotic lesion in animals given vitamin E. We have studied the uptake of LDL by the atherosclerotic plaque of patients undergoing endoarterectomy [68]. Radiolabeled LDL intravenously injected have been localized in foam cells of the carotid specimen obtained from endoarterectomy. The uptake of LDL was almost completely suppressed in patients treated for 4 weeks with vitamin E (900 mg/day).

The observation of a tendency to thrombosis in vessels of vitamin E-deficient animals has suggested an influence of Vitamin E on clotting system. The mechanism by which vitamin E affects the clotting system is not known. Experimental evidence suggests that vitamin E might modulate both transcriptional and post-transcriptional events of the coagulation system. At post-transcriptional level, vitamin E has been reported to modulate the assembly of prothrombin complex and thrombin generation [69]. Influence of vitamin E at transcriptional level can be deduced by the well known effect of oxidant stress on the expression of several genes, such as c-fos and c-myc, translocation of nuclear factor kB, from cytoplasm into the nucleus, and prevention of these events by antioxidants. [70] Several studies pointed out the influence of antioxidants on the expression of monocyte Tissue Factor (TF). Crutchley and Que [71] demonstrated an increased monocyte expression of TF by exposing THP-1 cells to 5 to 10 μM Cu. Based on Fenton chemistry, this effect should be attributed to the formation of oxygen-free radicals generated by copper ions. Vitamin E has been also shown to inhibit monocyte expression of TF and thrombin generation at concentration as low as 50 μM. [72]

Vitamin E exerts also an inhibitory effect on platelet function. Several studies demonstrated that vitamin E, in a range of concentration between 50 and 500 μM, inhibits ex vivo platelet aggregation induced by phorbole myristate, arachidonic acid and collagen. With oral supplementation to healthy volunteers and patients at risk of atherosclerosis Freedman et al [73] demonstrated that a daily dosage between 400 and 1200 IU of vitamin E for 14 days inhibits platelet aggregation elicited by phorbol myristate and arachidonic acid by interfering with platelet protein kinase C activity. interfering with platelet protein kinase C activity. Calzada et al. [74] administered 300 mg/day vitamin E for 8 weeks and demonstrated an inhibitory effect on PA induced by ADP, collagen and arachidonic acid. Finally, Pignatelli et al. [75] showed that 600 mg/day vitamin E for four weeks inhibited collagen-induced PA by interfering with platelet H_2O_2 formation and Ca^{++} mobilization.

Antioxidants and CHD

Observational Studies

Relationship between Coronary Heart Disease and Dietary Intake of Antioxidants

A large number of observational epidemiologic studies have evaluated potential relationships between antioxidants and coronary heart disease (CHD). To this purpose in the past 10 years studies to assess the relationship between coronary heart disease and dietary intake of antioxidants were performed (Table 1). One of them was the First National Health and Nutrition Examination Survey (NHANES I) Epidemiologic Follow-up Study cohort. This cohort was based on a representative sample of 11,348 non-institutionalized U.S. adults age 25-74 years who were nutritionally examined during 1971-1974 and followed up for mortality (1,809 deaths) through 1984, a median of 10 years. An index of vitamin C intake had been formed from detailed dietary measurements and use of vitamin supplements. Among those with the highest vitamin C intake, males had an standardized mortality ratio (SMR) of 0,65 for all causes and 0.58 for all cardiovascular diseases; females have an SMR of 0.90 for all causes and 0.75 for all cardiovascular diseases. [76]

The Nurses' Health study, [77] included over 87,000 female nurses 34 to 59 years of age, who completed dietary questionnaires that assessed their consumption of a wide range of nutrients, including vitamin E.. During follow-up of up to eight year there 552 cases of major coronary disease were documented. As compared with women in the lowest fifth of the cohort with respect to vitamin E intake, those in the top fifth had a relative risk of major coronary disease of 0.66 after adjustment for age and smoking. Further adjustment for a variety of other coronary risk factors and nutrients, including other antioxidants, had little effect on the results.

Similarly, the Health Professionals' Follow-up study, among almost 40,000 male 40 to 75 years, followed up for four years showed a lower risk of coronary disease among men with higher intakes of vitamin E. In contrast, a high intake of vitamin C was not associated with a lower risk of coronary disease [78]

Kushi et al. studied over 34000 postmenopausal women with no cardiovascular disease who in early 1986 completed a questionnaire that assessed, among other factors, their intake of vitamins A, E, and C from food sources and supplements. After seven years of follow-up results suggested that in postmenopausal women the intake of vitamin E from food was inversely associated with the risk of death from coronary heart disease. This association was particularly striking in the subgroup of 21,809 women who did not consume vitamin supplements (relative risks from lowest to highest quintile of vitamin E intake, 1.0, 0.68, 0.71, 0.42, and 0.42; P for trend = 0.008). After adjustment for possible confounding variables, this inverse association remained (relative risks from lowest to highest quintile, 1.0, 0.70, 0.76, 0.32, and 0.38; P for trend = 0.004). By contrast, the intake of vitamins A and C was not associated with lower risks of dying from coronary disease. [79]

Table 1. Observational studies Dietary Intake of antioxidant vitamins

Observational studies	Patients' characteristics	Year	Data analyzed	Results
NHANES I [76]	11,348 U.S. adults age 25-74 years followed up for, a median of 10 years	1992	Mortality and vit C intake	↓ *risk by vitamin C* (among those with the highest vitamin C intake, males had an standardized mortality ratio of 0,65 for all causes and 0.58 for all cardiovascular diseases; females of 0.90 for all causes and 0.75 for all cardiovascular diseases)
Nurses' Health study [77]	87,245 female nurses 34 to 59 years of age, followed-up for 8 years	1993	Death from CHD and vitamin E intake	↓ *risk by vitamin E* (highest vs lowest quintile: relative risk of 0.66)
Health Professionals' Follow-up study [78]	Male, health professionals 40 to 75 years, followed-up for 4 years	1993	Death from CHD vitamins intake	↓ *risk by vitamin E* (highest vs lowest quintile: relative risk of 0.59). No ↓ risk by vitamin C
Kushi et al. [79]	34000 postmenopausal women, followed-up for 7 years	1996	Death from CHD and vit intake	↓ *risk by vitamin E* (relative risks from lowest to highest quintile, 1.0, 0.70, 0.76, 0.32, and 0.38). No ↓ risk by vitamin C
Rotterdam Study [80]	4802 participants aged 55–95 years, 4-years follow-up	1999	Myocardial Infarction and vitamins intake	No ↓ *risk by vitamin C or E*
Chicago Western Electric Study [81]	1,843 middle-aged men	1997	Stroke and vitamin C intake.	↓ *risk by vitamin C* (highest vs lowest quartile: relative risk of 0,71)
Nurses' Health study and the Health Professionals' Follow-up Study[82]	75596 women followed up for 14 years, 38683 men followed up for 8 years	1999	Stroke and vitamin C intake	↓ risk by vitamin C (highest vs lowest quintile of intake: relative risk of 0,69)

On the other hand a negative result come from the Rotterdam Study in which 4802 participants aged 55–95 years, who were free of MI at baseline and for whom dietary data assessed by a semi-quantitative food frequency questionnaire were available., were followed up for 4 years: an association between vitamin C or vitamin E and MI. was not observed. [80]

Intriguingly vitamin C seems also to have some protective effect against stroke. The Chicago Western Electric Study, among 1,843 middle-aged men, during a period of 30 years, showed a little inverse relationship between dietary vitamin C intake and stroke incidence. [81] In a study based on both the Nurses' Health Study and the Health Professionals' Follow-up Study an inverse relationship between fruit and vegetables rich in vitamin C and ischemic stroke risk was found [82]

Coronary Heart Disease and Antioxidants Plasma Levels

Other studies evaluated plasma levels of different antioxidants, such as vitamin E, C and β-carotene in populations affected or not by CHD (Table 2).

Table 2. Observational studies Plasma levels of antioxidant vitamins and CHD

Observational studies	Patients' characteristics	Year	Data analyzed	Results
WHO/Monica project [83]	More than 100000 middle-aged men	1991	CHD mortality and vitamin E plasma levels	↓ *risk by vitamin E* (with low and medium coronary mortality 26-28 µM, with most frequent CHD 20-21,5 µM)
Riemersma RA et al. [86]	110 cases of angina 394 controls	1991	History of angina and plasma concentrations of vitamins A, C, E and β-carotene	↓ *risk by vitamin E* (patients with a history of angina had a lower vitamin E/cholesterol ratio -3,66 vs 3,86 µmol/mmol, p < 0.01-) Minor ↓ risk by vitamin C
Singh RB et al. [87]	cross-sectional survey within a random sample of 595 elderly people (72 with CHD)	1995	Coronary artery disease and plasma levels of vitamins A, C, E and β-carotene	↓ *risk by vitamin C and E* (relative risks of CHD between the lowest and the highest quintiles of vitamin E levels were 2,53 and 2,21)
Nyyssonen K et al. [87]	1605 randomly selected men without CHD, followed up for 8 years	1997	Myocardial infarction and vitamin C plasma levels	↓ *risk by vitamin C* (men who had vitamin C deficiency had a relative risk of acute myocardial infarction of 3.5)
Vita JA et al. [89]	149 CHD patients undergoing cardiac catheterization	1998	Extent of atherosclerosis activity of coronary artery disease and plasma antioxidant status.	↓ risk by vitamin C (presence of an unstable coronary syndrome). No↓ risk by vitamin C (extent of atherosclerosis)
Feki at al. [90]	62 angiographically confirmed coronary atherosclerotic patients and 65 age and sex-matched controls	2000	Coronary artery disease and vitamin E plasma levels	↓ risk by vitamin E (vitamin E/Cholesterol concentrations were significantly lower in coronary patients than in controls)

Mezzetti A et al. [91]	102 apparently healthy subjects age 80 and older, followed-up for 47.4 months	2002	Cardiovascular events and vitamin E plasma levels	↓ risk by vitamin E (highest vs lowest quartile: risk of cardiovascular events of 0,16
Iannuzzi et al. [92]	310 women examined by B-mode ultrasound to detect early signs of carotid atherosclerosis	2002	Atherosclerotic plaques at the carotid bifurcation and vitamin E levels	↓ risk by vitamin E (an inverse association was found between both the intake amount and plasma concentration of vitamin E and preclinical carotid atherosclerosis No ↓ risk by vitamin C
Gale CR et al. [95]	730 elderly people followed up for 20 years	1995	Stroke and CHD mortality and vitamin C plasma levels	↓ risk of mortality from stroke by vitamin C (highest vs lowest tertiles: relative risk of 0,7) No ↓ risk of mortality from CHD
Kurl S et al. [96]	2419 middle-aged men with no history of stroke followed up for 10 years	2002	Stroke and vitamin C plasma levels	↓ risk by vitamin C (lowest vs highest quartile: 2,1 fold risk of stroke

The WHO/Monica project has been one of the largest studies that analyzed the behavior of these vitamins in populations with different incidence of CHD mortality. [83] In populations with similar values of serum cholesterol and blood pressure an inverse correlation between CHD mortality and vitamin E plasma levels was observed; conversely, no relation existed between CHD mortality and other vitamins. In areas with low and medium coronary mortality plasma levels of vitamin E were 26-28 μM, while at sites with most frequent CHD mortality plasma levels were 20-21,5 μM. The Authors estimated also that the threshold risk for cardiovascular disease would be < 25 μM, that, in this particular population, corresponds to < 4,3 μmol vitamin E/mmol cholesterol.

This finding is consistent with other studies showing an inverse correlation between vitamin E plasma levels and cardiovascular mortality [84]. It was noticed, in particular, that in persons with high risk for cardiovascular mortality the vitamin E/cholesterol ratio was 3.5 while in persons with low risk the ratio was almost 5. [85] The inverse correlation between vitamin E levels and CHD was also noted in another observational study in which 110 patients with angina were compared to 394 control. [86] The study demonstrated that patients with a history of angina had a lower vitamin E/cholesterol ratio than controls (3,66 vs. 3,86 μmol/μmol, p < 0.01) with a significant adjusted odds ratio for angina between patients in the lowest and highest quartile. An inverse relation between angina and low plasma vitamin C existed but it was substantially reduced after adjustment for smoking.

In a cross-sectional survey within a random sample of a single urban setting in India, the relation between risk of coronary artery disease (CAD) and plasma levels of vitamins A, C, E and β-carotene was examined in 595 elderly subjects. Plasma levels of vitamins C and E appeared significantly inversely related to CAD. The adjusted odds ratios for CAD between the lowest and the highest quintiles of vitamin E and C levels were 2,53 and 2,21 after adjustment for confounding variables. [87]

A prospective population study of 1605 randomly selected men in Eastern Finland, followed up for 8 years showed that vitamin C deficiency, as assessed by low plasma ascorbate concentration, was a risk factor for coronary heart disease. [88]Vita JA and colleagues advanced the hypothesis that beneficial effects of vitamin C in coronary artery disease may result, in part, by an influence on lesion activity rather than a reduction in the overall extent of fixed disease. In plasma samples from 149 patients undergoing cardiac catheterization (65 with stable angina, 84 with unstable angina or a myocardial infarction within 2 weeks) the antioxidants didn't correlate with the extent of atherosclerosis, but lower plasma ascorbic acid concentration predicted the presence of an unstable coronary syndrome by multiple logistic regression. [89]

Another study, designed to assess the degree of association between vitamin E and CHD in a sample of the Tunisian population, included sixty-two angiographically confirmed coronary atherosclerotic patients and 65 age- and sex-matched controls. A trend toward a meaningful decrease of plasma tocopherol was observed in affected patients compared with controls (P = 0.06). Vitamin E concentrations standardized for cholesterol and lipid concentrations were significantly lower (P <0.02) in coronary patients than in controls (4.35 ± 1.03 vs. 4.82 ± 1.23 mmol/mol for cholesterol-adjusted vitamin E. This association between vitamin E and CHD remained unchanged independent of age, sex, smoking habit, hypertension, and diabetes. [90]

These findings have been further corroborated by another study in which 102 apparently healthy subjects were followed-up for 47.4 months. [91] A higher risk of cardiovascular events in subjects in the lowest quartile of vitamin E plasma levels compared to those in the highest was showed.

In a recent study the association between preclinical carotid atherosclerosis, and both the intake and plasma concentrations of antioxidant vitamins was evaluated. Among 5062 participants in Progetto Atena, a population-based study on the etiology of cardiovascular disease and cancer in women, 310 women were examined by B-mode ultrasound to detect early signs of carotid atherosclerosis. The participants answered a food-frequency questionnaire, and their plasma concentrations of vitamin E, vitamin A, and carotenoids were measured. The occurrence of atherosclerotic plaques at the carotid bifurcation was inversely associated with tertiles of vitamin E intake. Similarly, the ratio of plasma vitamin E to plasma cholesterol was inversely related to the presence of plaques at the carotid bifurcation. No association was found between the intake of other antioxidant vitamins (vitamins A and C and carotenoids) or their plasma concentrations and the presence of carotid plaques. [92] The results of a few similar previous studies were instead unclear. [93,94]

The association between vitamin C and stroke, shown in the previous dietary assessment studies, has been confirmed. In a 20 year follow up study of a cohort of randomly selected elderly people (730 men and women who had completed a seven day dietary record and who had no history or symptoms of stroke, cerebral arteriosclerosis, or coronary heart disease when examined) vitamin C concentration was strongly related to subsequent risk of death from stroke but not from coronary heart disease. [95]

A 10.4-year prospective population-based cohort study of 2419 randomly selected middle-aged men with no history of stroke at baseline examination showed that men with the lowest levels of plasma vitamin C had a 2.1-fold risk of any stroke compared with men with highest levels of plasma vitamin C, after adjustment for confounding factors. [96]

More recently a little study that compared 15 patients with ischemic stroke and 24 control showed that stroke patients had significantly lower plasma levels of vitamin C and higher levels of inflammatory markers than did controls. Interestingly, a significant differences in total vitamin C intake between groups was not present, suggesting that brain injury was associated to antioxidant depletion. [97]

Taken together these data suggest that vitamin E is an important predictor of CHD and may represent an independent risk factor for atherosclerosis and its complication.. Vitamin C appear a less strong predictor of CHD. Nevertheless vitamin C low plasma concentrations appear strongly associated with stroke and classical risk factors for CHD, like smoking and diabetes.

Due to the lack of standardization and a somewhat large dispersion of vitamin E/cholesterol ratio values, accurate analysis of vitamin E levels in patients and healthy subjects is crucial in order to have a reliable use of this variable in clinical practice and interventional trials. Very recently, for instance, healthy subjects [98] were shown to have values of vitamin E of 3.6 μmol/mmol cholesterol that is much less than that reported in control population. [99] Ascorbic acid is an unstable compound and is easily oxidized even in blood samples obtained from healthy volunteers. Oxidation of vitamin C in the test tube may produce erroneously low values and could account for some of these findings. [100] The increasing interest for both vitamins in the assessment of risk for cardiovascular disease strongly suggest the need of standardization assay of both vitamins.

Interventional Trials

While most epidemiologic studies demonstrated that dietary intake of vitamin E is inversely related to coronary heart complications, supplementation studies gave conflicting results. Clinical trials with antioxidants have been done in patients with or without previous history of cardiovascular disease. Surrogate end-points, such as analysis of atherosclerosis progression, or hard end-points, such as vascular death and myocardial infarction, have been examined for evaluating the clinical benefit of antioxidant vitamins (Table 3). The Alpha-Tocopherol-Beta-Carotene-Cancer (ATBC) [101] prevention study was a randomized, double-blind, placebo-controlled primary-prevention trial to determine whether daily supplementation with alpha-tocopherol, beta carotene, or both reduced the incidence of lung cancer and other cancers. A total of 29,133 male smokers 50 to 69 years of age were randomly assigned to one of four regimens: α-tocopherol (50 mg per day) alone, β-carotene (20 mg per day) alone, both α-tocopherol and β-carotene, or placebo for five to eight years of follow-up. The results of this trial showed no beneficial effect of supplemental vitamin E (α-tocopherol) or β-carotene in terms of the prevention of lung cancer, but the authors observed a reduction for death due to cardiovascular events in the group treated with α-tocopherol. For this reason, the authors made a sub-analysis analyzing to study the clinical efficacy of 50 mg/day vitamin E in a population suffering from coronary heart disease, and showed no changes of cardiovascular events during the follow-up. [102]

Table 3. Randomized trials of vitamin E treatment

Trial	Patients' characteristics	Location of study population	Number in treatment group. Antioxidant Control		Dose	Follow up (years)	Results
ATBC [101]	1862 man, smokers aged between 50 and 69 years, who had a previous MI	Finland	963	799	Vit E 50 mg	5,3	Vitamin E showed no effect
CHAOS [103]	Median age 62 years; angiographically proven CAD; 84% male (n=2002)	UK, single centre	1035	967	Vit E 400–800 IU	1,4	Vitamin E treatment substantially reduced the rate of non-fatal MI
GISSI [105]	Survivors of recent MI (<3 months); 85% male (n=11 324)	Italy, multicentre	5660	5664	Vit E 300 mg	3,5	Vitamin E showed no effect
HOPE [107]	Mean age 66 years; known cardiovascular disease or diabetes 73% male (n=9541)	Canada, USA, Europe, South America	4761	4780	Vit E 400 IU	4,5	Vitamin E showed no effect
SPACE [108]	Haemodialysis patients with pre-existing cardiovascular disease (n=196) aged 40-75 years	Israel, single centre	97	99	Vit E 800 IU	1,4	Vitamin E reduced composite cardiovascular disease endpoints and myocardial infarction
HPS [111]	Age range 40–80 years; known vascular disease or at-risk of vascular disease; 75% male (n=20 536)	UK, multicentre	10269	10267	Vit E 600 mg Vit C 250 mg	5	Vitamin E showed no effect
PPP [112]	primary prevention in patients with at least one risk factor age range 55–80 years; (n=4495)	Italy, multicentre	2231	2264	Vit E 300 mg	3,6	The results on vitamin E are not conclusive
Fang JC [113]	40 patients (0–2 years after cardiac transplantation)	USA, single centre	19	21	Vit E 800 IU Vit C 1 g	1	Supplementation with antioxidant retarded the early progression of transplant-associated coronary arteriosclerosis
ASAP [114]	520 men and postmenopausal women aged 45 to 69 years with serum cholesterol > or =5.0 mmol/L	Finland	390	130	Vit E 272 IU Vit C 500 mg	6	Vitamins C and E slows down atherosclerotic progression in hypercholesterolemic persons

The Cambridge Heart Antioxidant Study (CHAOS) tested the hypothesis if treatment with a high dose of alpha-tocopherol would reduce subsequent risk of myocardial infarction (MI) and cardiovascular death in patients with established ischemic heart disease. In this double-blind, placebo-controlled study with stratified randomization, 2002 patients with angiographically proven coronary atherosclerosis were enrolled and followed up for a median of 510 days (range 3-981). 1035 patients were assigned alpha-tocopherol (capsules containing 800 IU daily for first 546 patients; 400 IU daily for remainder); 967 received identical placebo capsules. The primary endpoints were a combination of cardiovascular death and non-fatal MI as well as non-fatal MI alone. This trial showed that in patients with symptomatic coronary atherosclerosis, alpha-tocopherol treatment substantially reduced the rate of non-fatal MI, with beneficial apparent effects after 1 year of treatment. No significant reduction in fatal myocardial infarction was recorded; on the contrary, a non-significant increase in cardiovascular death was detected in patients receiving vitamin E. [103] In a further analysis of mortality, however, it became clear that only six of 72 cardiovascular-disease deaths occurred in patients compliant with vitamin E treatment. [104]

The GISSI-Prevenzione trial [105] assessed the efficacy of vitamin E and n-3 polyunsaturated fatty acids (PUFA) on cardiovascular death, non-fatal MI, or stroke in patients with recent MI. 11 324 patients surviving recent (<3 months) myocardial infarction were randomly assigned supplements of n-3 PUFA (1 g daily, n=2836), vitamin E (300 mg daily, n=2830), both (n=2830), or none (control, n=2828) for 3.5 years. The primary combined efficacy endpoint was death, non-fatal myocardial infarction, and stroke. Intention-to-treat analyses were done according to a factorial design (two-way) and by treatment group (four-way).

Treatment with n-3 PUFA significantly lowered the risk of the primary endpoint in the two and four way analysis. By contrast with n-3 PUFA, the results for vitamin E did not support the evidence of its efficacy, although it was possible to see a significant decrease of cardiovascular deaths in the four-way analysis. Moreover 300 mg/day of synthetic vitamin E daily (which is equivalent to about 150 mg natural vitamin E [106]) is below the range in which clinical trials report positive results.

Similarly the Heart Outcomes Prevention Evaluation (HOPE) Study was a double-blind, randomized trial with a two-by-two factorial design, conducted to evaluate the effects of ramipril and vitamin E in 9541 patients at high risk for cardiovascular events. Patients were randomly assigned to receive either 400 IU of vitamin E from natural sources or an equivalent placebo daily for 4 to 6 years. The primary outcome of this study was represented by myocardial infarction, stroke or death from cardiovascular causes. Secondary and other outcomes were death from any cause; unstable angina; hospitalization for heart failure with clinical and radiological signs of congestion; revascularization or limb amputation; the development of overt nephropathy; and the development of heart failure In this study vitamin E did not reduce the incidence of cardiovascular events, as compared with the incidence among patients assigned to placebo, during the follow-up period. There were also no significant differences in the incidence of secondary cardiovascular outcomes or in death from any cause. There were no significant adverse effects of vitamin E. The investigators believed that perhaps longer follow-up was needed to detect benefit of vitamin E, although their data do not suggest a trend in that direction. [107] The SPACE trial [108] investigated the effect of high-dose vitamin E supplementation on cardiovascular disease outcomes in haemodialysis patients with pre-existing cardiovascular disease. This population was chosen because it is well established that patients undergoing chronic haemodialysis are exposed to increased oxidative stress induced by the membranes used in dialysis. [109,110] 196 patients were enrolled and randomized to receive 800 IU/day vitamin E or matching placebo. Patients were followed for a median 519 days. The primary endpoint was a composite variable consisting of: myocardial infarction (fatal and non-fatal), ischemic stroke, peripheral vascular disease and unstable angina. Among haemodialysis patients treated with high-dose vitamin E a 54% reduction was attained in the primary endpoint, contributed to largely by the reduction in total myocardial infarction (70%). The study was small, but the results are suggestive. Antioxidant therapy would be expected to have a greater treatment effect on patients in greater oxidative stress, and haemodialysis patients are in greater oxidative stress than other patient groups. [108] The accelerated cardiovascular-disease event rate observed in haemodialysis patients, contributed to by increased oxidative stress, showed to be reduced by antioxidant therapy.

A negative result came from the HPS trial, in which 20536 UK adults (aged 40–80) with coronary disease, other occlusive arterial disease, or diabetes were randomly allocated to receive antioxidant vitamin supplementation (600 mg vitamin E, 250 mg vitamin C, and 20 mg β-carotene daily) or matching placebo. Intention-to-treat comparisons of outcome were conducted between all vitamin-allocated and all placebo-allocated participants. Allocation to this vitamin regimen approximately doubled the plasma concentration of α-tocopherol, increased that of vitamin C by one-third, and quadrupled that of β-carotene. Primary outcomes were major coronary events (for overall analyses) and fatal or non-fatal vascular events (for subcategory analyses), with subsidiary assessments of cancer and of other major morbidity. After a 5 year treatment period there were no significant differences in all cause mortality or in deaths due to vascular on non vascular causes, in non fatal myocardial infarction or coronary death, in non-fatal or fatal stroke between the two groups of participants. [111]

In addiction to secondary prevention studies (that included patients with documented or known vascular disease) the Primary Prevention Project (PPP) studied the efficacy of vitamin E among patients who had one or more cardiovascular risk factors (hypertension, diabetes, or early family history of coronary disease). 4495 people were randomly allocated to receive aspirin (100 mg) or no aspirin, and vitamin E or no vitamin E. The main combined efficacy endpoint was the cumulative rate of cardiovascular death, non-fatal myocardial infarction, and non-fatal stroke. After a mean follow-up of 3,6 years the trial was prematurely stopped on ethical grounds when newly available evidence from other trials documented the benefit of aspirin in primary prevention. Vitamin E showed no effect on any prespecified endpoint. Even if the findings for vitamin E could be regarded as a false negative result, because of the inadequate power of a prematurely interrupted trial. [112]

The effect of antioxidant vitamins were also investigated using surrogate end-points such as carotid atherosclerotic progression.

Fang JC et al. [113] tested the effect of vitamin E (400UI x 2) plus vitamin C (500 mg x 2) in a 40 patients 0-2 years after cardiac transplantation. The primary endpoint was the change in average intimal index (plaque area divided by vessel area) measured by intravascular ultrasonography (IVUS). During 1 year of treatment, the intimal index increased in the placebo group by 8% (SE 2) but did not change significantly in the treatment group. Despite the small sample size due to the limited number of patients that undergo this procedure, the study was of particular interest because cardiac transplantation is associated to oxidative stress, which may contribute to the development of accelerated coronary arteriosclerosis.

The ASAP study [114] demonstrated that a combination of 136 IU vitamin E plus 250 mg of slow-release vitamin C twice daily slows down atherosclerotic progression in hypercholesterolemic patients. The subjects were 520 smoking and non-smoking men and postmenopausal women aged 45 to 69 years with serum cholesterol <5.0 mmol/L. The progression of common carotid artery (CCA) atherosclerosis was carried out by high resolution ultrasonography. After 6 years of follow-up in covariance analysis in both sexes, supplementation reduced the main study outcome, the slope of mean CCA intimal-media thickness by 26%. It was of note that the treatment was more effective in patients with low baseline values of vitamin C.

Most trials with antioxidants used vitamin E likely because epidemiological studies documented that regular assumption of this vitamin reduced the risk of cardiovascular events. [115] Patient selection of these trials was therefore based on the hypothesis that all patients at risk of cardiovascular disease could have benefits from supplementation with this vitamin, therefore many primary and secondary interventional trials, such the GISSI-Prevenzione, the HOPE and the PPP studies, did not consider the antioxidant status as entry criterion and did not report any data inherent to bioavailability of vitamin E. [105,107,112] The lack of this information renders of difficult interpretation the results of these trials also because the serious issue related to vitamin E bioavailability has been completely ignored. We demonstrated, in fact, that about 30 % of subjects did not have any increase of vitamin E plasma levels unless vitamin E was assumed after food intake. [85] This finding has been recently supported by Carrol et al. [116] showing a significant increment of plasma vitamin E when supplement was given immediately before meal. Among antioxidant trials, five reported plasma values of vitamin E in control population. Patients included in these trials suffered from cardiovascular disease or had classic risk factors for atherosclerosis [102,103,111] or renal insufficiency [108] or underwent heart transplantation. [113] In four of these trials a combination of vitamins was given: the ATBC [101] and the HPS [111] studies administered vitamins E, C and beta-carotene, the ASAP [114] and the study including patients undergoing heart transplantation [113] vitamin C and E. Vitamin E values of study populations were extremely wide ranging from 5.6 (the CHAOS and the HPS studies) to 4.3 (heart-transplant atherosclerosis). Assuming that values of vitamin E <5 μmol/mmol cholesterol identify patients at risk for cardiovascular disease, [106] we argue that only three studies included patients with low antioxidant status. Among these trails the ATBC provided negative results while the other two studies demonstrated that vitamin E alone or in combination with vitamin C significantly reduced cardiovascular events.

Conclusion

On the basis of these considerations we can conclude that there is compelling evidence that enhanced oxidative stress is detectable in patients with classic risk factors for atherosclerosis but its impact in the context of atherosclerosis progression is still unclear. The reason for this uncertainty is due to the lack of clear prospective study indicating that markers of oxidative stress, such as blood lipid peroxides or urinary F2-isoprostane, are of some value for predicting the progression of atherosclerosis, even if there some evidence suggesting that antibodies against oxidized LDL may be of some utility. [117] Conversely epidemiologic studies seem to indicate that low antioxidant status increases the risk for cardiovascular disease. Clinical characteristics of patients with low antioxidant status have not been defined and should be studied in the next future. So far clinical trials with antioxidants included patients without evaluating either oxidative stress or antioxidant status and such indiscriminate enrolment could perhaps account for the negative results of antioxidant trials recently emphasized by meta-analysis. [118] A recent report by Meagher et al [119] is highly relevant to this discussion. They fed normal subjects doses of vitamin E ranging from 200 to 2000 mg/d for 8 weeks. The highest dose increased plasma vitamin E levels 5-fold, but urinary excretion of isoprostanes and 4-hydroxynonenal (breakdown products of fatty acid auto-oxidation) was unaffected. The results suggest that in normally nourished subjects, additional vitamin E will not necessarily confer any additional antioxidant protection. Earlier studies in cigarette smokers, in contrast, did show a vitamin E effect on plasma isoprostane levels, suggesting that only in subjects under some oxidative stress antioxidant effect will be obtained. [120] Protective effect of vitamin E against coronary events in the SPACE study may reflect the fact that the subjects were under the oxidant stress known to accompany haemodialysis. [110] In the some way other patients under increased oxidative stress (such us smokers, diabetics) could be also constitute a population more likely to benefit from antioxidants..

Moreover, as Steinberg and Witzum focused, [6] the antioxidants might be effective in inhibiting the initial stages of human atherosclerosis and yet ineffective or much less effective in reducing plaque instability and rupture. If this were the case, it might be necessary to find some way to assess early stages of lesion development (e.g., high resolution ultrasound or MRI) rather than relying on the usual late clinical end points. Of course if the development of early lesions were successfully inhibited, there should eventually be a decrease in the frequency of clinical events, but in that case, the trials might need to extend beyond the conventional 5 years.

Another issue that deserves further attention is the choice of appropriate antioxidant treatment. So far several mechanisms, including enzymatic and non enzymatic oxidation of LDL, have been proposed but the exact process leading to LDL accumulation within vessel wall is still unclear. This fact creates uncertainty in the type of antioxidants that could be relevant for inhibiting atherosclerotic progress. Thus future trials with antioxidant should not be discouraged; conversely better identification of criteria identifying potential candidates for antioxidant treatment, together with the choice of an adequate daily regimen of antioxidants should be studied.

References

[1]   Frei B. On the role of vitamin C and other antioxidants in atherogenesis and vascular dysfunction. *Proc. Soc. Exp. Biol. Med.* 1999;222(3):196-204

[2]   Henriksen T, Mahoney EM, Steinberg D. Enhanced macrophage degradation of low-density lipoprotein previously incubated with cultured endothelial cells - recognition by receptors for acetylated low density lipoproteins. *Proc. Natl. Acad. Sci. USA* 1981, 78; 6499-6503.

[3]   Gotto AM. Antioxidants, statins, and atherosclerosis. *J. Am. Coll. Cardiol.* 2003; 41(7):1205-10.

[4]   Steinberg D, Parthesarathy S, Carew TE, et al. Beyond cholesterol: modifications of low-density lipoprotein that increase its atherogenicity. *N. Engl. J. Med.* 1989;320:915–24.

[5]   Palinski W, Rosenfeld ME, Yla-Herttuala S, et al. Low-density lipoprotein undergoes oxidative modification in vivo. *Proc. Natl. Acad. Sci. USA* 1989;86:1372–6.

[6]   Steinberg D, Witztum JL. Is the Oxidative Modification Hypothesis Relevant to Human Atherosclerosis? Do the Antioxidant Trials Conducted to Date Refute the Hypothesis? *Circulation* 2002;105:2107-2111.

[7]   Violi F, Micheletta F, Iuliano L. How to select patient candidates for antioxidant treatment? *Circulation* 2002;106(24):e195.

[8]   Ross R. Atherosclerosis--an inflammatory disease. *N. Engl. J. Med.* 1999;340(2):115-26.

[9]   Pearson TA. New tools for coronary risk assessment: what are their advantages and limitations? *Circulation* 2002; 9;105(7):886-92

[10]   Natoli S., Violi F. Oxidative stress and hypercholesterolemia: increase of hydroxyl radical in patients with hypercholesterolemia. *Cardiologia*, 1999;44(2):187-190.

[11]   Touyz R.M. Oxidative stress and vascular damage in hypertension. *Curr. Hypertens Rep.* 2000;2(1):98-105.

[12]   Bennefon T., Rousselot D., Bastard J.P., Jaudon M.C., Delattre J. Consequences of the diabetic status on the oxidant-antioxidant balance. *Diabetes Metab.* 2000; 26 (3): 163-176.

[13]   Celermajer D.S. et al. Passive smoking and impaired endothelium-dependent arterial dilation in healthy young men. *N. Engl. J. Med;* 334: (3): 150-154.

[14]   Loscalzo J. The oxidant stress of hyperhomocyst(e)inemia. *J. Clin. Invest* 1996;98(1):5-7.

[15]   Shepelev AP, Kornienko IV, Shestopalov AV, Antipov A. [Role of free radical oxidation processes in the pathogenesis of infectious diseases]. *Vopr. Med. Khim.* 2000; 46(2):110-6.

[16]   Bloodsworth A, O'Donnell VB, Freeman BA. Nitric oxide regulation of free radical- and enzyme-mediated lipid and lipoprotein oxidation. *Arterioscler. Thromb. Vasc. Biol.* 2000; 20:1707-15.

[17]   Griendling KK, Minieri CA, Ollerenshaw JD, Alexander RW. Angiotensin II stimulates NADH and NADPH oxidase activity in cultured vascular smooth muscle cells. *Circ. Res.* 1994;74(6):1141-8.

[18] Taddei S, Virdis A, Ghiadoni L, Magagna A, Salvetti A. Vitamin C improves endothelium-dependent vasodilation by restoring nitric oxide activity in essential hypertension. *Circulation* 1998:97:2222-2229.

[19] Iuliano L, Signore A, Violi F. Uptake of oxidized LDL by human atherosclerotic plaque. *Circulation* 1997;96(6):2093-4.

[20] Mezzetti A, Cipollone F, Cuccurullo F. Oxidative stress and cardiovascular complications in diabetes: isoprostanes as new markers on an old paradigm. *Cardiovasc. Res.* 2000;47:475-88.

[21] Timimi FK, Ting HH, Haley EA, Roddy MA, Ganz P, Creager MA. Vitamin C improves endothelium-dependent vasodilation in patients with insulin-dependent diabetes mellitus. *J. Am. Coll. Cardiol.* 1998;31:552-7.

[22] Paolisso G, Giugliano D. Oxidative stress and insulin action: is there a relationship? *Diabetologia* 1996;39:357-63.

[23] Davì G, Ciabattoni G, Consoli A, Mezzetti A, Falco A, Santarone S, Pennese E, Vitacolonna E, Bucciarelli T, Costantini F, Capani F, Patrono C. In vivo formation of 8-iso-prostaglandin f2alpha and platelet activation in diabetes mellitus: effects of improved metabolic control and vitamin E supplementation. *Circulation* 1999; 99(2): 224-9.

[24] TaguchiJ, Ikari Y, Umezu M, Watanabe T, Miyata T, Kurokawa K, Kimura T, Ohno M. Advanced glycation end products enhanced the aggregation of human platelets in vitro. *Circulation* 1997; 96 (suppl I):I-665.

[25] Cosentino F, Hishikawa K, Katusic ZS, Lüscher TF. High Glucose Increases Nitric Oxide Synthase Expression and Superoxide Anion Generation in Human Aortic Endothelial Cells. *Circulation* 1997;96:25-28.

[26] Wolin MS. Interactions of Oxidants With Vascular Signaling Systems. *Arterioscler. Thromb Vasc. Biol.* 2000;20:1430-1442.

[27] Guzik TJ, Mussa S, Gastaldi D, Sadowski J, Ratnatunga C, Pillai R, Channon KM. Mechanisms of Increased Vascular Superoxide Production in Human Diabetes Mellitus: Role of NAD(P)H Oxidase and Endothelial Nitric Oxide Synthase. *Circulation* 2002; 105: 1656-1662.

[28] Davì G, Alessandrini P, Mezzetti A, Minotti G, Bucciarelli T, Costantini F, Cipollone F, Bittolo-Bon G, Ciabattoni G, Patrono C. In Vivo Formation of 8-Epi-Prostaglandin F2ɪʏ is Increased in Hypercholesterolemia. *Arterioscler. Thromb Vasc. Biol.* 1997;17: 3230-3235.

[29] Ohara Y, Peterson TE, Sayegh HS, Subramanian RR, Wilcox JN, Harrison DG. Dietary Correction of Hypercholesterolemia in the Rabbit Normalizes Endothelial Superoxide Anion Production. *Circulation* 1995;92:898-903.

[30] Ting HH, Timimi FK, Haley EA, Roddy MA, Ganz P,Creager MA. Vitamin C Improves Endothelium-Dependent Vasodilation in Forearm Resistance Vessels of Humans With Hypercholesterolemia. *Circulation* 1997;95:2617-2622.

[31] Sanguigni V, Pignatelli P, Caccese D, Pulcinelli FM, Lenti L, Magnaterra R, Martini F, Lauro R, Violi F. Increased superoxide anion production by platelets in hypercholesterolemic patients. *Thromb Haemost.* 2002; 87:796-801.

[32] Takemoto M, Liao JK. Pleiotropic effects of 3-hydroxy-3-methylglutaryl coenzyme a reductase inhibitors. *Arterioscler. Thromb Vasc. Biol.* 2001; 11:1712-9.

[33] Ferro D, Parrotto S, Basili S, Alessandri C, Violi F. Simvastatin Inhibits the Monocyte Expression of Proinflammatory Cytokines in Patients With Hypercholesterolemia. *J. Am. Coll. Cardiol.* 2000;36:427-31.

[34] De Caterina R, Cipollone F, Filardo FP, Zimarino M, Bernini W, Lazzerini G, Bucciarelli T, Falco A, Marchesani P, Muraro R, Mezzetti A, Ciabattoni G. Low-density lipoprotein level reduction by the 3-hydroxy-3-methylglutaryl coenzyme-A inhibitor simvastatin is accompanied by a related reduction of F2-isoprostane formation in hypercholesterolemic subjects: no further effect of vitamin E. *Circulation* 2002; 106 (20): 2543-9.

[35] Pronai L, Hiramatsu K, Saigusa Y, Nakazawa H. Low superoxide scavenging activity associated with enhanced superoxide generation by monocytes from male hypertriglyceridemia with and without diabetes. *Atherosclerosis* 1991;90:39-47.

[36] Esterbauer H, Gebicki J, Puhl H, Jurgens G. The role of lipid peroxidation and antioxidants in oxidative modification of LDLLevine M, Rumsey SC, Daruwala R, Park JB, Wang Y. Criteria and recommendations for vitamin C intake. *Jama* 1999; 281(15):1415-23.

[37] Padayatty SJ, Katz A, Wang Y, et al. Vitamin C as an antioxidant: evaluation of its role in disease prevention. *J. Am. Coll. Nutr.* 2003;22(1):18-35.

[38] Padayatty SJ, Levine M. New insights into the physiology and pharmacology of vitamin C. *Cmaj* 2001;164(3):353-5.

[39] Martin A, Frei B. Both intracellular and extracellular vitamin C inhibit atherogenic modification of LDL by human vascular endothelial cells. *Arterioscler. Thromb Vasc. Biol.* 1997; 17:1583–1590.

[40] Carr AC, Tijerina T, Frei B. Vitamin C protects against and reverses specific hypochlorous acid- and chloramine-dependent modifications of low-density lipoprotein. *Biochem. J.* 2000;346:491– 499.

[41] Carr AC, Zhu BZ, Frei B. Potential antiatherogenic mechanisms of ascorbate (vitamin C) and alpha-tocopherol (vitamin E). *Circ. Res.* 2000;87(5):349-54.

[42] Hatta A, Frei B. Oxidative modification and antioxidant protection of human low density lipoprotein at high and low oxygen partial pressures. *J. Lipid Res.* 1995; 36(11): 2383-93.

[43] Retsky KL, Chen K, Zeind J, Frei B. Inhibition of copper-induced LDL oxidation by vitamin C is associated with decreased copper binding to LDL and 2-oxo-histidine formation. *Free Radic. Biol. Med.* 1999:26:90-98.

[44] Retsky KL, Frei B. Vitamin C prevents metal ion-dependant initiation and propagation of lipid peroxidation in human low-density lipoprotein. *Biochim. Biophys. Acta* :1257: 279-287.

[45] Upston JM, Terentis AC, Stocker R. Tocopherol-mediated peroxidation of lipoproteins: implications for vitamin E as a potential antiatherogenic supplement. *Faseb J* 1999; 13(9): 977-94.

[46] Packer, J. E., Slater, T. F., and Willson, R. L. Direct observation of a free radical interaction between vitamin E and vitamin C. *Nature* 1979;278:737–738.

[47] Sharma, M. K., and Buettner. G. R. Interaction of vitamin C and vitamin E during free radical stress in plasma: an ESR study. *Free Rad. Biol. Med.* 1993;14:649–653.

[48] Bowry, V. W., and Stocker, R. Tocopherol-mediated peroxidation. The pro-oxidant effect of vitamin E on the radical-initiated oxidation of human low-density lipoprotein. *J. Am.. Chem. Soc.* 1993; 115:6029–6044.

[49] Beckman JA, Goldfine AB, Gordon MB, Creager MA. Ascorbate restores endothelium-dependent vasodilation impaired by acute hyperglycemia in humans. *Circulation* 2001; 103(12): 1618-23.

[50] Nappo F, De Rosa N, Marfella R, et al. Impairment of endothelial functions by acute hyperhomocysteinemia and reversal by antioxidant vitamins. *Jama* 1999;281(22):2113-8.

[51] Kugiyama K, Motoyama T, Hirashima O, Ohgushi M, Soejima H, Misumi K, Kawano H, Miyao Y, Yoshimura M, Ogawa H, Mat-sumura T, Sugiyama S, Yasue H. Vitamin C attenuates abnormal vasomotor reactivity in spasm coronary arteries in patients with coronary spastic angina. *J. Am. Coll. Cardiol.* 1998:32:103-109.

[52] Hornig B, Arakawa N, Kohler C, Drexler H. Vitamin C improvesendothelial function of conduit arteries in patients with chronic heart failure. *Circulation* 1998;97:363-368.

[53] Solzbach U, Hornig B, Jeserich M, Just H. Vitamin C improves endothelial dysfunction of epicardial coronary arteries in hypertensive patients. *Circulation* 1997;96:1513-1519.

[54] Jackson TS, Xu A, Vita JA, Keaney JF, Jr. Ascorbate prevents the interaction of superoxide and nitric oxide only at very high physiological concentrations. *Circ. Res.* 1998; 83(9):916-22.

[55] Jonas E, Dwenger A, Hager A. In vitro effect of ascorbic acid on neutrophil-endothelial cell interaction. *J Biolumin Chemilumin* 1993;8:15-20.

[56] Lehr HA, Frei B, Arfors KE. Vitamin C prevents cigarette smoke-in duced leukocyte aggregation and adhesion to endothelium in vivo. *Proc. Natl. Acad. Sci. USA* 1994; 91: 7688-7692.

[57] Weber C, Wolfgang E, Weber K, Weber PC. Increased adhesiveness of isolated monocytes to endothelium is prevented by vitamin C intake in smokers. *Circulation* 1996; 93:1488-1492.

[58] Lehr HA, Frei B, Olofsson AM, Carew TE, Arfors KE. Protection from oxidized LDL-induced leukocyte adhesion to microvascular and macrovascular endothelium in vivo by vitamin C but not by vitamin E. *Circulation* 1995;91:1525–1532.

[59] Machlin LJ.Vitamin E. In: Machlin LJ, ed . Handbook of Vitamins: Nutritional, Biochemical and Clinical Aspects. New York, N.Y., Marcel Dekker, Inc., 1984; 99-145.

[60] Marchioli R. Vitamin E and cardiovascular disease. *Thromb Haemost* 2001;85(5):758-60.

[61] Violi F, Micheletta F, Iuliano L. Vitamin E, atherosclerosis and thrombosis. *Thromb Haemost* 2001;85(5):766-70.

[62] Palinski W, Ord VA, Plump AS, Breslow JL, Steinberg D, Witztum JL. ApoE-deficient mice are a model of lipoprotein oxidation in atherogenesis. Demonstration of

oxidation-specific epitopes in lesions and high titers of autoantibodies to malondialdehyde-lysine in serum. *Arterioscler. Thromb* 1994;14(4):605-16.

[63] Calara F, Dimayuga P, Niemann A, et al. An animal model to study local oxidation of LDL and its biological effects in the arterial wall. *Arterioscler. Thromb Vasc. Biol.* 1998; 18(6):884-93.

[64] Freyschuss A, Stiko-Rahm A, Swedenborg J, et al. Antioxidant treatment inhibits the development of intimal thickening after balloon injury of the aorta in hypercholesterolemic rabbits. *J. Clin. Invest* 1993;91(4):1282-8.

[65] Sparrow CP, Doebber TW, Olszewski J, et al. Low density lipoprotein is protected from oxidation and the progression of atherosclerosis is slowed in cholesterol-fed rabbits by the antioxidant N,N'-diphenyl-phenylenediamine. *J. Clin. Invest* 1992; 89(6): 1885-91.

[66] Pratico D, Tangirala RK, Rader DJ, Rokach J, FitzGerald GA. Vitamin E suppresses isoprostane generation in vivo and reduces atherosclerosis in ApoE-deficient mice. *Nat. Med.* 1998;4(10):1189-92.

[67] Iuliano L, Mauriello A, Sbarigia E, Spagnoli LG, Violi F. Radiolabeled native low-density lipoprotein injected into patients with carotid stenosis accumulates in macrophages of atherosclerotic plaque : effect of vitamin E supplementation. *Circulation* 2000;101(11):1249-54.

[68] Rota S, McWilliam NA, Baglin TP, Byrne CD. Atherogenic lipoproteins support assembly of the prothrombinase complex and thrombin generation: modulation by oxidation and vitamin E. *Blood* 1998;91(2):508-15.

[69] Schreck R, Meier B, Mannel DN, Droge W, Baeuerle PA. Dithiocarbamates as potent inhibitors of nuclear factor kappa B activation in intact cells. *J. Exp. Med.* 1992; 175(5):1181-94.

[70] Crutchley DJ, Que BG. Copper-induced tissue factor expression in human monocytic THP-1 cells and its inhibition by antioxidants. *Circulation* 1995;92(2):238-43.

[71] Ferro D, Basili S, Pratico D, Iuliano L, FitzGerald GA, Violi F. Vitamin E reduces monocyte tissue factor expression in cirrhotic patients. *Blood* 1999;93(9):2945-50.

[72] Freedman JE, Farhat JH, Loscalzo J, Keaney JF, Jr. alpha-tocopherol inhibits aggregation of human platelets by a protein kinase C-dependent mechanism. *Circulation* 1996; 94(10):2434-40.

[73] Calzada C, Bruckdorfer KR, Rice-Evans CA. The influence of antioxidant nutrients on platelet function in healthy volunteers. *Atherosclerosis* 1997;128(1):97-105.

[74] Pignatelli P, Pulcinelli FM, Lenti L, Gazzaniga PP, Violi F. Vitamin E inhibits collagen-induced platelet activation by blunting hydrogen peroxide. *Arterioscler. Thromb Vasc. Biol.* 1999;19(10):2542-7.

[75] Enstrom JE, Kanim LE, Klein MA. Vitamin C intake and mortality among a sample of the United States population. *Epidemiology* 1992;3(3):194-202.

[76] Stampfer MJ, Hennekens CH, Manson JE, Colditz GA, Rosner B, Willett WC. Vitamin E consumption and the risk of coronary disease in women. *N. Engl. J. Med. 1993*; 328(20):1444-9.

[77] Rimm EB, Stampfer MJ, Ascherio A, Giovannucci E, Colditz GA, Willett WC.
      Vitamin E consumption and the risk of coronary heart disease in men. *N. Engl. J. Med.*
      1993;328(20):1450-6.

[78] Kushi LH, Folsom AR, Prineas RJ, Mink PJ, Wu Y, Bostick RM. Dietary antioxidant
      vitamins and death from coronary heart disease in postmenopausal women. *N. Engl. J.
      Med.* 1996 May 2;334(18):1156-62.

[79] Klipstein-Grobusch K, Geleijnse JM, den Breeijen JH, Boeing H, Hofman A, Grobbee
      DE, Witteman JC. Dietary antioxidants and risk of myocardial infarction in the elderly:
      the Rotterdam Study. *Am. J. Clin. Nutr.* 1999;69(2):261-6.

[80] Daviglus ML, Orencia AJ, Dyer AR, et al. Dietary vitamin C, beta-carotene and 30-
      year risk of stroke: results from the Western Electric Study. *Neuroepidemiology* 1997;
      16(2):69-77).

[81] Joshipura KJ, Ascherio A, Manson JE, et al. Fruit and vegetable intake in relation to
      risk of ischemic stroke. *Jama* 1999;282(13):1233-9.

[82] Gey KF, Puska P, Jordan P, Moser UK. Inverse correlation between plasma vitamin E
      and mortality from ischemic heart disease in cross-cultural epidemiology. *Am. J. Clin.
      Nutr.* 1991;53(1 Suppl):326S-334S.

[83] Gey, K. F. Vitamin E and other essential antioxidants regarding coronary heart disease:
      risk assessment studies. Epidemiological basis of the antioxidant hypothesis of
      cardiovascular disease. In: Packer, L.; Fuchs, J., eds. *Vitamin E in health and disease.*
      New York, NY: Marcel Dekker, Inc.; 1993:589–633.

[84] Iuliano L, Micheletta F, Maranghi M, Frati G, Diczfalusy U, Violi F. Bioavailability of
      vitamin E as function of food intake in healthy subjects: effects on plasma peroxide-
      scavenging activity and cholesterol-oxidation products, *Arterioscler. Thromb. Vasc.
      Biol.* 2001;21:E34-7.

[85] Riemersma RA, Wood DA, Macintyre CC, Elton RA, Gey KF, Oliver MF. Risk of
      angina pectoris and plasma concentration of vitamins A, C, and E and carotene. *Lancet*
      1991;337:1-5.

[86] Singh RB, Ghosh S, Niaz MA, Singh R, Beegum R, Chibo H, Shoumin Z, Postiglione
      A. Dietary intake, plasma levels of antioxidant vitamins, and oxidative stress in relation
      to coronary artery disease in elderly subjects. *Am. J. Cardiol.* 1995;76(17):1233-8.

[87] Nyyssonen K, Parviainen MT, Salonen R, Tuomilehto J, Salonen JT. Vitamin C
      deficiency and risk of myocardial infarction: prospective population study of men from
      eastern Finland. *Bmj* 1997;314(7081):634-8.

[88] Vita JA, Keaney JF, Jr., Raby KE, et al. Low plasma ascorbic acid independently
      predicts the presence of an unstable coronary syndrome. *J. Am. Coll. Cardiol.* 1998;
      31(5): 980-6.

[89] Feki M, Souissi M, Mokhtar E, Hsairi M, Kaabachi N, Antebi H, Alcindor LG,
      Mechmeche R, Mebazaa A. Vitamin E and coronary heart disease in Tunisians. *Clin.
      Chem.* 2000;46(9):1401-5.

[90] Mezzetti A, Zuliani G, Romano F, Costantini F, Pierdomenico SD, Cuccurullo F, Fellin
      R. Vitamin E and lipid peroxide plasma levels predict the risk of cardiovascular events
      in a group of healthy very old people. *J. Am. Geriatr. Soc.* 2001;49:533-7.

[91] Iannuzzi A, Celentano E, Panico S, Galasso R, Covetti G, Sacchetti L, Zarrilli F, De Michele M, Rubba P. Dietary and circulating antioxidant vitamins in relation to carotid plaques in middle-aged women. *Am. J. Clin. Nutr.* 2002;76(3):582-7.

[92] McQuillan BM, Hung J, Beilby JP, Nidorf M, Thompson PL. Antioxidant vitamins and the risk of carotid atherosclerosis. The Perth Carotid Ultrasound Disease Assessment study (CUDAS). *J. Am. Coll. Cardiol.* 2001;38(7):1788-94.

[93] Gale CR, Ashurst HE, Powers HJ, Martyn CN. Antioxidant vitamin status and carotid atherosclerosis in the elderly. *Am. J. Clin. Nutr.* 2001 Sep;74(3):402-8.

[94] Gale CR, Martyn CN, Winter PD, Cooper C. Vitamin C and risk of death from stroke and coronary heart disease in cohort of elderly people. *Bmj* 1995;310(6994):1563-6.

[95] Kurl S, Tuomainen TP, Laukkanen JA, et al. Plasma vitamin C modifies the association between hypertension and risk of stroke. *Stroke* 2002;33(6):1568-73.

[96] Sanchez-Moreno C, Dashe JF, Scott T, Thaler D, Folstein MF, Martin A. Decreased levels of plasma vitamin C and increased concentrations of inflammatory and oxidative stress markers after stroke. *Stroke* 2004;35(1):163-89.

[97] Hodis HN, Mack WJ, LaBree L, Mahrer PR, Sevanian A, Liu CR, Liu CH, Hwang J, Selzer RH, Azen SP.. Alpha-tocopherol supplementation in healthy individuals reduces low-density lipoprotein oxidation but not atherosclerosis: the Vitamin E Atherosclerosis Prevention Study (VEAPS). *Circulation* 2002;106:1453-9.

[98] Violi F, Micheletta F, Iuliano L. Vitamin E supplementation. *Lancet* 2000;357:632-3.

[99] Padayatty SJ, Levine M: Vitamin C and myocardial infarction: the heart of the matter. *Am. J. Clin. Nutr.* 2000;71:1027–1028.

[100] The Alpha-Tocopherol Beta Carotene Cancer Prevention Study Group. The effect of vitamin E and beta carotene on the incidence of lung cancer and other cancers in male smokers. *N. Engl. J. Med.* 1994; 330: 1029–35.

[101] Rapola JM, Virtamo J, Ripatti S, Huttunen JK, Albanes D, Taylor PR, Heinonen OP. Randomized trial of alpha-tocopherol and betacarotene supplements on incidence of major coronary events in men with previous myocardial infarction. *Lancet* 1997;349: 1715-20.

[102] Stephens NG, Parsons A, Schofield PM, Kelly F, Cheeseman K, Mitchinson MJ. Randomized controlled trial of vitamin E in patients with coronary disease: Cambridge Heart Antioxidant Study. *Lancet* 1996;347(9004):781-6.

[103] Mitchinson MJ, Stephens NG, Parsons A, Bligh E, Schofield PM, Brown MJ. Mortality in the CHAOS trial. *Lancet* 1999; 353: 381–82.

[104] GISSI-Prevenzione Investigators. Dietary supplementation with n-3 polyunsaturated fatty acids and vitamin E after myocardial infarction: results of the GISSI-Prevenzione trial. *Lancet* 1999;354:447-55.

[105] Pryor WA. Vitamin E and heart disease: basic science to clinical interventions trials. *Free Radic. Biol. Med.* 2000; 28: 141–64).

[106] The Heart Outcomes Prevention Evaluation Study Investigators. Vitamin E supplementation and cardiovascular events in high-risk patients. *N. Eng. J. Med.* 2000; 342:154-60.

[107] Boaz M, Smetana S, Weinstein T, et al. Secondary prevention with antioxidants of cardiovascular disease in endstage renal disease (SPACE): randomised placebo-controlled trial. *Lancet* 2000;356(9237):1213-8.

[108] Loughrey CM, Young IS, McEneny J, et al. Oxidation of low density lipoprotein in patients on regular haemodialysis. *Atherosclerosis* 1994;110(2):185-93.

[109] Boaz M, Matas Z, Biro A, et al. Serum malondialdehyde and prevalent cardiovascular disease in hemodialysis. *Kidney Int.* 1999;56(3):1078-83.

[110] MRC/BHF Heart Protection Study of antioxidant vitamin supplementation in 20536 high risk individuals: a randomised placebo-controlled trial. *Lancet* 2002;360:23-33.

[111] De Gaetano G. Low-dose aspirin and vitamin E in people at cardiovascular risk: a randomised trial in general practice. Collaborative Group of the Primary Prevention Project. *Lancet* 2001;357(9250):89-95.

[112] Fang JC, Kinlay S, Beltrame J, Hikiti H, Wainstein M, Behrendt D, Suh J, Frei B, Mudge GH, Selwyn AP, Ganz P. Effect of vitamins C and E on progression of transplant associated arteriosclerosis: a randomised trial. *Lancet* 2002;359:1108-13.

[113] Salonen RM, Nyyssonen K, Kaikkonen J, et al. Six-year effect of combined vitamin C and E supplementation on atherosclerotic progression: the Antioxidant Supplementation in Atherosclerosis Prevention (ASAP) Study. *Circulation* 2003; 107(7): 947-53.

[114] Jha P, Flather M, Lonn E, Farkouh M, Yusuf S. The antioxidant vitamins and cardiovascular disease. A critical review of epidemiologic and clinical trial data. *Ann. Intern. Med.* 1995;123(11):860-72.

[115] Carroll MF, Schade DS. Timing of antioxidant vitamin ingestion alters postprandial proatherogenic serum markers. *Circulation* 2003;108(1):24-31.

[116] Inoue T, Uchida T, Kamishirado H, Takayanagi K, Morooka S. Antibody against oxidized low density lipoprotein may predict progression or regression of atherosclerotic coronary artery disease. *J. Am. Coll. Cardiol.* 2001;37(7):1871-6.

[117] Vivekananthan DP, Penn MS, Sapp SK, Hsu A, Topol EJ. Use of antioxidant vitamins for the prevention of cardiovascular disease: meta-analysis of randomised trials. *Lancet* 2003; 361(9374):2017-23.

[118] Meagher EA, Barry OP, Lawson JA, et al. Effects of vitamin E on lipid peroxidation in healthy persons. *JAMA* 2001; 285: 1178–1182.

[119] Morrow JD, Frei B, Longmire AW, et al. Increase in circulating products of lipid peroxidation (F2-isoprostanes) in smokers: smoking as a cause of oxidative damage. *N. Engl. J. Med.* 1995; 332: 1198–1203.

In: Handbook of Cardiovascular Research
Editors: Jorgen Brataas and Viggo Nanstveit

ISBN 978-1-60741-792-7
© 2009 Nova Science Publishers, Inc.

Chapter XXI

Exercise-Induced Cardiovascular Adjustments by Muscle Receptors Stimulation

Antonio Crisafulli [*] *and Alberto Concu*
Department of Sciences applied to Biological Systems,
section of Human Physiology, School of Sports Medicine,
University of Cagliari, Italy

Abstract

During exercise cardiovascular apparatus operates some adjustments which aim at meeting the metabolic needs of exercising muscle. Both mechanical (skeletal-muscle and respiratory pumps) and nervous (centrally and peripherally originating) mechanisms contribute to regulate blood pressure and flow to the metabolic demand.

Concerning the nervous component of this regulation, there are several inputs of both central/cortical and peripheral/intravascular origin that converge to the brain-stem neurons controlling cardiovascular activity and regulate the hemodynamic responses to exercise on the basis of the motor strategy. Furthermore, evidences support the concept that also nervous signals of extravascular origin, i.e. arising from muscle mechano- and/or metabo- receptors, activate the same control areas on the basis of the muscle mechanical and metabolic involvement.

This review focuses on inputs arising from exercising muscles which modulate cardiovascular system in order to connect blood pressure and flow with the actual muscle mechanical status (muscle length and strain, and tissue deformation due to muscle movements) and metabolic condition (concentration of catabolites in the extra-cellular compartment produced by muscle activity).

It was reported that the stimulation of type I afferent nervous fibers from muscle receptors increases blood pressure through a mechanism of peripheral origin. Among

---

[*] Via Porcell 4, 09124 Cagliari (Italy); Phone: +390706758918; Fax: +390706758917; e-mail: crisaful@unica.it/ concu@unica.it.

sub-groups of type I afferents, indirect findings suggest that type Ib from Golgi tendon organs may contribute to the muscle-induced cardiovascular reflex. On the contrary, it appears that group Ia from muscle spindle primary ending and group II afferents are not involved in this reflex. Opposite, it seems ascertained that type III and IV afferent nervous fibers can be activated by exercise-induced mechanical and chemical changes in the extracellular environment into they are scattered. It is believed that type III afferents act mainly as "mechanoreceptors", as they respond to muscle stretch and compression occurring during muscle contraction, while type IV fibres act as "metaboreceptors", since they are stimulated by end-products of muscle metabolism. The activity of both type III and IV afferents can reflexely increase heart rate and systemic vascular resistance which, in turn, lead blood pressure to raise. Moreover, there are several growing evidences that also myocardial contractility, stroke volume and cardiac pre-load can be modulated by the activity of these reflexes of muscular origin.

These findings suggest that signals arising from exercising muscle act to regulate cardiovascular adjustments during exercise so that blood flow can be set to meet the muscle metabolic request.

Introduction

The main task of the cardiovascular apparatus is to provide the blood flow needed to serve the contracting skeletal muscles. This activity is particularly emphasized during strenuous physical exertions such as running or cycling, when heart rate, cardiac contractility, and sympathetic nerve activity increase and cardiac output can reach and even exceed values of 30 liters•min^{-1}, which is about six folds higher than the normal resting value of human beings [Mitchell et al. 1983(a), Lewis et al. 1983, Nishiyasu et al. 2000, Ichinose et al. 2004]. At the same time, vasodilatory substances released by working muscles greatly decrease peripheral vascular resistance and counteract the effect of the elevated cardiac output upon blood pressure. Inasmuch as arterial blood pressure is the product of cardiac output by peripheral vascular resistance, the resulting effect is that mean arterial pressure is kept stable or slightly increased with respect to rest. This fact indicates that mechanisms controlling the circulatory system can defend blood pressure homeostasis in spite of the cardiovascular stress caused by exercise and that some adjustments must be made to achieve a balance between cardiac output and peripheral vascular resistance, i.e. working muscles must be supplied of blood flow without inducing great changes in arterial blood pressure.

Several mechanisms are believed to be responsible for this cardiovascular regulation: mechanical mechanisms, which include the muscle pump and the respiratory pump activity [Higginbotham et al.1986, Laughlin 1987, Carter et al. 1999, Crisafulli et al. 2003(b)], and neural mechanisms. Mechanical mechanisms act as facilitator of cardiac filling and their activity is testified by the increase in stroke volume that takes place at the beginning of muscle activity, i.e. when muscle and respiratory pump start working. Clearly, the isolated effect of muscle and respiratory pumps would be to raise blood pressure through a flow-increased mechanism if vasodilation did not contemporary lower systemic vascular resistance.

Concerning the neural component, its action is essential for a normal blood pressure regulation during exercise, as testified by subjects with spinal cord injuries who develop a marked hypotension in response to muscle vasodilation during electrically-induced exercise because of the absence of neural feedback [Dela et al. 2003]. There are strong evidences that both central and peripheral control mechanisms operate the cardiovascular adjustments of neural origin occurring during exercise [Mitchell et al. 1983(a)]. In the central mechanism, commonly known as "central command", the activation of regions of the brain responsible for motor unit recruitment also activates the cardiovascular control areas located in the medulla [Goodwin et al. 1972, Strange et al. 1993]. It is thought that the central command establishes at the onset of exercise a basal level of sympathetic and parasympathetic efferent activity tightly linked to the intensity of the effort. This basic pattern of autonomic activity is then modulated by peripheral signals which reflexly activate the cardiovascular control centers. The peripheral reflexogenic areas considered important for the cardiovascular regulation during exercise are the arterial baroreceptors and the receptors within muscle. In particular, baroreceptors operate in order to maintain blood pressure and counteract any mismatch between vascular resistance and cardiac output by controlling muscle vasodilation and cardiac chronotropism through sympathetic modulation. On the other hand, receptors within muscle can activate afferent nerves and, in turn, induce sympathetic-mediated cardiovascular adjustments in response to the mechanical and the metabolic condition of the contracting muscle [Mitchell et al. 1983(b), Stebbins et al. 1988, Rowell et al. 1990, Shi et al. 1995, Iellamo et al. 1997]. Thus, the balance between cardiac output and peripheral resistance is governed by an interplay between influence on the heart, released vasodilatory substances, and sympathetic vasoconstriction.

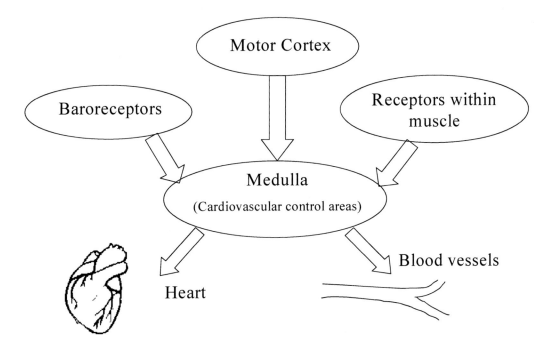

Figure 1. schematic representation of nervous inputs and outputs to the cardiovascular control areas of the Medulla.

In short, the autonomic nervous outputs to the cardiovascular system depend on the inputs to the cardiovascular control areas from cerebral motor cortex and from the peripheral reflexogenic areas (figure 1). Central and peripheral neural mechanisms probably work together and are not mutually exclusive in the regulation of cardiovascular response to exercise. Moreover, it would exist some redundancy between the two mechanisms and neural occlusion may be operative [Rybicky et al. 1989]. The system manages to regulate cardiac output and vascular conductance in order to defend blood pressure against changes in arterial resistance induced by vasodilatory substances produced during muscle contraction and to provide sufficient blood flow to working muscle.

This article focuses on the role played by the nervous peripheral inputs arising from exercising muscle; in the first part, the effects of mechanical stimulation of muscle receptors and nerve fibers are discussed, while in the second part we analyze reflexes of chemical origin and their possible involvement in the regulation of cardiovascular apparatus during exercise.

Cardiovascular Reflexes Arising from Mechanical Stimuli within Muscle

Afferent fibers from skeletal muscle are classically subdivided in four groups (I to IV) on the basis of their anatomical and electro-physiological characteristics [Mathews 1972]. Group I fibers have diameters of 12-20 μm and conduct impulses at 72-120 m sec^{-1}; group II have diameter of 2-16 μm and conduct impulses at 12-72 m sec^{-1}; group III have diameter of 1-6 μm and conduct impulses at 3-30 m sec^{-1}; finally, group IV, which, opposite to the first three groups are unmyelinated fibers, have diameters of 1μm or less and conduct impulses at 2.5 m sec^{-1} or less.

Almost all these fibers are susceptible of changing their firing rates towards the spinal cord when mechanical stimuli are applied to their endings and, in this way, they may contribute to the modulation related to muscle mechanical status made by the autonomic nervous system upon cardiovascular apparatus during exercise.

Type I Nervous Fibers and the Proprioceptive Cardiovascular Reflex

Decandia et al. [1991] found that electrically-stimulated group I afferent fibers of anaesthetized cats induced and increase in both systolic left ventricle pressure and systolic arterial pressure. Propanolol did not eliminate this reflex, thus excluding sympathetic heart activation as a cause of the phenomenon. Opposite, Phentolamine, which is a sympathetic alfa-receptor antagonist, blocked this blood pressure response, indicating that this muscle reflex acts by vasoconstricting blood vessels and by increasing peripheral vascular resistance to which follows a Starling-mediated increase in systolic left ventricular pressure and in systolic arterial pressure [Orani and Decandia 1994].

The above results followed a very accurate experiment, made by Orani et al. [1990] on anaesthetized cats, in which the effect of group I afferents stimulation on cardiovascular activity was clearly elucidated. After lumbo-sacral laminectomy the ventral roots were cut on both sides from L_5 to S_2 to avoid either spontaneous or reflex movements of both hind limbs. Thus, the nerves of the lateral gastrocnemius-soleus and medial gastrocnemius muscles were isolated on the left side and placed on a pair of silver stimulating electrodes. All other sciatic trunk nerves on the same side were also cut and gastrocnemius nerve endings were stimulated by connecting electrodes to a constant current stimulation unit. During two consecutive respiratory cycles continuous trains of electrical stimuli of 0.1 ms were applied with a frequency ranging from 200 to 300 Hz. Stimuli intensity was set at a value which ranged from 1 x to 2 x threshold (T) for the most excitable afferent fibers which, as it is known, are those comprised in the I group of the Matthews classification [Mathews 1972]. From the distal end of a small rootlet disconnected from the spinal cord, the afferent volleys were assessed during the gastrocnemius stimulation, in order to individuate the T stimuli intensity for group I fibers. It was also individuated the maximal intensity to excite group I fibers, which ranged from 1.8 to 2.0 x T. At near-maximal intensities stimulation, also small volleys attributable to group II afferents appeared after the first rapid volley due to group I firing. Increasing the intensity of stimuli up to 4 x T a third volleys appeared after those corresponding to group I and II afferents. These volleys were attributable to the most excitable group III afferent fibers. In brief, thanks to this technique, cardiovascular effects of different mechanoreceptor afferent fibers could be distinguished on the basis of the intensity of electrical stimulation. Inasmuch as in this experiment the stimuli intensity did not overcame 2.0 x T for group I fibers, it was unlikely that group III and IV afferents were stimulated.

Results showed that, at the start of the gastrocnemius stimulation, mean arterial blood pressure suddenly increased and, within two respiratory cycles which lasted the stimulation, it reached a value significantly higher (+6%) with respect to a control condition. Mean arterial pressure control values were reached between the first and the second breath following the stimuli cessation.

Subsequently, stimulation tests were repeated during anodal block of the most excitable afferent fibers (i.e. group I fibers) by applying a continuous electrical current at the site of stimulation. During a 50 ηA anodal block the volleys from gastrocnemius terminations to spinal cord of group I afferents were selectively blocked without having any effect on the amplitude and duration in the volleys of the group II fibers. Stimulation of gastrocnemius during anodal block was ineffective in eliciting the arterial pressure increase previously observed. When anodal block was removed, group I volleys reappeared and arterial pressure increased as it did during the test before the block. These results clearly indicate that excitation of group I afferents from muscle proprioceptors (i.e. anulospiral endings of Ia fibers in the muscle spindles and Ib endings in the Golgi tendon organs) and not of group II fibers from other mechanoreceptors were capable to evoke an arterial pressure response.

Inasmuch as the raise in systolic arterial pressure could be also explained by the fact that gastrocnemius stimulation induced an increase in pulmonary ventilation which in turn, through enhanced ventricle pre-load, caused a Starling-mediated increase in left ventricular systolic pressure and, consequently, in systolic arterial pressure, the muscle stimulation was repeated after curarisation while animals breathed at a constant artificial ventilation. In this setting, gastrocnemius stimulation during controlled ventilation produced the same arterial pressure response as in non-curarised animals, thus demonstrating that the raise in ventilation could not be responsible for the evoked pressor response. The results of the aforementioned experiment were interpreted by the authors through a sudden cardiovascular modulation of nervous origin (i.e. a reflex) at the start of physical exercise which preceded the chemically-mediated vasodilatation due to end-products of muscle metabolism.

However, it should be noticed that these results did not agree with those of some other experiments in which the effect on cardiovascular function of stimulation of group I fibers was investigated [Sato et al. 1981, Mitchell et al. 1983(a), Terui and Koizumi 1984]. In particular, McCloskey and Mitchell [1972] reported arterial pressure increases during the contraction of the hind limb muscles in cats and during simultaneous anodal block of group I afferents. From these results they deduced that these fibers were not involved in the evocation of the pressor reflex. However, the possibility that group I fibers may be effective cannot be excluded since their inefficacy would be definitely proved only if their selective stimulation did not produce excitatory effects. But Decandia et al. [1990] experiments, in which group I fibers were selectively stimulated, strongly support the effectiveness of these afferents in eliciting a pressor reflex, even if the specific importance of their involvement in the overall blood pressure response to exercise may be small and deserves to be better investigated.

Nevertheless, it must be considered that group I fibers contain both Ia and Ib contingents, the former of which concern afferent volleys from muscle spindle primary endings while the second concern the afferent volleys from Golgi tendon organ endings. Selective stimulation of muscle spindles, as it does the muscle vibration or the succinylcholine administration (a drug which specific excites muscle spindle primary endings) were utilized to elucidate possible effects of these proprioceptors on cardiovascular apparatus. McCloskey et al. [1972] applied mechanical vibration of 100-300 Hz (amplitude of vibration of 100-200 μ) along the length of the muscles of both hind limbs of anaesthetized cats and they did not discover any appreciable change in arterial pressure. On the other hand, Gautier et al. [1969] showed a very slight increase in heart rate after succinylcholine administration to anaesthetized cats. However, Kidd and Kucera [1969] demonstrated that this drug can also excite the endings of smaller myelinated fibers, so that cardiovascular responses to succinylcholine does not need to be necessarily attributed to Ia volleys.

Stimuli which are considered putative for muscle spindle excitation are also the passive muscle stretches. In conscious men, by means of a calf ergometer, Baum et al. [1995] produced a passive stretch of plantar flexor muscles. The stretch lasted 10 min and the increase reached in the angle joint of the ankle was of about 20 degrees. During the test electromiograms (EMG) of both the stretched soleus and gastrocnemius muscles were assessed to ensure that no active or reflex contractions did occur in these muscles. A Borg scale was also utilized to evaluate subjective ratings of pain sensations during the muscle stretching (values from 6 = painless to 20 = extremely painful). It was found that, during the stretching, no EMG changes took place, thus indicating that in the stretched muscles no active or reflex contraction occurred. This meant that, among the I group fibers, only the group Ia from primary ending of muscle spindles and not Ib from Golgi tendon organs were excited. On the other and, the Borg scale subjective ratings of pain at the end of the test gave a maximum value of 9. This fact indicated a very low pain sensation due to the ankle stretch and, consequently, not significant excitation of slow conducting nerve fibers of groups III and IV. Therefore, this muscle stretching protocol reasonably excited only group Ia fibers from primary endings of muscle spindles. No changes in arterial pressure were detectable during the test, thus the authors concluded that volleys in group Ia fibers were ineffective in eliciting any cardiovascular effect when muscles were stretched.

Similar conclusions can be deduced from the experiments made by Concu [1988] in which a passive sequence of alternative plantar and dorsal flexion of both ankles were applied in seated conscious men by an oscillating foot-board driven by an electromechanical apparatus. Heart rate, cardiac output, and stroke volume did not change when passive ankle oxillations were applied along the time corresponding to 3 respiratory cycles.

It is suggestive to consider that, in anaesthetized cats in which group I fibers were electrically stimulated, Carcassi et al. [1983] individuated Ib contingent as the hyperventilation eliciting fibers, whereas Ia contingent were ineffective in eliciting any ventilatory response. Considering that in almost all the experiments concerning the effects on pressor reflex from nervous muscle fibers, both respiratory and cardiovascular apparata were excited when these fibers were stimulated, it may be speculated that Golgi tendon organs rather than muscle spindles are responsible for the arterial blood pressure increase shown during the group I afferents stimulation. Indeed, active muscle contraction, which excites Golgi tendon organs, rather than passive muscle stretch, which excites muscle spindles, is probably more effective in reflecting the increased demand of blood from exercising muscles. It is our speculation that Ib fiber group should be suitable for sending this kind of information to nervous controllers of the cardiovascular system in order to correct any mismatch between cardiac output and vascular conductance, i.e. the blood pressure error that activates the arterial blood pressure response.

In any case, even if some cardiovascular effect can be produced by stimulation of group I fibers, the role played by these afferents on the arterial pressure adjustments during muscle activity appears the least if compared with that played by slow conducting nerve fibers of groups III and IV.

Type II Nervous Fibers Effect on Cardiovascular Activity

Group II afferent fibers effects on cardiovascular activity are scarcely investigated. However, Waldrop et al. [1984] failed to demonstrate any effectiveness of these afferents in eliciting heart rate and arterial blood pressure responses when they were selectively stimulated by succinylcholine injected into aorta of anaesthetized cats. After succinylcholine injection, these authors recorded the afferent impulse activity of fibers filaments dissected from either the L_7 and S_1 dorsal roots, among which afferent fibers arising from hind limb muscles, joints, and skin are comprised. They found that this drug induced high frequency volleys in group II but not in group III and IV fibers, both in paralyzed and non paralyzed condition. They also found that, when muscle fasciculation due to succinylcholine injection was abolished by paralysis induced with gallamine, succinylcholine-induced increase in firing activity of group II fibers did not produce any increase in heart rate and/or arterial pressure. Moreover, passive sequence of alternative plantar and dorsal flexion of both ankles, applied by Concu [1988] in conscious men, which along with group I afferents also produced group II fibers excitation from joint mechanoreceptor, did not produce any detectable cardiovascular effect. The fact that group II fibers excitation had no effect on cardiovascular apparatus has been demonstrated also by Decandia et al. in anaesthetized cats [1990]. When group I fibers volleys were selectively eliminated by anodal block, the remaining volleys from the group II fibers did not elicit any cardiovascular response.

It may be concluded that the secondary endings of muscle spindles or the corpuscolate endings inserted in muscles, joints, and skin, most of which send mechanocetive informations to spinal cord by means of group II afferent fibers, seem not to be involved in inducing cardiocirculatory changes when their respective receptive fields are stimulated.

Type III and IV Nervous Fibers and their Respective Influence on Cardiovascular Activity on the Basis O their Specific Sensibility to Mechanical Stimuli

Slow conducing nerve fibers of groups III and IV are thought to be excitable by mechanical stimulation. However, group III rather than group IV seems to be more sensible to this kind of stimulation [Kaufman et al. 1984, Leshnower et al. 2001]. Difficulties do exist in discriminating purely ergoreceptor from nociceptor function among group III and IV muscle afferents. Classically, ergoreceptors are considered those fibers in which muscle contraction induces an almost instantaneous increase in the firing rate of the corresponding afferents proportional to the intensity of the contraction. Moreover, often ergoreceptors transduce the touch sensation. On the contrary, nociceptors are considered those fibers that are stimulated by vigorous pinching of the muscle and transduce pain sensation. These latter fibers may be stimulated also by algesic chemicals such as bradykinin, serotonin, potassium, capsaicin, and hyperosmolar lactate an phosphate [Mitchell et al. 1983(b)].

In anaesthetized cats, Kaufman et al. [1983] induced gastrocnemius muscle static contraction by electrical stimulation of the cut peripheral end of L_7 ventral root which lasted 30-45 s, and selectively recorded group III and IV volleys from L_7-S_1 dorsal roots. During muscle contraction, an increase in arterial pressure was found which started on average about 6 s after the onset of the ventral root stimulation and reached a value 13% greater than control. These findings suggest that mechanical stimulation of skeletal muscle associated with contraction may stimulate afferents nerve endings and evoke cardiovascular reflexes. The discharge pattern of the most of the group III fibers excited during the muscle contraction (53%) was characterized by a sudden increase, with a short onset latency (about 0.8 s), in the firing frequency, which was proportional to the developed muscle tension. However, almost all of these fibers adapted their discharge rates to low values before the end of the muscle stimulation. On the contrary, muscle static contraction induced in 63% of excited group IV fibers a firing rate increase with an average onset latency of about 3.8 s. In the half of these fibers this firing rate was maintained throughout the contraction and they continued to fire for 10-12 s after the end of the contraction. The rapid response to contraction shown by many of the group III afferents suggest that they contribute to the initiation of the exercise pressor reflex [Matsukawa et al. 1994]. On the contrary, the firing behavior found in several fibers of group IV appeared especially well suited to function as the metabolic receptors, which are believed to signal a mismatch between blood supply and demand in contracting skeletal muscle [Haouzi et al. 1999, Gallagher et al. 2001]. In fact, their onset latency is a period of time compatible to allow the metabolic product of contraction to accumulate in a muscle undergoing static contraction. Moreover, the firing rate of these group IV fibers gradually increased as the contraction lasted, due to buildup of metabolites in the contracting muscles. However, it has been reported that a sub-population of group III/IV afferent fibers are polymodal, i.e. they respond to both mechanical and chemical stimuli [Kaufman et al. 1983, Matsukawa et al. 1994].

From the above results it seems clear that receptors within muscles gather information concerning the mass and the mechanical condition (muscle length and strain as well as tissue compression and deformation due to contractions) of the muscles involved in the exercise being performed. Mechanical information is then provided to the cardiovascular controlling areas which operate the hemodynamic adjustments in order to regulate blood flow on the basis of muscle status.

Type III and IV Nervous Fibers and the "Metaboreflex"

In this section we focus on the reflex cardiovascular response generated by nerve fibers which can be activated by the accumulation of end-products of muscle metabolism, i.e. the "metaboreceptors". As stated in the previous chapter, group III and IV are small slow-conducting nerves which are thought to be nociceptors [Mense 1993] and to be sensitive to mechanical distortion [Kaufman et al. 1983, Kaufman et al. 1987] as well as to end-products of muscle metabolism such as lactic acid, potassium, bradykinin, arachidonic acid products, and adenosine [Kniffki et al. 1978, Mense et al. 1983]. Both are composed of fine nerve fibers with either a myelin sheath (group III) or without myelin sheath (group IV). All group IV and most group III fibers terminate as free endings within muscle. The majority of group III fibers are mechano-sensitive and respond to mechanical events during muscle contraction such as stretch and compression, whereas group IV afferents are probably insensitive to mechanical stimuli but are activated by muscle metabolite accumulation [Kniffki et al. 1978, Mense et al. 1983, Leshnower et al. 2001]. Indeed, group III afferent fibers discharge at the onset of contraction and their firing rates tend to adapt if the muscle tension is maintained, which is coherent with the behavior of mechano-receptors; differently, group IV afferents discharge with latency after the beginning of muscle contraction and this pattern has been related with muscle metabolite production [Kaufman et al. 1983, Mense et al. 1983]. However, as previously stated, it has been reported that a sub-population of groups III/IV fibers responds to both mechanical and chemical stimuli [Kaufman et al. 1983, Mense et al. 1983]. Thus, group IV and at least in part group III afferents act as "metaboreceptors" and are involved in the cardiovascular chemoreflex originating in working muscle.

The presence of a controlling neural signal linked to metabolic events occurring within active muscle has been several times postulated and its contribution to the hemodynamic and autonomic response to exercise is now accepted [Rowell et al. 1990, O'Leary 1993, Strange et al. 1993, Piepoli et al. 1995]. The current thinking is that, when O_2 delivery does not suffice to meet the metabolic needs of contracting muscle, by-products accumulate because of a mismatch between metabolism and blood flow. This in turn causes activation of muscle metaboreceptors (free endings of group IV and perhaps III afferents) which leads to a reflex-increase in arterial blood pressure. Since this blood pressure response is abolished when group III and IV affernts are blockade, it could be stated that it is a nervous reflex, which is commonly called "metaboreflex" [Rowell et al. 1990, Piepoli et al. 1995, O'Leary et al. 1998]. It is believed that the metaboreflex-induced increase in blood pressure aims at restoring blood flow to the hypoperfused muscle. Nevertheless, it should be noted that this restoring effect has been demonstrated in dogs [Sheriff et al. 1987, O'Leary et al. 1995, O'Leary et al. 1999] whereas controversy exists whether or not it exists also in humans [Joyner 1991, Rowell et al. 1991]. In any case, the stimulation of group III and/or IV afferents appears to be essential for the normal hemodynamic response to exercise, since its absence abolishes the normal increase in blood pressure [Strange et al. 1993].

Little is known about the central projection of the afferent arms and the central pathways of integration of metaboreflex response. Most group III and IV fibers enter the spinal cord via the dorsal root and distribute in the dorsal horn of the segment of entry and for several segments up and down the spinal cord. Inputs from these fibers may have several levels of integration. The reflex seems not to require the rostral brain even if it a supraspinal level of integration may exist. In particular, the lateral reticular nucleus may be important for its expression and integration. It was proposed that the medulla is the area controlling the cardiovascular response during metaboreflex activation, while the spinal cord seems not to be operative in the intact animal [Mitchell et al. 1983 (a)]. Figure 2 is a schematic simplified picture of the putative mechanism of how metaboreflex works. Briefly, free endings of group IV and possibly III afferents are activated by end-products of muscle metabolism generated within muscle during contraction. These afferents, in turn, activate the cardiovascular control areas (probably located in the medulla) which operate the reflex response consisting in an increase in arterial blood pressure.

It is not clear whether or not a threshold for metaboreceptors stimulation by muscle end-products exists, i.e. whether metaboreflex operates only at moderate-high exercise intensities, when metabolites accumulate within working muscle, or even at mild muscle strain, when probably there is not a mismatch between muscle blood supply and demand and metabolites do not accumulate. It was reported in humans that the muscle metaboreflex has a threshold around a pH of 6.9 units and that mean arterial pressure increases linearly with decreasing muscle pH [Nishiyasu et al. 1994(b)]. Besides, studies employing ^{31}P nuclear magnetic resonance spectroscopy found that decrements in intramuscular pH were coupled to the rise of sympathetic nerve activity, thus suggesting that an event associated with glycolysis and lactate production may be important in activating the reflex [Victor et al. 1988, Sinoway et al. 1989, Cornett et al. 2000].These findings are consistent with the concept that the metaboreflex is activated whenever blood flow to contracting muscle is insufficient to warrant both oxygen delivery and metabolite washout [Rowell et al. 1990, Piepoli et al. 1995, Cornett et al. 2000]. According to this viewpoint, the metaboreflex acts to correct any mismatch between muscle blood flow and metabolism by superimposing to the central command activity.

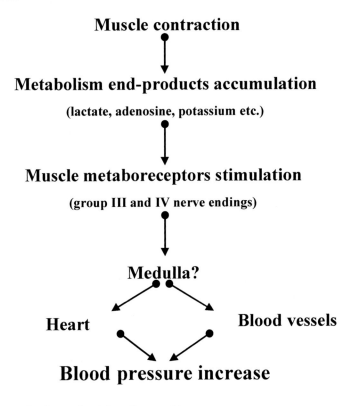

Figure 2. putative mechanisms of metaboreflex working.

However, it was also demonstrated that group IV fibers of cat muscle were responsive to a low level of exercise, i.e. when there was not a mismatch between blood delivery and metabolic needs of working muscle [Andreani et al. 1997]. The response at low level stimulation was interpreted with the fact that the metaboreflex plays a role in the cardiovascular regulation even when there is not an insufficient O_2 delivery to muscle and a mismatch between muscle flow and metabolism is not yet detectable. This is in accordance with the findings of Strange and co-workers [1993] who demonstrated in humans the essential role of the metaboreflex for reaching a normal blood pressure response even for mild exercise eliciting heart rate below 100 bpm. Therefore, it is possible that the metaboreflex is evoked even at low workloads, without any apparent accumulation of end-products of metabolism. According to this viewpoint, metaboreflex is responsible for a tonically active feedback to the cardiovascular control areas that starts working whenever the metabolism is activated by muscle contraction.

Hemodynamic Effects of Metaboreflex Activation

The typical hemodynamic feature of metaboreflex activation is the raise in arterial blood pressure [Mitchell et al. 1983 (a), Rowell et al. 1990, Piepoli et al. 1995]. With regard to the mechanisms responsible for the blood pressure response, it is commonly believed that it is achieved primarily by an increase in systemic vascular resistance caused by peripheral sympathetic vasoconstriction [Rowell et al. 1990, Piepoli et al. 1995]. The reflex effect on heart rate is supposed to be small or absent, and this fact led some authors to speculate that metaboreflex has little or no effect on cardiac output. However, it should be noticed that the effect on heart rate strongly depends on the setting of metaboreflex activation. In fact, two approaches have been used to study the relationship between hemodynamics and metaboreflex: 1) reducing muscle blood flow during effort, or 2) reducing blood flow at the cessation of effort by post-exercise ischemia in order to trap metabolites produced during previous muscle contraction [O'Leary 1993, Clark et al. 1995, Piepoli et al. 1995]. This latter study protocol is used in order to isolate central command and muscle mechanoreflexes from metaboreflex. While the activation of muscle metaboreflex during exercise can elicit some heart rate response through an increase in sympathetic activity towards sinus node, during post-exercise ischemia the rise of sympathetic activity is masked by the concomitantly enhanced parasympathetic outflow due to the loss of central command. The parasympathetic tone during post-exercise ischemia can be further increased by the arterial baroreflex, which responds to the metaboreflex-induced increase in blood pressure by buffering the elevated sympathetic drive to the heart and arteriolar vessels [Iellamo et al. 1999]. Thus, if metaboreflex is activated by post-exercise ischemia, the elevated sympathetic activity to sinus node is counteracted by enhanced parasympathetic tone due to the withdraw of central command and to the sympathetic-buffering effect of baroreflex activation. The resulting effect is that heart rate decreases despite the sympathetic tone to the heart is kept high [O'Leary 1993, Nishiyasu et al. 1994(a)]. Furthermore, it should be also considered that acetylcholine and norepinephrine have complex interaction at the pre-synaptic and post-synaptic level of sinus node [Levy 1971] and that the heart rate behavior may become remarkably unstable during situations resulting in accentuated sympatho-vagal antagonism. A characteristic aspect of sympathetic-parasympathetic interaction is represented by the "accentuated antagonism", which consists in a more pronounced bradycardia in response to vagal stimulation when sympathetic activity is elevated, as it occurs when metaboreflex is evoked [Stramba-Badiale et al. 1991, Tullpo et al. 1998]. Therefore, the lack of heart rate response to metaboreflex during post-exercise ischemia reported by several papers is not unexpected and can be explained through the elevated parasympathetic tone that takes place in this setting which accompanies the metaboreflex-induced increase in sympathetic drive [O'Leary 1993, Piepoli et al. 1995, Crisafulli et al. 2003(a)].

While the effect of metaboreflex upon systemic vascular resistance and heart rate is well established and accepted, less is known about its action upon central hemodynamics, i.e. cardiac output, stroke volume, myocardial contractility, and cardiac pre-load. As stated above, metaboreflex is considered to raise blood pressure primarily through an increase in systemic vascular resistance rather than through a flow-increase mechanism. This concept is based upon the fact that metaboreflex is supposed to induce little changes in cardiac output since it exerts little effects upon heart rate. However, as cardiac output is the product of heart rate and stroke volume, the lack of heart rate response to metaboreflex engagement does not necessary rule out a response in cardiac output, i.e. to detect any flow response the knowledge of both heart rate and stroke volume is necessary. In fact, several lines of evidence suggest that the activation of metaboreflex can actually affect also central hemodynamics. In particular, it was found in dogs that the muscle metaboreflex was capable to increase ventricular performance which, in turn, kept stroke volume constant despite the concomitant increase in heart rate and the consequent reduction in diastolic time and cardiac filling [O'Leary et al. 1998]. Similarly, it was reported in humans that myocardial contractility and stroke volume can be increased during metaboreflex activation caused by post-exercise ischemia [Bonde-Petersen et al. 1978, Bonde Petersen et al. 1982, Crisafulli et al. 2003(a)]. This hemodynamic responses aim at maintaining cardiac output despite the raise in after-load that takes place in this condition as a consequence of vasoconstriction. Indeed, stroke volume and consequently cardiac output would drop in response to any raise in after-load if myocardial contractility did not increase. Clearly, this occurrence could be detrimental since would reduce blood flow to contracting muscle and further impair the mismatch between metabolic demand and need. The importance of increasing cardiac contractility and stroke volume appears particularly when the metaboreflex is evoked during post-exercise ischemia, i.e. when bradycardia occurs, since in this circumstance the cardiovascular apparatus can rely only on the enhanced myocardial contractility to keep stroke volume and cardiac output constant in response to vasoconstriction [Crisafulli et al. 2003(a)].

It was also proposed that the muscle metaboreflex is capable of increasing cardiac filling pressure through splanchnic vasoconstriction and venoconstriction which expel blood volume into the central circulation [Sheriff et al. 1998, Gouvêa Bastos et al. 2000]. The rationale behind this blood volume "centralization" relies on the fact that any increase in cardiac output produced by improvement in heart rate and/or cardiac performance increases also pressure in the peripheral vascular bed and, as blood vessels are distensible, blood volume tends to accumulate in the periphery. Actually, there is a reciprocal relationship between cardiac output and ventricular filling pressure and increases in cardiac output will decrease central venous pressure and cardiac pre-load and this fact, in turn, will produce a drop in cardiac output, especially if muscle pump is not operating [Sheriff et al. 1993]. Thus, any increase in cardiac output must be accompanied by blood flow redistribution towards the central circulation to be effective since increases in heart rate or contractility, either alone or together, cannot effectively induce any flow improvement if they are not supported by an enhanced pre-load. It was speculated that the modulation of central venous pressure and cardiac filling are important mechanisms which accompany the rise in heart rate and cardiac contractility in order to increase cardiac output during metaboreflex response [Sheriff et al. 1998].

Therefore, from the above results it appears that metaboreflex can induce peripheral vasoconstriction as well as affect central hemodynamics by modulating cardiac contractility and pre-load. So, at least in the normal heart, the blood pressure response elicited by metaboreflex can be reached by adjusting both peripheral and central hemodynamics. Figure 3 shows the putative mechanisms through metaboreflex acts to increase blood pressure.

It is noteworthy that the strategy chosen to achieve the blood pressure response appears to depend on the intensity of exercise. It was reported both in humans and in animals that the cardiovascular response to metaboreflex relies mainly on cardiac output during mild exercise, whereas peripheral vasoconstriction becomes more important as exercise intensity rises [Augustyniak et al. 2001, Crisafulli et al. 2003(a)]. This behavior was attributed to the fact that the ability of increasing cardiac output depends on the presence of a cardiac reserve, which represents the heart possibility of increasing contractility and in turn stroke volume. If the cardiac reserve can be still used (i.e. if the contractility was not fully used during exercise), then the metaboreflex-induced pressure response relies mainly on cardiac output; differently, if there is not cardiac reserve further available for increasing stroke volume and cardiac output, as it is during and/or after strenuous efforts, then the response relies on peripheral vasoconstriction and systemic vascular resistance increase. These findings suggest that the intensity of exercise possibly dictates the mechanism by which the blood pressure response is elicited by metaboreflex [Fadel 2003]. If this concept was correct, then it would be no surprising that some human studies, which employed moderate and/or heavy rather than mild exercise, did not provide any changes in stroke volume during metaboreflex response [Bonde-Petersen et al. 1978, Gouvêa Bastos et al. 2000]. Moreover, these results indicate that the hemodynamic response to metaboreflex is complex and not merely constituted by a peripheral vasoconstriction. Further studies are needed to better clarify the role played by stroke volume and contractility responses in achieving the metaboreflex-induced raise in blood pressure.

In summarizing, it would seem that the cardiovascular apparatus operates with plasticity in order to regulate cardiovascular response to exercise and that the metaboreflex-induced increase in blood pressure can be reached even through the contractility reserve of myocardium.

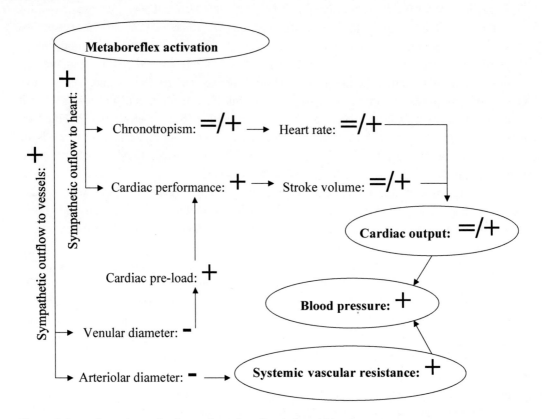

Figure 3. hemodynamic mechanisms of metaboreflex-induced blood pressure response.

Metaboreflex and its Possible Involvement in the Genesis of Heart Failure Exercise Intolerance

The hallmark symptom of congestive heart failure is exercise intolerance, which can severely limit the normal daily activities of patients such as working, going up a stair, or simply walking. In this disease a reduction in cardiac function induces a condition where the cardiovascular apparatus fails to meet the flow demand of exercising muscle and, in response to this situation, changes in sympathetic activity and alterations of mechanisms controlling the cardiovascular system also develop [Wilson et al. 1986, Van Der Borne et al. 1997, Shoemaker et al. 1999, Smith et al. 2003]. It was reported that an excessive vasocontriction in the splanchnic beds occurs and even active skeletal muscle may become vasoconstricted due to overactive sympathetic activity [Leimbach et al. 1986, Wilson et al. 1986, Sullivan et al. 1990, Floras 1993]. Yet, blood pressure response to exercise is more elevated than in normal individuals and this occurrence further worsens the myocardium performance, although what causes this altered cardiovascular response is not completely understood yet.

There are several clues that also the metaboreflex is involved in this abnormal blood flow dynamic. In particular, it is thought that one possible explanation of sympathetic overdrive is an exaggerated metaboreflex activity that takes place in response to under-perfusion of contracting muscle. This phenomenon, in turn, leads to vasoconstriction and exaggerated blood pressure response and, at least in part, this situation is responsible for the exercise intolerance shown by these patients [Piepoli et al. 1996, Shoemaker et al. 1998, Notarius et al. 2001]. Thus, according to this hypothesis, in chronic heart failure the metaboreflex activation does not effectively improve blood flow to exercising muscle; rather it would appear that metaboreflex engagement contributes to vasoconstrict the active muscle.

The origin of the overactive metaboreflex may be related to the progressive atrophy of skeletal muscle probably due to the chronic physical de-conditioning often observed in heart failure patients. Such condition increases the accumulation of end product of metabolism during effort because of the reduced oxidative capacity of muscle cells [Wilson et al. 1985, Massie et al. 1987, Drexler et al. 1992]. This causes over-activation of muscle metaboreceptors which, in turn, induces sympathetic vasocostriction and elevated blood pressure response to exertion. Moreover, inasmuch as physical training has been associated to attenuated blood pressure responses to metaboreflex [Mostoufi-Moab et al. 1998], it is possible to speculate that the chronic inactivity of subjects suffering from heart failure exerts an opposite effect, i.e. leads to a more pronounced blood pressure response during metaboreflex engagement. However, this scenario is not universally accepted and some authors reported blunted metaboreflex response in heart failure [Sterns et al. 1991, Negrão et al. 2001].

Moreover, it is conceivable to hypothesize that, together with the over-activation of the reflex, also the inability of increasing myocardial contractility and, consequently, stroke volume in response to metaboreflex may be in part responsible for the exaggerated vasoconstriction during exercise that occurs in heart failure. In fact, these patients can not rely on cardiac reserve to achieve the blood pressure response and, in absence of this mechanism, they can only utilize reflex vasoconstriction. Thus, heart failure causes a functional shift from cardiac output to vasoconstriction in order to achieve the blood pressure response to metaboreflex. This scenario has been demonstrated in an animal model, where the raise in blood pressure during metaboreflex activation was reached by reflex vasoconstriction rather than by a flow increase [Hammond et al. 2000, O'Leary et al. 2004], thus demonstrating that when the cardiac reserve can not be further utilized, then the vasoconstriction becomes the main mechanism through which a blood pressure raise can be reached. Nevertheless, the accentuated vasoconstriction that occurs in this setting leads to detrimental hemodynamic consequence. Indeed, vasoconstriction, by inducing an after-load increase, can further impair the myocardial performance of the already failing heart and this, in turn, may further worsen the skeletal muscle perfusion. Therefore, heart failure may be considered as a disease which disrupts the normal plasticity of cardiovascular response to exercise; in this condition the metaboreflex engagement may be responsible for accentuated vasoconstriction in the active muscle, which is opposite to the flow restoring effect supposed to be in the normal individuals.

Conclusion

The regulation of circulation during exercise implies various levels of control which include central and peripheral mechanisms. There are growing evidences that a peripheral signal of muscular origin acts as regulator of the cardiovascular response to exercise by modulating the basic pattern of autonomic activity established by central command. This mechanism works in response to the mechanical and the metabolic condition of the contracting muscle and it appears to be essential for the normal blood pressure response to muscular work. However, there is still the need to expand our understanding of the mechanisms through which the mechano-metaboreflexes operate. The effects upon central hemodynamics in normal humans are not completely understood yet, and further studies are needed to better elucidate the role of reflex-mediated myocardial contractility and stroke volume response. Moreover, research focusing on central hemodynamics during metaboreflex engagement in heart failure would help to further clarify the origin of exercise intolerance in this cardiac disease.

References

Andreani CM, Hill JM, Kaufman MP (1997). Responses of group III and IV afferents to dynamic exercise. *J. Appl. Physiol.* 82: 1811-1817.

Augustyniak RA, Collins HL, Ansorge EJ, Rossi NF, O'Leary DS (2001). Severe exercise alters the strength and mechanisms of the muscle metaboreflex. *Am. J. Physiol. 280 (Heart Circ. Physiol):* H1645-H1652.

Baum K, Selle K, Leyk D, Essfeld D (1995). Comparison of blood pressure and heart rate responses to isometric exercise and passive muscle stretch in humans. *Eur. J. Appl. Physiol.* 70 : 240-245.

Bonde-Petersen F, Rowell LB, Murray RG, GG Blomqvist, R White, E Karlsson, W Campbell, JH Mitchell (1978). Role of cardiac output in the pressor responses to graded muscle ischemia in man. *J. Appl. Physiol.* 45: 574-580.

Bonde-Petersen F, Suzuki Y (1982). Heart contractility at pressure loads induced by ischemia of exercised muscle in humans. *J. Appl. Physiol.* 52: 340-345.

Carcassi AM, Concu A, Decandia M, Onnis M, Orani GP, Piras MB (1983). Respiratory responses to stimulation of large fibers afferent from muscle receptors in cats. *Pflugers Arch.* 399: 309-314.

Carter III R, Watenpaugh DE, Wasmund WL, Wasmund SL, Smith ML (1999). Muscle pump and central command during recovery from exercise in humans. *J. Appl. Physiol.* 87: 1463-1469.

Clark AL, Piepoli M, Coats AJS (1995). Skeletal muscle and the control of ventilation on exercise: evidence for metabolic receptors. *Eur. J. Clin. Invest.* 25: 299-305.

Concu A (1988). Respiratory and cardiac effects of passive limb movements in man. *Pflugers Arch.* 412: 548-550.

Cornett JA, Herr MD, Gray KS, Smith MB, Yang QX, Sinoway LI (2000). Ischemic exercise and the muscle metaboreflex. *J. Appl. Physiol.* 89: 1432-1436.

Crisafulli A, Scott AC, Wensel R, Davos CH, Francis DP, Pagliaro P, Coats AJS, Concu A, Piepoli MF (2003a). Muscle metaboreflex-induced increases in stroke volume. *Med. Sci. Sports Exerc.* 35: 221-228.

Crisafulli A, Orrù V, Melis F, Tocco F, Concu A (2003b) Hemodynamics during active and passive recovery from a single bout of supramaximal exercise. *Eur. J. Appl. Physiol.* 89 : 209-216.

Decandia GF, Decandia M, Orani GP (1991). Group I fibers: pressor reflex and cardiac activity. *Cardioscience* 2: 189-192.

Dela F, Mohr T, Jensen CMR, Haahr HL, Secher NH, Biering-Sørensen F, Kjær M (2003). Cardiovascular control during exercise. Insight from spinal cord-injured humans. *Circulation* 107: 2127-2133.

Drexler H, Riede U, Munzel T, Konig H, Funke E, Just H (1992). Alterations of skeletal muscle in chronic heart failure. *Circulation* 85: 1751-1759.

Fadel PJ (2003). Muscle metaboreflex-induced increases in stroke volume. Commentary to accompany. *Med. Sci. Sports Exerc.* 35: 229.

Floras JS (1993). Clinical aspects of sympathetic activation and parasympathetic withdrawal in heart failure. *J. Am. Coll. Cardiol.* 4 (suppl. A): 72A-84A.

Gallagher KM, Fader PJ, Smith SA, Norton KH, Querry RG, Olivencia-Yurvati A, Raven PB (2001). Increases in pressure raise arterial blood pressure during dynamic exercise. *J. Appl. Physiol.* 91: 2351-2358.

Gautier H, Lacaisse A, Djours P (1969). Ventilatory response to muscle spindle stimulation by succinylcholine in cats. *Respiration Physiol.* 7: 383-88.

Goodwin GM, McCloskey DI, Eckberg DL (1972). Cardiovascular and respiratory responses to changes in central command during isometric exercise at constant muscle tension. *J. Physiol. (Lond.)* 226: 173-190.

Gouvêa Bastos B, Williamson JW, Harrelson T, Nôbrega ACL (2000). Left ventricular volumes and hemodynamic responses to postexercise ischemia in healthy humans. *Med. Sci. Sports Exerc.* 32: 1114-1118.

Hammond RL, Augustyniak RA, Rossi NF, Churchill PC, Lapanowsky K, O'Leary DS (2000). Heart failure alters the strength and mechanisms of the muscle metaboreflex. *Am. J. Physiol. 278 (Heart Circ. Physiol)*: H818-H828.

Haouzi P, Hill JM, Lewis BK, Kaufman MP (1999). Responses of group III and IV muscle afferents to distension of the peripheral vascular bed. *J. Appl. Physiol.* 87: 545-553.

Higginbotham MB, Morris KG, Williams RS, McHale PA, Coleman RE, Cobb FR (1986). Regulation of stroke volume during submaximal and maximal upright exercise in normal man. *Circ. Res.* 58: 281-291.

Ichinose M, Saito M, Wada H, Kitano A, Kondo N, Nishiyasu T (2004). Modulation of arterial baroreflex control of muscle sympathetic nerve activity by muscle metaboreflex in humans. *Am. J. Physiol.286 (Heart Circ. Physiol.)*: H701-H707.

Iellamo F, Legramante JM, Raimondi G, Peruzzi G (1997). Baroreflex control of sinus node during dynamic exercise: effect of central command and muscle reflexes. *Am. J. Physiol. 272 (Heart Circ. Physiol.)* : H1157-H1164.

Iellamo F, Pizzinelli P, Massaro M, Raimondi G, Peruzzi G, Legramante JM (1999). Muscle metaboreflex contribution to sinus node regulation during static exercise. *Circulation* 100: 27-32.

Joyner MJ (1991). Does the pressor response to ischemic exercise improve blood flow to contracting muscles in humans? *J. Appl. Physiol.* 71: 1496-1501.

Kaufman MP, Longhurst JC, Rybicki KJ, Wallach JH, Mitchell JH (1983). Effect of static muscular contraction on impulse activity of group III and IV afferents in cats. *J. Appl. Physiol.* 55: 105-112.

Kaufman MP, Waldrop TG, Rybicki KJ, Ordway GA, Mitchell JH (1984). Effects of static and rhytmic twitch contractions on the discharge of group III and IV muscle afferents. *Cardiovasc. Res.* 18: 663-668.

Kaufman MP, Rybicki KJ (1987). Discharge properties of group III and IV muscle afferents: their responses to mechanical and metabolic stimuli. *Circ. Res.* 61 *suppl.*: 160-165.

Kidd GL, Kucera J (1969). The excitation by suxamethonium of non proprioceptive afferents from caudal muscles of the rat. *Experientia* 25: 158-160.

Kniffki KD, Mense S, Schmidt RF (1978). Responses of group IV afferent units from skeletal muscle to stretch, contraction, and chemical stimulation. *Exp. Brain Res.* 31: 511-522.

Laughlin MH (1987). Skeletal muscle blood flow capacity: role of muscle pump in exercise hyperemia. *Am. J. Physiol. 253 (Heart Circ. Physiol.)*: H993-H1004.

Leimbach WN, Wallin BG, Victor RG, Aylward PE, Sundlof G, Mark AL (1986). *Circulation* 73: 913-919.

Leshnower BG, Potts JT, Garry MG, Mitchell JH (2001). Reflex cardiovascular responses evoked by selective activation of skeletal muscle ergoreceptors. *J. Appl. Physiol.* 90: 308-316.

Levy MN (1971). Sympathetic-parasympathetic interactions in the heart. *Circ. Res.* 29: 437-445.

Lewis SF, Taylor RM, Graham RM, Pettinger WA, Schutte JE, Blomqvist CG (1983). Cardiovascular responses to exercise as functions of absolute and relative work load. *J. Appl. Physiol.* 54: 1314-1323.

Massie BM, Conway M, Yonge R, Frostick S, Sleight P, Ledingham J, Radda G, Raiagopalan B (1987). $_{31}$P nuclear magnetic resonance evidence of abnormal skeletal muscle metabolism in patients with congestive heart failure. *Am. J. Cardiol.* 60: 309-315.

Mathews PB (1972). *Muscle receptors and their central actions.* London; Arnold.

Matsukawa K, Wall PT, Wilson LB, Mitchell JH (1994). Reflex stimulation of cardiac sympathetic nerve activity during static muscle contraction in cats. *Am. J. Physiol. 267 (Heart Circ. Physiol.):* H821-H827.

McCloskey DI, Matthews PBC, Mitchell JH (1972). Absence of appreciable cadiovascular and respiratory responses to muscle vibration. *J. Appl. Physiol.* 33: 623-626.

McCloskey DI, Mitchell JH (1972). Reflex cardiovascular and respiratory responses originating in exercising muscle. *J. Physiol. London* 224: 173-186.

Mense S, Stahnke M (1983). Responses in muscle afferent fibers of slow conduction velocity to contractions and ischemia in cat. *J. Physiol. (Lond.)* 342: 383-397.

Mense S. Nociception from skeletal muscle in relation to clinical muscle pain (1993). *Pain* 54: 241-289.

Mitchell JH, Kaufman MP, Iwamoto GA (1983a). The exercise pressor reflex: its cardiovascular effects, afferent mechanisms, and central pathways. *Ann. Rev. Physiol.* 45: 229-242.

Mitchell JH, Schmidt RF (1983b). Cardiovascular reflex control by afferent fibers from skeletal muscle receptors. In *Handbook of Physiology* vol. III, part 2, ed. Shepherd JT & Abboud FM, pp. 626-658. *American Physiological Society*, Bethesda USA.

Mostoufi-Moab S, Widmaier EJ, Cornett JA, Gray K, Sinoway LI (1998). Forearm training reduces the exercise pressor reflex during rhythmic handgrip. *J. Appl. Physiol.* 84: 277-283.

Negrão CE, Brandão Rondon MUP, Tinucci T, Alves MJN, Roveda F, Brage AMW, Reis SF, Nastari L, Barretto ACP, Krieger EMK, Middlekauff HR (2001). Abnormal neurovascular control during exercise is linked to heart failure severity. *Am. J. Physiol. 280 (Heart Circ. Physiol.)*: H1286-H1292.

Nishiyasu T, Nobusuke T, Morimoto K, Nishiyasu M, Yamaguchi Y, Murakami N (1994a). Enhancement of parasympathetic cardiac activity during activation of muscle metaboreflex in humans. *J. Appl. Physiol.* 77: 2778-2783.

Nishiyasu T, Ueno H, Nishiyasu M, Tan N, Morimoto K, Morimoto A, Deguchi T, Murakami N (1994b). Relationship between mean arterial pressure and muscle pH during forearm ischemia after sustained handgrip. *Acta Physiol. Scand.* 151: 143-148.

Nishiyasu T, Nagashima K, Nadel ER, Mack GW (2000). Human cardiovascular and humoral responses to moderate muscle activation during dynamic exercise. *J. Appl. Physiol.* 88: 300-307.

Notarius CF, Atchinson DA, Floras JS (2001). Impact of heart failure and exercise capacity on sympathetic response to handgrip exercise. *Am. J. Physiol. 280 (Heart Circ. Physiol.)*: H969-H976.

O'Leary DS (1993). Autonomic mechanisms of muscle metaboreflex control of heart rate. *J. Appl. Physiol.* 74: 1748-1754.

O'Leary DS, Sheriff DD (1995). Is the muscle metaboreflex important in control of blood flow to ischemic active skeletal muscle in dogs? *Am. J. Physiol. 268 (Heart Circ. Physiol. 37)* H980-H986.

O'Leary DS, Augustyniak RA (1998). Muscle metaboreflex increases ventricular performance in conscious dogs. *Am. J. Physiol. 275 (Heart Circ. Physiol. 44)*: H220-H224.

O'Leary DS, Augustyniak RA, Ansorge EJ, Collins H (1999). Muscle metaboreflex improves O_2 delivery to ischemic active skeletal muscle. *Am. J. Physiol. 276 (Heart Circ. Physiol.45)*: H1399-H1403.

O'Leary DS, Sala-Mercado JA, Augustyniak RA, Hammond RL, Rossi NF, Ansorge EJ (2004). Impaired muscle metaboreflex-induced increases in ventricular function in heart failure. *Am. J. Physiol 287 (Heart Circ. Physiol.)*: H2612-H2618.

Orani GP, Decandia M (1990). Group I afferent fibers: effects on cardiorespiratory system. *J. Appl. Physiol.* 68: 932-937.

Orani GP, Decandia M (1994). Role of the heart and peripheral resistance in the reflex effect of group I afferent fibers on blood pressure. *Cardioscience* 5: 25-30.

Piepoli M, Clark AL, Coats AJS (1995). Muscle metaboreceptors in hemodynamic, autonomic, and ventilatory responses to exercise in men. *Am. J. Physiol. 269 (Heart Circ. Physiol. 38)*: H1428-H1436.

Piepoli M, Clark AL, Volterrani M, Adamopoulos S, Sleight P, Coats AJS (1996). Contribution of muscle afferents to hemodynamic, autonomic, and ventilatory responses to exercise in patients with chronic heart failure. *Circulation* 93: 940-952.

Rowell LB, O'Leary DS (1990). Reflex control of the circulation during exercise: chemoreflexes and mechanoreflexes. *J. Appl. Physiol.* 69: 407-418.

Rowell LB, Savage MV, Chambers J, Blackmon JR (1991). Cardiovascular responses to graded reductions in leg perfusion in exercising humans. *Am. J. Physiol. 261 (Heart Circ. Physiol. 30)* H1545-H1553.

Rybicki KJ, Stremel RW, Iwamoto GA, Mitchell JH, Kaufman MP (1989). Occlusion of pressor responses to posterior diencephalic stimulation and static muscular contraction. *Brain Res. Bull.* 22: 305-312.

Sato A, Sato Y, Schmidt RF (1981). Heart rate changes reflecting modifications of afferent crdiac sympathetic outflow by cutaneous and muscle afferent volleys. *J. Auton. Nerv. Syst.* 4: 231-247.

Sheriff DD, Wyss C, Rowell L, Scher A (1987). Does inadequate oxygen delivery trigger pressor response to muscle hypoperfusion during exercise? *Am. J. Physiol. 253 (Heart Circ. Physiol.)*: H1199-H1207.

Sheriff DD, Zhou XP, Scher AM, Rowell LB (1993). Dependence of cardiac filling pressure on cardiac output during rest and dynamic exercise in dogs. *Am. J. Physiol. 265 (Heart Circ. Physiol. 34)* H316-H322.

Sheriff DD, Augstyniak RA, O'Leary DS (1998). Muscle chemoreflex-induced increases in right atrial pressure. *Am. J. Physiol. 275 (Heart Circ. Physiol. 44)*: H767-H775.

Shi X, Potts JT, Raven PB, Foresman BH (1995). Aortic-cardiac reflex during dynamic exercise. *J. Appl. Physiol.* 78: 1569-1574.

Shoemaker JK, Kunselman AR, Silber DH, Sinoway LI (1998). Maintained exercise pressor response in heart failure. *J. Appl. Physiol.* 85: 1793-1799.

Shoemaker JK, Naylor HL, Hogeman CS, Sinoway LI (1999). Blood flow dynamics in heart failure. *Circulation* 99: 3002-3008.

Sinoway L, Prophet S, Gorman I, Mosher T, Shenberger J, Dolecki M, Briggs R, Zelis R (1989). Muscle acidosis during static exercise is associated with calf vasoconstriction. *J. Appl. Physiol.* 66: 429-436.

Smith SA, Mammen PPA, Mitchell JH, Garry MG (2003). Role of the exercise pressor reflex in rats with dilated cardiomyopathy. *Circulation* 108: 1126-1132.

Stebbins CL, Brown B, Levin D, Longhurst JC (1988). Reflex effect of skeletal muscle mechanoreceptor stimulation on the cardiovascular system. *J. Appl. Physiol.* 65: 1539-1547.

Sterns DA, Ettinger SM, Gray KS, Whisler SK, Mosher TJ, Smith MB, Sinoway LI (1991). Skeletal muscle metaboreceptors exercise responses are attenuated in heart failure. *Circulation* 84: 2034-2039.

Stramba-Badiale M, Vavoli E, DE Ferrari GM, Cerati D, Foreman RD, Schwartz PJ (1991). Sympathetic-parasympathetic interaction and accentuated antagonism in conscious dogs. *Am. J. Physiol.260 (Heart Circ. Physiol.)*: H335-H340.

Strange S, Secher NH, Pawelczyk JA, Karpakka J, Christensen NJ, Mitchell JH, Saltin B (1993). Neural control of cardiovascular responses and of ventilation during dynamic exercise in man. *J. Physiol. (Lond.)* 470: 693-704.

Sullivan MJ, Green HJ, Cobb FR (1990). Skeletal muscle biochemistry and hystology in ambulatory patients with chronic heart failure. *Circulation* 81: 518-527.

Terui N, Koizumi K (1994). Responses of cardiacvagus and sympathetic nerves to excitation of somatic and visceral nerves. *J. Auton. Nerv. Invest.* 10: 73-91.

Tulppo MP, Makikallio TH, Sepanen T, Airaksinen JKE, Huikuri H (1998). Heart rate dynamics during accentuated sympathovagal interaction. *Am. J. Physiol. 274 (Heart Circ. Physiol.)*: H810-H816.

Van Der Borne P, Montano N, Pagani M, Oren R, Somers VK (1997). Absence of low-frequency variability of sympathetic nerve activity in severe heart failure. *Circulation* 95: 1449-1454.

Victor RG, Bertocci LA, Pryor SL, Nunnally RL (1988). Sympathetic nerve discharge is coupled to muscle cell pH during exercise in humans. *J. Clin. Invest.* 82: 1301-1305.

Waldrop TG, Rybicki KJ, Kaufman MP (1984). Chemical activation of group I and II muscle afferents has no cardiocirculatory effects. *J. Appl. Physiol.* 56: 1223-1228.

Wilson JR, Fink L, Maris J, Ferraro N, Power-Vanwart J, Eleff S, Chance B (1985). Evaluation of energy metabolism in skeletal muscle of patients with heart failure with gated phosphorus-3 I nuclear magnetic resonance. *Circulation* 71: 57-62.

Wilson JR, Falcone R, Ferraro N, Egler J (1986). Mechanisms of skeletal muscle underperfusion in a dog model of low-output heart failure. *Am. J. Physiol. 251 (Heart Circ. Physiol.)*: H227-H235.

In: Handbook of Cardiovascular Research
Editors: Jorgen Brataas and Viggo Nanstveit

ISBN 978-1-60741-792-7
© 2009 Nova Science Publishers, Inc.

Index

C

I

J

K

L

M

N

O

Q

R

S

T

U